CRC Desk Reference
of CLINICAL PHARMACOLOGY

CRC Desk Reference Series

Series Editor
Gerald Kerkut
University of Southampton
Southampton, England

Published Titles

CRC Desk Reference for Nutrition
Carolyn Berdanier, University of Georgia, Athens, Georgia

CRC Desk Reference of Clinical Pharmacology
Manuchair Ebadi, University of Nebraska, Omaha, Nebraska

Forthcoming Titles

CRC Desk Reference for Hematology
N. K. Shinton, University of Warwick, Coventry, United Kingdom

CRC Desk Reference
of CLINICAL PHARMACOLOGY

Manuchair Ebadi, Ph.D.

Professor of Pharmacology, Neurology and Psychiatry
University of Nebraska College of Medicine
Omaha, Nebraska

Fellow, American College of Clinical Pharmacology

CRC Press
Boca Raton Boston London New York Washington, D.C.

Library of Congress Cataloging-in-Publication Data

Ebadi, Manuchair S.
    CRC desk reference of clinical pharmacology / Manuchair Ebadi.
          p. cm. -- (CRC desk references)
      Includes index.
      ISBN 0-8493-9683-2 (alk. paper)
      1. Clinical pharmacology--Handbooks, manuals, etc.   I. Title.
    II. Series.
      [DNLM: 1. Drugs--administration & dosage--handbooks.   2. Drug
    Therapy--handbooks.   3. Pharmacokinetics--handbooks.
    4. Pharmacology, Clinical--handbooks.   QV 735 E15c 1997]
    RM301.12.E23   1997
    615′.1--dc21
    DNLM/DLC
    for Library of Congress   97-29883
                                                      CIP

No claim to original U.S. Government works
International Standard Book Number 0-8493-9683-2
Library of Congress Card Number 97-29883
Printed in the United States of America 1 2 3 4 5 6 7 8 9 0
Printed on acid-free paper

THE AUTHOR

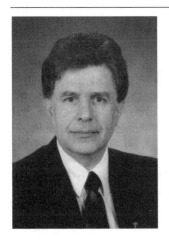

Manuchair Ebadi earned a B.S. degree in Chemistry from Park College (Parkville, MO, 1960), an M.S. degree in Pharmacology from the University of Missouri College of Pharmacy (Kansas City, MO, 1962), and a Ph.D. degree in Pharmacology from the University of Missouri College of Medicine (Columbia, 1967). He completed his postdoctoral training at the Laboratory of Preclinical Pharmacology, the National Institute of Mental Health (Washington, DC, 1970). He served as the Chairman of the Department of Pharmacology at the University of Nebraska College of Medicine from 1970 until 1988.

During his academic career, Professor Ebadi has received thirty-two awards including the Burlington Northern Faculty Achievement Award (1987), the University of Nebraska's system-wide Outstanding Teaching and Creative Activity Award (1995); and was inducted into the Golden Apple Hall of Fame (1995) for having received eleven Golden Apple awards. He is a member of sixteen research and scholarly societies including Alpha Omega Alpha Honor Medical Society.

In 1976, he became the Mid-America State Universities Association (MASUA) Honor Lecturer; in 1987, from the University of Missouri Alumni Association he received an award for Meritorious Contributions to Pharmaceutical Sciences; in 1995 he was honored by a Resolution and Commendation of the Board of Regents of the University of Nebraska for having developed a sustained record of excellence in teaching, including creative instructional methodology; and in 1996 he received the Distinguished Alumni Award from Park College, his alma mater.

Dr. Ebadi serves on the Editorial Board of several journals including *Toxicology* and *Applied Pharmacology*.

*This book is humbly and reverently dedicated
to the honored memory of my beloved parents,
Ali Ebadi Shahmirzadi and Rogieh Djavadi Ebadi Shahmirzadi.*

In books lie the soul of the whole past time, the articulate audible voice of the past when the body and material substances of it has altogether vanished like a dream.

Thomas Carlyle

SERIES PREFACE

This series of volumes will form a set of concise medical science encyclopedias.

Very few people read a medical or science book right through from cover to cover. They tend to dip into the book, reading a few pages here and a few pages there. More often they look up subjects in the index at the back of the book and with a finger in the index page, they look up the different page references, often having difficulty in finding the reference subject on the given page. This is partly because an index usually gives the page references in numerical order (though the more important references are often printed in bold) and partly because the indexer likes to give every possible reference, major, minor, and minuscule.

The present book is in effect an annotated index. The topics are arranged in alphabetical order, so that they are easy to find. The intention is that each topic should be concise so that after having read it, the reader will be able to remember the important information in that topic. There is a "take away message." Too often in larger encyclopedias, the item has to be read several times to get the key information, i.e., they are discursive instead of being didactic. The intention in the present book is to give the time-pressed reader the necessary data quickly and concisely.

On the other hand, some subjects have to be discussed in more detail to provide the background information necessary to provide a fuller understanding of the subject.

In addition the book contains "orientation" subjects that give the background and bring the reader up to date. Medicine and science advance very quickly these days and although recent graduates can be assumed to have the modern information, even those graduating five years ago can sometimes find themselves unsure about new facts, ideas, and terminology that are now currently mentioned in the news and have come into vogue.

It is difficult to get a correct balance between being sufficiently informative so as to be useful, being too concise so that the required information is not present, and being so long that the reader can't find the time to read the item.

It is hoped that these Desk References get near the correct balance and will be useful sources of information for the reader.

Gerald Kerkut
Series Editor

PREFACE

Hippocrates (460-377 B.C.) lamented, "Life is short, and the art long; the occasion fleeting; experience fallacious; and judgment difficult." New drugs and novel avenues of treatment are emerging rapidly, requiring constant vigilance to remain informed.

The *CRC Desk Reference of Clinical Pharmacology,* designed and prepared specifically for physicians and other members of the health-care delivery team, contains more than 2000 entries appearing under three broad categories:

I. **Short reviews** (1%) dealing with important topics of clinical pharmacology such as the pharmacokinetic basis of therapeutics, pharmacodynamic principles, and drug-drug interactions. In addition, major areas of therapeutics such as antiemetic drugs, antihistaminics, calcium channel blocking agents, and nonsteroidal antiinflammatory agents have been reviewed. The ninety-nine diagrams and twenty-six tables not only cover major areas of therapeutics but also deal with multiple medications. For example, Table 1 summarizes the pharmacological properties of acetohexamide, chlorpropamide, glipizide, glyburide, tolazomide, and tolbutamide, the orally effective hypoglycemic agents. Table 2 summarizes the analgesic, antipyretic, antiinflammatory, and uricosuric properties of all nonsteroidal antiinflammatory agents. Figure 1 deals with pharmacokinetic principles such as absorption, distribution, tissue binding, biotransformation, and elimination of drugs. Figure 2 deals with 5-fluorouracil, dacarbazine, cytarabine, methotrexate, vincristine, vinblastine, bleomycin, actinomycin D, and doxorubicin exerting their effects at G_1 phase, S phase, G_2 phase, and miotic phase of the cell cycle, respectively.

II. **Abstract-length entries** (39%) providing a short description of every medication in use today.

III. **Short dictionary-style entries** (60%) describing in one sentence the exact therapeutic use of a medication. For example — Halcinonide, a topical adrenocorticoid with antiinflammatory properties is indicated in inflammation of acute and chronic corticosteroid-responsive dermatoses.

Each entry gives the name of the drug, its classification, its dosage, its indications, its mechanism of action, its pharmacokinetic properties if appropriate, its side effects, and its signs and symptoms of overdosage. The section on pharmacokinetics has been designed to be meaningful in nature. For example, if a drug is mainly eliminated unchanged, it is noted that its dose should be adjusted downward in renal failure.

Another unique feature of the book is that items of information have been given in a comprehensive fashion. For example, Table 21 provides information to be used in the treatment of hypertensive emergics. This includes provision of pharmacological properties of sodium nitroprusside, diazoxide, labetalol, nitroglycerin, phentolamine, trimethaphan, hydralazine, and nicardipine. All these drugs have their own separate entries but have also been assembled in a meaningful fashion in one place.

The author expresses his heart-felt appreciation and gratitude to Professor Gerald A. Kerkut of the University of Southampton and Mr. David Grist of CRC Press LLC for the confidence rendered and for the kind invitation to prepare a volume on clinical pharmacology. Their valuable guidance, direction, and support have been immense and are gratefully acknowledged.

The author also acknowledges the contribution of the members of the international advisory board in the process of designing, writing, and completing this desk reference. They are:

Thomas E. Andreoli, M.D.
Professor and Chairman
Department of Medicine
University of Arkansas
College of Medicine
Little Rock, Arkansas

Franco Frashini, M.D.
Director
Department of Pharmacology &
  Chemotherapy
University Degli Studi di Milano
Milan, Italy

Alfred M. Freedman, M.D.
Professor & Chairman of Psychiatry
Director of Psychiatric Services
Metropolitan & Flower & Fifth
Hospitals & Chairman, Dept. of Psychiatry,
  Grasslands Hospital
Valhalla, New York

Robert H. Handschumacher, Ph.D.
Professor of Pharmacology
Yale University School of Medicine
New Haven, Connecticut

Ronald F. Pfeiffer, M.D.
Professor of Neurology
Director, Division of Neurodegenerative
  Diseases
University of Tennessee
College of Medicine
Memphis, Tennessee

Alan C. Sartorelli, Ph.D.
Alfred Gilman Professor of Pharmacology
  & Epidemiology
Yale University School of Medicine
New Haven, Connecticut

Arnold Schwartz, Ph.D.
Professor and Chairman
Department of Pharmacology & Cell
  Biophysics
University of Cincinnati
College of Medicine
Cincinnati, Ohio

Howard M. Spiro, M.D.
Department of Internal Medicine
Yale University School of Medicine
New Haven, Connecticut

Elliot S. Vesell, M.D.
Evan Pugh Professor & Chairman
  Department of Pharmacology
Pennsylvania State University
College of Medicine
Hershey, Pennsylvania

The author also expresses his everlasting admiration to Mrs. Margaret McCall and to Mrs. Lori Ann Clapper for their magnificent dedication, uncompromising diligence, and competent skills in typing the entire manuscript and to Mr. John Enrique Mata for designing and drawing the art work. The exceptional and rare talent, skills, and expertise of Ms. Gail Renard, the project editor, and Ms. Kathy Johnson, the typesetter, in refining this volume, are gratefully and respectfully acknowledged. Thanks are also due to Cindy Carelli, Carolyn Lea, Julie Haydu, and Becky McEldowney — all of CRC — for their help and professionalism.

The author hopes that by providing simple and unique diagrams, comprehensive tables, and more than 2000 entries, the *CRC Desk Reference of Clinical Pharmacology* will become a valuable and essential reference book for physicians and other members of the medical profession in their quest to alleviate the mental and physical sufferings of their fellow human beings.

M. Ebadi
July 1997
Omaha

NOTICE

The indications and dosages of all drugs in this book have been recommended in the medical literature and conform to the practices of the general medical community. The medications described do not necessarily have specific approval by the U.S. Food and Drug Administration for use in the diseases and dosages for which they are recommended. The package insert for each drug should be consulted for use and dosage as approved by the FDA. Because standards for usage change, it is advisable to keep abreast of revised recommendations, particularly concerning new drugs.

HOW TO USE THIS BOOK

This book may be used as an encyclopedia of medications in which compounds appear under their generic names in alphabetical order from Abortifacient, which lists diversified drugs such as aminopterin, azothioprine, carboprost tromethamine, cyclophosphamide, and mercaptopurine, to Zopiclone, the first compound of the cyclopytolone class possessing anticonvulsant, anxiolytic, muscle relaxant, and sedative properties. Furthermore, in the index, all drugs, including their generic names and multiple trade names, appear in alphabetical order.

This book may also be used as a textbook bearing introductory materials such as the pharmacokinetic basis of therapeutics, the pharmacodynamic basis of therapeutics, and adverse reactions and drug-drug interactions, which have been presented in a review format. In addition, many important and often-used medications such as androgens, antacids, antiemetic agents, antihistamines, barbiturates, benzodiazepine derivatives, calcium channel blockers, cathartics, cephalosporins, chemoprotectants, corticosteroids, cytokines, digitalis, folic acid antagonists, general anesthetics, insulin preparations, iron preparations, laxatives, levodopa-carbidopa, nitrates-nitrites, penicillins, salicylates and allied medications, tetracyclines, thiazide diuretics, and vitamins, have been described in more detail. The 26 tables and 99 figures summarize and illustrate in an attractive fashion information about major areas of therapeutics. In addition, medications have been covered under multiple headings to make the search for them simple and to make their descriptions informative. For example, aspirin is found in the sections on acetylsalicylic acid, nonsteroidal antiinflammatory agents, and salicylates and allied compounds.

The orientation articles, which the reader will find enclosed in boxes throughout the text, summarize the treatments of common disorders/diseases including Alzheimer's disease, arrhythmias, arthritis, asthma, congestive heart failure, constipation, Crohn's disease, duodenal ulcer, erectile dysfunction, fungal infections, Gaucher's disease, Gilles de la Tourette syndrome, glaucoma, gonorrhea, gout, heart failure, human immunodeficiency virus (HIV) infection, Huntington's disease, hypertension, insomnia, Legionnaire's disease, mania, migraine, multiple sclerosis, mycoses, narcolepsy, obesity, osteoporosis, otitis media, panic disorder, parasitic infections, Parkinson's disease, peptic ulcer, seizure disorders, sinusitis, syphilis, upper respiratory tract infections, urinary tract infections, uveitis, vaginal candidiasis, and Wilson's disease.

Orientation articles provide an encyclopedic listing of medications dealing with aminoglycoside antibiotics, analgesics, androgens, angiotensin-converting enzyme inhibitors, antianxiety agents, antibacterial drugs, antidepressants, antidiarrheal medications, antidotes, antiemetics, antipsychotics, antiviral agents, diuretics, estrogen preparations, expectorants, laxatives, lipid lowering drugs, orphan drugs, radiopaque agents, sulfonamides, tetracyclines, thrombolytic agents, and many others.

In many cases, newly introduced medications, such as the use of melatonin for sleep disorders, have been introduced. Discussion of some novel medications, such as tizanmidine for the treatment of spasticity or urapidel for the treatment of hypertension, has been provided. Discussion on the rapidly growing family of peptides, such as trefoil peptides, with a possible healing factor for peptic ulcers and inflammatory bowel diseases, and many other novel avenues of therapeutics have been introduced. Whenever possible, the descriptions of medications have been given in concise form and in a nugget fashion.

LIST OF
ORIENTATION ARTICLES

These will be found in the book in their alphabetical position.

LIST OF TABLES

LIST OF FIGURES

CONTENTS

The Pharmacokinetic Basis of Therapeutics

The primary objectives of therapy should be to prevent and cure disease. If these goals are not achievable, the secondary objectives should be to use drugs that mitigate the progressive, devastating, or disabling aspects of disease. The nature of the disease then determines the amount of drug or drugs to be given and the duration of therapy.

Pharmacokinetic principles, which deal with the fate of drugs, embrace the absorption, distribution, binding, biotransformation, and excretion of drugs and their metabolites in the body (Figure 1).

ABSORPTION OF DRUGS

Multiple physical and chemical factors influence the rate and extent of absorption of drugs. These include:

Drug Particle Size

The rate of dissolution of a drug increases significantly as the size of the drug particle decreases. For example, the reduction in particle size of **digoxin** from 3 to 1 mm^3 increases the surface area of drug particles exposed to solution by as much as 300%. The more soluble drugs are absorbed faster and more completely than are the relatively insoluble ones. The oral bioavailability of numerous drugs has been increased by a reduction in particle size.

Buccal and Sublingual Absorption

Compared with other routes of administration, different mucosa that line the oral cavity (buccal and sublingual sites of drug administration) offer advantages that include: (1) being noninvasive, (2) producing a rapid onset of action, (3) providing high blood levels, (4) avoiding first-pass effects, and (5) circumventing the exposure of drugs to the acidic and digestive fluid of the stomach. In addition, drugs may be easily applied (checked), sufficiently localized, and, if necessary, readily retrieved.

Intranasal Delivery

The intranasal route of administration is best for those drugs that either undergo extensive degradation or are poorly absorbed after oral administration.

Drugs that are routinely administered intranasally include peptides such as **vasopressin** and its analog **desmopressin, luteinizing hormone-releasing hormone, buserelin, leuprolide, nafarelin,** and **oxytocin**.

Rectal Administration

The oral administration of drugs, which is the route of choice, is impractical or impossible to use under certain circumstances such as in conditions causing nausea and vomiting, in patients with convulsions, just before surgery, and in uncooperative patients. The rectal route is also desirable for inducing anesthesia in children.

Degree of Ionization

The degree of dissociation of drugs and the pH of the internal medium play important roles in the transfer of drugs across biologic membranes. Most drugs are either weak acids or bases. Therefore, in solution, they exist in nonionized and ionized forms. The nonionized forms of various compounds are more lipid soluble and can penetrate the cellular membranes. The rate of passage of many drugs across various membranes becomes a function of the

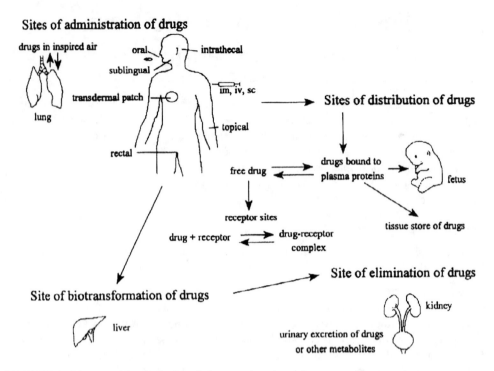

FIGURE 1 Pharmacokinetic basis of therapeutics. im = intramuscular; iv = intravenous; sc = subcutaneous. (Adapted from Ebadi, M., *Pharmacology, An Illustrated Review with Questions and Answers*, 3rd Edition, Lippincott-Raven Press, Philadelphia, 1996.)

negative logarithm of the dissociation constant (pK_a) of the drug and the pH of the internal medium. For example, phenytoin (an acid with a pK_a of 8.3) is insoluble at the pH of gastric juice (pH 2.0) and is absorbed from the upper part of the intestinal tract. Aspirin (pK_a of 3.0) is best absorbed when the pH of the stomach is highly acidic in nature.

Surface Area

Because both ionized and nonionized drugs are absorbed from subcutaneous and intramuscular sites of injection, ionization does not appear to play as important a role in the passage of drugs across the capillary wall. Finally, although drugs such as **acetylsalicylic acid** are best absorbed from an acidic medium, such as that in the stomach, most of the **aspirin** is nevertheless absorbed in the upper small intestine, which has a considerably greater absorptive surface. Similarly, the perfusion rate of the intestine is considerably greater than that of the stomach. In fact, most drugs, whether nonionized or ionized and whether acidic, basic, or neutral, are absorbed mostly from the small intestine. Consistent with this is the observation that buffered acetylsalicylic acid preparations are dissolved faster and absorbed better mostly in the intestine. Similarly, patients with achlorhydria or those who have undergone gastrectomy have little difficulty with the absorption of orally ingested drugs.

Blood Flow

The absorption of drugs in solution from intramuscular and subcutaneous sites of injection is limited by the perfusion rate. Increasing the blood flow enhances the absorption of drugs, whereas decreasing the blood flow reduces absorption. Massaging the site where a drug has been administered therefore increases the rate of absorption. Placing an ice pack on the site retards it. One may take advantage of this concept and deliberately retard the absorption of drugs by reducing the peripheral circulation. For instance, **local anesthetics** are often combined with a vasoconstricting substance such as **epinephrine** and injected as a mixture. The epinephrine causes vasoconstriction, hence producing a bloodless field of operation. Epinephrine prevents the rapid absorption of local anesthetics and thus both enhances their duration of action and prevents systemic toxicity (see Figure 72).

Gastric Emptying Time

Because drugs are mostly absorbed from the upper part of the small intestine, the rate of gastric emptying time plays a crucial role in drug absorption. If rapid absorption is desired, drugs should be taken on an empty stomach. Meals, especially those with a high fat content, retard absorption. The desire for rapid absorption of drugs necessitates that the interactions between food and drugs be monitored carefully.

Hepatic First-Pass Effect

There are several possible mechanisms responsible for an inadequate plasma concentration of a drug and/or its active metabolites following oral administration. By far the most important reason for an inadequate plasma concentration following the oral or parenteral administration of a drug is the first-pass effect, which consists of the loss of a drug as it passes through the liver for the first time. For example, nitroglycerin, which is used in the management of patients with angina pectoris, is given sublingually. Taken orally, nitroglycerin is rapidly inactivated in the liver and the resulting concentration is inadequate to be of immediate value to the patient. Sublingually administered nitroglycerin bypasses the liver and enters the superior vena cava, whereupon it perfuses the coronary circulation (see Figure 60).

Binding of Various Drugs to Plasma Proteins

In an ideal therapeutic regimen, a sufficient amount of the drug should reach the locus of action (receptor site) in order to bring about the desired effect, but not so much as to produce toxicity. Furthermore, the drug should not disappear too rapidly from the locus of action, or the therapeutic effects will be transient and hence of limited value. The binding of drugs to plasma proteins and various subcellular components tends to accomplish these objectives. Human plasma contains over sixty different proteins, and the most abundant one is albumin.

The percentage of protein binding of drugs at therapeutic levels varies dramatically. Some drugs such as allopurinol, heparin, and isoniazid do not become bound. Other drugs such as antipyrine, ethambutol, and theophylline become bound to the extend of only 4 to 15%. Several drugs such as ampicillin (25%) and digoxin (23%) show low protein binding; some such as atropine (50%) and meperidine (40%) show moderate protein binding; and some drugs such as carbamazepine (72%), furosemide (75%), nitrofurantoin (70%), and rifampin (85%) show high degrees of protein binding. Some drugs such as dicumarol (97%), diazepam (96%), phenylbutazone (98%), and diazoxide (96%) bind extensively to plasma proteins.

The binding sites of proteins are not unlimited and are subject to saturation. When this occurs, toxicity may develop following further drug administration, since the later portion of the drug remains free. Consistent with this view is the observation that toxic manifestations of drugs are quite frequent and considerably higher in individuals suffering from hypoalbuminemia or altered plasma and tissue protein concentrations, or both.

Drugs may alter the protein binding of other agents. For instance, aspirin decreases the binding of **thyroxine** and the binding of **bilirubin** is hindered by many pharmacologic agents. The more tightly bound drugs can displace the less firmly bound agents. The intensity of the effect of displaced drug on the patient will simply depend on the blood level of the free drug and its nature. At times, the effect may be highly undesirable and even fatal. Only the slight displacement of a highly bound drug such as **dicumarol** (an oral anticoagulant) by **phenylbutazone**, which has such greater affinity for binding sites, can cause serious hemorrhage. Because only 3% of the anticoagulant is free, an additional displacement of 3% increases its effects by 100%.

The Site of Action of Drugs

It is generally accepted that most, but not all, drugs (e.g., antiseptics) exert their potent and specific effects by forming a bond, generally reversible, with a cellular component called a receptor site, which should be differentiated from acceptor or silent sites where drugs are stored. Drugs that interact with a receptor and elicit a response are called agonists. Drugs that interact with receptors and prevent the action of agonists are termed antagonists. For example, **acetylcholine**, which causes bradycardia, is an agonist; **atropine**, which blocks the action of acetylcholine and prevents bradycardia, is an antagonist. The relative effects of drugs are often judged in terms of their potency, which is a measure of the dosage required to bring about a response, and their efficacy, which is a measure of their inherent ability to exert an effect.

When the pharmacologic properties of two compounds are compared, one may prove to be more potent and efficacious than the other. For instance, as an analgesic, **morphine** is more potent and efficacious than **acetylsalicylic acid**. On the other hand, two compounds may be equally efficacious but one could be more potent. Haloperidol and chlorpromazine are both efficacious neuroleptics in the management of schizophrenia but haloperidol is more potent.

A drug's affinity and intrinsic activity also need to be differentiated. Intrinsic activity refers to a drug's ability to bind to the receptor, which results in pharmacologic actions. Affinity is a measure of the degree to which a drug binds to the receptor — whether it exerts a pharmacologic action (as an agonist) or simply blocks the receptor (as an antagonist).

Physiologic and Pharmacologic Antagonism

If two drugs, one an agonist and another an antagonist, bind to an identical receptor site, either producing or preventing an effect, this association is called pharmacologic antagonism. **Naloxone, atropine,** and **diphenhydramine** are pharmacologic and specific antagonists of morphine, acetylcholine, and histamine at their respective receptor sites. In physiologic antagonism, the drugs do not bind to the same receptor sites but produce functionally opposite results. For example, histamine produces vasodilation, whereas epinephrine produces vasoconstriction; however, they interact with two separate receptor sites. Physiologic antagonism is utilized extensively in medicine, especially in overcoming the toxicity of pharmacologic agents. For instance, diazepam (Valium) may be used to overcome the CNS excitation produced by **physotigmine**, an acetylcholinesterase inhibitor, which results in an increased acetylcholine concentration. Diazepam overcomes the acetylcholine-mediated CNS excitation by enhancing the activity of GABA, an inhibitory neurotransmitter.

Biotransformation

Biotransformation may be defined as the enzyme-catalyzed alteration of drugs by the living organism. Although few drugs are eliminated unchanged, urinary excretion is a negligible means of terminating the action of most drugs or poisons in the body. As a matter of fact, the urinary excretion of a highly lipid-soluble substance such as pentobarbital would be so slow that it would take the body a century to rid itself of the effect of a single dose of the agent. Therefore, through evolutionary adaptations, mammalian and other terrestrial animals have developed systems that allow the conversion of most lipid-soluble substances to water-soluble ones, so that they may be easily excreted by the kidney.

FACTORS THAT MODIFY THE METABOLISM OF DRUGS

Many environmental factors and pathophysiologic conditions inhibit or stimulate the activity of drug-metabolizing enzymes, and hence may alter the outcome of a therapeutic regimen. Pharmacogenetics, the immaturity of drug-metabolizing enzyme systems, and drug-drug interactions, are a few of the factors that have been shown to alter drug metabolism.

Pharmacogenetics

Pharmacogenetics represents the study of the hereditary variation in the handling of drugs. Pharmacogenetic abnormalities may be entirely innocuous until the affected individual is challenged with particular drugs. The alterations in the handling of a drug may be attributed to abnormalities at either an anatomic or molecular level. For example, patients with inherited subaortic stenosis may experience an adverse drug reaction to **digitalis**. Molecular abnormalities may be due to an alteration in the receptor sites or the absence or deficiency of a particular enzyme. The hyposensitivity and resistance of certain individuals to **coumarin** anticoagulants and the hypersensitivity of patients with Down's syndrome to **atropine** most probably stem from abnormalities in their respective receptor sites. Acatalasia and the decrease in the activities of pseudocholinesterase, acetylase, and glucose 6-phosphate dehydrogenase are a few examples of enzymatic deficiencies that can lead to mild to very severe adverse reactions.

Liver Disease

The liver is the principal metabolic organ, and hepatic disease or dysfunction may impair drug elimination. Any alteration in the serum albumin or bilirubin levels and in the prothrombin time indicates impaired liver function. Similarly, skin bruising and bleeding tendency indicate decreased production of clotting factors by the liver.

The Influence of Age

Drug metabolism is qualitatively and quantitatively very deficient in newborns. For example, chloramphenicol, when used injudiciously, may cause gray syndrome, which is characterized by vomiting, refusal to suck, irregular and rapid respiration, abdominal distention, periods of cyanosis, passage of large green stools, cardiovascular collapse, and death. The mechanism of chloramphenicol toxicity is apparently the failure in the newborn to conjugate chloramphenicol with glucuronic acid, due to inadequate activity of hepatic glucuronyl transferase. This, in combination with inadequate renal excretion of the drug in the newborn, results in a higher than expected plasma level of chloramphenicol. Therefore, a newborn should receive doses of chloramphenicol not greater than 25 to 50 mg per kilogram of body weight.

The elderly are prone to toxicity from numerous drugs, including cardiac glycosides. A dose of digitoxin, which may be totally therapeutic and innocuous for a patient at age 60, may produce severe toxicity and even death in the same patient at age 70. The ability of the liver to metabolize drugs and of the kidney to excrete drug metabolites declines with age.

Enzyme Induction and Inhibition

The activities of microsomal drug-metabolizing enzymes in humans can be enhanced by altering the levels of endogenous hormones such as androgens, estrogens, progestational steroids, glucocorticoids, anabolic steroids, norepinephrine, insulin, and thyroxine. This effect can also be elicited by the administration of exogenous substances such as drugs, food preservatives, coloring agents, insecticides, volatile oils, urea herbicides, and polycyclic aromatic hydrocarbons.

Clinical Implications of Enzyme Induction and Inhibition

Patients are often given several drugs at the same time. The possibility that one drug may accelerate or inhibit the metabolism of another should always be kept in mind. When this phenomenon occurs, the removal of an enzyme inducer could be hazardous. The following examples reveal the consequence of enzyme induction.

Phenylbutazone is an analgesic, antipyretic, uricosuric, and antiinflammatory agent. Among its side effects are activation of peptic ulcer and gastrointestinal hemorrhage. If one gives a dog large amounts of phenylbutazone, side effects such as vomiting and diarrhea with bloody stool ensue. However, if phenylbutazone treatment is continued for several days, these side effects disappear. In this case, phenylbutazone "induces" its own hydroxylation, which results in a lower plasma level of the drug and ultimately the absence of the side effects. Long-term treatment with phenylbutazone and many other drugs, such as **chlorpromazine, pentobarbital, phenobarbital, chlordiazepoxide,** and the like, which stimulate their own metabolism, should be expected to result in decreased effectiveness and toxicity.

Patients who are on anticoagulant therapy may suffer severe hemorrhage several days after discharge from the hospital. Often these patients are sedated with barbiturates during their hospitalization, which tends to stimulate the enzymes that metabolize dicumarol. The abrupt withdrawal of barbiturates after discharge tends to revert the activity of the drug-metabolizing enzymes to their prebarbiturate stage, which raises the free circulating level of the anticoagulant and results in hemorrhage. Obviously, treatment with phenobarbital should prompt altering the maintenance dosage of anticoagulants.

Renal Excretion of Drugs

An orally administered drug will gradually begin to be absorbed. As the amount of drug in the body increases by 50%, the amount of the drug at the absorption site should decrease by the same amount. The absorbed drug will gradually be metabolized or excreted mostly by the kidneys. Besides their renal elimination, drugs and their metabolites are eliminated in bile, breast milk, perspiration, and by the lungs. The excretion of drugs into breast milk may be a significant concern in breast-fed children, and the excretion of drugs, especially gaseous anesthetics, from the lungs also becomes important in specialized circumstances.

Rate of Excretion of Drugs by the Kidneys

The amount of a drug (and/or its metabolites) that appears in the urine depends on the amount of drug undergoing glomerular filtration, tubular secretion, and tubular resorption. **Metabolism** plays a major role in drug excretion, since the metabolites are more water-soluble substances, which are excreted. Drugs are excreted when they are in their free form, but plasma protein-bound drugs and tissue-stored drugs are not excreted.

The excretion of drugs from the kidneys, like the absorption of drugs from the gastrointestinal tract, depends on lipid solubility, the degree of ionization of drugs, and the pH of the urine. Nonionized lipid-soluble drugs are resorbed and not eliminated. Generally, drugs that are bases are excreted when the urine is acidic, whereas acidic compounds are excreted in greater quantities if the urine is alkaline. For example, in phenobarbital (weak acid pK_a of 7.3) poisoning, alkalinization of the urine with **sodium bicarbonate** is helpful in eliminating the phenobarbital. In amphetamine toxicity, acidification of the urine with **ammonium chloride** is required.

Drugs that undergo both glomerular filtration and active tubular secretion have a very short half-life. **Penicillin** is one such compound, but its half-life is prolonged by the coadministration of **probenecid**, a uricosuric drug that inhibits the tubular secretion of penicillin. Most drugs, however, have half-lives that are relatively longer than penicillin's because they undergo glomerular filtration, partial tubular resorption, and no active tubular secretion.

Significance of Blood Flow on Drug Clearance

In general, the rate of extraction of drug from blood and the rate of clearance by the kidney depend on blood flow and the ability of the kidney to extract the drug (the extraction ratio). If all of the drug is removed from the blood as it traverses through the kidneys, the extraction ratio is one. The higher the blood flow, the higher is the rate of excretion of that drug, and the clearance is said to be perfusion-rate limited. For example, the extraction ratio of **digoxin,** one of the cardiac glycosides, is low, and toxicity is likely to occur in renal failure. Similarly, the hepatic extraction ratio of **digitoxin** is low, and toxicity is likely to occur in hepatic failure. Consequently, cardiologists have long recognized that digitoxin and digoxin should be avoided in patients suffering from liver and renal failure, respectively.

Half-Life of a Drug

The half-life of a drug, or its elimination half-life, is the time required for its concentration in the blood to be reduced by one-half. For **penicillin G**, the half-life is 20 minutes, indicating that only 50% of it remains in the blood 20 minutes after its intravenous administration. Both the intravenously and orally administered identical drugs have the same half-lives once they reach the general circulation. When given at regular intervals, a drug or its metabolite reaches a plateau concentration after approximately four to five half-lives. This plateau changes only if the dose or frequency of administration, or both, are altered.

The Pharmacodynamic Basis
of Therapeutics

Appropriate drug therapy can improve the quality of life, whereas injudicious drug therapy may be harmful. Medications are given for a variety of diagnostic, prophylactic, and therapeutic purposes. These prescribed medications bring about the desired effects in most patients, but they may also prove to be inert and ineffective in some. They may even evoke totally unexpected responses and precipitate serious reactions in others.

The use of drugs in the treatment of a disease is termed **pharmacotherapeutics**. However, the use of drugs is not always necessary in managing a disease. A drug may be used substitutively, supportively, prophylactically, symptomatically, diagnostically, or correctively. For instance, in juvenile-onset diabetes mellitus (type I, insulin-dependent diabetes mellitus) and Addison's disease, insulin and cortisone acetate are used, respectively, as substitutes or supplements for substances that were either never produced or are not now produced by the body. In adult-onset diabetes mellitus, oral antidiabetic agents support the physiologic function of the body by stimulating the synthesis and release of insulin.

Oral contraceptive tablets are used to prevent pregnancy. Isoniazid may be used to prevent the development of active tuberculosis in those individuals who have been exposed to the disease but show no evidence of infection, in those who test positively for it but have no apparent disease, and in those with once active but now inactive disease.

Drugs may eliminate or reduce the symptoms of a disease without influencing the actual pathology. For example, fever may be associated with respiratory tract infection, bacterial endocarditis, biliary tract disorders, tuberculosis, carcinoma, cirrhosis of the liver, collagen diseases, encephalitis, glomerulonephritis, Hodgkin's disease, hysteria, malaria, leukemia, measles, mumps, and plague, to name a few. Aspirin can reduce the fever in these disorders but cannot alter the disease processes themselves.

A drug may also be used to diagnose a disease. Histamine has been used to assess the ability of the stomach to secrete acid and to determine parietal cell mass. If anacidity or hyposecretion occurs in response to histamine administration, this may indicate pernicious anemia, atrophic gastritis, or gastric carcinoma; a hypersecretory response may be observed in patients with duodenal ulcer or with the Zollinger-Ellison syndrome.

In most cases, drugs do not **cure** diseases, but do ease or eliminate the associated symptoms. For example, no drugs exist that cure essential hypertension, but there are some that lower blood pressure. In reducing symptoms, drugs never create new functions. They can only stimulate or depress the functions already inherent to the cells.

In alleviating symptoms, drugs may also induce adverse effects, which may or may not be acceptable to patients. For instance, numerous agents with anticholinergic properties cause dry mouth, which is easily correctable and hence is acceptable to patients. Conversely, some antihypertensive medications cause impotence in male patients, which they may find unacceptable, and this side effect may thus lead to lack of compliance with the prescribed medication.

Pharmacodynamics may be defined as the study of the actions and effects of drugs on organ, tissue, cellular, and subcellular levels. Therefore, pharmacodynamics provides us with information about how drugs bring about their beneficial effects and how they cause their side effects. By understanding and applying the knowledge gained in studying pharmacodynamics, physicians and other members of the health-care delivery team are able to provide effective and safe therapeutic care to their patients.

Pharmacodynamics considers the sites, modes, and mechanisms of actions of drugs. For example, if a patient with multiple fractures receives a subcutaneous injection of 10 to 15 mg of morphine sulfate, analgesia, sedation, respiratory depression, emesis, miosis, suppression of the gastrointestinal tract, and oliguria may ensue. These diversified effects occur at multiple peripheral and central sites and through the influence of numerous modes and mechanisms of action.

Site of Action

The receptor sites where a drug acts to initiate a group of functions is that drug's site of action. For example, the central sites of action of morphine include the cerebral cortex, hypothalamus, and medullary center.

Mode of Action

The character of an effect produced by the drug is called the **mode of action** of that drug. Morphine, by depressing the function of the cerebral cortex, hypothalamus, and medullary center, is responsible for decreasing pain perception (analgesia), inducing narcosis (heavy sedation), depressing the cough center (antitussive effect), initially stimulating then depressing the vomiting center, and depressing respiration.

Mechanism of Action

The identification of molecular and biochemical events leading to an effect is called the mechanism of action of that drug. For instance, morphine causes respiratory depression by depressing the responsiveness of the respiratory center to carbon dioxide.

Cellular Sites of Actions of Drugs

Because drugs are very reactive, many elicit their effects or side effects, or both, by interacting with coenzymes, enzymes, or nucleic acids, as well as other macromolecules and physiologic processes such as transport mechanisms. To gain an appreciation of the complex interactions between drugs and physiologic parameters, some examples are cited.

Drug-Coenzyme Interactions

Isoniazid and Pyridoxal Phosphate

The primary drugs, first-line agents that combine the greatest level of efficacy with an acceptable degree of toxicity, in the treatment of **tuberculosis** are isoniazid, ethambutol, pyrazinamide, and rifampin. **Isoniazid** is prescribed orally in doses of 4 to 5 mg per kilogram of body weight. If pyridoxine is not given along with the isoniazid, peripheral neuritis is the most common side effect to arise. In toxic doses, optic neuritis, muscular twitching, dizziness, ataxia, paresthesias, and convulsions may occur, especially in malnourished patients. These neuropathies are thought to result from a chemical interaction between isoniazid and **pyridoxal phosphate**, and the reduced level of this important coenzyme in the body. The coadministration of **pyridoxine** averts these side effects.

L-Dopa and Pyridoxal Phosphate

L-Dopa, given orally on a long-term basis, is effective in combating the pathophysiologic effects of parkinsonism, which are thought to result in part from dopamine deficiency in the striatum. The administration of pyridoxine to a parkinsonian patient benefiting from L-dopa therapy nullifies its therapeutic effects. The mechanism responsible for this is thought to be due to pyridoxal phosphate-stimulated **dopa decarboxylase** and the conversion of a higher than ordinary amount of L-dopa to dopamine in the periphery, resulting in the reduced formation of dopamine in the striatum. At the present time, most patients are treated concurrently with levodopa and a dopa decarboxylase inhibitor, such as **carbidopa**, which circumvents this problem.

Folic Acid and Trimethoprim-Sulfamethoxazole

In acute and chronic urinary tract infection, the combination of **trimethoprim** and **sulfamethoxazole** (Bactrim, Septra) exerts a truly synergistic effect on bacteria. The sulfonamide inhibits the utilization of p-aminobenzoic acid in the synthesis of folic acid, while trimethoprim, by inhibiting dihydrofolic acid reductase, blocks the conversion of dihydrofolic acid to tetrafolic acid reductase, which is essential to bacteria in the *de novo* synthesis of purines, pyrimidines, and certain amino acids. Because mammalian organisms do not synthesize **folic acid**, but require it as a vitamin in their daily diets, trimethoprim-sulfamethoxazole does not interfere with the metabolism of mammalian cells.

Dicumarol and Vitamin K

Phytonadione (vitamin K_1; phylloquinone) is identical to naturally occurring vitamin K_1, which is required for the synthesis of blood coagulation factors such as prothrombin (II), proconvertin (VII), Christmas factor or plasma thromboplastin component (IX), and Stuart-Prower factor (X) in the liver. Dicumarol and ethylbiscoumacetate act as competitive antagonists of vitamin K and interfere with the synthesis of these factors in the liver. Similarly, hypoprothrombinemic-induced bleeding can be rectified by the administration of vitamin K.

Drug-Enzyme Interactions

Numerous drugs exert their effects and side effects by interacting with enzymes. Following are some examples of these interactions.

Allopurinol, Xanthine Oxidase, and Hyperuricemic States

Allopurinol is used to lower uric acid levels in the treatment of primary **gout**, as a prophylaxis in myeloproliferative neoplastic disease, for investigational purposes in **Lesch-Nyhan** syndrome, and as an adjunct with **thiazide diuretics** or **ethambutol**. The mechanism of action of allopurinol is the inhibition of xanthine oxidase, which converts hypoxanthine into xanthine and in turn becomes oxidized into uric acid.

$$\text{Hypoxanthine} \xrightarrow{\underset{\text{oxidase}}{\text{Xanthine}}} \text{xanthine} \xrightarrow{\underset{\text{oxidase}}{\text{Xanthine}}} \text{uric acid}$$

When xanthine oxidase is inhibited by allopurinol, the plasma level of uric acid and the size of the urate pool in the body both decrease (see Figure 5).

Drugs and Bronchial Asthma

Bronchial asthma is characterized by respiratory distress, apnea, wheezing, flushing, and cyanosis. Because bronchoconstriction seems to be the common denominator in the pathogenesis of asthma, bronchodilation is usually considered an effective pharmacologic intervention.

Aminophylline (theophylline ethylenediamine), given intravenously, is used in patients with **status asthmaticus** who do not respond to epinephrine. In addition, epinephrine may be administered subcutaneously for severe acute asthma attacks. Epinephrine may also be given along with theophylline. It is thought that the bronchodilation is associated with the enhanced concentration of cyclic AMP, which is metabolized according to the following scheme.

$$\text{ATP} \xrightarrow{\underset{\text{cyclase}}{\text{Adenylate}}} \text{cyclic AMP} \xrightarrow{\text{Phosphodiesterase}} 5' \text{ AMP}$$

Epinephrine stimulates the beta-adrenergic receptors in the bronchioles, which in turn activates membrane-bound adenylate cyclase to synthesize more cyclic AMP, whereas theophylline inhibits the activity of phosphodiesterase, conserving the previously synthesized cyclic AMP. In addition, recent evidence suggests that theophylline blocks the receptor for **adenosine**. The inhalation of adenosine can precipitate marked bronchoconstriction in asthmatic patients, but shows no appreciable effects in normal subjects (see Figure 19).

It is now recognized that adenosine receptors are linked through appropriate guanine nucleotide-binding regulatory proteins (G-proteins), not only to adenyl cyclase but also to other effector systems. Moreover, theophylline may inhibit the synthesis of prostaglandin and reduce the uptake or metabolism of catecholamines in nonneuronal tissues (see Figure 42).

Corticosteroids, which are also effective in the symptomatic treatment of certain types of asthma, exert their beneficial effects in part by enhancing the catecholamine effects, and also by antagonizing the cholinergic actions, one of which is bronchoconstriction.

Tranylcypromine and Endogenous Depression

Tranylcypromine (Parnate), a monoamine oxidase inhibitor, is effective in the symptomatic treatment of endogenous depression and certain phobic-anxiety states. In addition, it may be of value in the treatment of bulimia, posttraumatic reactions, and other obsessive-compulsive ruminative disorders. Monoamine oxidase, an enzyme found primarily in neurons, the liver, and the lungs, catalyzes the oxidative deamination of serotonin, dopamine, and norepinephrine (see Figure 27).

$$\text{Norepinephrine} \xrightarrow[\text{oxidase}]{\text{Monoamine}} 3\text{-methoxy-}4\text{-hydroxy-phenylethylene glycol}$$

As a monoamine oxidase inhibitor, **tranylcypromine** increases the monoamine concentrations in the body. The simultaneous administration of tranylcypromine and ingestion of food containing biogenic amines, such as cheese and wines that have a high tyramine content, may evoke a hypertensive crisis, characterized by marked hypertension, occipital headache, palpitation, dilated pupils, and, in some cases, intracranial and subsequently fatal hemorrhage. These side effects result from the accumulation of catecholamine released by the tyramine and by the inhibition of its catabolism imposed by tranylcypromine.

Drug-Nucleic Acid Interactions

Chemotherapeutic agents useful in the treatment of neoplastic diseases exert their therapeutic effects by modifying the synthesis or functions of nucleic acids. For example, **6-mercaptopurine** inhibits purine-ring biosynthesis, **cytarabine** inhibits DNA polymerase, alkylating agents crosslink DNA, and hydroxyurea inhibits the conversion of ribonucleotides into deoxyribonucleotides. However, other pharmacologic agents such as chlorpromazine, a neuroleptic, also modify nucleic acid synthesis. One of the side effects of chlorpromazine is mild to severe agranulocytosis. **Chlorpromazine** reduces the synthesis of DNA by inhibiting the activity of thymidine kinase according to the following scheme:

$$\text{Thymidine} + \text{ATP} \xrightarrow[\text{kinase}]{\text{Thymidine}} \text{thymidine } 5' \text{ phosphate} + \text{ADP}$$

In addition to chlorpromazine, phenylbutazone (an analgesic and antiinflammatory agent), sulfonamides (chemotherapeutic agents), chlorthiazide (a diuretic), thiouracil and methimazole (antithyroid drugs), phenytoin (an anticonvulsant), pyribenzamine (an antihistaminic), and chloramphenicol (an antimicrobial) may cause **agranulocytosis** in susceptible individuals. The incidence of this side effect is highest among those subjects with a lower than normal proliferative capacity of the bone marrow.

The Interactions of Drugs with Neuronal Elements

Neuropharmacology is the study of drugs that affect the nervous system and its neuronal components. The functions of the nervous system are intimately linked with the synthesis, storage, release, and uptake of many transmitters and their modulators. The beneficial effects or side effects of an extensive number of drugs are brought about through their interaction with these neurotransmitter-neuromodulator systems.

An example of this interaction is offered by **reserpine** (see Figure 27). Reserpine may be used in conjunction with a diuretic in the treatment of mild to moderate hypertension. It is thought that reserpine produces this antihypertensive effect by preventing the storage of norepinephrine and hence reducing the pool of this neurotransmitter in the body. This amine-depleting action of reserpine not only brings about its beneficial effects, but also causes its side effects. For instance, reserpine may tranquilize and lead to depression (by depleting the catecholamine content in the brain), and may cause bradycardia and miosis plus increase the motility of the gastrointestinal tract (all stemming from the enhanced cholinergic activity secondary to decreased sympathetic activity). Reserpine may also increase the atrioventricular conduction time resulting from an increase in the refractory period of the atrioventricular conduction system, due to depletion of myocardial norepinephrine stores.

Interaction of Drugs with the Endocrine System

The nervous system and the endocrine system are linked and interrelated functionally and exhibit pharmacologic cross-reactivities. The endocrine system, which is an effector arm of the nervous system, is, in part, adrenergic in character. A few examples of the interactions of drugs with the endocrine system follow.

Alpha-Methyldopa and Renin

Hypotension and decreased renal perfusion pressure promote the release of renin from the juxtaglomerular apparatus of the kidney. **Renin** converts angiotensin I to **angiotensin II**, a potent endogenously occurring vasoconstrictor (see Figure 21). Catecholamine can also release renin, and this effect is blocked by **propranolol**, a beta-adrenergic receptor blocking agent. Drugs that alter the renin level are able to alter blood pressure. Alpha-methyldopa suppresses renin release, whereas the oral contraceptive medications have the opposite effect. In addition, other antihypertensive medications such as **captopril** specifically inhibit angiotensin-converting enzyme, hence preventing the formation of angiotensin II (see Figure 21).

Drugs and Prolactin

The release of prolactin from the adenohypophysis is a centrally mediated event involving the **dopaminergic neurons**. Stimulation of these neurons blocks prolactin production, whereas blockade of dopaminergic function causes lactation. **Chlorpromazine**, which blocks dopamine receptors, **reserpine**, which depletes dopamine stores, and alpha-methyldopa, which forms a false transmitter such as alpha-methyldopamine, are all able to cause **inappropriate lactation** in a nonpregnant woman.

Alpha-Methyldopa and Hypertension

Alpha-methyldopa is used in the treatment of mild to moderate hypertension. The proposed mechanism of action is suppression of renin release, stimulation of central $alpha_2$-inhibitory adrenergic receptors ($alpha_2$-adrenergic receptors are presynaptic receptors and their stimulation results in inhibition of norepinephrine release), and possibly the formation of a false transmitter such as alpha-methylnorepinephrine. Substances activating beta-adrenergic receptor sites, such as angiotensin II, augment the release of norepinephrine, whereas substances activating alpha-adrenergic receptor sites, such as dopamine, acetylcholine, and prostaglandins (PGE_1 and PGE_2 but not PGF_2A), reduce the release of norepinephrine. Besides reducing blood pressure, alpha-methyldopa causes sedation (interference with norepinephrine), parkinsonism (interference with dopamine), psychosis (interference with serotonin), and decreased libido and impotence (interference with norepinephrine).

Diabetes Mellitus and Insulin Release

First-generation sulfonylureas such as tolbutamide, chlorpropamide, tolazamide, or acetohexamide, and **second-generation sulfonylureas** such as glyburide, glipizide (see Figure 44 and Table 1), or glipizide are used to control hyperglycemia in type II diabetics who cannot achieve appropriate control with changes in diet alone, and in diabetics who do not have complicating factors such as infections, ketosis, and acidosis for which crystalline zinc insulin may be required. The hypoglycemic effects of **tolazamide** appear to be elicited by stimulation of insulin secretion from the beta cells of the pancreatic islets, which is mediated via beta-adrenergic receptor sites. Pharmacological agents such as **isoproterenol**, which stimulates beta-adrenergic receptors, or **phentolamine**, which blocks alpha-adrenergic receptor sites (see Figure 27), promote the release of insulin. Examples of agents that may cause **hyperglycemia** under certain circumstances are aldosterone, caffeine, catecholamines, chlorpromazine, corticosteroids, ethacrynic acid, furosemide, glucagon, indomethacin, nicotine, oral contraceptives, and thiazide diuretics. Examples of drugs causing **hypoglycemia** are alcohol, isoniazid, methimazole, propranolol, and salicylate.

This discussion clearly emphasizes the fact that **drugs do not create functions, but merely stimulate or inhibit functions already inherent in the cells.** These pharmacodynamic-related interactions take place at various levels of cellular activities, including ion transport, enzymes, coenzymes, nucleic acids, and numerous other biochemical events yet to be delineated.

ADVERSE REACTIONS AND DRUG-DRUG INTERACTIONS

On medical services, it is common for a patient with multiple medical problems to be taking as many as 10 to 15 drugs concomitantly. It is also becoming increasingly obvious to physicians and other members of the health-care delivery team that many **drug combinations**, when used inappropriately and injudiciously, have the inherent potential to interact adversely, leading to side effects and even death. However, under certain circumstances, these drug interactions are beneficial because they actually enhance the therapeutic effectiveness or cause diminution of toxic reactions.

Whether drugs are given individually or in combination, some side effects or adverse reactions are inevitable and cannot be eliminated. For example, patients undergoing treatment with antineoplastic drugs will experience expected side effects, such as hair loss. Nevertheless, many adverse effects of the drugs, or **drug-drug interactions**, are either avoidable or may be substantially minimized.

The varied and complex mechanisms involved can be broadly classified as **pharmacokinetic interactions** or **pharmacodynamic interactions**. In pharmacokinetic interactions, drugs interfere with and/or alter the absorption, distribution, biotransformation, or excretion of other drugs. In pharmacodynamic interactions, drugs modify the intended and expected actions of other drugs. Before elaborating on the pharmacokinetic interactions, some terms will be defined.

DEFINITIONS

Iatrogenic Reactions

Iatrogenic reactions broadly refer to any adverse reactions produced unintentionally by physicians in their patients. For example, one of the side effects of many antihistaminic preparations (H_1 antagonists) such as ethanolamine derivatives (prototype: diphenhydramine) is heavy sedation. Although sedation may be desirable for some patients, it may interfere with daytime activities. Other antihistaminic preparations (also H_1 antagonists) such as piperidine derivatives (prototypes: **terfenadine** or **astemizole**) do not cross the blood-brain barrier and hence have no sedative properties.

Allergic Reactions

Drug allergy refers to those drug reactions occurring in a patient who was previously exposed to, sensitized with, and developed antibodies to that drug. The underlying immunologic mechanisms may be varied and complex, involving **anaphylactoid immediate reactions** (e.g., penicillin, due to formation of specific immunoglobulin E), **cytotoxic reactions** (e.g., drug-induced hemolytic anemias), and **delayed allergic reactions** (e.g., drug-induced contact dermatitis). By taking a careful history before the administration of drugs in conjunction with watchful monitoring of patients, the incidence of drug-induced allergic reactions can be lessened.

Idiosyncratic Reactions

Idiosyncrasy refers to an abnormal, unexpected, or peculiar reaction seen in only certain patients. For example, **succinylcholine** may cause prolonged apnea in patients with **pseudocholinesterase deficiency**, and **hemolytic anemia** may be seen following the administration of a number of drugs, including sulfonamides in patients with **glucose-6-phosphate dehydro-genase deficiency**. Idiosyncratic reactions, which may be explained in part by **pharmacogenetics** (i.e., the influence of heredity on the response to drugs or on their fate in the body), become manifest only in the presence of insulting drugs. Although these reactions are inevitable when they occur unexpectedly for the first time, they may be circumvented altogether in patients who have previously shown such abnormal reactions.

Tolerance and Tachyphylaxis

Tolerance refers to decreased responses following the long-term administration of drugs. For example, after repeated **morphine** use, tolerance to all of its effects occurs, except for miosis and constipation, which continue. Morphine also no longer causes respiratory depression as readily in a tolerant patient. Although it is generally accepted that tolerance may occur following the use of many depressant drugs such as alcohol, benzodiazepine, antianxiety agents, and barbiturates, it may also occur following the use of other agents such as clonazepam (an anticonvulsant), carbamazepine (an anticonvulsant and the drug of choice in the treatment of trigeminal and glossopharyngeal neuralgias), and chlorpromazine (a neuroleptic).

Tachyphylaxis refers to a quickly developing tolerance brought about by the rapid and repeated administration of drugs. For example, indirect-acting sympathomimetic agents such as **tyramine**, which exert their effects through the release of norepinephrine, are able to cause tachyphylaxis. If norepinephrine is not present, tyramine fails to exert its effect until the supply of norepinephrine in nerve terminals has been replenished.

Although tachyphylaxis is innocuous and not regarded as a major clinical problem, not appreciating tolerance as an entity may have devastating consequences. For example, respiratory depression is not seen in a morphine-tolerant patient, and a dosage that far exceeds the normal therapeutic level is required to induce an effect. However, tolerance is lost or lessened following the discontinued administration of morphine. Therefore, in a once tolerant patient, administering a dose of morphine that was quite innocuous prior to the occurrence of tolerance may prove fatal by causing severe respiratory depression.

Supersensitivity

Supersensitivity refers to the increased responsiveness to a drug that results either from denervation or following administration of a drug (a receptor antagonist) for a prolonged period. For example, the blocking of dopamine receptors by chlorpromazine may cause supersensitivity by up-regulating dopamine receptors.

Pharmacokinetic Interactions

Drugs may affect the absorption, distribution, metabolism, or excretion of other drugs. This includes those interactions in which the gastrointestinal absorption of a drug, plasma protein binding, drug metabolism, and urinary excretion are either enhanced or inhibited.

INTERACTION AT THE SITE OF ABSORPTION

The rate or extent of drug absorption from the gastrointestinal tract can be influenced in a number of ways. Following are examples of these various influences.

Alteration of Gastric pH

Iron poisoning is characterized by vomiting, abdominal pain, gastroenteritis, and shock, and, if not properly treated, severe metabolic acidosis, coma, and death eventuate. **Deferoxamine**, which binds iron, is used as the preferred chelator in treating iron poisoning. The metabolic acidosis may be appropriately treated with sodium bicarbonate. However, because deferoxamine chelates iron more effectively in an acidic medium, it should not be administered orally along with sodium bicarbonate. The ideal treatment of iron poisoning consists of gastric aspiration, followed by lavage with a phosphate solution to form insoluble iron salts. Deferoxamine should then be given intravenously or intramuscularly to chelate the iron that has been absorbed. Sodium bicarbonate may be administered intravenously. To absorb any residual iron remaining in the stomach, deferoxamine may then be instilled into the stomach.

Formation of Complexes

Tetracyclines, as broad-spectrum antibiotics, are the drugs of choice in treating *Mycoplasma pneumoniae* infections. Most tetracyclines are absorbed to various degrees (30 to 100%) from the gastrointestinal tract, primarily from the stomach and upper small intestine. The absorption of tetracyclines is hindered by milk and milk products, by numerous **antacids** such as aluminum hydroxide, sodium bicarbonate, and calcium carbonate, and by iron preparations such as ferrous sulfate. Therefore these and similar substances should not be administered orally together with tetracycline.

Alteration in Gastric Emptying Time

Agents that reduce gastrointestinal motility and prolong gastric emptying time, reduce the rate of absorption of drugs whose absorption takes place primarily in the duodenum. Furthermore, by prolonging the time poorly soluble drugs are kept in the stomach, their bioavailability may be altered. Hence, compounds with strong anticholinergic properties such as **propantheline** (for peptic diseases), **glycopyrrolate** (for asthma), **benztropine** (for parkinsonism), and **imipramine** (for depression) are potentially able to alter the absorption of other concomitantly administered drugs. The absorption of digoxin and dicumerol is altered by imipramine and other tricyclic antidepressants. On the other hand, some drugs such as antacids may speed the gastric emptying time.

Interactions at the Plasma Protein-Binding Sites

Drugs may **compete** for binding sites on the plasma or tissue protein, or may **displace** previously bound drugs. For example, **phenylbutazone** may compete with **phenytoin** for binding to albumin. Similarly, phenylbutazone (an antiinflammatory agent) is able to displace warfarin (an anticoagulant) from its binding site and enhance the free circulating concentration of the anticoagulant. Sulfonamides (chemotherapeutic agents) are able to displace sulfonylureas (oral antidiabetic agents) and cause hypoglycemia. Estradiol, by inhibiting the hepatic metabolism of proteins, may increase the amount of binding proteins. For example, women taking estrogen-containing oral contraceptives may demonstrate elevated levels of protein-bound iodine but remain euthyroid.

Interactions at the Stage of Drug Biotransformation

Drug biotransformation usually converts the nonpolar active drugs into more water-soluble, but pharmacologically inactive, products. Drugs may stimulate or inhibit the metabolism of other drugs. These interactions may be either innocuous or detrimental to the expected therapeutic objectives.

The prolonged ingestion of alcohol or phenobarbital induces drug biotransformation. The maximum inducing effects vary from drug to drug, usually occurring and subsiding within 7 to 10 days. The sudden withdrawal of an inducing agent in some circumstances can prove fatal. For example, hypnotic sedatives accelerate the rate of metabolism of **coumarin** anticoagulants. Increased doses of coumarin may therefore have to be given in order to achieve the desired prothrombin time and therapeutic effects. The sudden withdrawal of a hypnotic-sedative agent may cause the coumarin-catabolizing enzyme to revert to the pretreatment level, and, in the presence of large concentrations of free coumarin, **hemorrhage** may ensue. Because physicians anticipate that their patients may not require hypnotic-sedatives after being discharged from the hospital, the maintenance doses of coumarin anticoagulants are gradually reduced 2 to 3 days before discharge.

On the other hand, drugs may **inhibit** the metabolism of other drugs. For example, allopurinol (a xanthine oxidase inhibitor that inhibits the synthesis of uric acid) increases the effectiveness of anticoagulants by inhibiting their metabolism. Chloramphenicol (a potent inhibitor of microsomal protein synthesis) and cimetidine (an H_2-receptor blocker used in acid-pepsin disease) have similar properties. In addition, drugs may **compete** with each other for metabolism. In methyl alcohol (methanol) poisoning, ethyl alcohol may be given intravenously to avert methanol-induced **blindness** and minimize the severe **acidosis**. Ethyl alcohol competes with methyl alcohol for catabolism by liver alcohol dehydrogenase. The unmetabolized and less toxic methanol is excreted unchanged in the urine.

Interactions at the Site of Excretion

Numerous drugs are able to either enhance or inhibit the excretion of other drugs. For example, **sodium bicarbonate** enhances the excretion of **phenobarbital**. Probenecid interferes with the active secretion of **penicillin**, and hence prolongs its half-life. **Probenecid's** uricosuric effects are counteracted by acetylsalicylic acid, which also possesses a uricosuric effect. When given concomitantly, both are excreted.

A

ABORTIFACIENTS

Prostaglandins stimulate the myometrium of the gravid uterus to contract in a manner that is similar to the contractions seen in the term uterus during labor. **Carboprost tromethamine**, for IM use only, is administered in an initial dose of 250 mcg, with subsequent doses of 250 mcg at 2.0- to 4.0-hour intervals, and not exceeding a total dose of 12.0 mg. **Dinoprostone** (Prostaglandin E_2) is administered by vaginal suppository (20 mg), and the subject should remain in a supine position for 10 minutes following insertion. Additional suppositories may be given every four hours until abortion occurs. Prostaglandins stimulate the smooth muscle of the GI tract, causing vomiting or diarrhea. Aminopterin, mercaptopurine, azathioprine, and cyclophosphamide have been known to cause miscarriage.

ACEBUTOLOL

Acebutolol is a $beta_1$ selective adrenergic receptor blocking agent which has intrinsic sympathomimetic activity with a plasma half-life of 3 to 4 hours. It is indicated in **hypertension**, to be used alone or in combination with other antihypertensive medications. It is also indicated in the management of **ventricular premature beats**. The initial dose in uncomplicated mild to moderate hypertension is 400 mg. In ventricular arrhythmia, the initial dose of 200 mg twice daily may be increased gradually until optimal response is obtained (600 to 1200 mg/day), and the medication is decreased gradually in two weeks. The dose of acebutolol is lower in elderly patients (200 to 600 mg/day) and should be reduced in impairment of renal and hepatic functions.

ACENOCOUMAROL

The coumarin anticoagulants include dicumarol, warfarin sodium (coumadin sodium), warfarin potassium (Athrombin-K), acenocoumarol, and phenprocouman. Phenprocouman, acenocoumarol, and ethyl biscoumacetate are not generally available in the United States, but are prescribed in Europe and elsewhere. Phenprocouman (Marcumar) has a longer plasma half-life (5 days) than warfarin, as well as a somewhat slower onset of action and a longer duration of action (7 to 14 days). It is administered in daily maintenance doses of 0.75 to 6.0 mg. By contrast, acenocoumarol (Nicoumarlone; Sinthrome) has a shorter half-life (10 to 24 hours), a more rapid effect on the prothrombin time, and a shorter duration of action (2 days). The maintenance dose is 1 to 8 mg daily. Ethyl biscoumacetate (Tromexane) has a very short half-life of 2 to 3 hours and is seldom used.

ACETAMINOPHEN

(N-Acetyl-P-Aminophenol, APAP, Acephen, Anacin-3, Bromo-Seltzer, Datril, Datril 500, Tempra, Tylenol, Valadol, Valorin)

Acetaminophen is classified as a non-narcotic analgesic and antipyretic agent. Aspirin is superior to acetaminophen in treating pain of inflammatory origin. Acetaminophen is superior to aspirin in not affecting prothrombin response or producing GI ulceration. Therefore, acetaminophen is used in individuals who are allergic to aspirin; or in the presence of hemostatic disturbances, including bleeding diatheses, such as hemophilia, upper GI diseases, such as ulcer, gastritis, or hiatus hernia; or in patients who are taking anticoagulants. Acetaminophen reduces fever by acting on the hypothalamic heat-regulating centers, by blocking the actions of endogenous pyrogens, and by increasing heat dissipation through vasodilatation and sweating. Acetaminophen inhibits the activity of prostaglandin synthetase in the CNS, but not in the peripheral systems, which accounts for its lack of antirheumatic and antiinflammatory effects. Acetaminophen is metabolized in the liver and excreted by the kidneys mostly as glucuronate or sulfate conjugates. When given in larger than therapeutic doses (325 to 650 mg p.o. not exceeding 4 g daily) or in glutathione deficiency, acetaminophen may cause hepatic necrosis. Similarly, hepatotoxicity may occur in chronic alcoholics following therapeutic doses of acetaminophen. In addition, the potential hepatotoxicity of acetaminophen may increase by administration of large doses of barbiturates, hydantoins, sulfinpyrazone, carbamazepine, or rifampin when given for a prolonged period of time. Activated charcoal reduces the absorption of acetaminophen, and **N-acetylcysteine**, which provides sulfhydryl groups, is a specific antidote for acetaminophen toxicity.

ACETAZOLAMIDE

(Acetamide, Acetazolamide Sodium, AK-Zol, Albox, AK-Zol, Dehydratin, Diamox, Diamox Sequels, Diamox Sodium, Ederen, Glauconox, Glaupax, Inidrase, Ledamox, Nephramid, Ocu-zolamide, Oratrol, Storzolamide)

Acetazolamide is classified as an anticonvulsant, antiglaucomatous agent, and diuretic, and is a potent inhibitor of the enzyme carbonic anhydrase. The carbonic anhydrase inhibitors consist of **acetazolamide** (Diamox), **ethoxzolamide** (Cardrase), and **dichlorphenamide** (Daranide). Acetazolamide is an old agent, whereas ethoxzolamide and dichlorphenamide are newer preparations. Dichlorphenamide is the most potent carbonic anhydrase inhibitor in use today. The presence of SO_2NH_2 (sulfonamide) causes such compounds to inhibit carbonic anhydrase (CA), which catalyzes the hydration of carbon dioxide as follows:

$$CO_2 + H_2O \xrightarrow{\quad CA \quad} H_2CO_3 \rightleftharpoons H^+ + HCO_3^-$$

These agents inhibit carbonic anhydrase in the renal tubular cells in both the proximal and distal tubules (see Figures 4 and 89). When the rate of hydrogen generation is reduced, HCO_3^- is lost in urine, and the patient tends to become acidotic. However, the plasma concentration of HCO_3^- is lowered and less is filtered, so the diuresis becomes less effective. In addition, the sodium output is increased because its resorption in exchange for hydrogen is limited by the decreased availability of hydrogen. With less hydrogen available, the exchange of sodium for potassium predominates, and this fosters the loss of potassium. Chloride excretion is not altered significantly. Because the aqueous humor has a high concentration of bicarbonate, carbonic anhydrase inhibitors are primarily used in the treatment of **glaucoma**. They are no longer used as diuretics or as antiepileptic agents.

In **acute angle-closure glaucoma**, **dichlorphenamide** (100 to 200 mg, followed by 100 mg q. 12 hours) may be used with **miotics** and **osmotic agents** to rapidly reduce intraocular tension.

ACETIC ACID

(Domeboro Otic, Vosol Otic Solution)

Acetic acid (2 drops in each ear b.i.d.) is an antibacterial and antifungal agent, which is indicated in the treatment of external ear canal infection.

ACETOHEXAMIDE
(Dimelin, Dimelor, Dymelor, Gamadiabet, Ordimel, Toyobexin)

Acetohexamide is a blood glucose lowering drug of the sulfonylurea class. The first-generation oral hypoglycemic agents include tolbutamide (Orinase), acetohexamide (Dymelor), tolazamide (Tolinase), and chlorpropamide (Diabinese). The second-generation oral hypoglycemic agents include **glyburide** (DiaBeta, Micronase), and **glipizide** (Glucotrol) (see Table 1 and Figure 44). These agents exert their effects initially by enhancing the secretion of insulin by β cells of the pancreas. Following several months of continuous treatment, insulin levels return to pretreatment values, whereas glucose levels remain improved. Oral hypoglycemic agents reduce the rate of hepatic glucose production, and increase the sensitivity and number of insulin receptors. Acetohexamide is an intermediate-acting sulfonylurea with a maximum hypoglycemic effect in three hours and a duration of action of 12 to 18 hours. It is metabolized by the liver to an active metabolite which, like acetohexamide, exhibits diuretic and uricosuric effects. The recommended dose range is 250 to 1500 mg/day, and since it undergoes urinary excretion, it can accumulate in renal failure. Prolonged (4 to 10 days) hypoglycemia has been reported in neonates born to diabetic mothers who were receiving a long-acting drug at the time of delivery. Overdosage of acetohexamide causes severe hypoglycemia, which in turn may cause headache, weakness, confusion, dizziness, lethargy, convulsions, coma, or death. In elderly, debilitated, or malnourished patients, especially those with impaired renal or hepatic functions, the doses of acetohexamide should be adjusted carefully.

TABLE 1
Comparison of Orally Administered Sulfonylurea Hypoglycemic Agents

Characteristics	Tolbutamide	Acetohexamide	Tolazamide	Chlorpropamide	Glipizide	Glyburide
Relative potency	1	2.5	5	6	100	150
Duration of action (hr)	6–10	12–18	16–24	24–72	16–24	18–24
Extent of protein binding	>98	~90	>98	~95	>98	>98
Hepatic metabolism	Yes	Yes	Yes	Yes	Yes	Yes
Urinary excretion	Yes	Yes	Yes	Yes	Yes	Yes
Fecal excretion (% of dose)	Negligible	Negligible	Negligible	Negligible	12	50
Dose (mg) range	500–3,000	250–1,500	100–1,000	100–500	2.5–40	1.25–20
Diuretic	Yes	Yes	Yes	No	No	Yes
Antidiuretic	Yes	No	No	Yes	No	No
Disulfiram-like effects	No	No	No	Yes	No	No

ACETOHYDROXAMIC ACID
(Lithostat)

Acetohydroxamic acid (250 mg p.o. t.i.d.), an **antiurolithic agent**, is indicated as an adjunctive agent in treating chronic urinary tract infections caused by urease-producing bacteria. Acetohydroxamic acid, which inhibits urease and reduces the production of ammonia, is devoid of antibacterial activity.

ACETOPHENAZINE MALEATE
(Tindal)

Acetophenazine (20 mg tablet p.o. t.i.d.; not available in injectable form) is a neuroleptic which exerts its antipsychotic effects by blocking the hyperactivity of dopaminergic receptors in the mesocortical and mesolimbic systems. However, by blocking dopaminergic receptors in the nigrostriatal pathway, acetophenazine causes pseudoparkinsonism which is treated by anticholinergic drugs such as trihexyphenidyl or benztropine. Acetophenazine also possesses anticholinergic, antihistaminic, and alpha adrenergic blocking effects. It reduces the actions of sympathomimetic amines including phenylephrine, phenylpropanolamine, and ephedrine. Acetophenazine potentiates the effects of alcohol, narcotic analgesics and barbiturates, and general, spinal, or epidural anesthetics. The combination of magnesium sulfate and acetophenazine may cause oversedation, hypotension, and respiratory depression. Acetaphenazine potentiates the effects of antiarrhythmic agents (guanidine, disopyramide, or procainamide) by enhancing the incidence of cardiac arrhythmias and conduction defects; the effects of compounds possessing anticholinergic properties including amitriptyline and diphenhydramine by causing oversedation, paralytic ileus, visual disturbances, and constipation; the effects of nitrates causing hypotension; and the effects of metrizamide increasing the risk of seizures. Acetophenazine is absorbed orally, is bound to plasma protein to the extent of 90%, exerts its effects in 30 minutes, and the peak effect is seen in 2 to 4 hours. It is distributed widely in the body and its fluids, including appearing in breast milk. It is metabolized in the liver and the metabolites are eliminated mostly in the urine and through the biliary tract in the feces. For other effects or side effects, see also the section on phenothiazine derivatives and Table 23.

ACETYLCHOLINE

Acetylcholine, an ester of choline and acetic acid, is synthesized in cholinergic neurons according to the following scheme:

$$\text{Acetyl CoA + choline} \xrightarrow{\text{Choline acetyltransferase}} \text{acetylcholine}$$

The acetylcholine, in turn, is hydrolyzed by both acetylcholinesterase and plasma butyrylcholinesterase. Choline is actively transported into nerve terminals (synaptosomes) by a high-affinity uptake mechanism. Furthermore, the availability of choline regulates the synthesis of acetylcholine (Figure 18).

Hemicholinium blocks the transport of choline into synaptosomes, whereas **botulinum toxin** blocks the calcium-mediated release of acetylcholine. The released acetylcholine is hydrolyzed rapidly by acetylcholinesterase to choline and acetate.

Acetylcholine receptors are classified as either **muscarinic** or **nicotinic**. The alkaloid **muscarine** mimics the effects produced by stimulation of the parasympathetic system. These effects are postganglionic and are exerted on exocrine glands, cardiac muscle, and smooth muscle. The alkaloid **nicotine** mimics the actions of acetylcholine, which include stimulation of all autonomic ganglia, stimulation of the adrenal medulla, and contraction of skeletal muscle.

Dimethylphenylpiperazinium stimulates the autonomic ganglia; tetra-ethylammonium and **hexamethonium** block the autonomic ganglia; phenyltrimethylammonium stimulates skeletal motor muscle end plates; decamethonium produces neuromuscular blockade; and **d-tubocurarine** blocks both the autonomic ganglia and the motor fiber end plates.

Among the agents cited, only **d-tubocurarine** is useful as a drug (skeletal muscle relaxant); the rest are useful only as research tools. **Cholinesterase**, found in liver and plasma, can hydrolyze other esters such as **succinylcholine** (a skeletal muscle relaxant). Cholinergic peripheral receptors are located on: (1) postganglionic parasympathetic fibers, (2) postganglionic sympathetic fibers, (3) all autonomic ganglia, and (4) skeletal end plates.

In addition, cholinergic receptors are distributed extensively in the CNS and participate in diversified functions such as audition, vision, learning and memory, ingestive behaviors (thirst and hunger), thermoregulation, locomotor activity, diurnal rhythms, sleep, and sexual activity. Changes in cholinergic neurons have been observed in **neurologic syndromes** such as catalepsy, stereotypy, and tremor, and in psychiatric disorders such as depression.

Methacholine, carbachol, and **bethanechol** are all agents that mimic the effects of stimulation of cholinergic nerves. The two currently used derivatives of acetylcholine are **bethanechol** (Urecholine chloride) and **carbachol** (Miostat). Unlike acetylcholine, both agents are resistant to hydrolysis by cholinesterase. Both are muscarinic agonists. The **nicotinic action** of carbachol is greater than that of acetylcholine, whereas bethanechol is devoid of nicotinic action. The **cardiovascular actions** of acetylcholine are vasodilation and negative chronotropic and inotropic effects. The cardiovascular effects of **methacholine** are more pronounced than those of acetylcholine, which in turn are greater than those of carbachol or bethanechol. The **gastrointestinal effects** (increase in tone, amplitude of contractions, and peristalsis) of bethanechol and carbachol are equal but greater than those of acetylcholine. The effects of carbachol and bethanechol on the **urinary tract**, consisting of ureteral peristalsis, contraction of the detrusor muscle of the urinary bladder, and an increase in voluntary voiding pressure, are equivalent and exceed those produced by acetylcholine.

The **miotic effects** of carbachol and bethanechol are greater than those of acetylcholine. **Atropine** is able to antagonize all cholinergic (muscarinic) effects produced by acetylcholine, methacholine, carbachol, and bethanechol. However, this antagonism is least evident with carbachol. Bethanechol is of value in the management of postoperative abdominal distention, gastric atony or stasis, and urinary retention. Carbachol (0.25 to 3.0%) may be used for the long-term therapy of noncongestive wide-angle glaucoma.

ACETYLCYSTEINE
(Mucomyst, Mucosal)

As a mucolytic agent, acetylcysteine splits disulfide linkages between mucoprotein molecular complexes decreasing their viscosity. It is used as an adjunct therapy in emphysema with bronchitis, chronic asthmatic bronchitis, tuberculosis, bronchiectasis, primary amyloidosis of the lung, pneumonia, and tracheobronchitis. In addition, it is used in pulmonary complications of cystic fibrosis and those associated with anesthetics, surgery, or care following tracheostomy.

Acetylcysteine is also used to attenuate hepatic injury from overdosing (10 to 15 g) with acetaminophen. By maintaining the hepatic level of glutathione, acetylcysteine protects the liver by acting as an alternate substrate for conjugation and hence detoxification of the reactive metabolite of acetaminophen. It is given in a dose of 140 mg/kg orally as a loading dose and then 70 mg/kg orally every four hours until acetaminophen's level becomes nontoxic.

Acetylcysteine (Fluimucil) is being tested as an immunomodulator in acquired immune deficiency syndrome (AIDS).

N-ACETYLPROCAINAMIDE
(Acecainide HCl)

N-acetylprocainamide, a metabolite of procainamide, is classified as a Type III antiarrhythmic agent. It prolongs atrial and ventricular action potential durations and refractory period without depressing conduction velocity. When compared to procainamide, N-acetylprocainamide has distinct electrophysiologic and pharmacologic effects and does not cause lupus-like syndrome. The common side effects of N-acetylprocainamide are gastrointestinal disturbances, dizziness, lightheadedness, blurred vision, numbness, and tingling sensation. The majority of N-acetyl-procainamide is excreted unchanged in the urine.

ACETYLSALICYCLIC ACID
(Aspirin)

Acetylsalicylic acid possesses analgesic, antipyretic, antiinflammatory, and uricosuric properties (see Table 2). Unlike the narcotic analgesics such as morphine, aspirin does not depress respiration, is relatively nontoxic, and lacks addiction liability. Aspirin is a weak or mild analgesic that is effective for ameliorating short, intermittent types of pain such as neuralgia, myalgia, and toothache. It does not have the efficacy of morphine and cannot relieve the severe, prolonged, and lancinating types of pain associated with trauma such as burns or fractures. Like morphine, it produces analgesia by raising the pain threshold in the thalamus, but, unlike morphine, it does not alter the patient's reactions to pain. Because aspirin does not cause hypnosis or euphoria, its site of action has been postulated to be subcortical. In addition to **raising the pain threshold**, the antiinflammatory effects of aspirin may contribute to its analgesic actions. However, no direct association between the antiinflammatory and analgesic effects of these compounds should be expected. For example, aspirin has both analgesic and antiinflammatory properties, whereas, acetaminophen has analgesic but not antiinflammatory properties. Furthermore, potent antiinflammatory agents such as phenylbutazone have only weak analgesic effects. Aspirin does not alter the normal body temperature, which is maintained by a balance between heat production and dissipation. In a fever associated with infection, increased oxidative processes enhance heat production. Aspirin acts by causing cutaneous vasodilation, which prompts perspiration and enhances heat dissipation. This effect is mediated via the hypothalamic nuclei, as proved by the fact that a lesion in the preoptic area suppresses the mechanism through which aspirin exerts its antipyretic effects. The antipyretic effects of aspirin may be due to its inhibition of hypothalamic prostaglandin synthesis (Figure 11). Although aspirin-induced diaphoresis contributes to its antipyretic effects, it is not an absolutely necessary process, since antipyresis takes place in the presence of atropine.

Small doses (600 mg) of aspirin cause **hyperuricemia**, but large doses (>5 gm) have a uricosuric effect. Aspirin inhibits uric acid resorption by the tubules in the kidneys. However, because of the availability of more effective uricosuric agents, aspirin is no longer used for this purpose.

Aspirin has an **antiinflammatory** action as well as **antirheumatic** and **antiarthritic** effects, and may therefore be used in the treatment of rheumatic fever. Aspirin is extremely effective in managing rheumatoid arthritis and allied diseases involving the joints, such as ankylosing spondylitis and osteoarthritis. It is thought that aspirin and indomethacin exert their antiinflammatory effects by inhibiting **prostaglandin** synthesis through the inhibition of **cyclooxygenase** (Figure 11). The presynthesized prostaglandins are released during a tissue injury that fosters inflammation and pain. Furthermore, aspirin reduces the formation of prostaglandin in the platelets and leukocytes, which is responsible for the reported hematologic effects associated with aspirin.

The current thinking concerning the role of aspirin in the prevention of cardiovascular disease is that it is beneficial in the event of **myocardial infarction** and **stroke**. It is effective because, in platelets, small amounts of aspirin acetylate irreversibly and bind to the active site of **thromboxane A_2**, a potent promoter of **platelet aggregation** (see Figure 12).

The menstrual cycle is associated with two potentially incapacitating events: **dysmenorrhea** and the **premenstrual syndrome**. Substantial evidence indicates that the excessive production

TABLE 2
The Pharmacologic Efficacy of Various Compounds Possessing Analgesic, Antipyretic, Uricosuric, and Antiinflammatory Actions

Specific groups	Analgesic	Antipyretic	Antiinflammatory	Uricosuric
Salicylate derivatives				
Acetylsalicylic acid (aspirin)	*	*	*	*
Pyrazolone derivatives				
Phenylbutazone	*	*	*	*
Oxyphenbutazone	*	*	*	*
Sulfinpyrazone	0	0	0	*
Paraaminophenol derivatives				
Acetaminophen	*	*	0	0
Phenacetin	*	*	0	0
Propionic acid derivatives				
Ibuprofen	*	*	*	0
Naproxen	*	*	*	0
Fenoprofen	*	*	*	0
Flurbiprofen	*	*	*	0
Ketoprofen	*	*	*	0
Newer drugs				
Indomethacin	*	*	*	0
Sulindac	*	0	*	0
Mefenamic acid	*	0	*	0
Tolmetin	*	*	*	0
Diflunisal	*	0	*	0
Piroxicam	*	*	*	0
Diclofenac	*	*	*	0
Etodolac	*	0	*	0
Nabumetone	*	*	*	0

* = possesses the property assigned; 0 = lacks the property assigned.

of prostaglandin F_{2a} is the major source of painful menstruation. The nonsteroidal antiinflammatory drugs approved for the treatment of dysmenorrhea are **aspirin, ibuprofen, mefenamic acid**, and **naproxen**.

Aspirin both directly and indirectly stimulates respiration. In analgesic doses, aspirin increases **oxygen consumption** and **carbon dioxide production**. However, increased alveolar ventilation balances the increased carbon dioxide production, thus, the partial pressure of CO_2 (PCO_2) in plasma does not change. In the event of salicylate intoxication (e.g., 10 to 12 grams of aspirin given in 6 to 8 hours in adults, and an even smaller dosage in children whose brain is far more sensitive to salicylate intoxication), salicylate stimulates the medullary centers directly and this causes **hyperventilation** characterized by an increase in the depth and rate of respiration. The PCO_2 level declines, causing hypocapnia, and the blood pH increases, causing **respiratory alkalosis**. The low PCO_2 then decreases the renal tubular resorption of bicarbonate and compensates for the alkalosis.

If the salicylate level continues to rise, the respiratory centers become depressed, the PCO_2 level becomes elevated, and the blood pH becomes more acidic, causing **respiratory acidosis**.

Dehydration, reduced bicarbonate levels, and the accumulation of salicylic acid, salicyluric acid resulting from metabolism of aspirin, and lactic acid and pyruvic acid resulting from deranged carbohydrate metabolism may cause **metabolic acidosis**.

Although innocuous in most subjects, the therapeutic analgesic doses of aspirin may cause epigastric distress, nausea, vomiting, and bleeding. Aspirin can also exacerbate the symptoms of peptic ulcer, characterized by heartburn, dyspepsia, and erosive gastritis. An extensive number of salts have been synthesized from salicylate (e.g., calcium carbaspirin, choline salicylate, alloxipirin, and numerous buffered derivatives), and each has shown some ability to reduce the gastrointestinal toxicity of aspirin. However, other unknown factors may contribute to this undesirable gastrointestinal property of aspirin. In experimental animals, the intravenous administration of sodium salicylate or subcutaneous administration of methyl salicylate has produced petechial hemorrhage of the gastric mucosa. Furthermore, compounds possessing antiinflammatory properties (aspirin, phenylbutazone, and oxyphenbutazone) are associated with a higher incidence of gastrointestinal toxicity than those compounds devoid of antiinflammatory properties (phenacetin and acetaminophen).

Aspirin reduces the **leukocytosis** associated with acute rheumatic fever. When given on a long-term basis, it also reduces the hemoglobin level and the hematocrit. Aspirin use can cause reversible **hypoprothrombinemia** by interfering with the function of **vitamin K** in prothrombin synthesis. Therefore, aspirin should be used with caution in patients with vitamin K deficiency, preexisting hypoprothrombinemia, or hepatic damage; in patients taking anticoagulants; and in patients scheduled for surgery. Aspirin leads to **hemolytic anemia** in individuals with glucose 6-phosphate dehydrogenase deficiency. An **aspirin tolerance test** is used diagnostically in **von Willebrand's disease**, because it will further prolong the bleeding time if the disease exists. Aspirin prevents platelet aggregation and may be helpful in the treatment of thromboembolic diseases. In addition to aspirin, indomethacin, phenylbutazone, sulfinpyrazone, and dipyridamole prevent platelet aggregation (see Figures 12 and 84); whereas epinephrine, serotonin, and prostaglandins promote platelet aggregation and hence are procoagulants. The erythrocyte sedimentation rate is often elevated in infections and inflammations but aspirin therapy will yield a false negative. The supportive treatment of aspirin poisoning may include **gastric lavage** (to prevent the further absorption of salicylate), **fluid replenishment** (to offset the dehydration and oliguria), **alcohol and water sponging** (to combat the hyperthermia), the administration of **vitamin K** (to prevent possible hemorrhage), **sodium bicarbonate** administration (to combat acidosis), and, in extreme cases, **peritoneal dialysis** and **exchange transfusion**.

ACTINOMYCIN D

(Dactinomycin)

The antibiotics that bind to DNA are nonspecific to the cell-cycle phase. Actinomycin binds to double-stranded DNA and prevents RNA synthesis by inhibiting DNA-dependent RNA polymerase. It is administered intravenously in the treatment for pediatric solid tumors such as Wilms' tumor and rhabdomyosarcoma and for gestational choriocarcinoma. Dactinomycin causes skin reactions, gastrointestinal injury, and delayed bone marrow depression (see Figure 2).

ACTIVATED CHARCOAL

(Actidose-Aqua, Arm-A-Char, Charcoaide, Charcocaps, Insta-Char, Liquid-Antidose)

Activated charcoal (1000 mg p.o. t.i.d.), is indicated for the treatment of flatulence and dyspepsia. Activated charcoal, as an adsorbent (30 g in 250 ml water to make a slurry), is indicated

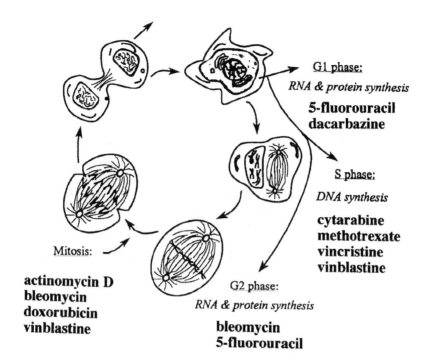

G1 phase:
RNA & protein synthesis

**5-fluorouracil
dacarbazine**

S phase:
DNA synthesis

**cytarabine
methotrexate
vincristine
vinblastine**

Mitosis:

**actinomycin D
bleomycin
doxorubicin
vinblastine**

G2 phase:
RNA & protein synthesis

**bleomycin
5-fluorouracil**

FIGURE 2   The actions of antineoplastic agents on different phases of the cell cycle.

in the treatment of overdosage from numerous medications. It absorbs intestinal gas causing discomfort, toxic and nontoxic irritants causing diarrhea, and drugs preventing their absorption, and hence toxicity.

ACUTE RESPIRATORY DISTRESS SYNDROME: TREATMENT OF
Acute respiratory distress syndrome (ARDS) or acute lung injury may be defined as a condition involving impaired oxygenation. The nonpharmacologic therapies include mechanical ventilation. The pharmacologic therapies include the use of exogenous surfactant, corticosteroids, acetylcysteine (antioxidant), ketoconazole, nitric oxide, eicosanoids and their inhibitors, sodium nitroprusside (vasodilator), pentoxifylline, antiendotoxin, and anticytokine therapy and antibiotics.

ACYCLOVIR

(Zovirax)

The herpes virus family includes the herpes simplex virus, varicella zoster virus, cytomegalovirus, and Epstein-Barr virus. Acyclovir (Zovirax), a synthetic acyclic purine neuroside analog, has antiviral activity against the herpes viruses, especially herpes simplex type 1. It inhibits viral replication by inhibiting DNA synthesis. It interacts with the virus-induced enzyme, especially thymidine kinase and DNA polymerase (see Figure 3). Mutations that lead to amino acid substitutions then give rise to resistance in either enzyme. Acyclovir is effective in the treatment of herpes simplex virus type 1 and type 2 infections, including chronic and recurrent mucocutaneous herpes in the immunologically impaired host, primary and secondary genital herpes, neonatal herpes, and herpes simplex encephalitis.

In genital herpes, oral acyclovir (200 mg every four hours, five times daily for 10 days) reduces the duration of acute infection, attenuates pain and new lesion formation, and decreases but does not eliminate the recurrence of episodes. Acyclovir is effective in localized cutaneous herpes zoster infection and chicken pox infection, lessening severe itching and lesion formation.

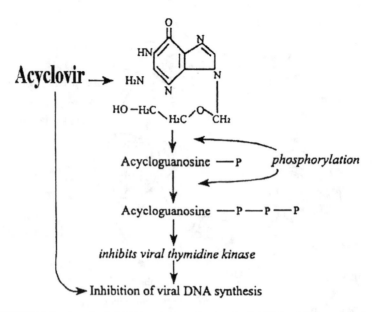

FIGURE 3   Acyclovir inhibits viral replication by inhibiting DNA synthesis.

Parenteral acyclovir (e.g., 5 mg/kg infused at a constant rate over one hour every eight hours for seven days) may be used in mucosal and cutaneous herpes simplex virus infections, and in varicella zoster infections (shingles) in immunocompromised patients and in herpes simplex encephalitis.

Acyclovir is available for topical application (Zovirax ointment 5% 50 mg/kg in a polyethylene glycol base), which may cause mucosal irritation and transient burning when applied to genital lesions.

Acyclovir is slowly absorbed from the GI tract, and peak effective plasma concentration is reached in 1.5 to 2 hours. It is widely distributed in tissues and body fluids, including brain, kidney, lung, liver, muscle, spleen, uterus, vaginal mucosa, vaginal secretions, CSF, and herpetic vesicular fluid. Acyclovir is eliminated by glomerular filtration and tubular secretion. It decreases the renal clearance of **methotrexate**, which is eliminated by active tubular secretion.

The side effects of oral acyclovir are nausea, diarrhea, rash, headache, and rarely nephrotoxicity or neurotoxicity. The principal dose-limiting toxicities of intravenous acyclovir are preexisting renal insufficiency, high doses (plasma level >25 microgram/hour), or both. Rapid infusion, dehydration, inadequate urine flow, or nephrotoxic agents increase the risk. Probenecid decreases the renal clearance of acyclovir and prolongs its half-life, and acyclovir decreases the renal clearance of methotrexate or other agents undergoing active tubular secretion. The combined use of zidovudine and acyclovir have caused severe somnolence and lethargy.

ADENOSINE

As an autacoid, adenosine possesses negative chronotropic and inotropic effects, is a vasodilator in almost all vascular beds, inhibits neurotransmitter release in the central nervous system, causes sedation, displays anticonvulsant activity, regulates renin release, inhibits platelet aggregation, modulates lymphocyte function, induces bronchospasm, and inhibits lipolysis.

Receptors for adenosine are referred to as **purinergic receptors** (P_1, which should be distinguished from the P_2 receptors that mediate the actions of ATP in the gastrointestinal tract and vascular endothelium). Adenosine is able to modulate **adenylate cyclase**, similar to acetylcholine.

To accomplish this, it interacts with ion channels to hyperpolarize and decrease the duration of the action potentials and activates phospholipase C in certain tissues.

ADRENOCORTICOTROPIC HORMONE (ACTH)

The adrenal steroids are divided into three major categories: **glucocorticoids, mineralocorticoids,** and **sex hormones**. The glucocorticoids mainly influence carbohydrate metabolism and, to a certain extent, protein and lipid metabolism. The main glucocorticoid is **cortisol**, with a daily secretion of 15 mg. The mineralocorticoids influence **salt and water metabolism** and in general conserve sodium levels. They promote the resorption of sodium and the secretion of potassium in the cortical collecting tubules and possibly the connecting segment. They also elicit hydrogen secretion in the medullary collecting tubules. The main mineralocorticoid is **aldosterone**, with a daily secretion of 100 micrograms. Small quantities of **progesterone, testosterone**, and **estradiol** are also produced by the adrenal gland. However, they play a minor role compared to the testicular and ovarian hormones.

Adrenal glucocorticoid and androgen production is controlled predominantly by the **hypothalamic-pituitary axis**, whereas the production of aldosterone by the zona glomerulosa is predominantly regulated by the **renin-angiotensin system** and potassium concentration. The hypothalamus, pituitary, and adrenal form a **neuroendocrine axis** whose primary function is to regulate the production of both cortisol and some of the adrenal steroids (Figure 28).

Corticotropin-releasing factor and **arginine vasopressin**, which are released predominantly by the paraventricular nucleus of the hypothalamus, are important regulators of corticotropin (ACTH) release, which in turn triggers the release of cortisol and other steroids by the adrenal gland. Both the administration of certain psychoactive agents and emotional arousal originating from the limbic system are able to modify the functions of the pituitary-adrenal axis and to stimulate the synthesis of cortisol.

ACTH elicits the following effects: It enhances the synthesis of pregnenolone, activates adenylate cyclase and elevates the cyclic adenosine monophosphate level, enhances the level of adrenal steroids, especially cortisol, and reduces the level of ascorbic acid.

The level of cortisol is thought to directly control the secretion of ACTH through a negative feedback mechanism that may be directed at both the hypothalamus and the anterior pituitary gland. Conversely, a reduced concentration of cortisol or cortisol-like substances eliminates the negative effect and enhances the release of ACTH (see Figure 28).

ADRENERGIC (SYMPATHOMIMETIC) COMPOUNDS	
Direct-acting Sympathomimetic Agents	
Albuterol	Mephentermine
Bitolterol	Metaproterenol
Dobutamine	Methoxamine
Dopamine	Norepinephrine
Epinephrine	Phenylephrine
Isoetharine	Ritodrine
Isoproterenol	Terbutaline
Indirect-acting Sympathomimetic Agents	
Amphetamine	Phenylpropanolamine
Ephedrine	Pseudoephedrine

ADRENERGIC (SYMPATHOMIMETIC) RECEPTOR BLOCKING AGENTS	
Alpha-adrenergic Blocking Agents	
Phenoxybenzamine	Prazosin
Phentolamine	Tolazoline
Beta-adrenergic Blocking Agents	
Acebutolol	Nadolol
Atenolol	Pindolol
Esmolol	Propranolol
Labetolol	Timolol
Metoprolol	

ADRENOCORTICOIDS
Topical Antiinflammatory Agents Available as Cream, Gel, Lotion, or Ointment

Alclometasone dipropionate	Diflucortolone valerate
Amcinonide	Flumethasone pivalate
Beclomethasone dipropionate	Fluocinolone acetonide
Betamethasone benzoate	Fluocinonide
Betamethasone dipropionate	Flurandrenolide
Betamethasone valerate	Halcinonide
Clobetasol propionate	Hydrocortisone
Clobetasone butyrate	Hydrocortisone acetate
Clocortolone pivalate	Hydrocortisone butyrate
Desonide	Hydrocortisone valerate
Desoximetasone	Methylprednisolone acetate
Dexamethasone	Mometasone furoate
Dexamethasone sodium phosphate	Triamcinolone acetonide
Diflorasone diacetate	

AGED PATIENTS: ALTERED PHARMACOKINETIC PROFILE	
Pharmacokinetic Profiles	**Parameters Affected**
Absorption	Elevated gastric pH Decreased gastrointestinal blood flow Decreased active transport mechanisms
Distribution	Decreased total body water Decreased lean body mass Increased body fat Decreased serum albumin
Metabolism	Decreased liver blood flow Decreased liver size Possibly decreased enzymatic activity
Excretion	Decreased glomerular filtration rate Decreased renal blood flow Decreased tubular function
Receptors	Diminished cholinergic, alpha-1 adrenergic, and opioid receptors

Statistical analysis has firmly established four isolated but interrelated facts about the aged population.

Longevity is increasing.

The aged population of the world is expanding.

The aged population may have multiple diseases and may be taking multiple medications.

The potential of drug–drug interactions and adverse drug reactions is a conspicuous problem among the elderly.

The appreciation and application of concepts involved in geriatric pharmacology will not only reduce the incidence of potential drug-related toxicities but will also enhance the quality of life for this group of patients. As in the pediatric population, the pharmacokinetic parameters are distinct for the older age groups. Because the plasma albumin level decreases with aging, the binding of drugs to plasma protein also diminishes. Furthermore, because the total body fat increases with aging, the storage of lipid-soluble substances (silent sites) also varies. Since the total water in the body also decreases, this alters the volumes of distribution of the drugs. The metabolism of some drugs is reduced, and thus their half-lives are increased. Because the glomerular filtration rate and the tubular excretion rate are diminished by the aging process, the excretion of most drugs and their metabolites is below the standard for younger patients. Consequently, the very old patient behaves pharmacokinetically very much like the very young one. However, to further complicate the situation, unlike pediatric patients, the elderly may have several diseases, including cardiovascular ones, and may be taking several agents, especially those with very narrow margins of safety (e.g., digitalis and the tricyclic antidepressants). Therefore, it is imperative that these pharmacokinetic principles be taken into consideration when prescribing medications for older patients in order to avoid undue toxicities.

AGGREGIN

Platelets circulate in blood without adhering to other platelets or to the endothelium. However, when the endothelial cells are perturbed, the platelets adhere and undergo a change in shape, and aggregate. ADP is known to induce the platelet shape change, aggregation, and exposure of fibrinogen binding sites (see Figure 84).

The platelet surface contains **aggregin**, a membrane protein with a molecular weight of 100 kDa, with physical and immunochemical properties that differ from those of platelet glycoprotein IIIa.

Binding to aggregin is required in order for epinephrine-induced platelet aggregation to take place. In turn, **epinephrine** increases the affinity of ADP for its receptor. **Thrombin** stimulates platelet aggregation independent of ADP, but by raising the level of calcium in the cytoplasm, it activates platelet **calpain**, which in turn cleaves aggregin.

AGMATINE

Agmatine, an endogenous vasodilating substance, has recently been identified as an endogenous clonidine-displacing substance (CDS) in mammalian brain. Agmatine, like CDS, binds to imidazoline receptors (I receptors) and alpha$_2$-adrenoceptors which stimulate the release of catecholamines from adrenal chromaffin cells in a dose-dependent manner. Although arginine decarboxylase, the enzyme which forms agmatine, has been localized in endothelial cells and endothelial cells storing agmatine, the effects of agmatine on systemic hemodynamics are unknown.

AGRANULOCYTOSIS: DRUG-INDUCED			
Acetaminophen	Clozapine	Imipramine	Phenylbutazone
Acetazolamide	Dapsone	Indomethacin	Phenytoin
Acetylsalicylic acid	Desipramine	Isoniazid	Primidone
Allopurinol	Doxycycline	Levamisole	Procainamide
β-Lactam antibiotics	Ethacrynic acid	Lincomycin	Propranolol
Benzodiazepines	Ethosuximide	Meprobamate	Propylthiouracil
Brompheniramine	Fenoprofen	Methazolamide	Pyrimethamine
Carbamazepine	Flucytosine	Methimazole	Quinine
Captopril	Ganciclovir	Metronidazole	Rifampin
Ceftriaxone	Gentamicin	Nitrofurantoin	Streptomycin
Chloramphenicol	Gold salts	Oxyphenbutazone	Sulfa antibiotics
Chlorpropamide	Griseofulvin	Para-aminosalicyclic acid	Tocainide
Chlorpromazine	Hydralazine	Penicillamine	Tolbutamide
Cimetidine	Hydroxychloroquine	Pentazocine	Vancomycin
Clindamycin	Ibuprofen	Phenothiazines	Zidovudine
Clomipramine			

A number of mechanisms may produce drug-induced agranulocytosis. For example, chlorpromazine and other phenothiazine derivatives (perphenazine, prochlorperazine, thioridazine, and triflupromazine) *may* cause agranulocytosis. The incidence of this is higher among female and elderly patients whose bone marrow has lower proliferative potential. These agents inhibit DNA polymerase, thymidylate kinase, and the incorporation of [^{3}H]thymidine into DNA. Because the phenothiazine-induced agranulocytosis is a toxic reaction, it may be prevented by carefully monitoring the status of peripheral blood.

AIDS DRUGS

See *Protease inhibitors, Stavudine, Zalcitabine, Zidovudine.*

ALBUMIN

(Albuminar-5, Albutein 5%, Bumianate 5%, Plasbumin-5)

Plasma albumin (molecular weight, 66,400), the most abundant protein in the plasma, exerts 80% of the colloid osmotic pressure of blood. Albumin has two binding sites: **Site I** binds structurally unrelated substances (e.g., warfarin, phenytoin, and sulfonamides), and **Site II**, which is more selective, binds a smaller number of drugs (i.e., diazepam, phenylbutazone, and ibuprofen).

The **percentage of protein binding** of drugs at therapeutic levels varies dramatically. Some drugs such as allopurinol, heparin, and isoniazid do not become bound. Other drugs such as antipyrine, ethambutol, and theophylline become bound to the extent of only 4 to 15%. Several drugs such as ampicillin (25%) and digoxin (23%) show low protein binding; some drugs such as atropine (50%) and meperidine (40%) show moderate protein binding; and some drugs such as carbamazepine (72%), furosemide (75%), nitrofurantoin (70%), and rifampin (85%) show high degrees of protein binding. Some such as dicumarol (97%), diazepam (96%), phenylbutazone (98%), and diazoxide (96%) bind extensively to plasma proteins.

The binding sites of the protein are not unlimited and are subject to saturation. When this occurs, toxicity may develop following further drug administration, since the later portion of the drug remains free. Consistent with this view is the observation that toxic manifestations of drugs are quite frequent and considerably higher in individuals suffering from hypoalbuminemia or altered plasma and tissue protein concentrations, or both.

Drugs may alter the protein binding of other agents. For instance, aspirin decreases the binding of thyroxine, and the binding of bilirubin is hindered by many pharmacologic agents. The more tightly bound drugs can displace the less firmly bound agents. The intensity of the effect of displaced drug on the patient will simply depend on the blood level of the free drug and its nature. At times, the effect may be highly undesirable and even fatal. Only the slight displacement of a highly bound drug such as dicumarol (an oral anticoagulant) by phenylbutazone, which has greater affinity for binding sites, can cause serious hemorrhage. Because only 3% of the anticoagulant is free, an additional displacement of 3% increases its effects by 100%. The serum albumin and total protein concentrations are lower in infancy and increase to adult values by the age of 10 to 12 months.

Normal serum albumin (5% containing 130 to 160 mEq/L sodium) may be used in the treatment of a patient in **shock** with greatly reduced blood volume, after a **burn injury**, and in acute but not chronic **hypoproteinemia**. The use of albumin in transfusion (1 g/kg 1 to 2 hours before transfusion) is effective in hyperbilirubinemia and erythroblastosis fetalis, increasing the amount of bilirubin removed with each transfusion.

ALBUTEROL SULFATE

(Proventil, Ventolin)

Albuterol sulfate is available as a tablet (2 mg, 4 mg), solution (2 mg/5 ml), and aerosol inhaler (90 mcg/metered spray).

Albuterol selectively stimulates beta-adrenergic receptors in the lungs causing relaxation of bronchial smooth muscles which in turn relieves bronchospasm and reduces airway resistance. The selective beta$_2$-adrenergic stimulants cause bronchodilation without cardiac acceleration (see Figure 86). **Metaproterenol** and **terbutaline** are available in tablet form, and terbutaline is also available for subcutaneous injection. Metaproterenol and **albuterol** are available in metered-dose inhalers.

Inhalational selective beta$_2$-adrenergic receptor agonists (**albuterol, terbutaline, fenoterol,** and **bitolterol**) have a rapid onset of action and are effective for 3 to 6 hours. **Formoterol** and **salmeterol** are longer-acting agents (12 hours) and may prove useful in treating nocturnal symptoms.

Albuterol is used to relieve and prevent bronchospasm in patients with reversible obstructive airway disease and in individuals with exercise-induced bronchospasm. The onset of action of albuterol is 5 to 15 minutes, peak of action is 0.5 to 2 hours, and duration of action is 3 to 6 hours. Albuterol does not cross the blood-brain barrier. It must be used cautiously in patients with hyperthyroidism, diabetes mellitus, coronary insufficiency, and hypertension. The concomitant use of albuterol with monoamine oxidase inhibitors or tricyclic antidepressants should be discouraged. Glucocorticoids (beclomethasone, dexamethasone, flunisolide, or triamcinolone) may be used 15 minutes after inhalational albuterol.

ALCLOMETASONE DIPROPIONATE

(Aclovate)

Alclometasone (0.05% ointment) is a topical adrenocorticoid with antiinflammatory properties which is indicated in inflammation of corticosteroid-responsive dermatoses.

ALCURONIUM

Neuromuscular blocking agents may be used to diagnose myasthenia gravis, facilitate endotracheal intubation, relieve laryngeal spasm, provide relaxation during brief, diagnostic, and surgical procedures, prevent bone fracture in electroconvulsive therapy, produce apnea and controlled ventilation during thoracic surgery and neurosurgery, reduce muscular spasticity in neurologic diseases (multiple sclerosis, cerebral palsy, or tetanus), and reduce the muscular spasm and pain resulting from sprains, arthritis, myositis, and fibrositis.

Skeletal muscle relaxants can be classified into four categories of depolarizing or competitive blocking agents (e.g., tubocurarine), direct-acting relaxants (e.g., Dantrolene sodium), and centrally acting muscle relaxants (e.g., diazepam). Alcuronium is about twice as potent as *d*-tubocurarine, but it has a shorter duration of action. Muscular relaxation occurs 2 to 4 minutes after the injection of 0.2 mg/kg and lasts about 15 to 20 minutes. Like *d*-tubocurarine, it may lower blood pressure but does not cause histamine release. There is no evidence for any significant metabolism of alcuronium, and most of the drug is excreted unchanged in the urine, so it should be used cautiously in the presence of impaired renal function.

ALDESLEUKIN

(Interleukin-2, IL-2) (Proleukin)

Aldesleukin (600,000 IU/kg IV q. 8 hours for 5 days) is a lymphokine with immunoregulatory properties which is indicated in metastatic renal cell carcinoma. In addition, interleukin-2 is used in cell transfer therapy in cancer patients. Cell transfer therapy is a new approach to strengthening the innate ability of the immune system to fight against cancer. In this therapy, lymphocytes are isolated and cultured with **interleukin-2** for three days to yield **lymphokine-activated killer cells**, which are then administered to patients along with interleukin-2 (see Figure 53).

ALDOSTERONE

It is generally assumed that the intracellular content of sodium in vascular smooth muscle is increased in essential hypertension. Although the major role of aldosterone (see Figure 4) in

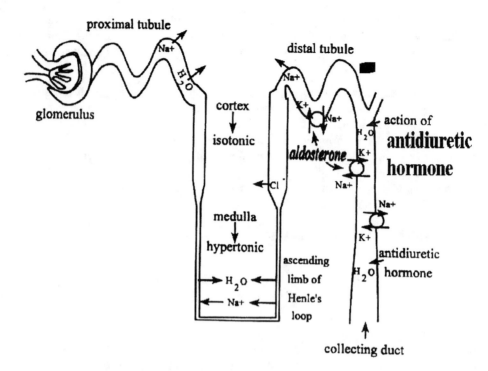

FIGURE 4 The main mineralocorticoid is **aldosterone**, which is synthesized from 18-hydroxycorti-costerone by a dehydrogenase. The consequence of 18-hydroxycorticosterone dehydrogenase deficiency is diminished secretion of aldosterone, and the clinical manifestations consist of sodium depletion, dehydration, hypotension, potassium retention, and enhanced plasma renin levels.

the regulation of blood pressure is a renal one, it may also be involved in some extrarenal effects responsible for the regulation of body fluid and blood pressure. Recent studies have suggested that vascular walls specifically bind to aldosterone and that aldosterone has a direct vasoconstrictive effect on vascular smooth muscle *in vitro*. Indeed, **canrenoate potassium** (Soldactone S), an **aldosterone antagonist**, reduces blood pressure (see Figure 21).

ALENDRONATE SODIUM
(Fosamax)

Alendronate sodium (10 mg/day) is indicated for the treatment of osteoporosis in postmeno-pausal women and of Paget's disease. It acts as a specific inhibitor of osteoclast-mediated bone resorption. The osteoclasts adhere normally to the bone surface but lack the ruffled border that is indicative of active resorption. Alendronate does not interfere with osteoclast recruitment or attachment, but it does inhibit osteoclast activity. Bones examined 6 and 49 days after (³H)alendronate administration showed that normal bone was formed on top of the alendronate, which was incorporated in bone matrix. Alendronate is not pharmacologically active, thus, it must be continuously administered to suppress osteoclasts on newly formed resorption sur-faces. Calcium supplements, antacids, and other oral medications will interfere with absorption of Fosamax. Therefore, patients must wait at least one hour before taking Fosamax.

ALFENTANIL HYDROCHLORIDE
(Alfenta)

Alfentanil, an opiate analgesic (8 to 50 mcg/kg IV), is indicated as an adjunct to general anesthetic in the maintenance of general anesthesia with barbiturate, nitrous oxide, and oxygen.

In addition, it is used as a primary anesthetic for induction of anesthesia when endotracheal intubation and mechanical ventilation are required.

ALGLUCERASE

(Glucocerebrosidase, Glucosylceramidase, Glucocerebrosidase-Beta-Glucosidase [Ceredase])

Alglucerase (initially 60 units/kg by infusion) is indicated for long-term endogenous enzyme (glucoslyceramidase) replacement in confirmed Type I **Gaucher's disease**.

ALLERGIC RHINITIS: TREATMENT OF	
Agents	**Properties**
Acrivastine	Nonsedating antihistamine
Azelastine	Antihistamine
Budesonide	Topical corticosteroid
Fenoterol	β_2-Adrenergic agonist
Fluocortin butyl	Topical corticosteroid
Ketotifen	Mast cell stabilizer
Mequitazine	
Nedocromil sodium	
Oxatomide	
Avoiding the offending allergens is the best preventative treatment. The aforementioned medications are symptomatic in nature.	

ALLOPURINOL SODIUM

(Zyloprim)

Allopurinol reduces the synthesis of uric acid by inhibiting the activity of xanthine oxidase (Figure 5). The reduction in the uric acid pool occurs slowly. Because xanthine and hypoxanthine are more soluble than uric acid, they are easily excreted.

Gout is a hyperuricemic state (>6 mg/dl) that is effectively diagnosed through the detection of monosodium urate crystals in the synovial fluid of the involved joint. Conditions causing hyperuricemia include: the excessive synthesis of uric acid, the excessive synthesis of purine — precursor to uric acid — a high dietary intake of purine (shellfish, organ meat, anchovies, and wild game), diminished renal excretion of uric acid, and tissue destruction following injury or therapeutic irradiation.

Numerous agents, when used in therapeutic doses, can also cause hyperuricemia. This includes an analgesic dose of aspirin, thiazide diuretics, nicotinic acid, chronic consumption of alcohol, and antineoplastic agents.

If left untreated, the hyperuricemic state may precipitate an acute attack of gout, which first appears in metatarsal phalangeal joints. Ultimately, tophaceous deposits form in the joints and soft tissues such as the kidneys. The hyperuricemic state may be corrected either by inhibiting the synthesis of uric acid by allopurinol or by enhancing the elimination of uric acid by uricosuric agents.

Allopurinol not only is used in treating the hyperuricemia associated with gout, but also in the secondary hyperuricemia associated with the use of antineoplastic agents. Therefore, allopurinol may be used in the management of patients with leukemia, lymphoma, and solid tumor malignancies who are receiving cancer therapy that causes elevations of serum and

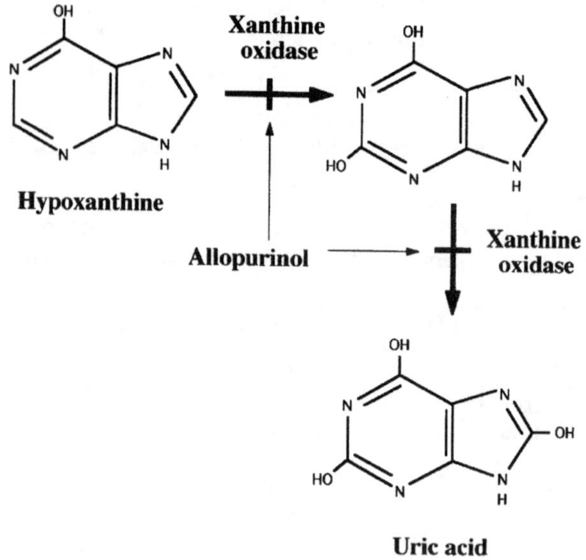

FIGURE 5 Allopurinol reduces the synthesis of uric acid by inhibiting the activity of xanthine oxidase. Not only is it used in treating the hyperuricemia associated with gout, but also in the secondary hyperuricemia associated with the use of antineoplastic agents. Allopurinol may interfere with the metabolism of antineoplastic agents such as **azathioprine** and **6-mercaptopurine**.

urinary uric acid levels. Allopurinol may interfere with the metabolism of antineoplastic agents such as **azathioprine** and **6-mercaptopurine**.

Allopurinol and oxipurinol have plasma half-lives of 1 to 2 hours and 15 hours, respectively. Allopurinol is cleared by glomerular filtration, whereas oxipurinol and uric acid are reabsorbed in the kidney tubules in a similar fashion. Therefore, the addition of uricosuric drugs increases the excretion of oxipurinol and hence may reduce the effectiveness of allopurinol.

Allopurinol may cause a cutaneous reaction (3%) which is predominantly pruritic and maculopapular in nature, is accompanied by fever, malaise, or muscle ache, and the incidence increases with renal impairment. Since the onset of skin rash may be followed by severe hypersensitivity reactions, allopurinol should be discontinued by patients who develop such rashes. Patients with impaired renal function require less drug and careful observation.

ALPHA-METHYLDOPA

(Aldomet)

The **catecholamine-synthesizing enzymes** are not only able to synthesize dopamine and norepinephrine from a physiologically occurring substrate such as L-dopa, but also from exogenous substrates such as **alpha-methyldopa**, which is converted to alpha-methyldopamine and in turn to alpha-methylnorepinephrine. Alpha-methyldopamine and alpha-methylnorepinephrine are called false transmitters and, in general (except for alpha-methylnorepinephrine), are weaker agonists (see Figure 27).

Alpha-methyldopa is used in the treatment of mild to moderate hypertension. The proposed mechanism of action is suppression of renin release, stimulation of central alpha$_2$-inhibitory adrenergic receptors (alpha$_2$-adrenergic receptor sites) such as dopamine, acetylcholine, and prostaglandins (PGE_1 and PGE_2 but not PGF_2A), reduction of the release of norepinephrine. In addition, alpha-methyldopa reduces the peripheral vascular resistance without altering the heart rate or cardiac output. Postural hypotension is mild and infrequent. Besides reducing blood pressure, alpha-methyldopa causes sedation (interference with norepinephrine), parkinsonism (interference with dopamine), psychosis (interference with serotonin), and decreased libido and impotence (interference with norepinephrine). Alpha-methyldopa has a long onset and a short duration of action. It is especially useful in the management of hypertension complicated by renal dysfunction, since it does not alter either renal blood flow or the glomerular filtration rate. It is contraindicated in patients with liver disease and may produce hepatitis-like symptoms.

ALPHA-PROTEINASE INHIBITOR

(Human) (Alpha₁-PI) (Prolastin)

Alpha$_1$ proteinase inhibitor (60 mg/kg IV once weekly), is indicated for chronic replacement of alpha$_1$-antitrypsin in patients with clinically demonstrable panacinar emphysema and PIZZ, PIZ (null), or Pi (null) (null) phenotype.

ALPRAZOLAM

(Xanax)

Alprazolam is effective in the management of anxiety disorders, of panic disorder with or without agoraphobia, and of anxious depression with a dosage regimen which must be individualized for each patient. Similar to benzodiazepine derivatives, alprazolam causes a dose-dependent CNS depression from mild sedation to hypnosis. Alprazolam is absorbed orally, is bound to plasma protein to the extent of 70 to 80%, possesses a half-life of 14 to 16 hours, and a volume of distribution of 1.02 to 1.20 L/kg. Both the half-life and volume of distribution are markedly increased in obese subjects. Alprazolam is metabolized to alpha-hydroxyalprazolam derivative which is inactive (see Table 8). Alprazolam crosses the placental barrier and is found in the human milk. The manifestations of overdosage include somnolence, confusion, impaired coordination, diminished reflexes, and coma. Death has been reported with large doses of alprazolam (LD50 in rats 500 to 2000 mg/kg) especially when taken with ethanol. Flumazenil (Mazicon), a specific benzodiazepine receptor antagonist, is effective in reversing the alprazolam-induced CNS depression, and should be complemented with other supportive therapy to aid respiration (Figure 40). The use of flumazenil is associated with the risk of precipitating seizures in susceptible individuals.

ALPRENOLOL

Alprenolol, which possesses dual beta-adrenergic receptor blocking effects and intrinsic sympathomimetic activity, has been used widely and successfully in the treatment of hypertension, angina pectoris, and cardiac arrhythmias. The levo isomer of alprenolol has approximately one hundred times greater affinity for the beta-adrenoreceptors than the dextro isomers but has equal efficacy for their membrane-stabilizing properties. Because of this action, both isomers of alprenolol may produce a direct cardio depressant effect, including an antiarrhythmic effect unrelated to their beta-adrenergic receptor blocking activity. Alprenolol (4 to 20 mg IV) reduces sinus tachycardia, diminishes the ventricular rate in patients with atrial fibrillation, and suppresses ventricular ectopic beats. It reduces lipolysis and, hence, free fatty acid production in hypotensive patients.

Alprenolol is completely absorbed from the gastrointestinal tract, rapidly distributed to various extravascular sites, and metabolized to 4-hydroxyalprenol, an active metabolite. Alprenolol has additive effects when used in combination with saluretic diuretics or hydralazine. Alprenolol prevents sudden death in postinfarction patients, reduces persistent ventricular ectopic beats, ventricular premature beats occurring in acute myocardial infarction, and diminishes digitalis-induced ventricular arrhythmias. Therefore, alprenolol may be used with greater safety than other beta-adrenoceptor antagonists in patients with bradycardia and prolonged interval, in patients with Raynaud's phenomenon, intermittent claudication, and cold extremities. The reported side effects for alprenolol are CNS disorders such as insomnia and nightmares, gastrointestinal disorders such as esophageal stricture ulcer, and bronchospasm.

ALPROSTADIL

(Prostin VR Pediatric)

Alprostadil (0.05 to 0.1 mcg/kg/minute via infusion pump) is indicated for temporary maintenance of patency of ductus arteriosus until surgery can be performed (see Figure 51).

ALTEPLASE

(Recombinant Alteplase, Tissue Plasminogen Activator [Activase])

Alteplase (6 to 10 mg IV bolus over the first 1 to 2 minutes, then 20 mg/hour for an additional 2 hours) is indicated for lysis of thrombi obstructing coronary arteries in management of acute myocardial infarction (see Figure 35).

ALTRETAMINE

(Hexamethylmelamine, Hexalen)

Altretamine, an alkylating agent with antineoplastic properties (260 mg/m^2 day/p.o.), is indicated as a palliative treatment of persistent or recurrent ovarian cancer after first-line therapy with cisplatin, or alkylating agent combination, single agent therapy.

Altretamine is a sym-triazine cytotoxic agent which is structurally related to the alkylating agents. Its precise mechanism of action is unknown but hydroxymethyl intermediates in the metabolism process are possibly the reactive species, and may act as alkylating agents. However, altretamine is not directly cross-resistant with classical alkylating agents.

Subgroup analysis suggests that the addition of altretamine or the combination of altretamine and doxorubicin to cyclophosphamide and cisplatin may confer survival advantages in patients with limited residual disease following debulking surgery.

ALUMINUM HYDROXIDE

(Alagel, AlternaGEL, Alu-cap, Aluminett, Alu-Tab, Amphojel, Dialume, Hydroxal, Nephrox, Nutrajel)

Aluminum hydroxide, an antacid with hypophosphatemic properties (500 to 1800 mg p.o.), is indicated in acid pepsin disease and in hyperphosphatemia in renal failure (see Table 7).

ALUMINUM PHOSPHATE

(Phosphaljel)

Aluminum phosphate (233 mg/5 ml to be used in 15 to 30 ml q. 2 hours between meals), by decreasing the fecal extraction of phosphate, is used as a phosphate replacement regimen.

ALZHEIMER'S DISEASE: TREATMENT OF

Alzheimer's disease (AD), with or without comorbid conditions, is by far the leading cause of dementia. Dementia can be defined as the acquired and sustained deterioration of intellectual functions in an alert patient. It thus is distinguished from conditions such as mental retardation and delirium. Operationally, because of diminished cognitive ability, a demented person conducts everyday activities less well in relation to past performance. Formal criteria for dementia include the development of multiple cognitive deficits that include memory impairment and at least one of the following cognitive disturbances: aphasia, apraxia, agnosia, or a disturbance in executive functioning defined as the ability to think abstractly and to plan, initiate, sequence, monitor, and stop complex behavior. These disturbances must be sufficiently severe to cause significant impairment in social or occupational functioning and represent a decline from a previous level of functioning. Criteria also have been proposed that do not require the presence of memory loss to accommodate disorders, such as vascular dementia in which memory may be spared.

Following the introduction of tacrine hydrochloride (Cognex®) in the United States and several other countries, researchers are pursuing two broad therapeutic strategies for AD. The first involves identifying agents or combinations of agents whose actions can compensate for the considerable cerebral damage that has typically occurred by the time the diagnosis of AD is made. Such therapeutic approaches include the development of additional cholinesterase inhibitors, agents that work on the receptors of other systems damaged by the disease process, and antiinflammatory and immunomodulatory agents. The second and ultimately more promising strategy involves the development of approaches to retard, halt, or even prevent disease progression. Such protective approaches, which depend on the development of more effective methods for predicting and diagnosing AD, include the administration of nerve growth factor and other neurotrophins and the use of pharmacologic or genetic interventions to limit amyloid deposition and the formation of neurofibrillary tangles.

Over 30% of patients with dementia develop a group of secondary behavioral disturbances, including depression, hallucinations and delusions, agitation, insomnia, and wandering. Because these secondary symptoms impair patients' functions, increase their need for supervision, and often influence the decision to institutionalize them, the control of these symptoms is a priority in managing AD.

Drugs used in the treatment of depression in Alzheimer's disease are:

Monoamine Oxidase Inhibitors (MAOI)
Phenelzine
Tranylcypromine

Tricyclic Antidepressants
Desipramine
Nortriptyline

**Selective Serotonin
Reuptake Inhibitors (SSRI)**
Fluoxetine
Paroxetine
Sertraline

Drugs used in the treatment of psychosis and agitation in Alzheimer's disease are:	**Drugs used in the treatment of insomnia in Alzheimer's disease are:**
Classical Antipsychotics	**Tricyclic Antidepressants**
Chlorpromazine	Nortriptyline
Haloperidol	Trazodone
Thioridazine	**Benzodiazepines**
Atypical Antipsychotics	Lorazepam
Clozapine	Oxazepam
Risperidone	Triazolam
Benzodiazepines	**Antipsychotics**
Lorazepam	Chlorpromazine
Oxazepam	Haloperidol
Triazolam	Thioridazine

Although it is the most common form of dementia, AD-related dementia may be associated with other dementing illnesses including vascular dementia and Parkinson's disease. Other less common causes of dementia, including progressive supranuclear palsy, Huntington's disease, Pick's disease, Creutzfeldt-Jakob disease, and a variety of rare metabolic disorders, can usually be distinguished from AD by distinctive physical signs and symptoms that appear before or in tandem with the onset of cognitive impairment.

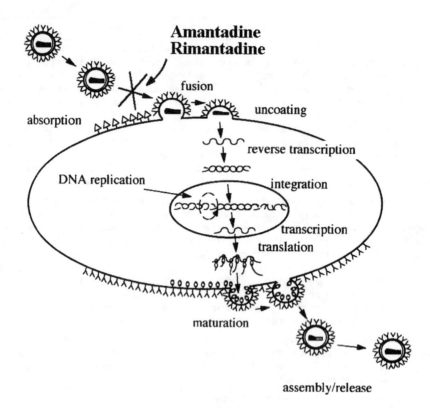

FIGURE 6 Amantadine and rimantadine, effective against RNA virus, exert their effects by preventing the penetration and uncoating of the virus.

AMANTADINE
(Symmetrel)

Amantadine is 70% to 90% effective in preventing illnesses caused by circulating strains of Type A influenza viruses, when administered 24 to 48 hours after onset of illness. It exerts its effects by preventing the penetration and uncoating of the virus (Figure 6). Amantadine is also useful in the treatment of mild parkinsonism, hemiparkinsonism, and drug-induced parkinsonism. Although the actions of amantadine are still not fully understood, there is some evidence that the drug inhibits the uptake of dopamine into the synaptosomes. In addition, amantadine has an indirect amphetamine-like effect, in that it releases dopamine. Amantadine augments the actions of anticholinergic medications used in patients with Parkinson's disease, and the doses of one or both should be reduced. Amantadine, which releases catecholamine, may cause insomnia, nervousness, dizziness, and ataxia when taken in toxic doses.

AMBENONIUM CHLORIDE
(Mytelase)

Ambenonium, a cholinesterase inhibitor (5 to 25 mg p.o. t.i.d.), is indicated in the symptomatic treatment of myasthenia gravis. Ambenonium results in accumulation of acetylcholine stimulating cholinergic receptors at the myoneural junction (see Figure 18).

AMCINONIDE

(Cyclocort)

Amcinonide, a topical adrenocorticoid with antiinflammatory properties (0.1% cream, ointment, or lotion), is indicated in the treatment of inflammation of corticosteroid-responsive dermatoses.

AMIFOSTINE

One of the goals of cancer chemotherapy is to enhance the efficacy of antineoplastic agents and at the same time protect the nonmalignant tissues using chemoprotective agents. A few of the chemoenhancers and chemoprotectors are listed below:

Chemoenhancers	Chemoprotectors
Acridines	Amifostine
Amiodarone	Bismuth salts
Buthionine sulfoximine	Dexrazoxane
Calcium channel blockers	Diethyldithiocarbamate
Cyclosporine	Diuretics, phorbol esters
Ethacrynic acid	Glutathione esters
Phenothiazines	Metallothionein
Phorbol esters	Oxothiazolidine-4-carboxylate
Progesterone	Steroids
Streptozocin	Thiosulfate
Tamoxifen	
Triparanol	

Anthracycline antibiotics (e.g., doxorubicin) cause unique cardiomyopathies. An acute form is characterized by abnormal electrocardiographic changes including ST-T wave alterations and arrhythmias. This is brief and rarely a serious problem. Cineangiographic studies have shown an acute, reversible reduction in ejection fraction 24 hours after a single dose. An exaggerated manifestation of acute myocardial damage, the **"pericarditis-myocarditis syndrome,"** may be characterized by severe disturbances in impulse conduction and frank congestive heart failure, often associated with pericardial effusion. Chronic cumulative dose-related toxicity of anthracycline antibiotics is manifested by congestive heart failure that is unresponsive to digitalis. Cardiac irradiation or administration of high doses of cyclophosphamide or another anthracycline may increase the risk of cardiotoxicity. There is evidence that cardiac damage is reduced by the concomitant administration of the iron chelator **dexrazoxane** (ADR-529) or by **amifostine** (WR-2721) or its active metabolite (WR-1065).

AMIKACIN SULFATE

(Amikin, Elkins-Sinn, Apothecon)

Among the aminoglycosides (see Figure 80), amikacin has the broadest antimicrobial spectrum of action, and, for this reason, it is usually reserved for the treatment of serious infections due to susceptible strains of Gram-negative bacteria, including *Pseudomonas sp., Escherichia coli, Proteus sp., Providencia sp., Klebsiella sp., Enterobacter sp., Serratia sp.,* and *Acinetobacter (Mima-Herellea) sp.* Amikacin is effective in bacterial septicemia including neonatal sepsis, in infections of the respiratory tract and CNS including meningitis, in intraabdominal infection including peritonitis, and in postoperative infections. Amikacin (up to 15 mg/kg/day) is given for 7 to 10 days. The patient's renal status and vestibular or auditory functions must be monitored carefully.

AMILORIDE
(Midamor)

Triamterene (Dyrenium, Maxzide) and amiloride are potassium-sparing diuretics which inhibit renal epithelial Na⁺ channels. Triamterene, amiloride, and spironolactone (Alactone), which is an aldosterone antagonist, all act in the distal tubule, where the resorption of sodium is accompanied by the transfer of potassium into the lumen contents (see Figure 4). When sodium resorption is hindered, potassium excretion is correspondingly reduced such that more potassium is retained. The potassium-sparing diuretics are not very efficacious, as they affect only 1 to 2% of the filtered load of sodium. All are given orally and eliminated in the urine, mostly by glomerular filtration, though some active tubular secretion may occur.

Molecular cloning studies recently have revealed that the amiloride-sensitive Na⁺ channel consists of three subunits (alpha, beta, gamma). Although the alpha subunit is sufficient for channel activity, maximal Na⁺ permeability is induced when all three subunits are coexpressed in the same cell, suggesting a minimal oligomeric structure in which one copy of each subunit is associated in a heterotrimeric protein.

Amiloride is used with thiazide or loop diuretics in hypertension, in congestive heart failure, in digitalis-induced hypokalemia, and in arrhythmias resulting from hypokalemia. Inappropriate use of amiloride may cause hyperkalemia (potassium >5.5 mEq/L) which may be fatal if not corrected, and may be more deleterious in elderly individuals and in patients with diabetes mellitus and renal impairment. The symptoms of hyperkalemia include fatigue, flaccid paralysis of the extremities, paresthesias, bradycardia, ECG abnormalities, and shock. Amiloride is not metabolized, but is contraindicated in anuria, acute or chronic renal insufficiency, or in diabetic nephropathy. Amiloride should not be used with potassium preparations, and should be used cautiously with ACE inhibitors since these agents cause hyperkalemia.

AMINO ACID SOLUTIONS
(Aminosyn, Aminosyn with Dextrose, Aminosyn with Electrolytes, Aminosyn-PF, Aminosyn (pH6), Aminosyn II, Aminosyn II in Dextrose, Aminosyn II with Electrolytes, Aminosyn II with Electrolytes in Dextrose, FreAmine III, FreAmine III with Electrolytes, Novamine, Novamine without Electrolytes, ProcalAmine, Travasol with Electrolytes, Travasol without Electrolytes, TrophAmine)

Amino acid solutions (1 to 1.5 g/kg IV daily) will provide nutritional support in patients with renal failure, high metabolic stress, or hepatic encephalopathy with cirrhosis or hepatitis. Amino acid injection and solution provide a substrate for protein synthesis in the protein-depleted patient or enhance conservation of body protein.

AMINOGLUTETHIMIDE
(Cytadren)

Aminoglutethimide (250 mg p.o. q.i.d.) is indicated in the treatment of adrenal hyperplasia from ectopic ACTH-producing tumors (see Figure 28). In addition, it has been used in medial adrenalectomy in postmenopausal metastatic breast cancer and prostate cancer; and in suppression of adrenal function in Cushing's syndrome.

Aminoglutethimide interferes with the conversion of cholesterol to delta-5-pregnenolone, effectively inhibiting the synthesis of corticosteroids, androgens, and estrogens. Therefore, by suppressing the adrenals, aminoglutethimide inhibits the growth of tumors that need estrogen to thrive.

AMINOGLYCOSIDE ANTIBIOTICS	
Amikacin	Paromomycin
Gentamicin	Streptomycin
Kanamycin	Tobramycin
Netilmicin	

AMINOPHYLLINE
(Theophylline Ethylenediamine)

The methylxanthines consist of aminophylline, dyphylline, enprofylline, and pentoxifylline. Aminophylline is the most widely used of the soluble theophyllines.

Epinephrine stimulates the beta-adrenergic receptors in the bronchioles, which in turn activates membrane-bound adenylate cyclase to synthesize more cyclic AMP, whereas theophylline inhibits the activity of phosphodiesterase, conserving the previously synthesized cyclic AMP (see Figure 10). In addition, recent evidence suggests that theophylline blocks the receptor for adenosine. The inhalation of adenosine can precipitate marked bronchoconstriction in asthmatic patients, but shows no appreciable effects in normal subjects.

It is now recognized that adenosine receptors are linked through appropriate guanine nucleotide-binding regulatory proteins (G-proteins), not only to adenyl cyclase but also to other effector systems. Moreover, theophylline may inhibit the synthesis of prostaglandin and reduce the uptake or metabolism of catecholamines in nonneuronal tissues (see Figure 42).

Corticosteroids, which are also effective in symptomatic treatment of certain types of asthma, exert their beneficial effects in part by enhancing catecholamine effects and also by antagonizing the cholinergic actions, one of which is bronchoconstriction. Aminophylline also causes central nervous system stimulation, cardiac acceleration, diuresis, and gastric secretion. Aminophylline is available in an oral, rectal (pediatric), or intravenous solution, which is used in the treatment of status asthmaticus. Although aminophylline is a less effective bronchodilator than beta-adrenergic agonists, it is particularly useful in preventing nocturnal asthma.

AMINOSALICYLATE SODIUM
(Para-Aminosalicylate, P.A.S.) (Nemasol Sodium, Sodium P.A.S., Tubasal)

Aminosalicylate sodium (3.3 to 4 g p.o. q. 8 hours) is indicated as adjunctive treatment of tuberculosis. It inhibits the formation of folic acid and hence suppresses the growth and reproduction of *Mycobacterium tuberculosis.*

AMIODARONE HCL
(Cordarone)

Amiodarone is a structural analog of thyroid hormone, is highly lipophilic, is concentrated in many tissues, and is eliminated very slowly. Following discontinuation of chronic oral therapy, amiodarone has a biphasic elimination with an initial one-half reduction of plasma levels after 2.5 to 10 days. A much slower terminal plasma elimination phase shows a half-life of the parent compound ranging from 26 to 107 days (mean 53 days), with most patients in the 40 to 55 day range. Steady-state plasma concentrations would therefore be reached between 130 and 535 days (average 265 days).

Amiodarone (plasma concentration of 0.5 to 2.0 microgram/ml) decreases conduction velocity by blocking Na^+ channels, inhibits abnormal automaticity, and prolongs the duration of action potential. Prolongation of PR, QRS, and QT intervals and sinus bradycardia are frequent during chronic therapy. Oral amiodarone is indicated in patients with **recurrent ventricular tachycardia** or fibrillation resistant to other drugs. In addition, it is effective in maintaining sinus rhythm in patients with atrial fibrillation. Amiodarone is metabolized to desthyl-amiodarone, an active antiarrhythmic agent.

Amiodarone may cause asymptomatic corneal microdeposits and inhibit the conversion of thyroxine (T4) to triiodothyronine (T3). Amiodarone has caused pulmonary toxicity (hypersensitivity pneumonitis or interstitial/alveolar pneumonitis). Amiodarone is embryotoxic in that it increases fetal resorption and causes growth retardation. It is excreted in breast milk.

AMIODIPINE BESYLATE
(Norvasc)

Amiodipine, a calcium channel blocking agent (5 mg p.o. daily), is indicated in the treatment of chronic stable angina, vasospastic angina (Prinzmetal's or variant angina) (see also Figure 95 and Table 20).

AMITRIPTYLINE
(Elavil)

The **dibenzapine derivatives** are called **tricyclic antidepressants** and include **imipramine** (Tofranil), **desipramine** (Norpramin), **amitriptyline** (Elavil), **nortriptyline** (Aventyl), **protriptyline** (Vivactil), and **doxepin** (Adapin). Amitriptyline is indicated in depression; major depression with melancholia or psychotic symptoms; depressive phase of bipolar disorder; depression associated with organic disease, alcoholism, schizophrenia, or mental retardation; anorexia or bulimia associated with depression (see Figure 7).

Tricyclic antidepressants resemble the phenothiazine antipsychotics such as chlorpromazine in structure and function. Like the phenothiazine derivatives (e.g., chlorpromazine), tricyclic antidepressants (e.g., amitriptyline) may reduce the seizure threshold and precipitate seizures in epileptic patients, cause cholestatic jaundice, movement disorders, and hematologic side effects. Unlike the phenothiazine derivatives, the tricyclic antidepressants may increase motor activity, have a very slow onset and long duration of action, have a relatively narrow margin of safety and a strong anticholinergic effect. In fact, dry mouth is the most common side effect, and other anticholinergic effects such as tachycardia, loss of accommodation, constipation, urinary retention, and paralytic ileus have been reported following amitriptyline.

Imipramine is demethylated to **desipramine**, and **amitriptyline** is demethylated to **nortriptyline**. Both metabolites are active antidepressants. Tricyclic antidepressants bind to plasma proteins to the extent of 90%, and, because of their extensive first-pass metabolism in the liver, they have very low and variable bioavailability. In those circumstances when it is desirable to measure the plasma concentrations of these drugs, the concentrations of their active metabolites should also be measured.

Tricyclic antidepressants, like some of the phenothiazine derivatives, are **sedative in nature**. Those compounds containing **tertiary amines** (imipramine, amitriptyline, and doxepin) are the most sedative. Those compounds containing a **secondary amine** (nortriptyline and desipramine) are less so, and protriptyline has no sedative effect (see Table 3). Tricyclic antidepressants, like some of the phenothiazine derivatives (e.g., thioridazine), have an **anticholinergic property. Amitriptyline** is the strongest in this regard and **desipramine** is the weakest (see Tables 3 through 5).

The tricyclic antidepressants also have **cardiovascular actions**. In particular, they cause orthostatic hypotension by obtunding the various reflex mechanisms involved in maintaining

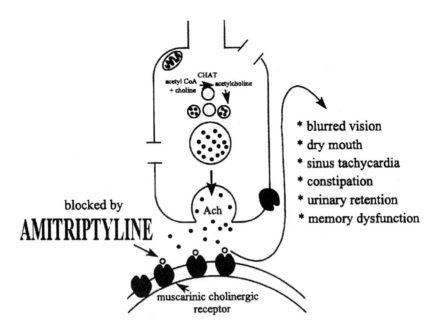

FIGURE 7 Amitriptyline, a tricyclic antidepressant, causes sedation and orthostatic hypotension. In addition, possesses strong anticholinergic properties. (Adapted from Ebadi, M., *Pharmacology, An Illustrated Review with Questions and Answers*, 3rd Edition, Lippincott-Raven Press, Philadelphia, 1996.)

blood pressure (see Table 3). Antidepressants block the uptake of norepinephrine, serotonin, or dopamine (see Table 4) and block several receptor sites (see Table 5), causing beneficial effects as well as side effects. For example, amitriptyline blocks muscarinic cholinergic receptors causing blurred vision, dry mouth, sinus tachycardia, constipation, urinary retention, and memory dysfunction (see Figure 7). Therefore, because of its pronounced anticholinergic and potential arrhythmogenic effects, amitriptyline is contraindicated in the acute recovery phase of myocardial infarction, congestive heart failure, angina, prostatic hypertrophy, paralytic ileus, and urinary retention, and in patients undergoing surgery with general anesthetics which may cause arrhythmias (e.g., Halothane) (see Tables 3 through 5, and 15).

AMMONIUM CHLORIDE

Ammonium chloride, an acid-forming salt (4 to 12 g p.o. daily), is indicated in metabolic alkalosis. In addition, as an acidifying agent, it has been used as an expectorant.

AMOBARBITAL

(Amytal)

Amobarbital, a barbiturate, is used as a sedative to treat insomnia and as a preanesthetic medication. The barbiturates were used extensively in the past as hypnotic-sedatives, but have been replaced by the much safer benzodiazepine derivatives (see Table 8). They do continue to be used as anesthetics (e.g., thiopental) and anticonvulsants (e.g., phenobarbital). The primary mechanism of action of barbiturates is to increase inhibition through the **gamma-aminobutyric acid** (GABA) **system** (see Figure 40). Anesthetic barbiturates also decrease excitation via a decrease in calcium conductance. The most commonly used barbiturates are thiopental (Pentothal), methohexital (Brevital), secobarbital (Seconal), pentobarbital (Nembutal), amobarbital (Amytal), and phenobarbital (Luminal).

TABLE 3
Side Effects of Antidepressant Drugs

Drugs	Sedation	Insomnia	Anticholinergic Effects	Nausea	Orthostatic Hypotension
A. Tricyclic antidepressants					
Amitriptyline	+++	0	+++	0	+++
Trimipramine	+++	0	+++	0	++
Desipramine	+	+	+	0	+
Doxepin	+++	0	++	0	+++
Imipramine	++	0	++	0	++
Nortriptyline	++	0	+	0	+
Protriptyline	+	++	++	0	+
B. Second-generation antidepressants					
Amoxapine	++	0	+	0	++
Fluoxetine	0	++	0	++	0
Maprotiline	++	0	+	0	++
Trazodone	++++	0	0	+	++
Bupropion	0	++	0	+	0

0 = no side effect; + = minor side effect; ++ = moderate side effect; +++ = major side effect.

TABLE 4
The Inhibition of Monoamine Uptake by Antidepressants

Drugs	Norepinephrine	Serotonin	Dopamine
A. Tricyclic antidepressants			
Amitriptyline	±	++	0
Nortriptyline	++	±	0
Imipramine	+	+	0
Desipramine	+++	0	0
Clomipramine	+	+++	0
Trimipramine	+	0	0
Doxepine	++	+	0
B. Second-generation antidepressants			
Maprotiline	++	0	0
Amoxapine	++	0	0
Fluoxetine	0	+++	0
Bupropion	±	0	++
Mianserin	0	0	0
Trazodone	0	+	0

0 = no effect; ± = an equivocal effect; + = slight effect; ++ = moderate effect; +++ = large effect.

Barbiturates are classified according to their **duration of action**; these are: **ultra short-acting** (thiopental and methohexital), **short- to intermediate-acting** (pentobarbital, secobarbital, and amobarbital), and **long-acting** (phenobarbital). The selection of a barbiturate is in part determined by the duration of action desired and by the clinical problems at hand. An ultra short-acting drug is used for inducing anesthesia. For treating epilepsy, a long-acting drug is used, whereas, in a sleep disorder, a short-acting or an intermediate-type drug is used,

TABLE 5

The Affinity of Antidepressants for Various Receptors

Drugs	Alpha$_1$ Adrenergic Blockade	Alpha$_2$ Adrenergic Blockade	Histaminergic (H$_1$) Blockade	Muscarinic Blockade	Dopaminergic (D$_2$) Blockade
			Receptor Affinity		
A. **Tricyclic antidepressants**					
Amitriptyline	+++	±	++++	++++	0
Nortriptyline	+	0	+	++	0
Imipramine	++	0	+	++	0
Desipramine	+	0	0	+	0
Clomipramine	++	0	+	++	0
Trimipramine	++	±	+++	++	+
Doxepin	++	0	+++	++	0
B. **Second-generation antidepressants**					
Maprotiline	+	0	++	+	0
Amoxapine	++	±	±	0	++
Fluoxetine	0	0	0	0	0
Trazodone	++	±	±	+	0
Bupropion	0	0	0	0	0
Mianserin	++	++	+++	0	0

0 = no effect; ± = an equivocal effect; + = slight effect; ++ = moderate effect; +++ = large effect; ++++ = maximal effect.

depending on whether patients have difficulty falling asleep or if they have difficulty staying asleep.

In general, the more **lipid soluble** a barbiturate derivative is, the greater is its plasma and tissue binding capacity, the extent of its metabolism, and its storage in adipose tissues. In addition, very lipid-soluble substances have a faster onset of action and a shorter duration of action.

Barbiturates do not raise the **pain threshold** and have no analgesic property. In anesthetic doses, they depress all areas of the CNS, including the hypothalamic thermoregulatory system, respiratory center, and vasomotor centers, as well as the **polysynaptic pathways** in the spinal column. In addition, some, such as phenobarbital, but not all, are anticonvulsants. In toxic doses, barbiturates cause oliguria. Barbiturates are absorbed orally and distributed widely throughout the body. They are metabolized in the liver by aliphatic oxygenation, aromatic oxygenation, and N-dealkylation.

The inactive metabolites are excreted in the urine. The administration of **bicarbonate** enhances the urinary excretion of barbiturates that have a pK$_a$ of 7.4 (**phenobarbital** and **thiopental**). This generalization is not true of other barbiturates. The long-term administration of barbiturates activates the cytochrome P-450 drug metabolizing system.

Acute barbiturate toxicity is characterized by **automatism**, or a state of drug-induced confusion, in which patients lose track of how much medication they have taken and take more. Death results from **respiratory failure**. The treatment of poisoning consists of support respiration, prevention of hypotension, diuresis, hemodialysis, and in the event of phenobarbital poisoning, the administration of **sodium bicarbonate**. Tolerance does not develop to lethal doses. The abrupt withdrawal from barbiturates may cause tremors, restlessness, anxiety, weakness, nausea and vomiting, seizures, delirium, and cardiac arrest.

AMODIAQUINE
(Camoquin)

Amodiaquine is a congener of chlorquine that is no longer recommended for chemoprophy-laxis of fulciparum malaria. It causes agranulocytosis and hepatic toxicity.

AMOXAPINE
(Asendin)

Amoxapine (50 mg p.o. t.i.d.) is a second-generation antidepressant with indications in depression associated with melancholia or psychotic symptoms; depressive phase of bipolar disorder; depression associated with organic disease or alcoholism; psychoneurotic anxiety; mixed symptoms of anxiety or depression. Amoxapine is absorbed orally, is bound to plasma proteins to the extent of 92%, is distributed widely throughout the body and its fluids including milk, is metabolized to 8-hydroxyamoxapine (an active metabolite) and is also excreted in the urine. Amoxapine causes mild to moderate degrees of sedation, orthostatic hypotension, and anticholinergic effects. In addition, since it blocks dopaminergic receptors in the striatum, it causes movement disorders (see Tables 3 through 5).

AMOXICILLIN
(Amoxil)

Amoxicillin is a penicillinase-susceptible semisynthetic penicillin which resembles ampicillin (see Table 22). Amoxicillin is stable in acidic pH of the stomach, and is more rapidly and completely absorbed from the gastrointestinal tract than is ampicillin, which is the major difference between the two. The antimicrobial spectrum of amoxicillin is essentially identical to that of ampicillin, with the important exception that amoxicillin appears to be less effective than ampicillin for shigellosis. **Clavulanic acid** is a beta-lactam structurally related to the penicillins that inactivates beta-lactamase enzymes commonly found in microorganisms resistant to penicillin. The combination of amoxicillin/clavulanic acid extends the antibiotic spectrum of amoxicillin to include bacteria normally resistant to amoxicillin and other beta-lactam antibiotics. Amoxicillin is indicated in infections caused by *Philus influenzae, E. coli, P. mirabilis,* and *N. gonorrhoeae,* Gram-positive-streptococci (including *S. faecalis), S. pneumoniae,* and nonpenicillinase-producing staphylocci.

The **broad-spectrum penicillins**, such as **ampicillin** and **amoxicillin**, may cause gastrointestinal irritation. Occasionally, the overgrowth of staphylococci, *Pseudomonas, Proteus,* or yeasts may be responsible for causing **enteritis**. Because amoxicillin is more completely absorbed from the gastrointestinal tract, it causes less diarrhea than ampicillin.

AMPHETAMINE SULFATE
(Dexedrine)

Amphetamines are sympathomimetic amines with CNS stimulant activity which are used in narcolepsy (5 to 60 mg/day in individual doses) and in attention deficit disorder in children (2.5 mg to not more than 40 mg daily). Amphetamine releases norepinephrine and in high doses also dopamine. It is absorbed from the gastrointestinal tract, metabolized in the liver, and is excreted unchanged in the urine. Acidification of urine shortens amphetamine's half-life, whereas alkalinization of urine prolongs it. The accumulation of hydroxy metabolite of amphetamine has been thought to cause amphetamine-induced psychosis. Therapeutic doses of amphetamine may cause insomnia, tremor, and restlessness; and toxic doses of amphetamine may cause mydriasis, hypertension, and arrhythmia. **Chlorpromazine** is an excellent antidote in amphetamine toxicity. The continuous use of amphetamine causes tolerance requiring higher doses, and hence there exists a high potential for its abuse. Amphetamine should not be used with a monoamine oxidase A inhibitor such as **tranylcypromine**, since the chance of inducing hypertension is magnified. Similar caution should be exercised with biogenic amine uptake blockers such as **tricyclic antidepressants**. Amphetamine is contraindicated in advanced arteriosclerosis; symptomatic cardiovascular disease; moderate to severe hypertension; hyperthyroidism; hypersensitivity or idiosyncrasy to the sympathomimetic amines; glaucoma; agitated states; history of drug abuse; during or within 14 days following administration of MAO inhibitors (see Figure 27).

AMPHOTERICIN B

(Fungizone)

Amphotericin B (fungizone), which is ineffective in curing infections caused by bacteria, *Rickettsia*, or viruses, is either fungicidal or fungistatic, depending on the drug concentration used or the sensitivity of the particular fungus. Numerous pathogenic yeasts (*Cryptococcus neoformans*), pathogenic yeast-like organisms (*Monilia*), dimorphic fungi (*Blastomyces*), filamentous fungi (*Cladosporosium*), and other fungi are highly sensitive to amphotericin B. Furthermore, the antifungal actions of amphotericin B are enhanced by flucytosine, minocycline, or rifampin, agents otherwise devoid of antifungal activity.

Amphotericin B imposes its antifungal effects by binding to the **sterol moiety** of the membrane and damaging its structural and functional integrity (Figure 8). Amphotericin B is available in the form of a sterile lyophilized powder. Because it is insoluble in water, it is marketed with sodium deoxycholate for dispersal in sterile water and 5% dextrose. The polyene antibiotics, amphotericin B, nystatin, and candicidin, are all poorly absorbed from the gastrointestinal tract. In the plasma, amphotericin B binds to lipoproteins including cholesterol. It is extensively metabolized and the inactive metabolite, or metabolites, are slowly excreted in the urine.

Amphotericin B is the only polyene antibiotic given **parenterally**. When the intravenous route is contemplated, amphotericin B is dispersed fresh and infused slowly. Amphotericin B should not be administered rapidly because this causes cardiac toxicity. Heparin (1,000 units) is often added to the infusion suspension to avert the risk of thrombophlebitis. Amphotericin B can also precipitate normocytic or normochromic anemia, leukopenia, and thrombocytopenia.

During the infusion of amphotericin B, the patient's temperature will rise, which may or may not be accompanied by hypotension and delirium. Often hydrocortisone sodium succinate is added to the infusion during the initial but not the succeeding alternate-day treatment with amphotericin B.

Amphotericin B is **nephrotoxic** in most patients and often causes a permanent reduction in the glomerular filtration rate. Furthermore, **hypokalemia** may occur, requiring the oral administration of potassium chloride.

Amphotericin B has been used intrathecally in patients with **coccidioidal** or **cryptococcal meningitis**. The side effects associated with this route of administration are headache, paresthesia, nerve palsy, and visual impairment. To treat **coccidioidal arthritis**, amphotericin B may be injected intramuscularly, or directly into the joint (see Figure 9).

AMPICILLIN

(Amcill, Omnipen, Polycillin)

The aminopenicillins, including ampicillin, amoxicillin, and their congeners, are bactericidal for both Gram-positive and Gram-negative bacteria. They are somewhat less active than

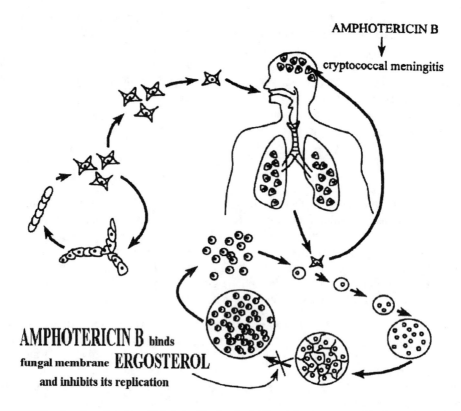

AMPHOTERICIN B

cryptococcal meningitis

AMPHOTERICIN B binds
fungal membrane **ERGOSTEROL**
and inhibits its replication

FIGURE 8 Amphotericin B, which is ineffective in ridding infections caused by bacteria, *Rickettsia*, or viruses, is either fungicidal or fungistatic, depending on the drug concentration used or the sensitivity of the particular fungus.

penicillin G against Gram-positive cocci sensitive to the latter agent. Ampicillin is stable in acidic pH of the stomach and is absorbed well when given orally, but its absorption is hindered by food (see Table 22). Ampicillin appears in bile, undergoes enterohepatic circulation, and is excreted in the feces. Renal impairment prolongs the half-life of ampicillin, and its doses should be adjusted. Ampicillin is indicated in infections caused by susceptible strains of *Shigella, Salmonella* (including *S. typhosa*), *Escherichia coli, Hemophilus influenzae, Proteus mirabilis, Neisseria gonorrhoeae,* and enterococci. It is also effective in the treatment of meningitis due to *N. meningitidis* and in infections caused by susceptible Gram-positive organisms, penicillin G-sensitive staphylococci, streptococci, and pneumococci. Ampicillin with probenecid is indicated in the treatment of uncomplicated urethral, endocervical, or rectal infections in adults caused by *Neisseria gonorrhoeae*. Ampicillin sodium and sulbactam sodium are indicated in **skin and skin structure infections** caused by beta-lactamase producing strains of *Staphylococcus aureus, Escherichia coli, Klebsiella sp.* (including *K. pneumoniae*), *Proteus mirabilis, Bacteroides fragilis, Enterobacter sp.,* and *Acinetobacter caloacticus;* **intra-abdominal infections** caused by beta lactamase-producing strains of *E. coli, Klebsiella sp.* (including *K. pneumoniae*), *Bacteroides* (including *B. fragilis*), and *Enterobacter sp.;* **gynecological infections** caused by beta lactamase-producing strains of *E. coli* and *Bacteroides sp.* (including *B. fragilis*). High concentration of beta-lactam may cause convulsive seizures.

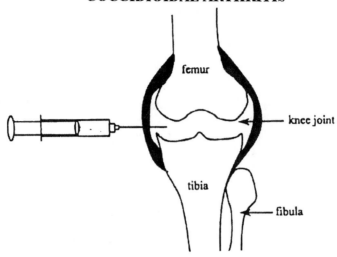

AMPHOTERICIN B injected intra-articularly to treat

COCCIDIOIDAL ARTHRITIS

FIGURE 9   Numerous pathogenic yeasts (*Cryptococcus neoformans*), pathogenic yeast-like organisms (*Monilia*), dimorphic fungi (*Blastomyces*), filamentous fungi (*Cladosporosium*), and other fungi are highly sensitive to amphotericin B.

AMRINONE LACTATE
(Inocor)

Agents with **positive inotropic actions** that may be used in the management of congestive heart failure include the **cardiac glycosides** (e.g., digoxin and digitoxin), **dopaminergic analogs** (e.g., dobutamine), **phosphodiesterase inhibitors** (e.g., amrinone and milrinone), **angiotensin antagonists** (e.g., captopril, enalapril, and lisinopril), and **vasodilators** (nitrates and hydralazine). Amrinone and milrinone are bipyridine derivatives and relatively selective inhibitors of the cyclic GMP-inhibited, cyclic AMP phosphodiesterase (PDE Type III) family (Figure 10). They cause vasodilation with a consequent fall in systemic vascular resistance, and increase both the force of contraction and velocity of relaxation of cardiac muscle. Both drugs are effective when given either as single agents or more commonly, in combination with other oral and/or intravenous drugs for short-term treatment of patients with severe heart failure due to systolic right or left ventricular dysfunction. The elimination half-lives of amrinone (0.5 microgram/kg) and milrinone (50 micrograms/kg) are 2 to 3 hours and 30 to 60 minutes, respectively. Thrombocytopenia occurs in 10% of patients receiving amrinone but is rare with milrinone.

AMYL NITRITE
Amyl nitrite possesses the following molecular structure:

$$CH_3 \diagdown$$
$$\qquad\qquad CH - CH_2 - CH_2 - NO_2$$
$$CH_3 \diagup$$

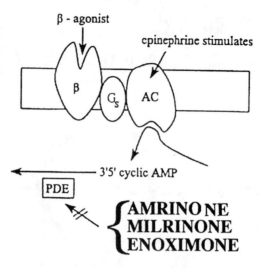

FIGURE 10 **Amrinone, milrinone,** and **enoximone** differ from aminophylline in that they exhibit a certain degree of selectivity for peak III phosphodiesterase, which is found predominantly in myocardial and vascular tissues. These agents exert both **positive inotropic** and **direct vasodilating actions**.

Amyl nitrite is a highly volatile liquid which is sold in fragile glass ampules packaged in a protective cloth covering. The ampule can be crushed, which causes the rapid release of inhalable vapors. Amyl nitrite has a rapid onset of action, and its duration of action is 8 to 10 minutes. The pronounced vasodilation causes tachycardia, enhanced cardiac output, and vasoconstriction. Amyl nitrite is no longer used for the control of angina.

ANALGESICS: NARCOTICS	
Methadone-like Agonists	**Morphine-like Agonists**
Methadone	Codeine
Propoxyphene	Hydrocodone
Meperidine-like Agonists	Hydromorphone
Alfentanil	Levorphanol
Fentanyl	Morphine
Meperidine	Oxycodone
Sufentanil	Oxymorphone
Mixed Agonist-Antagonists	**Narcotic Antagonists**
Buprenorphine	Naloxone
Butorphanol	Naltrexone
Dezocine	
Nalbuphine	
Pentazocine	

ANALGESICS: NON-NARCOTIC AGENTS	
Acetaminophen	Fenoprofen
Aspirin	Magnesium salicylate
Choline salicylate	Meclofenamate
Diflunisal	Mefenamic acid
Etodolac	Naproxen
Ibuprofen	Naproxen sodium
Ketoprofen	Sodium salicylate
Ketorolac (intramuscular)	

TABLE 6
Examples of Anabolic and Androgenic Steroids

Steroids with anabolic activities
Dromostanolone propionate (Drolban)
Ethylestrenol (Maxibolin)
Methandrostenolone (Dianabol)
Nandrolone decanoate (Deca-Durabolin)
Nandrolone phenpropionate (Durabolin)
Oxandrolone (Anavar)
Oxymetholone (Adroyd)
Stanozolol (Winstrol)
Testolactone (Teslac)

Steroids with androgenic properties
Fluoxymesterone (Halotestin)
Methyltestosterone (Metandren)
Testosterone (Android-T)
Testosterone propionate cypionate (Depotestosterone)
Testosterone enanthate (Delatestryl)

ANDROGENS

Testosterone, the male sex hormone, is responsible for the development and maintenance of the **male sex organs** (the penis, prostate gland, seminal vesicle, and vas deferens) and **secondary sex characteristics**. In addition, testosterone has **anabolic effects**. Similar to progesterone, testosterone is metabolized very rapidly in the liver by the first-pass mechanism, and hence requires **structural modifications** in order to be effective. For example, the 17–OH group of testosterone may be modified by the addition of propionic acid, which yields testosterone propionate; cyclopentylpropionic acid, which yields testosterone cypionate; or enanthate, which yields testosterone enanthate. In addition, the 17 position may be methylated to yield methyltestosterone, or a fluorine and a methyl group may be inserted to yield fluoxymesterone. In general, these agents are more effective when given orally and have a longer duration of action than testosterone itself (Table 6).

Testosterone and its derivatives are used in the treatment of hypogonadism (eunuchoidism), hypopituitarism, accelerated growth, aging in men, osteoporosis, anemia, endometriosis, promotion of metabolism, suppression of lactation, and breast carcinoma.

Hormonal therapy with testosterone should be reserved primarily for patients with **hypogonadal disorders**. There are two important warnings about the indiscriminate use of intramuscular testosterone in patients with serum testosterone levels in the normal range. First, many impotent patients are older and may have adenocarcinoma of the prostate, thus exogenous testosterone may accelerate the growth of the neoplasm. Second, although testosterone may induce a marked increase in libido, patients may still be unable to achieve adequate erection.

One of the side effects of testosterone compounds is **masculinization in women** (such as hirsutism, acne, depression of menses, and clitoral enlargement) and of their female offspring. Therefore, androgens are contraindicated in pregnant women. **Prostatic hypertrophy** may occur in males, which leads to urinary retention. Therefore androgens are contraindicated in men with prostatic carcinoma.

Cyproterone inhibits the action of androgens, and **gossypol** prevents spermatogenesis without altering the other endocrine functions of the testis (Figure 87).

ANDROGENIC STEROIDS	
Danazol	Oxandrolone
Dromostanolone propionate	Oxymetholone
Fluoxymesterone	Stanozolol
Metandren	Testosterone
Methyltestosterone	Testosterone cypionate
Nandrolone decanoate	Testosterone enanthate
Nandrolone phenpropionate	Testosterone propionate

ANESTHETICS: INHALATIONAL	
Desflurane	Isoflurane
Enflurane	Nitrous oxide
Halothane	Sevoflurane

ANGIOTENSIN

In studying the role of the renin-angiotensin system in the development of hypertension, it has become apparent that there are two systems: a tissue and a circulating renin angiotensin. The control of hypertension is focused primarily on the renin-angiotensin system in the cardiovascular system and the brain. **Angiotensin-converting enzyme** (ACE) is found in the lung, plasma, the brush borders of the proximal renal tubule, the endothelium of vascular beds, the brain, and the testis (see Figure 21). Its two most important actions are the **inactivation of bradykinin** and the **conversion of angiotensin I to angiotensin II.**

Receptors for angiotensin II are found in the medulla oblongata in neurons involved in the regulation of **baroreceptor activity**. Because studies in hypertensive patients have indicated that **ACE inhibitors** reduce sympathetic activity and enhance baroreceptor sensitivity, it is possible that the primary hypotensive mechanism of these agents is mediated through the blockade of angiotensin II formation in the cardiovascular centers of the brain. The relationship of the renin-angiotensin-aldosterone system to **bradykinin** and **prostaglandin** production is shown in Figure 19.

ANGIOTENSIN-CONVERTING ENZYME (ACE) INHIBITORS FOR HYPERTENSION			
Drugs	**Initial Daily Dosages**	**Drugs**	**Initial Daily Dosages**
Benazepril	10 mg	Moexipril	7.5 mg once
Captopril	25 mg bid or tid	Monopril	20 mg
Enalapril	5 mg	Perindopril	4 mg
Fornopril	10 mg	Quinapril	10 mg
Fosinopril	10 mg	Ramipril	2.5 mg
Lisinopril	10 mg	Trandolapril	1 or 2 mg once

The adverse effects of ACE inhibitors are excessive hypotension associated with volume or salt depletion. All ACE inhibitors commonly cause a dry cough and rarely may cause angioedema. Renal failure can occur in patients with bilateral renal artery stenosis. Hyperkalemia may occur in patients with renal insufficiency, diabetics with even mild renal impairment, and patients taking potassium supplements or potassium-sparing diuretics. ACE inhibitors are fetotoxic and are not recommended for use during pregnancy.

ANISINDIONE

(Miradon)

The **coumarin anticoagulants** include dicumarol, warfarin sodium (coumadin sodium), warfarin potassium (Athrombin-K), acenocoumarol (Sintrom), and phenprocouman (Liquamar). The **inanedione derivatives** are **phenindione** (Hedulin), **diphenadione** (Dipaxin), and **anisindione** (Miradon). Anisindione is available in a 50 mg tablet, and is used in 300 mg dosage the first day, 200 mg the second day, 100 mg the third day, and thereafter 25 to 250 mg daily for maintenance.

ANISTREPLASE

(Anisoylated Plasminogen-Streptokinase Activator Complex; APSAC) (Eminase)

Anistreplase, a thrombolytic enzyme (30 units by direct IV injection over 2 to 5 minutes), is indicated in the treatment of acute coronary arterial thrombosis (see Figure 35).

ANOREXIA NERVOSA AND BULIMIA NERVOSA: TREATMENT OF
In most patients, intense dieting and compulsive exercising are the earliest signs of anorexia nervosa. In addition to amenorrhea, patients with anorexia nervosa, or bulimia nervosa, frequently complain of constipation, stomach bloating, and abdominal pain suggestive of abnormalities in gastrointestinal motility.
Although restoration of body weight and normal eating usually result in a return to normal times for gastric emptying, the short-term use of prokinetic agents such as cisapride or domperidone is indicated.
One of the most serious, and possibly irreversible, consequences of anorexia nervosa is osteoporosis, and estrogen supplementation has been advocated for its treatment.
In addition to psychotherapy, fluoxetine has offered promising results. On the other hand, serotonin uptake inhibitors, tricyclic antidepressants, and monoamine oxidase inhibitors have been shown to reduce the frequency of binge eating and vomiting, and to improve dysphoria and disturbed attitudes toward body weight and shape in patients with bulimia nervosa. Despite this, there is little knowledge regarding the mechanisms and specificity of action of these agents in bulimia nervosa.
A 24-week clinical trial of desipramine combined with individual cognitive therapy produces the best outcome.

ANTACIDS

The medical treatment of esophageal, gastric, and duodenal ulcer includes relieving the symptoms, accelerating healing, preventing complications, and preventing recurrence. **Drug treatment** includes the use of antacids, anticholinergic drugs, histamine H_2-receptor antagonists, and inhibitors of $H^+K^+ATPase$ (see Figures 24 and 63).

Because acid-pepsin disease rarely occurs in the absence of gastric acid and pepsin, antacids are highly effective in its overall management. Antacids consist of a mixture of magnesium, aluminum, and calcium compounds (see Table 7). Their efficacy is based on their inherent ability to **react with and neutralize gastric acid**. **Sodium bicarbonate**, which may leave the stomach rapidly, can cause alkalosis and sodium retention. **Calcium salts** may produce hypercalcemia, which can be detrimental in patients with impaired renal function. **Aluminum salts** may decrease the absorption of tetracyclines and anticholinergic drugs.

ANTACIDS					
Solid Preparations					
Product	Al(OH)$_3$		Mg(OH)$_2$	CaCO$_3$	SIMETHICONE
Gelusil II	400		400	0	30
Maalox TC	600		300	0	0
Mylanta II	400		400	0	40
Riopan Plus II		Magaldrate	1080		20
Rolaids		NaAlCO$_3$(OH)$_2$	325		0
Tums Ex	0		0	750	0
Liquid Preparations					
Gelusil II	400		400	0	30
Kudrox	500		450	0	40
Maalox TC	600		300	0	0
Milk of Magnesia	0		390	0	0
Mylanta II	400		400	0	40
Riopan Plus II		Magaldrate	1080		30

TABLE 7
Composition and Acid-Neutralizing Capacity of Nonprescription Antacid Preparations (Suspensions)

Product	Content (mg/5 ml)				Acid-neutralizing capacity (per 5 ml)
	A1(OH)$_3$	Mg(OH)$_2$	CaCO$_3$	Simethicone	
Maalox TC	600	300	0	0	27
Mylanta-II	400	400	0	40	25
Kudrox	500	450	0	40	25
Gelusil-II	200	200	0	25	24
Camalox	225	200	250	0	18
Di-Gel	200	200	0	20	—
Marblen	400 MgCO$_3$ + 520 CaCO$_3$	=		0	18
Alternagel	600	0	0	—	16
Silain-Gel	282	285	0	25	15
Riopan	540 magaldrate			0	15
Gelusil-M	300	200	0	25	15
Milk of Magnesia	0	390	0	0	14
Aludrox	307	103	0	—	12
Basaljel	AL(OH)CO$_3$ equivalent to 400			—	12
Gelusil	200	200	0	25	12
Wingel	180	160	0	0	10
Kolantyl Gel	150	150	0	0	10
Amphojel	320	0	0	—	10
Gaviscon	31.7A1(OH)$_3$ + 137 MgCO$_3$ I Na alginate			0	4

ANTHRALIN
(Anthra-Derm, Drithocreme, Drithocreme HP 1%, Dritho-Scalp, Lasan)

Anthralin, a germicide (ointment 0.1%, 0.25%, 0.4%, 0.5% 1%; cream 0.1%, 0.25%, 0.4%, 0.5%, 1%), is indicated in the treatment of quiescent or chronic psoriasis.

ANTIANXIETY AGENTS		
Benzodiazepine Derivatives		
Alprazolam Chlordiazepoxide Clonazepam	Clorazepate Diazepam Halazepam	Lorazepam Oxazepam Prazepam
Azaspirodecanedione Derivatives		
	Buspirone Gepirone Ipsapirone	

The neurochemical basis for anxiety is only partially understood. Various manifestations of anxiety, such as palpitations and tremulousness, may be viewed as hyperactivity of the adrenergic system, and beta-adrenergic receptor-blocking agents are effective for the treatment of acute stress reactions, adjustment disorders, generalized anxiety, panic disorder, and agoraphobia. The discovery of the benzodiazepine-GABA receptor-chloride ionophore complex furnished additional evidence that this complex participates in the etiology and manifestation of anxiety. The fact that certain benzodiazepine receptor inverse agonists, such as beta-carboline carboxylate ethyl ester, cause anxiety substantiates the involvement of benzodiazepine-GABA receptors in the etiology and manifestations of anxiety disorders.

The introduction of novel anxiolytic agents such as buspirone, which interacts with the serotoninergic system, has suggested that serotoninergic fibers may be the final pathway through which anxiolytic effects are expressed.

Buspirone has a chemical structure that is distinct from that of the benzodiazepines. Without this structural homology, it is not surprising that buspirone does not interact with the GABA receptors. Furthermore, the clinical profile of buspirone appears to be anxioselective, with a much reduced potential for abuse.

ANTIBACTERIAL DRUGS OF CHOICE		
Infecting Organisms	Drug of First Choice	Alternative Drugs
Gram-Positive Cocci		
Enterococcus		
endocarditis or other severe infection	penicillin G or ampicillin + gentamicin or streptomycin	vancomycin + gentamicin or streptomycin; teicoplanin; quinupristin/dalfopristin
uncomplicated urinary tract infection	ampicillin or amoxicillin	nitrofurantoin; a fluoroquinolone
Staphylococcus aureus or *epidermidis* non-penicillinase producing	penicillin G or V	a cephalosporin; vancomycin; imipenem; clindamycin; a fluoroquinolone
penicillinase-producing	a penicillinase-resistant penicillin	a cephalosporin; vancomycin; amoxicillin/clavulanic acid; ticarcillin/clavulanic acid; piperacillin/tazobactam; ampicillin/sulbactam; imipenem; clindamycin; a fluoroquinolone
methicillin-resistant	vancomycin ± gentamicin ± rifampin	trimethoprim-sulfamethoxazole; a fluoroquinolone; minocycline
Streptococcus pyogenes (group A) and groups C and G	penicillin G or V	clindamycin; erythromycin; a cephalosporin; vancomycin; clarithromycin; azithromycin
Streptococcus, group B	penicillin G or ampicillin	a cephalosporin; vancomycin; erythromycin
Streptococcus, viridans group	penicillin G ± gentamicin	a cephalosporin; vancomycin
Streptococcus bovis	penicillin G	a cephalosporin; vancomycin
Streptococcus, anaerobic or *Peptostreptococcus*	penicillin G	clindamycin; a cephalosporin; vancomycin
Streptococcus pneumoniae (pneumococcus)	penicillin G or V	a cephalosporin, erythromycin; vancomycin ± rifampin; trimethoprim-sulfamethoxazole; azithromycin; clarithromycin; clindamycin; chloramphenicol; a tetracycline; quinupristin/dalfopristin
Gram-Negative Cocci		
Moraxella (Branhamella) catarrhalis	trimethoprim-sulfamethoxazole	amoxicillin/clavulanic acid; erythromycin; clarithromycin; azithromycin; a tetracycline; cefuroxime; cefotaxime; ceftizoxime; ceftriaxone; cefuroxime axetil; cefixime; a fluoroquinolone
Neisseria gonorrhoeae (gonococcus)	ceftriaxone or cefixime	cefotaxime; a fluoroquinolone; spectinomycin; penicillin G
Neisseria meningitidis (meningococcus)	penicillin G	cefotaxime; ceftizoxime; ceftriaxone; chloramphenicol; a sulfonamide

Infecting Organisms	Drug of First Choice	Alternative Drugs
Gram-Positive Bacilli		
Bacillus anthracis (anthrax)	penicillin G	an erythromycin; a tetracycline
Bacillus cereus, subtilis	vancomycin	imipenem; clindamycin
Clostridium perfringens	penicillin G	clindamycin; metronidazole; imipenem; a tetracycline; chloramphenicol
Clostridium tetani	penicillin G	a tetracycline
Clostridium difficile	metronidazole	vancomycin; bacitracin
Corynebacterium diphtheriae	an erythromycin	penicillin G
Corynebacterium, JK group	vancomycin	penicillin G + gentamicin; erythromycin
Listeria monocytogenes	ampicillin ± gentamicin	trimethoprim-sulfamethoxazole
Enteric Gram-Negative Bacilli		
Bacteroides		
oropharyngeal strains	penicillin G or clindamycin	cefoxitin; metronidazole; chloramphenicol; cefotetan; ampicillin/sulbactam
gastrointestinal strains	metronidazole	clindamycin; imipenem; ticarcillin/clavulanic acid; piperacillin/tazobactam; cefoxitin; cefotetan; ampicillin/sulbactam; piperacillin; chloramphenicol; ceftizoxime; cefmetazole
Campylobacter fetus	imipenem	gentamicin
Campylobacter jejuni	a fluoroquinolone or erythromycin	a tetracycline; gentamicin
Enterobacter	imipenem	cefotaxime, ceftizoxime, ceftriaxone or ceftazidime; gentamicin, tobramycin or amikacin; trimethoprim-sulfamethoxazole; ticarcillin, mezlocillin or piperacillin; aztreonam; a fluoroquinolone
Escherichia coli	cefotaxime, ceftizoxime, ceftriaxone, or ceftazidime	ampicillin ± gentamicin, tobramycin or amikacin; carbenicillin, ticarcillin, mezlocillin or piperacillin; gentamicin, tobramycin or amikacin; amoxicillin/clavulanic acid; ticarcillin/clavulanic acid; piperacillin/tazobactam; ampicillin/sulbactam; trimethoprim-sulfamethoxazole; imipenem; aztreonam; a fluoroquinolone; another cephalosporin
Helicobacter pylori	tetracycline HCl + metronidazole + bismuth subsalicylate	tetracycline HCl + clarithromycin + bismuth subsalicylate; amoxicillin + metronidazole + bismuth subsalicylate
Klebsiella pneumoniae	cefotaxime, ceftizoxime, ceftriaxone or ceftazidime	imipenem; gentamicin, tobramycin or amikacin; amoxicillin/clavulanic acid; ticarcillin/clavulanic acid; piperacillin/tazobactam; ampicillin/sulbactam; trimethoprim-sulfamethoxazole; aztreonam; a fluoroquinolone; mezlocillin or piperacillin; another cephalosporin

Proteus mirabilis	ampicillin	a cephalosporin; ticarcillin, mezlocillin, or piperacillin; gentamicin, tobramycin, or amikacin; trimethoprim-sulfamethoxazole; imipenem; aztreonam; a fluoroquinolone; chloramphenicol
Proteus, indole-positive (including *Providencia rettgeri, Morganella morganii*, and *Proteus vulgaris*)	cefotaxime, ceftizoxime, ceftriaxone, or ceftazidime	imipenem; gentamicin, tobramycin, or amikacin; carbenicillin, ticarcillin, mezlocillin, or piperacillin; amoxicillin/clavulanic acid; ticarcillin/clavulanic acid; piperacillin/tazobactam; ampicillin/sulbactam; aztreonam; trimethoprim-sulfamethoxazole; a fluoroquinolone
Providencia stuartii	cefotaxime, ceftizoxime, ceftriaxone, or ceftazidime	imipenem; ticarcillin/clavulanic acid; piperacillin/tazobactam; gentamicin, tobramycin, or amikacin; carbenicillin; ticarcillin, mezlocillin, or piperacillin; aztreonam; trimethoprim-sulfamethoxazole; a fluoroquinolone
Salmonella typhi	a fluoroquinolone or ceftriaxone	chloramphenicol; trimethoprim-sulfamethoxazole; ampicillin; amoxicillin
other *Salmonella*	cefotaxime or ceftriaxone or a fluoroquinolone	ampicillin or amoxicillin; trimethoprim-sulfamethoxazole; chloramphenicol
Serratia	cefotaxime, ceftizoxime, ceftriaxone, or ceftazidime	gentamicin or amikacin; imipenem; aztreonam; trimethoprim-sulfamethoxazole; carbenicillin; ticarcillin; mezlocillin or piperacillin; a fluoroquinolone
Shigella	a fluoroquinolone	trimethoprim-sulfamethoxazole; ampicillin; ceftriaxone
Yersinia enterocolitica	trimethoprim-sulfamethoxazole	a fluoroquinolone; gentamicin, tobramycin or amikacin; cefotaxime or ceftizoxime
Other Gram-Negative Bacilli		
Acinetobacter	imipenem	amikacin, tobramycin, or gentamicin; ticarcillin, mezlocillin, or piperacillin; ceftazidime; trimethoprim-sulfamethoxazole; a fluoroquinolone; minocycline; doxycycline
Aeromonas	trimethoprim-sulfamethoxazole	gentamicin or tobramycin; imipenem; a fluoroquinolone
Bartonella		
Agent of bacillary angiomatosis (*Bartonella henselae* or *quintana*)	an erythromycin	doxycycline
Cat scratch bacillus (*Bartonella henselae*)	ciprofloxacin	trimethoprim-sulfamethoxazole; gentamicin; rifampin
Bordetella pertussis (whooping cough)	an erythromycin	trimethoprim-sulfamethoxazole; ampicillin
Brucella	a tetracycline + streptomycin or gentamicin	a tetracycline + rifampin; chloramphenicol ± streptomycin; trimethoprim-sulfamethoxazole ± gentamicin; rifampin + a tetracycline; ceftazidime; chloramphenicol
Burkholderia cepacia	trimethoprim-sulfamethoxazole	ceftazidime; chloramphenicol

Infecting Organisms	Drug of First Choice	Alternative Drugs
Calymmatobacterium granulomatis (granuloma inguinale)	a tetracycline	streptomycin or gentamicin; trimethoprim-sulfamethoxazole; erythromycin
Eikenella corrodens	ampicillin	an erythromycin; a tetracycline; amoxicillin/clavulanic acid; ampicillin/sulbactam; ceftriaxone
Francisella tularensis (tularemia)	streptomycin	gentamicin; a tetracycline; chloramphenicol
Fusobacterium	penicillin G	metronidazole; clindamycin; cefoxitin; chloramphenicol
Gardnerella vaginalis (bacterial vaginosis)	oral metronidazole	topical clindamycin or metronidazole; oral clindamycin
Haemophilus ducreyi (chancroid)	erythromycin or ceftriaxone or azithromycin	a fluoroquinolone
Haemophilus influenzae		
meningitis, epiglottitis, arthritis, and other serious infections	cefotaxime or ceftriaxone	cefuroxime (but not for meningitis); chloramphenicol
upper respiratory infections and bronchitis	trimethoprim-sulfamethoxazole	cefuroxime; amoxicillin/clavulanic acid; cefuroxime axetil; cefaclor; cefotaxime; ampicillin or amoxicillin; a tetracycline; clarithromycin; azithromycin; a fluoroquinolone
Legionella species	erythromycin ± rifampin	clarithromycin; azithromycin; ciprofloxacin; trimethoprim-sulfamethoxazole
Leptotrichia buccalis	penicillin G	a tetracycline; clindamycin; erythromycin
Pasteurella multocida	penicillin G	a tetracycline; a cephalosporin; amoxicillin/clavulanic acid; ampicillin/sulbactam
Pseudomonas aeruginosa		
urinary tract infections	a fluoroquinolone	carbenicillin, ticarcillin, piperacillin or mezlocillin; ceftazidime; imipenem; aztreonam; tobramycin; gentamicin; amikacin
other infections	ticarcillin, mezlocillin, or piperacillin + tobramycin, gentamicin or amikacin	ceftazidime, imipenem or aztreonam + tobramycin, gentamicin, or amikacin; ciprofloxacin
Pseudomonas mallei (glanders)	streptomycin + a tetracycline	streptomycin + chloramphenicol
Pseudomonas pseudomallei (melioidosis)	ceftazidime	chloramphenicol + doxycycline + trimethoprim-sulfamethoxazole; amoxicillin/clavulanic acid; imipenem
Spirillum minus (rat bite fever)	penicillin G	a tetracycline; streptomycin
Stenotrophomonas maltophilia (*Pseudomonas maltophilia*)	trimethoprim-sulfamethoxazole	minocycline; ceftazidime; a fluoroquinolone
Streptobacillus moniliformis (rat bite fever; Haverhill fever)	penicillin G	a tetracycline; streptomycin
Vibrio cholerae (cholera)	a tetracycline	trimethoprim-sulfamethoxazole; a fluoroquinolone
Vibrio vulnificus	a tetracycline	cefotaxime
Yersinia pestis (plague)	streptomycin	a tetracycline; chloramphenicol; gentamicin

Acid Fast Bacilli

Mycobacterium tuberculosis	isoniazid + rifampin + pyrazinamide ± ethambutol or streptomycin	ciprofloxacin or ofloxacin; cycloserine; capreomycin or kanamycin or amikacin; ethionamide; clofazimine; aminosalicylic acid
Mycobacterium kansasii	isoniazid + rifampin ± ethambutol or streptomycin	clarithromycin; ethionamide; cycloserine
Mycobacterium avium complex	clarithromycin or azithromycin + one or more of the following: ethambutol; rifabutin; ciprofloxacin	rifampin; clofazimine; amikacin
prophylaxis	rifabutin or clarithromycin	azithromycin
Mycobacterium fortuitum complex	amikacin + doxycycline	cefoxitin; rifampin; a sulfonamide
Mycobacterium marinum (balnei)	minocycline	trimethoprim-sulfamethoxazole; rifampin; clarithromycin; doxycycline
Mycobacterium leprae (leprosy)	dapsone + rifampin ± clofazimine	minocycline; ofloxacin; sparfloxacin; clarithromycin

Actinomycetes

Actinomyces israelii (actinomycosis)	penicillin G	a tetracycline; erythromycin; clindamycin
Nocardia	trimethoprim-sulfamethoxazole	sulfisoxazole; amikacin; a tetracycline; imipenem; cycloserine

Chlamydiae

Chlamydia psittaci (psittacosis; ornithosis)	a tetracycline	chloramphenicol
Chlamydia trachomatis (trachoma)	azithromycin	a tetracycline (topical plus oral); a sulfonamide (topical plus oral)
(inclusion conjunctivitis)	erythromycin (oral or IV)	a sulfonamide
(pneumonia)	erythromycin	a sulfonamide
(urethritis, cervicitis)	doxycycline or azithromycin	erythromycin; ofloxacin; sulfisoxazole; amoxicillin
(lymphogranuloma venereum)	a tetracycline	erythromycin
Chlamydia pneumoniae (TWAR strain)	a tetracycline	erythromycin; clarithromycin; azithromycin

Ehrlichia

Ehrlichia chaffeensis	a tetracycline	
Agent of human granulocytic ehrlichiosis	a tetracycline	

Mycoplasma

Mycoplasma pneumoniae	erythromycin or a tetracycline	clarithromycin; azithromycin
Ureaplasma urealyticum	erythromycin	a tetracycline; clarithromycin
Rickettsia — Rocky Mountain spotted fever, endemic typhus (murine), epidemic typhus (louse-borne), scrub typhus, trench fever, Q fever	a tetracycline	chloramphenicol; a fluoroquinolone

Infecting Organisms	Drug of First Choice	Alternative Drugs
Spirochetes		
Borrelia burgdorferi (Lyme disease)	doxycycline or amoxicillin	cefuroxime axetil; ceftriaxone; cefotaxime; penicillin G; azithromycin; clarithromycin
Borrelia recurrentis (relapsing fever)	a tetracycline	penicillin G
Leptospira	penicillin G	a tetracycline
Treponema pallidum (syphilis)	penicillin G	a tetracycline; ceftriaxone
Treponema pertenue (yaws)	penicillin G	a tetracycline

ANTIDEPRESSANTS

Tricyclic Antidepressants	
Tertiary Amines Amitriptyline Doxepin Imipramine Trimipramine	**Tetracyclic** Maprotiline
	Bicyclic Fluoxetine
	Triazolopyridine Trazodone
Secondary Amines Desipramine Nortriptyline Protriptyline	**Aminoketone** Bupropion
	Monoamine Oxidase Inhibitors Isocarboxazide Phenelzine Tranylcypromine
Dibenzoxazepine Amoxapine	

ANTIDIARRHEAL MEDICATIONS

Antimotility Agents
Atropine
Diphenoxylate
Loperamide
Opium tincture
Paregoric

Adsorbents
Kaolin-pectin mixture
Polycarbophil

Antisecretory Agent (bismuth subsalicylate)

Enzymes (lactase)

Bacterial Replacement
(*Lactobacillus acidophilus, L. bulgaricus*)

ANTIDIURETIC HORMONE

Analogs	Descriptions
Desmopressin acetate	1-deamino-8-D-arginine-vasopressin acetate
Lypressin	8-lysine vasopressin
Ornipressin	8-ornithine-vasopressin
Terlipressin	triglycyl-lysine-vasopressin (inactive prodrug)
Vasopressin (argipressin)	8-arginine vasopressin

ANTIDOTES		
Acetylcysteine	for	Acetaminophen
Amyl Nitrite Sodium Nitrite Sodium Thiosulfate	for	Cyanide
Anticholinesterases Edrophonium Cl Neostigmine Pyridostigmine Br	for	Cholinergic agents: Organophosphates, carbamates, pilocarpine, physostigmine, or isoflurophate
Deferoxamine Mesylate	for	Iron
Digoxin Immune Fab	for	Digoxin
Dimercaprol (BAL)	for	Arsenic, gold, mercury, lead
Edetate Calcium Disodium	for	Lead
Edetate Disodium	for	Hypercalcemia, digitalis toxicity
Glucagon	for	Insulin-induced hypoglycemia
Hydroxocobalamin	for	Cyanide poisoning from nitroprusside
Leucovorin Calcium	for	Folic acid antagonists (e.g., methotrexate)
Methylene Blue	for	Cyanide
Naloxone	for	Opioids
Physostigmine Salicylate	for	Drugs with anticholinergic actions
Pralidoxime Chloride	for	Anticholinesterases, organophosphates
Protamine Sulfate	for	Heparin
Vitamin K	for	Oral anticoagulants

ANTIEMETIC AGENTS

The physiologic purpose of **nausea** is to discourage food intake, and **vomiting** is meant to expel food or other toxic substances present in the upper part of the gastrointestinal tract. **Protracted vomiting** may not only cause electrolyte imbalance, dehydration, or a malnutrition syndrome, but also lead to mucosal laceration and upper gastrointestinal hemorrhage (**Mallory-Weiss syndrome**).

Nausea and vomiting may occur when the stomach is overly irritated, stimulated, or distended (from overeating). In addition, nausea and vomiting may occur when the **chemoreceptor trigger zone for emesis** or the **vomiting center**, or both, are directly stimulated.

Pharmacologic agents such as aspirin and levodopa may cause vomiting by directly irritating the stomach. Agents such as aminophylline, isoniazid, reserpine, antiinflammatory steroids, and caffeine may also elicit vomiting in susceptible individuals by causing the release of hydrochloric acid. This drug-induced emesis may be avoided by having patients take the drugs with meals. Antiemetics are not effective in rectifying these conditions, and their use is not justified.

In addition to agents that stimulate or irritate the stomach, many other factors may be responsible for inducing emesis centrally. The central control of vomiting is vested in two areas:

1. The **vomiting center**, which is located in the lateral reticular formation in the midst of a group of cells governing activities such as salivation and respiration.
2. The **chemoreceptor trigger zone**, which is a narrow strip along the floor of the fourth ventricle located close to the vomiting center.

The functions of these two areas are distinct but interdependent. The vomiting center is activated by impulses that originate from the gastrointestinal tract and other peripheral structures. In addition, there are unidentified tracts that extend from the cerebral cortex to the vomiting center, such that emotional trauma and unpleasant olfactory and visual stimuli may cause nausea and vomiting.

Stimulation of the **vestibular apparatus** that responds to movements of the head, neck, and eye muscles may also cause nausea and vomiting by stimulating the vomiting center. On the other hand, circulating chemicals, toxins, viruses, and ions may provoke nausea and vomiting by first stimulating the **chemoreceptor zone for emesis**, which in turn stimulates the vomiting center.

The nausea and vomiting associated with circulating physical agents (radiation therapy and virus particles) and chemical agents (toxins and cancer chemotherapeutic agents) are treated with phenothiazine derivatives such as chlorpromazine, perphenazine, prochlorperazine, promethazine, triethylperazine, and trifluopromazine. These agents block the dopamine receptors in the **area postrema** (see Figures 64 through 72).

A new class of antiemetic agents, the serotonin receptor antagonists, has been identified. These agents could be clinically useful in a wide range of areas. Selective antagonists of the serotonin (5-hydroxytryptamine) type 3 ($5-HT_3$) receptor such as **batanopride, granisetron, ondansetron,** or **zacopride** have proved in early clinical trials to be potent antiemetic agents in patients undergoing cytotoxic chemotherapy. Their efficacy has been shown to be comparable or superior to that of conventional phenothiazine antiemetics. The toxic effects observed so far with these agents have been modest (see Figures 64 through 72).

The specific and rational use of antiemetic agents depends on the nature of the emesis-inducing problem. **Psychogenically induced vomiting** is best controlled by sedatives and antianxiety agents such as

- Phenobarbital
- Buclizine (Softran) (also has antihistaminic properties)
- Hydroxyzine (Atarax) (also has antihistaminic properties)

The nausea and vomiting produced by **motion sickness** are best treated with antihistaminic agents that have a considerable amount of anticholinergic activity. Examples include:

- Chlorpheniramine (Chlor-Trimeton)
- Diphenhydramine (Benadryl)
- Dimehydrinate (Dramamine)
- Cyclizine (Marizine)
- Meclizine (Bonamine)
- Promethazine (Phenergan), a phenothiazine derivative that has no antipsychotic properties and has a predominantly antihistaminic properties
- Diphenidol (Vontrol)
- Trimethobenzamide (Tigan)

The nausea and vomiting associated with chemicophysical agents that stimulate the chemoreceptor trigger zone for emesis are best treated with a phenothiazine derivative. With the exception of thioridazine (Mellaril), all have antiemetic effects, and the ones most often used are:

- Chlorpromazine (Thorazine)
- Fluphenazine (Prolixin, Permitil)
- Perphenazine (Trilafon)
- Promazine (Sparine)
- Promethazine (Phenergan)
- Thiethylperazine (Torecan)
- Triflupromazine (Vesprin)
- Prochlorperazine (Compazine)

Phenothiazine derivatives depress the chemoreceptor trigger zone for emesis, and large doses also inhibit the vomiting center. It has been reported that thiethylperazine depresses both the chemoreceptor trigger zone and the vomiting center (see Figure 73).

Radiation-induced emesis, or uncontrolled vomiting in patients undergoing radiation therapy, may necessitate either discontinuation of the treatment or prophylactic treatment with phenothiazine antiemetics.

Antineoplastic agents such as nitrogen-mustard or cisplatin may cause disabling nausea and severe vomiting. Triflupromazine has been shown to be more effective than chlorpromazine in controlling these symptoms. Recent studies have suggested that the naturally occurring cannabinoid (marijuana) or synthetic cannabinoids (Nabilone) are also effective in combating the vomiting associated with cancer chemotherapeutic agents. Besides their antiemetic effects, cannabinoids increase appetite, cause euphoria, and are analgesics. These properties are useful in a patient who is in the terminal stages of cancer.

Postoperative nausea and vomiting are directly related to the type and dose of the anesthetic used. It has been shown that the use of a muscle relaxant, which substantially reduces the amount of anesthetic needed, lessens the incidence and intensity of postoperative nausea and vomiting. However, most of the phenothiazines may be used to control postoperative emesis.

The nausea and vomiting associated with **the first trimester of pregnancy** are benign and self-limiting in nature. If at all possible, no medications should be used. If absolutely necessary, antihistaminics (meclizine and trimethobenzamide) may be effective. Pyridoxine (vitamin B_6) should not be prescribed, as it may predispose to vitamin B_6-dependent syndrome in the infant.

ANTIEMETIC PREPARATIONS			
Antacids (see Table 7)			
Antihistaminic-anticholinergic Agents			
Benzquinamide Buclizine Cyclizine	Dimenhydrinate Diphenhydramine Hydroxyzine	Meclizine Promethazine Pyrilamine	Scopolamine Trimethobenzamide
Benzodiazepines Diazepam Lorazepam			
Butyrophenones Droperidol Haloperidol			
Cannabinoids Dronabinol Nabilone			
Corticosteroids Dexamethasone Methylprednisolone			
Non-phenothiazine Dopamine Receptor Antagonist Metoclopramide			
Phenothiazine Dopamine Receptor Antagonists			
Chlorpromazine Fluphenazine Prochlorperazine	Promazine Thiethylperazine		
Serotonin Receptor Antagonists			
Batanopride Granisetron	Ondansetron Zacopride		

ANTIHEMOPHILIC FACTOR

(AHF, Hemoni M, Humate-P, Koāte-HP, Koāte-HS, Koāte-HT, Monoclate, Profilate OSD)

Antihemophilic factor, a blood derivative, is indicated for the treatment of hemophilia A (Factor VIII deficiency). Antihemophilic factor replaces deficient clotting factors that convert prothrombin to thrombin (see Tables 16 and 17 and Figure 35).

ANTIHISTAMINIC AGENTS

The diversified actions of histamine are brought forth through their interaction with different types of receptors, which are described in the following sections.

Histamine$_1$ Receptors

Histamine$_1$ (H$_1$) receptors mediate such actions as bronchoconstriction and the contraction of smooth muscle in the gastrointestinal tract. These effects are blocked by classic antihistaminics such as **pyrilamine**. Examples of other H$_1$-receptor blocking agents are:

Ethanolamine derivatives
> Diphenhydramine hydrochloride (Benadryl)
> Dimenhydrinate (Dramamine)
> Carbinoxamine maleate (Clistin)

Ethylenediamine derivatives
> Pyrilamine maleate
> Tripelennamine hydrochloride
> Tripelennamine citrate

Alkylamine derivatives
> Chlorpheniramine maleate (Chlor-Trimeton)
> Brompheniramine maleate (Dimetane)

Piperazine derivatives
> Hydroxyzine hydrochloride (Atarax)
> Hydroxyzine pamoate (Vistaril)
> Cyclizine hydrochloride (Marezine)
> Meclizine hydrochloride (Antivert)

Phenothiazine derivatives
> Promethazine hydrochloride (Phenergan)

Piperidine derivatives (Second-generation antihistaminics)
> Terfenadine (Seldane)
> Astemizole (Hismanal)

The pharmacologic characteristics of H$_1$-receptor antagonists are qualitatively similar in that they antagonize (competitive H$_1$ blockers) the histamine-mediated bronchoconstriction, vasodilation, and enhanced capillary permeability. Some of these agents also have **anticholinergic properties**. Diphenhydramine has strong atropine-like effects, whereas pyrilamine has weak anticholinergic effects (see Figure 49).

Some antihistaminics such as benztropine (Cogentin) are used in the treatment of **parkinsonism** and in controlling neuroleptic-induced **pseudoparkinsonism**. Furthermore, diphenhydramine is most effective in reversing neuroleptic-induced **dystonia**. The usefulness of these agents in the management of these extrapyramidal disorders is related to their anticholinergic effects. Some antihistaminics such as cyproheptadine (Periactin) also block serotonin-receptor sites. As a result they have been advocated for use in patients with allergic dermatitis characterized by urticaria or pruritus, or both.

Some antihistaminics, such as promethazine and diphenhydramine, have **local anesthetic properties**. They may be used substitutively in patients who are allergic to both amide and ester types of local anesthetics. Some phenothiazine antihistaminics, such as promethazine, have **alpha-adrenergic blocking effects**. Therefore, like phenothiazine neuroleptics, promethazine may cause **orthostatic hypotension**.

Besides the specific uses discussed, the general therapeutic uses of antihistaminics include allergic reactions such as urticaria, allergic rhinitis, motion sickness, vestibular disturbances, and the nausea and vomiting associated with pregnancy.

The most common side effect of the antihistaminics is sedation, and all of them cause it to varying degrees. For example, diphenhydramine, dimenhydrinate, and promethazine cause marked sedation, but pyrilamine produces only moderate sedation. Chlorpheniramine, meclizine, and cyclizine have mild sedative properties, while terfenadine, astemizole, loratadine, and cetirizine are nonsedating.

The acute poisoning that occurs with most antihistaminics does not cause severe central nervous system (CNS) depression as would be expected based on their sedative properties, but is manifested by mydriasis, fever, flushing, CNS excitement, hallucinations, ataxia, athetosis, and convulsions. Some of these effects, which resemble those of atropine poisoning, may be due to their anticholinergic properties. **Diazepam** is an effective antidote to poisoning and should be used to reverse the CNS excitement and convulsions.

Histamine$_2$ Receptors

Stimulation of the H$_2$ receptors elicits a variety of responses, the most widely studied of which is **gastric acid secretion** from the parietal cells of the gastric glands (see Figure 24). However, many other effects mediated by H$_2$ receptors are manifested in peripheral tissues. These include the positive chronotropic action in the auricular muscle, the inotropic action in the ventricular muscle, and the lipolytic effect in fat cells. In addition, the extensive use of **cimetidine** has led to the synthesis and marketing of more specific and efficacious analogs with pharmacologic properties that are outlined in Table 9 and Figure 24. Examples of the various H$_2$-receptor blocking agents are:

Imidazole derivatives
  Cimetidine and etintidine
Furan derivatives
  Ranitidine and nizatidine
Guanidinothiazole derivatives
  Famotidine
Piperidinomethylphenoxy derivatives
  Roxatidine acetate and roxatidine

Histamine$_3$ Receptors

H$_3$ receptors suppress **gastric acid secretion** and this is evoked by cholinergic stimuli. H$_3$ receptors exist outside the parietal cells and seem to be located on cholinergic and nonadrenergic noncholinergic neurons of the myenteric plexus, where they inhibit the release of neurotransmitters. The agonist and antagonist for H$_3$ receptors are **alpha-methylhistamine** and **thioperamide**, respectively.

ANTIHISTAMINES (H$_1$ RECEPTOR ANTAGONISTS)	
Alkylamine Class	**Phenothiazine Class**
Brompheniramine maleate	Methdilazine hydrochloride
Chlorpheniramine maleate	Promethazine hydrochloride
Dexchlorpheniramine maleate	Trimeprazine
Ethanolamine Class	**Piperidine Class**
Carbinoxamine maleate	Azatadine maleate
Clemastine fumarate	Cyproheptadine hydrochloride
Diphenhydramine hydrochloride	Diphenylpyraline hydrochloride
	Phenindamine tartrate

Ethylenediamine Class	Newer Products
Pyrilamine maleate	Astemizole
Tripelennamine hydrochloride	Terfenadine
	Loratadine

Astemizole, terfenadine, and loratadine are devoid of sedative or anticholinergic properties.

ANTIHYPERTENSIVE MEDICATIONS

Alpha-1 Adrenergic Receptor Blocking Agents
Doxazosin
Prazosin hydrochloride
Terazosin

Beta-1 Adrenergic Receptor Blocking Agents

Acebutolol	Nadolol
Atenolol	Penbutolol
Betaxolol	Pindolol
Carteolol	Propranolol hydrochloride
Metoprolol tartrate	Timolol maleate

Angiotensin-converting Enzyme Inhibitors

Benazepril	Lisinopril
Captopril	Ouinapril
Enalapril maleate	Ramipril
Fosinopril	

Calcium Channel Antagonists

Diltiazem hydrochloride	Nifedipine
Felodipine	Verapamil hydrochloride
Isradipine	
Nicardipine	

Diuretics

Thiazides and Related Sulfonamide Diuretics

Bendroflumethiazide	Indapamide
Benzthiazide	Methyclothiazide
Chlorothiazide sodium	Metolazone
Chlorthalidone	Polythiazide
Cyclothiazide	Quinethazone
Hydrochlorothiazide	Trichlormethiazide
Hydroflumethiazide	

Loop Diuretics
Bumetanide
Ethacrynic acid
Furosemide

Potassium-sparing Agents
Amiloride hydrochloride
Spironolactone
Triamterene

Central-acting Adrenergic Inhibitors
Clonidine hydrochloride
Guanabenz acetate
Guanfacine
Methyldopa

Peripheral-acting Adrenergic Antagonists
Guanadrel sulfate
Guanethidine monosulfate
Reserpine

Vasodilators
Hydralazine hydrochloride
Minoxidil

ANTINEOPLASTIC AGENTS			
Alkylating Agents (and Trade Names)			
Busulfan	(Myleran)	Lomustine	(CCNU)
Carmustine	(BCNU)	Mechlorethamine	(HN$_2$, nitrogen mustard)
Chlorambucil	(Leukeran)	Melphalan	(L-phenylalanine mustard)
Cyclophosphamide	(Cytoxan)	Semustine	(MeCCNU)
Hexamethylmelamine	(Hexastat)	Streptozocin	(Streptozotocin)
Ifosfamide	(Ifex)	Thiotepa	(Triethylenethiophosphoramide)
Antimetabolites (and Trade Names)			
Cladribine	(2-Chloro-	Methotrexate	(Amethopterin)
Cytarabine	deoxyadenosine)	PALA	(Sparfosate)
Floxuridine	(Ara-C)	Pentostatin	(2′-Deoxy-coformycin)
Fludarabine phosphate	(5-Fluorodeoxy-	Purinethol	(6-MP Mercaptopurine)
Fluorouracil	uridine)	Thioguanine	(6-TG 6-thioguanine)
	(F-ara-A fludara)		
	(5-Fu)		
Natural Products (and Trade Names)			
Asparaginase	(L-Asnase)	Idarubicin	(Mitomycin C)
Bleomycin	(Bleo)	Mitomycin	(Mithramycin)
Camptothecin		Plicamycin	(Paclitaxel)
Dactinomycin	(Actinomycin D)	Taxol	(VM-26)
Daunorubicin	(Daunomycin)	Teniposide	(Vincaleukoblastine velban)
Doxorubicin	(Adriamycin)	Vinblastine	(Oncovin)
Epirubicin		Vincristine	
Etoposide	(VP-16 VePesid)	Vindesine	
Homoharringtonine	(HHT)		
Miscellaneous (and Trade Names)			
Amsarcrine	(m-AMSA)	Hydrea	(Hydroxyurea)
Carboplatin	(Paraplatin)	Mitoxantrone	(Novantrone DHAQ)
Cisplatin	(CBDCA)	Procarbazine	(MIH Natulan)
Dacarbazine	(DDP)		
	(DIC DTIC)		
Hormones and Antagonists			
Adrenocorticosteroids			
Androgens			
Antiandrogen			
Antiestrogen			
Estrogens			
Gonadotropin-releasing hormone analog			
Progestins			

ANTIPARASITIC MEDICATIONS AND THEIR SIDE EFFECTS

Albendazole
Diarrhea; abdominal pain; migration of *ascaris* through mouth and nose; leukopenia; alopecia; increased serum transaminase activity

Benznidazole
Allergic rash; dose-dependent polyneuropathy; gastrointestinal disturbances; psychic disturbances

Bithionol
Photosensitivity reactions; vomiting; diarrhea; abdominal pain; urticaria; leukopenia; toxic hepatitis

Chloroquine HCl and Chloroquine Phosphate
Pruritus; vomiting; headache; confusion; depigmentation of hair; skin eruptions; corneal opacity; weight loss; partial alopecia; extraocular muscle palsies; exacerbation of psoriasis, eczema, and other exfoliative dermatoses; myalgias; photophobia; irreversible retinal injury (especially when total dosage exceeds 100 grams); discoloration of nails and mucus membranes; nerve-type deafness; peripheral neuropathy and myopathy; heart block; blood dyscrasias; hematemesis

Crotamiton
Rash; conjunctivitis; photosensitivity reactions; vomiting; diarrhea; abdominal pain; urticaria; leukopenia; toxic hepatitis

Dehydroemetine
Cardiac arrhythmias; precordial pain; muscle weakness; cellulitis as site of injection; diarrhea; vomiting; peripheral neuropathy; heart failure; headache; dyspnea

Diethylcarbamazine Citrate USP
Severe allergic or febrile reactions in patients with microfilaria in the blood or the skin; GI disturbances; encephalopathy

Diloxanide Furoate
Flatulence; nausea; vomiting; diarrhea; diplopia; dizziness; urticaria; pruritus

Eflornithine
Anemia; leukopenia; diarrhea; thrombocytopenia; seizures; hearing loss

Flubendazole - similar to mebendazole

Furazolidone
Nausea; vomiting; allergic reactions, including pulmonary infiltration; hypotension; urticaria; fever; vesicular rash; hypoglycemia; headache; hemolytic anemia in G-6-PD deficiency and neonates; disulfiram-like reaction with alcohol; MAO-inhibitor interactions; polyneuritis

Halofantrine
Diarrhea; abdominal pain; pruritus

Iodoquinol
Rash; acne; slight enlargement of the thyroid gland; nausea; diarrhea; cramps; anal pruritus; optic atrophy; loss of vision; peripheral neuropathy after prolonged use in high dosage (for months); iodine sensitivity

Ivermectin
Mazzotti-type reaction seen in onchocerciasis, including fever; pruritus; tender lymph nodes; headache; joint and bone pain; hypotension

Lindane
Eczematous rash; conjunctivitis; convulsions; aplastic anemia

Malathion
Local irritation

Mebendazole
Diarrhea; abdominal pain; migration of *ascaris* through mouth and nose; leukopenia; agranulocytosis; hypospermia

Mefloquine
Vertigo; lightheadedness; nausea; other gastrointestinal disturbances; nightmares; visual disturbances; headache; confusion; psychosis; hypotension; convulsions; coma

Meglumine Antimoniate - similar to stibogluconate sodium

Melarsoprol
Myocardial damage; albuminuria; hypertension; colic; Herxheimer-type reaction; encephalopathy; vomiting; peripheral neuropathy; shock

Metronidazole
Nausea; headache; dry mouth; metallic taste; vomiting; diarrhea; insomnia; weakness; stomatitis; vertigo; paresthesias; rash; dark urine; urethral burning; disulfiram-like reaction with alcohol; seizures; encephalopathy; pseudomembranous colitis; ataxia; leukopenia; peripheral neuropathy; pancreatitis

Niclosamide
Nausea; abdominal pain

Nifurtimox
Anorexia; vomiting; weight loss; loss of memory; sleep disorders; tremor; paresthesias; weakness; polyneuritis; convulsions; fever; pulmonary infiltrates and pleural effusion

Ornidazole
Dizziness; headache; gastrointestinal disturbances; reversible peripheral neuropathy

Oxamniquine

Headache; fever; dizziness; somnolence; nausea; diarrhea; rash; insomnia; hepatic enzyme changes; ECG changes; EEG changes; orange-red discoloration of urine; seizures; neuropsychiatric disturbances

Paromomycin

GI disturbances; eighth-nerve damage (mainly auditory); renal damage

Pentamidine Isethionate

Hypotension; hypoglycemia often followed by diabetes mellitus; vomiting; blood dyscrasias; renal damage; pain at injection site; GI disturbances; may aggravate diabetes; shock; hypocalcemia; liver damage; cardiotoxicity; delirium; rash; Herxheimer-type reaction; anaphylaxis; acute pancreatitis; hyperkalemia

Permethrin

Burning; stinging; numbness; increased pruritus; pain; edema; erythema; rash

Praziquantel

Malaise; headache; dizziness; sedation; abdominal discomfort; fever; sweating; nausea; eosinophilia; fatigue; pruritus; rash

Primaquine Phosphate USP

Hemolytic anemia in G-6-PD deficiency neutropenia; GI disturbances; methemoglobinemia in G-6-PD deficiency; CNS symptoms; hypertension; arrhythmias

Proguanil

Oral ulceration; hair loss; scaling of palms and soles; hematuria (with large doses); vomiting; abdominal pain; diarrhea (with large doses)

Pyrantel Pamoate

GI disturbances; headache; dizziness; rash; fever

Pyrethrins and Piperonyl Butoxide

Allergic reactions

Pyrimethamine

Blood dyscrasias; folic acid deficiency; rash; vomiting; convulsions; shock; possibly pulmonary eosinophilia

Quinacrine HCl

Dizziness; headache; vomiting; diarrhea; yellow staining of skin; toxic psychosis; insomnia; bizarre dreams; blood dyscrasias; urticaria; blue and black nail pigmentation; psoriasis-like rash; acute hepatic necrosis; convulsions; severe exfoliative dermatitis; ocular effects similar to those caused by chloroquine

Quinine Dihydrochloride and Sulfate

Cinchonism (tinnitus, headache, nausea, abdominal pain, visual disturbance); deafness; hemolytic anemia; other blood dyscrasias; photosensitivity reactions; hypoglycemia; arrhythmias; hypotension; drug fever; blindness; sudden death if injected too rapidly

Spiramycin

GI disturbances; allergic reactions

Stibogluconate Sodium

Muscle pain and joint stiffness; nausea; transaminase elevations; T-wave flattening or inversion; weakness; colic; liver damage; bradycardia; leukopenia; diarrhea; rash; pruritus; myocardial damage; hemolytic anemia; renal damage; shock; sudden death

Suramin Sodium

Vomiting; pruritus; urticaria; paresthesias; hyperesthesia of hands and feet; photophobia; peripheral neuropathy; kidney damage; blood dyscrasias; shock; optic atrophy

Thiabendazole

Nausea; vomiting; vertigo; leukopenia; crystalluria; rash; hallucinations; olfactory disturbance; erythema multi forme; Stevens-Johnson syndrome; shock; tinnitus; intrahepatic cholestasis; convulsions; angioneurotic edema

Tinidazole

Metallic taste; nausea; vomiting; rash

Trimetrexate (with "leucovorin rescue")

Rash; peripheral neuropathy; bone marrow depression; increased serum aminotransferase concentrations

Tryparsamide

Nausea; vomiting; impaired vision; optic atrophy; fever; exfoliative dermatitis; allergic reactions; tinnitus

ANTIPSYCHOTICS	
Butyrophenone	Loxapine
Haloperidol	Dihydroindolone
Dibenzoxapine	Molindone
Clozapine	
Phenothiazines (Alipathic)	
Chlorpromazine	
Phenothiazines (Piperazine)	
Acetophenazine	Prochlorperazine
Fluphenazine	Trifluoperazine
Perphenazine	
Phenothiazines (Piperidine)	
Mesoridazine	Chlorprothixene
Thioridazine	Thiothixen
Thioxanthenes	

ANTIVIRAL AGENTS	
Antiherpes Virus Agents	
Acyclovir	(ACV, acycloguanosine)
Famciclovir	(FCV)
Foscarnet	(PFA, phosphonoformate)
Ganciclovir	(GCV, DHPG)
Idoxuridine	(IDUR)
Sorivudine	(BV-ara-U, brovavir)
Trifluridine	(TFT, trifluorothymidine)
Valacyclovir	
Vidarabine	(ara-A, adenine arabinoside)
Antiretroviral Agents	
Didanosine	(ddI)
Stavudine	(d4T)
Zalcitabine	(ddC)
Zidovudine	(AZT, ZDV, azidothymidine)
Other antiviral agents	
Amantadine	Ribavirin
Interferon alpha (interferon alfa)	Rimantadine

ANTITHROMBIN III

(Heparin Cofactor I) (Antativ, Thrombate III)

Antithrombin III, an anticoagulant and antithrombotic agent (50 to 100 IU/min IV), is indicated for prophylaxis and adjunct treatment of thromboembolism associated with hereditary antithrombin III deficiency (see also Tables 16 and 17 and Figure 35).

APOMORPHINE HCL

Ipecac is a mixture of the alcohol-soluble alkaloid which is obtained from the South American plant *Cephaelis ipecacuanha*, and is used solely in the form of **syrup of ipecac. Apomorphine hydrochloride** (5 mg sc) and **copper sulfate** are also emetics. Syrup of ipecac and copper sulfate cause emesis by locally irritating the stomach, whereas apomorphine stimulates the **chemoreceptor trigger zone for emesis** located in the caudal portion of the fourth ventricle (area postrema), which in turn stimulates the vomiting center in the lateral reticular formation of the medulla (see Figure 73). Results are usually obtained within 5 to 10 minutes after parenteral administration. Apomorphine and other emetics should not be used in cases of poisoning with corrosive agents; in shock or coma; and in narcosis resulting from opiates, barbiturates, alcohol, or other CNS depressants. Overdosage with apomorphine may cause circulatory failure which is reversed by **naloxone**.

APRACLONIDINE HYDROCHLORIDE

(Iopidine)

Apraclonidine, an alpha-adrenergic receptor blocking agent which reduces intraocular pressure (1 drop in the eye 1 hour before initiation of laser surgery on the anterior segment, followed by 1 drop immediately upon completion of surgery), is indicated for prevention or control of intraocular pressure elevations after argon laser trabeculoplasty or iridotomy.

APROBARBITAL

(Alurate)

Aprobarbital, a barbiturate sedative-hypnotic (40 to 80 mg p.o. h.s.), is indicated in the management of mild-to-severe insomnia (see also **Barbiturates**).

APROTININ

(Trasylol)

Aprotinin, a protease inhibitor (10,000 units or 1.4 mg by IV injection), is indicated for a prophylactic reduction of preoperative blood loss and the need for blood transfusion in patients undergoing cardiopulmonary bypass during repeat coronary artery bypass graft surgery, or in selected patients undergoing initial coronary artery bypass graft surgery in whom the risk of bleeding is high because of impaired hemostasis or in whom transfusion in unavailable or unacceptable.

ARRHYTHMIAS: TREATMENT FOR	
Drugs	**Adverse effects**
Beta-Adrenergic Blockers	
Acebutolol	Hypotension, bradycardia, heart failure, bronchospasm, arthritis, myalgia, arthralgia, lupus-like syndrome, pulmonary complications
Esmolol	Hypotension, heart block, heart failure, bronchospasm, pain at infusion site
Propranolol	Fatigue, impotence, heart block, hypotension, heart failure, bronchospasm, depression
Calcium-Channel Blockers	
Diltiazem	Heart block, hypotension, asystole, heart failure, liver damage
Verapamil HCl	Heart block, heart failure, hypotension, asystole, dizziness, headache, fatigue, edema, nausea, constipation

Drugs	Adverse effects
Quinidine, Procainamide, Disopyramide	
Disopyramide	Anticholinergic effects (urinary retention, aggravation of glaucoma, constipation), hypotension, heart failure, tachyarrhythmias, torsades de pointes, heart block, nausea, vomiting, diarrhea, hypoglycemia, nervousness
Procainamide	Lupus-like syndrome, confusion, insomnia, GI symptoms, rash, hypotension, arrhythmias, torsades de pointes, blood dyscrasias, fever, hepatitis and hepatic failure, myopathy; IV: hypotension, heart block
Quinidine	Diarrhea and other GI symptoms, cinchonism, hepatic granulomas and necrosis, thrombocytopenia, rashes, hypotension, heart block, tachyarrhythmias, torsades de pointes, fever, lupus-like syndrome
Flecainide, Propafenone, Moricizine	
Flecainide	Bradycardia, heart block, new ventricular fibrillation, sustained ventricular tachycardia, heart failure, dizziness, blurred vision, nervousness, headache, GI upset, neutropenia
Moricizine	Bradycardia, heart failure, new ventricular fibrillation, sustained ventricular tachycardia, nausea, dizziness, headache
Propafenone	Bradycardia, heart block, new ventricular fibrillation, sustained ventricular tachycardia, heart failure, dizziness, lightheadedness, metallic taste, GI upset, bronchospasm, hepatic toxicity
Adenosine	
Adenosine	Facial flushing, transient dyspnea, chest discomfort, hypotension; may cause bronchoconstriction in patients with asthma
Lidocaine and Similar Agents	
Lidocaine	Drowsiness or agitation, slurred speech, tinnitus, disorientation, coma, seizures, paresthesias, cardiac depression (especially with excessive accumulation in heart failure or liver failure or infusions for more than 24 hours), bradycardia/asystole
Mexiletine	GI upset, fatigue, nervousness, dizziness, tremor, sleep upset, seizures, visual disturbances, psychosis, fever, blood dyscrasias, hepatitis
Tocainide	GI upset, paresthesias, dizziness, tremor, confusion, nightmares, psychotic reactions, coma, seizures, rash, fever, arthralgia, agranulocytosis, aplastic anemia, thrombocytopenia, hepatic granulomas, interstitial pneumonitis
Amiodarone, Sotalol, Ibutilide	
Amiodarone	Acute pulmonary toxicity, pulmonary fibrosis, bradycardia, heart block, new ventricular fibrillation, sustained ventricular tachycardia, torsades de pointes (unusual), hyper- or hypothyroidism, GI upset, alcoholic-like hepatitis, peripheral neuropathy, ataxia, tremor, dizziness, photosensitivity, blue-gray skin, corneal microdeposits
Ibutilide	Torsades de pointes, AV block
Sotalol	Heart block, hypotension, bronchospasm, bradycardia, torsades de pointes
Other Agents	
Bretylium	Initial hypertension, orthostatic hypotension, nausea and vomiting, increased sensitivity to catecholamines, initial increase in arrhythmias
Digoxin	Bradycardia, AV block arrhythmias, anorexia, nausea, vomiting, diarrhea, abdominal pain, headache, confusion, abnormal vision
Magnesium sulfate	Areflexia, apnea (very high doses)

ARTHRITIS AND DEGENERATIVE JOINT DISEASE: TREATMENT OF

Rheumatoid arthritis is an autoimmune disease. The antigen that stimulates the initial autoimmune response and the genetic mechanism that promotes its development are unknown. Once the disease process is under way, antigen–antibody complexes presumably activate the complement and elicit the release of various mediators, causing inflammation. The treatment of rheumatoid arthritis is aimed at reducing this inflammation, thereby decreasing the pain and attempting to slow the joint destruction.

In the management of arthritic conditions, drugs are chosen on an empirical basis, usually trying the least toxic substances first. The following schedule may be used in drug selection.

First choice—nonsteroidal antiinflammatory agents
Aspirin
Ibuprofen, tolmetin, naproxen, fenoprofen, or sulindac
Indomethacin or phenylbutazone

Second choice—disease-modifying agents
Gold salts
p-Penicillamine
Hydroxychloroquine

Third choice
Steroids
Immunosuppressive agents

Gold salt therapy is reserved for those patients with progressive disease who do not obtain satisfactory relief from therapy with aspirin-like drugs. The principle that underlies this therapy is that gold, which accumulates in lysosomes, decreases the migration and phagocytic activity of macrophages. Aurothioglucose, gold sodium thiomalate, or auranofin may cause toxic effects such as cutaneous reactions (from erythema to exfoliative dermatitis) as well as albuminuria, hematuria, and thrombocytopenia.

Besides the nonsteroidal antiinflammatory agents and gold, other drugs are also used for the treatment of rheumatoid arthritis. These include immunosuppressive agents, glucocorticoids, penicillamine, and hydroxychloroquine. With the exception of glucocorticoids, these drugs resemble gold salts in that they do not possess antiinflammatory or analgesic properties and their therapeutic effects become evident only after several weeks or months of treatment.

Nonsalicylate nonsteroidal antiinflammatory drugs for the treatment of rheumatoid arthritis and allied degenerative joint diseases

Drugs	Half-Life (hr)	Doses per Day
Propionic Acids		
Fenoprofen	2 to 3	3 to 4
Ibuprofen	1.8 to 2.5	3 to 4
Ketoprofen	2 to 4	3 to 4
Naproxen	12 to 15	2
Indoles		
Sulindac	16.4	2
Tolmetin	1.0 to 1.5	
Oxicams		
Piroxicam	30 to 86	1 to 2

ARTIFICIAL TEARS

(Adapettes, Adsorbotear, Artificial Tears, Hypotears, Isopto Alkaline, Isopto Plain, Isopto Tears, Lacril Artificial Tears, Lacrisert, Liquifilm Forte, Liquifilm Tears, Lyteers, Moisture Drops, Murocel Solution, Muro Tears Solution, Neotears, Tearisol, Tears Naturale, Tears Plus)

Artificial tears, a derivative of polyvinyl alcohol or cellulose (1 to 2 drops in eye t.i.d.), is indicated in conditions where the production of tears is insufficient, or in moderate to severe dry eye syndromes, including keratoconjunctivitis sicca.

ASCORBIC ACID (VITAMIN C)

(Arco-cee, Ascorbicap, Cebid, Timecelles, Cecon Solution, Cemil, Cetane, Cevalin, Cevi-Bid, Ce-Vi-Sol, Cevita, C-Long, C-Span, Dull-C, Flavorcee, Vitacee)

Ascorbic acid, a water soluble vitamin (100 to 250 mg p.o. daily), is indicated in the treatment of frank and subclinical scurvy; in extensive burns, delayed fracture or wound healing, postoperative wound healing, severe febrile or chronic disease states; and in prevention of ascorbic acid deficiency in those with poor nutritional habits or increased requirements. In addition, ascorbic acid has been used for potentiation of methenamine in urine acidification and as an adjunctive therapy in the treatment of idiopathic methemoglobinemia.

ASPARAGINASE

(Elspar, Kidrolase)

Asparaginase, an antineoplastic agent (200 IU/kg/day IV for 28 days), is used in the treatment of acute lymphocytic leukemia.

ASPIRIN

(A.S.A., A.S.A. Enseals, Ascriptin, Aspergum, Bayer Timed-Release, Bufferin, Buffinol, Easpirin, Ecotrin, Empirin, Encaprin, Entrophen, Measurin, Zorprin)

Aspirin is indicated in the treatment of mild pain, fever, arthritis, thromboembolic disorders, transient ischemic attacks, to reduce the risk of heart attack in patients with previous myocardial infarction or unstable angina, and treatment of Kawasaki (mucocutaneous lymph node) syndrome (see Table 2 and the section on **Acetylsalicylic acid**). Many of aspirin's pharmacological actions are thought to be mediated by inhibiting **prostaglandin** synthesis through the inhibition of **cyclooxygenase** (Figure 11).

The current thinking concerning the role of aspirin in the prevention of cardiovascular disease is that it is beneficial in the event of **myocardial infarction** and **stroke**. It is effective because, in platelets, small amounts of aspirin acetylate irreversibly and bind to the active site of **thromboxane A$_2$**, a potent promoter of **platelet aggregation** (see Figure 12).

ASTEMIZOLE

(Hismanal)

Astemizole, cetirizine, loratadine, and terfenadine are **second-generation** antihistaminic agents that are relatively **nonsedating**. Other H$_1$-receptor antagonists currently undergoing clinical trials are **azelastine, ebastine**, and **levocabastine**. Astemizole (10 to 30 mg p.o.) is a long-acting peripheral H$_1$ receptor antagonist, which does not pass across the blood-brain barrier and is devoid of anticholinergic properties. Astemizole is absorbed well from the

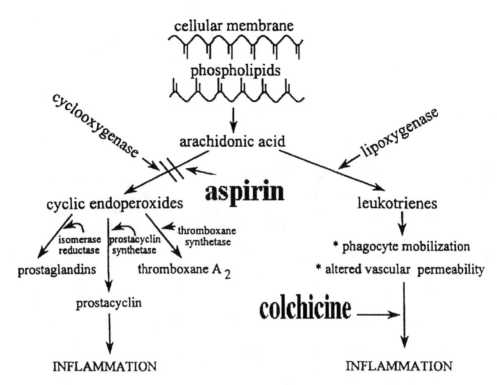

FIGURE 11 Aspirin and related compounds inhibit the enzyme **cyclooxygenase** and prevent the formation of prostaglandin endoperoxides, PGG_2 and PGH_2, which are normally formed from arachidonic acid. (Adapted from Ebadi, M., *Pharmacology, An Illustrated Review with Questions and Answers,* 3rd Edition, Lippincott-Raven Press, Philadelphia, 1996.)

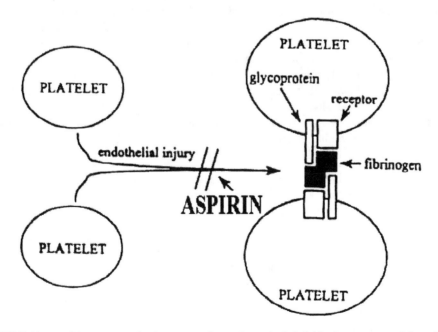

FIGURE 12 Aspirin prevents platelet aggregation and may be helpful in the treatment of thromboembolic disease. (Adapted from Ebadi, M., *Pharmacology, An Illustrated Review with Questions and Answers,* 3rd Edition, Lippincott-Raven Press, Philadelphia, 1996.)

gastrointestinal tract, is bound to plasma proteins to the extent of 96%, undergoes extensive first-pass metabolism, and the metabolites, including desmethylastemizole are excreted in the feces. The metabolism of astemizole is inhibited by erythromycin, ketoconazole, or itraconazole, resulting in elevated levels of astemizole and desmethylastemizole, which may cause cardiac arrhythmias (prolongation of QT intervals) in individuals with a history of cardiovascular disorders, or in patients who are electrolyte imbalanced.

ATENOLOL
(Tenormin)

Atenolol, introduced in 1976, is the most cardioselective beta-adrenergic blocking agent. The cardioselective beta-blockers are acebutolol, atenolol, and metoprolol; and the nonselective beta-blockers are alprenolol, nadolol, oxyprenolol, pindolol, propranolol, sotalol, and timolol (see Figures 14, 27, 33, 57, 61, and 75). Evidence suggests that atenolol is the most beta$_2$-receptor-selective of the beta-blocking agents; therefore, as long as the daily dose is sufficiently low, side effects related to blockade of beta$_2$-receptors — such as increased airway resistance, bronchospasm, prolongation of insulin-induced hypoglycemia, and cold extremities — are seen less frequently. Unlike pindolol, which has pronounced intrinsic sympathomimetic activity (ISA), atenolol is devoid of ISA activity. In contrast to beta-blockers without ISA, such as atenolol, beta-blockers with this property cause a reduction in peripheral vascular resistance with little change in cardiac output. This difference may be due to activation of peripheral beta$_2$-receptors by agents with ISA. This effect on peripheral vasculature offers advantages in the treatment of patients with peripheral vascular disease or obstructive airway disease.

Unlike propranolol, which has quinidine-like effects in that it impairs the capacity of excitable tissues to undergo depolarization, atenolol has no membrane-stabilizing effects. Most beta-adrenergic receptor blocking agents are lipid soluble, whereas atenolol, nadolol, and sotalol are water soluble. Therefore, atenolol has several advantages as an antihypertensive agent. Because it is water soluble, it is excreted relatively slowly by the kidney; therefore, it need be given no more than once daily in most cases. Furthermore, its hydrophilicity results in limited passage through the blood-brain barrier, thus resulting in fewer central nervous system-related side effects compared with lipophilic beta-blockers, such as acebutolol, alprenolol, metoprolol, oxyprenolol, pindolol, propranolol, and timolol. Atenolol reduces heart rate, cardiac index, and blood pressure. It has no effect on plasma volume, exchangeable sodium or potassium, or total body potassium. Like other beta-blocking agents, atenolol inhibits the release of renin, resulting in a decrease in angiotensin II production and aldosterone secretion. Atenolol reduces renal vascular resistance in hypertensive patients.

Atenolol is indicated in arteriosclerotic heart disease with angina pectoris, hypertension, cardiac arrhythmias and myocardial infarction; in hypertrophic obstructive cardiomyopathy, dissecting aneurysm of the aorta, pheochromocytoma, and in prevention of migraine headaches.

Atenolol is contraindicated in congestive heart failure, sinus bradycardia, and atrioventricular block greater than first degree. Atenolol has additive effects with drugs such as reserpine, causing depletion of catecholamine. It should be used cautiously with agents potentially exerting negative inotropic or chronotropic effects, such as calcium channel blockers. Because atenolol is excreted unchanged by the kidney, serum levels are increased in patients with impaired renal function.

ASTHMA: TREATMENT OF	
Drugs	**Formulations**
Newer Adrenergic Drugs	
Albuterol	metered-dose inhaler (90 µg/puff)
	powder inhaler (200 µg Rotacaps)
	nebulized solution (5 mg/ml)
	syrup or tablets
	extended-release tablets
	(Repetabs) (4 mg)
	(Volmax) (4 mg and 8 mg)
Bitolterol mesylate	metered-dose inhaler (370 µg/puff)
Metaproterenol	metered-dose inhaler (650 µg/puff)
	nebulized solution (5% solution)
	syrup or tablets
Pirbuterol	metered-dose inhaler (200 µg/puff)
Terbutaline	subcutaneous (1 mg/ml)
(*Brethaire*)	tablets
	metered-dose inhaler (200 µg/puff)
Corticosteroids	
Beclomethasone dipropionate	metered-dose inhaler (42 µg/puff)
Flunisolide	metered-dose inhaler (250 µg/puff)
Prednisone or Prednisolone	oral tablets (5, 10, 20 mg)
	oral liquid (*Liquid Pred, PediaPred, Prelone*)
Triamcinolone acetonide	metered-dose inhaler (100 µg/puff)
Cromolyn	*Spinhaler*, powder (20 mg/capsule)
	metered-dose inhaler (800 µg/puff)
	nebulized solution (10 mg/ml)
Theophylline, Oral	
Extended-release capsules or tablets	

ATHESIN

Athesin contains 9 mg of alfaxalone and 3 mg of alfadolone acetate per milliliter. Following intravenous administration, athesin produces sleep within 30 seconds and also causes respiratory depression and apnea. Athesin releases histamine and may cause hypersensitivity reactions such as bronchospasm.

ATOVAQUONE
(Mepron)

Atovaquone, an antiprotozoal agent (750 mg p.o. t.i.d for 21 days), is indicated in the treatment of mild to moderate *Pneumocystis carinii* pneumonia in patients who cannot tolerate trimethoprim-sulfamethoxazole.

ATRACURIUM BESYLATE
(Tracrium)

Atracurium is a nondepolarizing skeletal muscle relaxant. It binds to cholinergic receptor sites and antagonizes the action of acetylcholine. At a dose of 0.5 mg/kg, it releases less histamine and produces less hemodynamic alterations than either d-tubocurarine or metocurine (see also Figure 92). Atracurium is used as an adjunct to general anesthesia in order to facilitate endotracheal intubation and to relax skeletal muscles during either surgery or mechanical ventilation. The duration of action of atracurium (30 minutes) is shorter than those of d-tubocurarine, metocurine, and pancuronium. Halothane, enflurane, or isoflurane prolongs the duration of neuromuscular blockade by atracurium by 20 to 30%.

Atracurium-induced bradycardia is more common than that produced by other skeletal muscle relaxants. The neuromuscular blocking effects of atracurium are prolonged in hypokalemia and following administration of thiazide diuretics. Hypokalemia enhances the neuromuscular blockade, possibly by hyperpolarizing the end plate membrane, increasing resistance to depolarization. Similarly, the duration of action of atracurium is prolonged by antibiotics such as aminoglycosides, bacitracin, capreomycin, colistimethate, polymyxin B, clindamycin, and lincomycin. Atracurium has an acid pH and should not be mixed in the same syringe with drugs (e.g., barbiturates) having alkaline pHs.

ATRIAL NATRIURETIC FACTOR
(ANF)

The atria contain secretory granules that increase in quantity with sodium restriction and decrease with sodium loading. Atrial extracts possess both vasodilatory and natriuretic activity that is mediated by **atrial natriuretic factor**, which is also known as **cardionatrin, atriopeptin, atrin,** or **auriculin.**

Atrial natriuretic factor brings about these changes by:

- Increasing the glomerular filtration rate, plus increasing the renal excretion of water, sodium, chloride, magnesium, calcium, and phosphate ions
- Blunting renin release in response to a variety of stimuli
- Blocking the release of aldosterone
- Decreasing cardiac output
- Opposing the actions of catecholamines and angiotensin II
- Causing vasodilation (Figure 13).

ATROPINE

Atropine and scopolamine are cholinergic receptor blocking agents. They are obtained from belladonna alkaloids, as well as other synthetic anticholinergic drugs. They inhibit the actions of smooth muscle, heart, and exocrine glands (see Figures 14 and 18). In addition to these peripheral effects, anticholinergic drugs, by blocking the acetylcholine receptor sites in the CNS, have pronounced CNS effects such as restlessness, irritability, excitement, and hallucinations. Scopolamine, on the other hand, depresses the CNS and, in therapeutic doses, produces fatigue, hypnosis, and amnesia. Therefore, it is used extensively in numerous medications, often in combination with antihistamines.

The pharmacologic effects of atropine in general are dose dependent. For example, in small doses, atropine depresses sweating, elevates body temperature, decreases salivary and bronchial secretions, and relaxes bronchial smooth muscles. In somewhat larger doses (1 to 3 mg), it produces mydriasis (blockade of the iris sphincter muscle), cycloplegia (blockade of the ciliary muscle), and cardiovascular effects characterized by transient bradycardia (central vagal stimulation) and tachycardia (vagal blockade at the sinoatrial node). Lacking any significant effects on circulation, atropine is often used as a preanesthetic medication to depress bronchial secretion and prevent pronounced bradycardia during abdominal surgical procedures. In still larger doses, it depresses the tone and motility of the gastrointestinal tract,

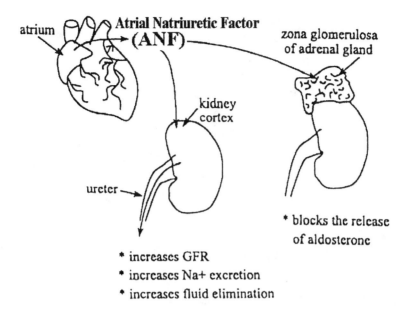

FIGURE 13   Atrial natriuretic factor (ANF) is a polypeptide hormone that is secreted mainly by the heart atria in response to increases in atrial pressure or atrial stretch.

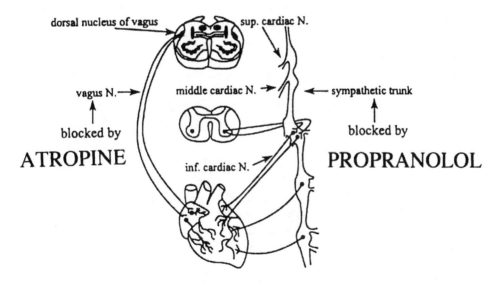

Actions of autonomic drugs in bradyarrhythmia/tachyarrhythmia

FIGURE 14   **Atropine** inhibits the actions of acetylcholine and cholinomimetic drugs at muscarinic receptors in smooth muscles, heart, and exocrine glands.

the tone of the urinary bladder, and gastric secretion. Therefore, the effective doses for use in acid-pepsin diseases are preceded by numerous side effects.

Atropine is absorbed orally and crosses the placental barrier, whereupon it causes fetal tachycardia. Atropine has been used to examine the functional integrity of the placenta.

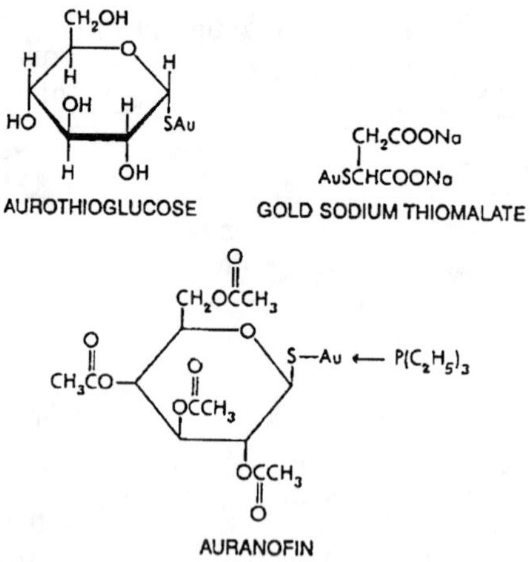

FIGURE 15 Auranofin, a gold salt with antiarthritic properties, reduces inflammation by altering the immune system.

Atropine toxicity is characterized by dry mouth, burning sensation in the mouth, rapid pulse, mydriasis, blurred vision, photophobia, dry and flushed skin, restlessness, and excitement.

Physostigmine, given intravenously, counteracts both the peripheral and central side effects of atropine and other anticholinergic drugs such as thioridazine (neuroleptic), imipramine (antidepressant), and benztropine (antiparkinsonian medication). Conditions that are contraindications to the use of atropine and related drugs are glaucoma and prostatic hypertrophy, in which they cause urinary retention (see Figure 50).

ATROPINE SULFATE

Atropine sulfate, an anticholinergic agent with antiarrhythmic and vagolytic properties (0.5 to 1 mg by IV push), is indicated in symptomatic bradycardia and bradyarrhythmia (functional or escape rhythm). It is used preoperatively for diminishing secretions and blocking cardiac vagal reflexes and as an antidote for anticholinesterase insecticide poisoning (see Figures 14 and 71).

AURANOFIN

(Ridauva)

Gold compounds (Figure 15) are able to prevent or suppress experimental arthritis produced by infections and chemical agents. They reduce the signs and symptoms of inflammation associated with rheumatoid arthritis. Therefore, auranofin is indicated in the management of rheumatoid arthritis in patients who have had insufficient therapeutic response to or are intolerant of nonsteroidal antiinflammatory drugs. Gold compounds inhibit the maturation and function of mononuclear phagocytes and of T cells, and hence suppress immune responsiveness. Decreased concentrations of rheumatoid factor and immunoglobulins are often observed in patients who are treated with gold. Unlike antiinflammatory agents, auranofin (6 mg/day) does not produce an immediate response, and beneficial effects are seen in 3 to 4 months. Steady-state concentrations of gold in plasma are proportional to the doses administered and are reached after 8 to 12 weeks of treatment. After cessation of treatment, the half-life of gold in the body is about 80 days. Auranofin is predominantly excreted in the feces. Auranofin may cause a fall in hemoglobin, leukopenia, thrombocytopenia, proteinuria, or hematouria. Therefore, it is contraindicated in patients with hematological disorders or renal impairment.

AUROTHIOGLUCOSE
(Solganal)

Chrysotherapy (gold therapy, see Figure 15) is employed in the treatment of progressive rheumatoid arthritis in patients who do not obtain satisfactory relief with nonsteroidal anti-inflammatory agents. Aurothioglucose and gold sodium thiomalate are absorbed erratically when given orally and hence are administered intramuscularly.

Aurothioglucose is bound to albumin to the extent of 95% and reaches high concentration in synovial fluid of affected joints. Gold is excreted mainly by the kidneys (40 to 90%), and 10 to 40% is found in the feces. Sulfhydryl agents, such as dismercaprol, penicillamine, and N-acetylcysteine increase the excretion of gold. The adverse effects of aurothioglucose include hematologic abnormalities (10%), including thrombocytopenia, leukopenia, or pancytopenia. Other adverse effects include stomatitis, a metallic taste in the mouth, skin pigmentation, enterocolitis, cholestatic jaundice, peripheral neuropathy, pulmonary infiltrates, and coroneal deposition of gold (Figure 15).

AUTONOMIC RECEPTORS*			
	Receptor Subtype	Agonists	Antagonists
Adrenergic Receptors			
	Alpha-1A	Epinephrine Norepinephrine Phenylephrine	Phentolamine Prazosin
	Alpha-1B	Epinephrine Norepinephrine Phenylephrine	Phentolamine Prazosin
	Alpha-2A	Epinephrine Norepinephrine Clonidine	Phentolamine Yohimbine Prazosin
	Alpha-2B	Epinephrine Norepinephrine Clonidine	Phentolamine Yohimbine
	Beta-1	Epinephrine Norepinephrine Isoproterenol	Propranolol Atenolol
	Beta-2	Epinephrine Isoproterenol Terbutaline	Propranolol
	Beta-3	Norepinephrine Epinephrine	Cyanopindolol
Cholinergic Receptors			
Muscarinic	M_1	Acetylcholine Muscarine Carbamylcholine	Atropine Pirenzepine
	M_2	Acetylcholine Muscarine Carbamylcholine	Atropine Methoctramine
Nicotinic	Ganglionic	Acetylcholine Nicotine	Hexamethonium Mecamylamine
	Skeletal muscle	Acetylcholine Nicotine	d-Tubocurarine Succinylcholine

*In addition to the adrenergic and cholinergic receptor subtypes listed, other autonomic receptor subtypes have been identified, but specific agonists or antagonists to be used in medical practice are unavailable.

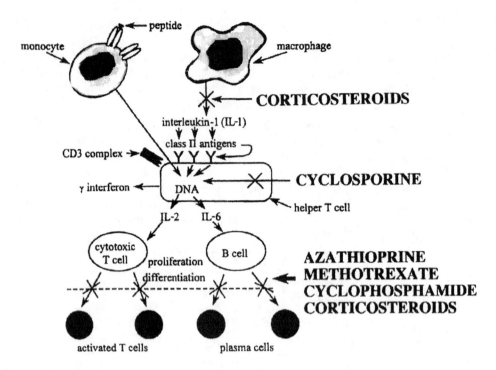

FIGURE 16 Azathioprine, a purine antagonist with immunosuppressive properties, inhibits RNA and DNA synthesis. (Adapted from Ebadi, M., *Pharmacology, An Illustrated Review with Questions and Answers*, 3rd Edition, Lippincott-Raven Press, Philadelphia, 1996.)

AZATADINE MALEATE

(Optimine)

Azatadine, a histamine receptor antagonist (1 to 2 mg p.o. b.i.d.), is indicated in the treatment of rhinitis, allergy symptoms, and chronic urticaria caused by histamine (see also Figure 49).

AZATHIOPRINE

(Imuran)

Azathioprine (3 to 10 mg/kg) prevents transplant rejection. It is reserved for patients deemed not to respond to cyclosporine and prednisone. Azathioprine is cleared to **6-mercaptopurine** which in turn can be converted to 6-mercaptopurine nucleotides leading to an inhibition of *de novo* purine synthesis or anabolism to thio-IMP, which, as a fraudulent nucleotide, can interfere with the salvage pathway of purine synthesis. Thio-IMP is subsequently converted to thio-GMP and eventually thio-GTP, leading to DNA damage upon intercalation of thio-GMP into the DNA backbone (see Figure 16). Azathioprine is a more effective immunosuppressant than is mercaptopurine (Purinethol).

Azathioprine is indicated in **renal homotransplantation** (five-year patient survival rate of 35%); in **rheumatoid arthritis** (for patients with severe, active, and erosive disease not responding to conventional therapies); and in chronic ulcerative colitis, myasthenia gravis, and Behcet's syndrome (adverse effects may offset its limited value). As with other cytotoxic drugs, azathioprine can affect rapidly growing cells, resulting in leukopenia, thrombocytopenia, and gastrointestinal toxicity. In addition, hepatotoxicity (cholestasis) has been reported.

Many of the general problems of immunosuppression, such as increased risk of infections, can also occur. In addition, there is some evidence of mutagenicity and possible carcinogenicity.

AZELASTINE

Terfenadine, astemizole, loratadine, and **cetirizine** are second-generation antihistaminic agents that are relatively nonsedating. Other H_1-receptor antagonists currently undergoing clinical trials are **azelastine, ebastine,** and **levocabastine.**

AZITHROMYCIN
(Zithromax)

Azithromycin, an azalide macrolide antibiotic (500 mg p.o. as a single dose on day 1, followed by 250 mg daily on days 2 to 5; total accumulation dose is 1.5 g), is indicated in the treatment of acute bacterial exacerbations of chronic obstructive pulmonary disease caused by *Haemophilus influenzae, Moraxella (Branhamella) catarrhalis,* or *Streptococcus pneumoniae;* mild community-acquired pneumonia caused by *H. influenzae* or *S. pneumoniae;* uncomplicated skin and skin-structure infections caused by *Staphylococcus aureus, Streptococcus pyrogenes,* or *S. agalactiae;* second-line therapy of pharyngitis or tonsillitis caused by *S. pyrogenes;* and in nongonococcal urethritis or cervicitis caused by *Chlamydia trachomatis.*

AZLOCILLIN

Carbenicillin cures serious infections caused by *Pseudomonas* species and *Proteus* strains resistant to ampicillin. It is not absorbed from the gastrointestinal tract, and therefore must be administered intraperitoneally. **Carbenicillin indanyl** is acid stable and hence can be given orally. **Ticarcillin** is four times more potent than carbenicillin in treating a *Pseudomonas aeruginosa* infection, and **azlocillin** is ten times more potent than carbenicillin against *Pseudomonas.* **Mezlocillin** and **piperacillin** are more active against *Klebsiella* infection than is carbenicillin (see Table 22).

AZTREONAM
(Azactam)

Aztreonam, a monobactam antibiotic (500 mg to 2 g IV or IM q. 8 to 12 hours), is indicated in the treatment of urinary tract, respiratory tract, intra-abdominal, gynecological, or skin infections; or septicemia caused by Gram-negative bacteria (see Figure 55).

B

BACAMPICILLIN HYDROCHLORIDE
(Spectrobid)

Bacampicillin, an aminopenicillin antibiotic (400 to 800 mg p.o. q. 12 hours), is indicated in the treatment of upper and lower respiratory tract, urinary tract, and skin infections caused by susceptible organisms, and gonorrhea.

BACILLUS CALMETTE-GUÉRIN (BCG), LIVE INTRAVESICAL
(TheraCys, Tice BCG)

Bacillus Calmette-Guérin, a bacterial agent with antineoplastic properties (three reconstituted and diluted vials are injected intravesically once weekly for six weeks), is used in the treatment of *in situ* carcinoma of the urinary bladder (primary or relapsed).

BACILLUS CALMETTE-GUÉRIN (BCG) VACCINE

This BCG vaccine (0.1 ml intradermally) is indicated in conditions where an individual has been exposed to tuberculosis, where immunity is not permanent.

BACITRACIN
(Baciquent)

Bacitracin, which inhibits cell wall synthesis, is active against Gram-positive bacteria. In combination with polymyxin and neomycin, it is often used in the treatment of topical infections as well as open infections such as infected eczema, dermal ulcers, and surgical wounds. The parenteral administration of bacitracin may cause nephrotoxicity.

BACLOFEN
(Lioresal)

Baclofen (40 to 80 mg daily) is indicated for the alleviation of signs and symptoms of spasticity from multiple sclerosis, and for the relief of flexor spasms and concomitant pain, clonus, and muscular rigidity. Baclofen is as effective as diazepam in reducing spasticity, but causes less sedation. Baclofen acts as a GABA agonist at $GABA_B$ receptors (see Figure 17). Activation of receptors in the brain by baclofen results in hyperpolarization, probably increased by K^+ conductance. It has been suggested that this hyperpolarization (in the cord as well as the brain) serves a presynaptic inhibitory function (Figure 17).

Baclofen is absorbed orally, reaching peak plasma concentration in 2 hours, having a half-life of 3 to 4 hours, and being excreted unchanged by the kidneys. The onset and duration of action of baclofen are 4 and 8 hours, respectively. Baclofen should be given cautiously in patients with renal impairment. The administration of baclofen via spinal catheter or lumbar puncture in a single bolus test dose of 50 to 100 mcg or via an implantable pump for administration into the intrathecal space has been approved for severe spasticity and pain in patients with cerebral palsy not responding to oral medications.

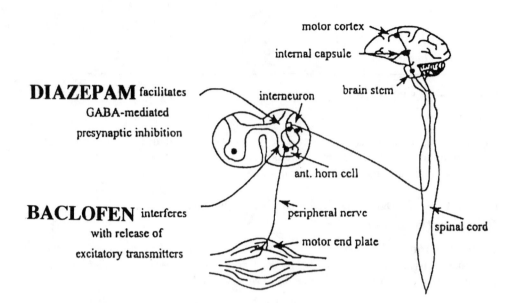

FIGURE 17   Baclofen, a skeletal muscle relaxant acts at the spinal cord level to inhibit transmission of monosynaptic and polysynaptic reflex. (Adapted from Ebadi, M., *Pharmacology, An Illustrated Review with Questions and Answers*, 3rd Edition, Lippincott-Raven Press, Philadelphia, 1996.)

BALSALAZINE

The idiopathic inflammatory bowel disease includes ulcerative colitis and granulomatous disease of the gastrointestinal tract (Crohn's disease). The newer derivatives of 5-aminosali-cylic acid, namely **balsalazine, sulfasalazine,** or **olsalazine**, may be effective for treating ulcerative colitis but not Crohn's disease.

BANTOPRIDE

A new class of antiemetic agents, the serotonin antagonists, has been identified. These agents could be clinically useful in a wide range of areas. Selective antagonists of the serotonin (5-hydroxytryptamine) type 3(5-HT$_3$) receptor such as **bantopride, granisetron, ondansetron**, or **zacopride** have proved in early clinical trials to be potent antiemetic agents in patients undergoing cytotoxic chemotherapy. Their efficacy has been shown to be comparable or superior to that of conventional phenothiazine antiemetics. The toxic effects observed so far with these agents have been modest (see Figures 64 and 73).

BARBITURATES

The barbiturates were used extensively in the past as hypnotic-sedatives but have been replaced by the much safer benzodiazepine derivatives. They do continue to be used as anesthetics and as anticonvulsants. The primary mechanism of action of barbiturates is to increase inhibition through the **gamma-aminobutyric acid** (GABA) **system**. Anesthetic barbiturates also decrease excitation via a decrease in calcium conductance (see Figure 40).

The most commonly used barbiturates are thiopental (Pentothal), methohexital (Brevital), secobarbital (Seconal), pentobarbital (Nembutal), amobarbital (Amytal), and phenobarbital (Luminal).

Barbiturates are classified according to their **duration of action.** These are: **ultra short-acting** (thiopental and methohexital), **short- to intermediate-acting** (pentobarbital, secobarbital, and amobarbital), and **long-acting** (phenobarbital).

In general, the more **lipid soluble** a barbiturate derivative is, the greater is its plasma- and tissue-binding capacity, the extent of its metabolism, and its storage in adipose tissues. In addition, very lipid-soluble substances have a faster onset of action and a shorter duration of action.

Barbiturates do not raise the **pain threshold** and have no **analgesic** property. In anesthetic doses, they depress all areas of the CNS, including the hypothalamic thermoregulatory system, respiratory center, and vasomotor centers, as well as the **polysynaptic pathways** in the spinal column. In addition, some, such as phenobarbital, but not all are anticonvulsants. In toxic doses, barbiturates cause oliguria.

Barbiturates are absorbed orally and distributed widely throughout the body. They are metabolized in the liver by aliphatic oxygenation, aromatic oxygenation, and N-dealkylation.

The inactive metabolites are excreted in the urine. The administration of **bicarbonate** enhances the urinary excretion of barbiturates that have a pK_a of 7.4 (**phenobarbital** and **thiopental**). This generalization is not true of other barbiturates. The long-term administration of barbiturates activates the cytochrome P-450 drug metabolizing system.

Acute barbiturate toxicity is characterized by **automatism**, or a state of drug-induced confusion, in which patients lose track of how much medication they have taken and take more. Death results from **respiratory failure**. The treatment of poisoning consists of supporting respiration, prevention of hypotension, as well as diuresis, hemodialysis, and in the event of phenobarbital poisoning, the administration of **sodium bicarbonate**. Tolerance does not develop from lethal doses. The abrupt withdrawal from barbiturates may cause tremors, restlessness, anxiety, weakness, nausea and vomiting, seizures, delirium, and cardiac arrest.

The selection of a barbiturate is in part determined by the duration of action desired and by the clinical problems at hand. An ultra short-acting drug is used for inducing anesthesia. For treating epilepsy, a long-acting drug is used, whereas, in a sleep disorder, a short-acting or an intermediate-type is used, depending on whether patients have difficulty falling asleep or if they have difficulty staying asleep.

BECLAMETHASONE DIPROPIONATE
(Beclovent, Vanceril)

Beclamethasone dipropionate inhaler (see Table 10) is indicated only for patients who require chronic treatment with corticosteroids for control of the symptoms of bronchial asthma. Patients require two inhalations, (84 mcg) 3 to 4 times/day.

Prednisone is available in oral form, and **beclomethasone** may be used as an aerosol, especially in children. The corticosteroids may exert their effects through multiple mechanisms, including: relaxing bronchospasm, decreasing mucous secretion, potentiating beta-adrenergic receptors, antagonizing cholinergic actions, stabilizing lysosomes, possessing antiinflammatory properties, inhibiting antibody formation, and antagonizing histamine actions.

Corticosteroids do not inhibit the release of mediators from mast cells or block the early response to allergens, but they do block the late response and the subsequent bronchial hyperresponsiveness.

Steroids such as **beclomethasone dipropionate, budesonide, triamcinolone acetonide**, and **flunisolide** are active when given topically and can control asthma without causing systemic effects or adrenal suppression. However, orally administered steroids such as **prednisone, prednisolone**, or **methylprednisolone** are still needed by some patients.

The **side effects** of high-dose inhalational steroids include oropharyngeal candidiasis and dysphonia. The orally administered steroids may produce osteoporosis, weight gain, hypertension, diabetes, myopathy, psychiatric disturbances, skin fragility, or cataracts.

BENAZEPRIL
(Lotensin)

Benazepril, an angiotensin-converting enzyme (ACE) inhibitor (10 mg p.o. daily), is indicated in the treatment of hypertension (see Figure 21 and Table 26).

BENDROFLUMETHIAZIDE
(Naturetin)

Bendroflumethiazide, a thiazide diuretic (2.5 to 20 mg p.o. daily), is indicated in edema and hypertension (see also Table 25).

BENTIROMIDE
(Chymex)

Bentiromide, a paraaminobenzoic acid (PABA) derivative (500 mg dose p.o.), is used as a screening test for pancreatic exocrine insufficiency. Following oral administration, bentiromide is cleaved by the pancreatic enzyme chymotrypsin, causing the release of PABA (para-aminobenzoic acid).

BENZOCAINE
(Americaine, Hurricaine, Orabase with Benzocaine, Orajel, Rid-A-Pain)

Benzocaine, an ester local anesthetic (20% topical gel), is indicated as a local anesthetic for dental pain or dental procedures and as a local anesthetic for pruritic dermatoses, pruritis, or other irritations.

BENZODIAZEPINE DERIVATIVES

The anxiolytic agents consist of **benzodiazepine** derivatives and **azaspirodecanedione** derivatives. For a long period of time, the drug treatment of anxiety disorders has been dominated by the **benzodiazepine derivatives** (Table 8). After the advent of **chlordiazepoxide** in the late 1950s, many derivatives were synthesized and introduced into clinical practice. This class of antianxiety agents shares the property of binding to a benzodiazepine receptor, part of the **gamma-aminobutyric acid (GABA) receptor-chloride channel complex** whose function it modulates allosterically (see Figures 40, 43, and 96). Not only the anxiolytic effects of the benzodiazepines, but also the other activities making up their pharmacologic profile, such as the **anticonvulsant, sedative**, or **muscle relaxant** effects, seem to be mediated by the GABA-related mechanism. In addition to the direct involvement of the GABA system, in parallel or more downstream to this, several other neurotransmitters such as **serotonin** have been suggested to participate in different aspects of benzodiazepine action. These **azaspirodecedione derivatives** include **buspirone, gepirone,** and **ipsapirone.**

Benzodiazepines are of value in the treatment of **anxious depressions** and anxiety-tension associated with schizophrenia, as well as in patients undergoing psychotherapy. They should be used only when the symptoms are disabling and not just to alleviate stress.

Benzodiazepines are of value in alleviating the symptoms of **cerebral palsy**, spasticity resulting from degenerative disorders such as **multiple sclerosis, tetanus, stiff-man syndrome**, and backache and muscle strain. The effective doses are generally large and may be increased as the disease progresses (e.g., multiple sclerosis).

To abort an epileptic seizure, **diazepam**, given intravenously, is a drug of choice. **Clonazepam** is also effective for achieving this.

During acute withdrawal from alcohol, the intravenous administration of **diazepam** is recommended, usually followed by **chlordiazepoxide** given orally.

TABLE 8
Summary of Benzodiazepine Derivatives

Drugs	Trade Names	Dose Range (mg)	Active Metabolites	Half-Life (hrs)
Chlordiazepoxide	Librium	5–200	Desmethylchlordiazepoxide, desmoxepam, desmethyldiazepam	>100
Diazepam	Valium, Valrelease	2–40	Desmethyldiazepam	>50
Oxazepam	Serax	30–120	None	5–14
Flurazepam	Dalmane	15–30	Flurazepam aldehyde, 1-hyroxyethylflurazepam, desalkylflurazepam	>100
Chlorazepate	Tranxene	15–60	Desmethyldiazepam	>100
Prazepam	Centrax	20–60	Desmethyldiazepam	>100
Lorazepam	Ativan	2–6	None	8–25
Halazepam	Paxipam	80–160	N-Desmethyldiazepam	>100
Alprazolam	Xanax	0.5–4	Alpha-hydroxyalprazolam	12–15
Temazepam	Restoril	15–30	Oxazepam	8–13
Triazolam	Halcion	0.125–0.5	Insignificant	1.5–5

Diazepam and **flunitrazepam** are often used as sedatives. In addition, these agents are also effective in controlling somnambulism, enuresis, and night terrors.

Preanesthetic, Premedication, and Diagnostic Procedures

Intravenously administered **diazepam** may be used for induction prior to maintaining anesthesia with other agents, in endoscopic procedures, and in cardioversion. In general these agents cause amnesia, relieve anxiety, and reduce or eliminate the use of narcotic analgesics. During labor and delivery, only short-acting benzodiazepines, such as **oxazepam,** should be used.

BENZODIAZEPINES: USES OF	
Agents	**Select Therapeutic Uses**
Alprazolam	Anxiety disorders, agoraphobia
Brotizolam	
Chlordiazepoxide	Anxiety disorders, management of alcohol withdrawal, anesthetic premedication
Clobazam	
Clonazepam	Seizure disorders, mania, movement disorders
Clorazepate	Anxiety disorders, seizure disorders
Demoxepam	
Diazepam	Anxiety disorders, status epilepticus, muscle relaxation, anesthetic premedication
Estazolam	Insomnia
Flumazenil	Antidote to benzodiazepines
Flurazepam	Insomnia
Halazepam	Anxiety disorders
Lorazepam	Anxiety disorders, preanesthetic medication
Midazolam	Preanesthetic and intraoperative medication
Nitrazepam	
Nordazepam	
Oxazepam	Anxiety disorders

Agents	Select Therapeutic Uses
Prazepam	
Quazepam	Insomnia
Temazepam	Insomnia
Triazolam	Insomnia

Agents for which no uses have been identified have not been studied extensively.

BENZONATATE
(Tessalon)

Benzonatate, an ester local anesthetic with antitussive properties (100 mg p.o. t.i.d.), is used for cough suppression.

BENZPHETAMINE HYDROCHLORIDE
(Didrex)

Benzphetamine, a sympathomimetic agent with anorexant properties (25 to 50 mg p.o. daily), is indicated as a short-term adjunct in the treatment of obesity (see **Amphetamine sulfate**).

BENZQUINAMIDE HYDROCHLORIDE
(Emete-Con)

Benzquinamide, a benzoquinolizine derivative (50 mg IM), is indicated in the management of nausea and vomiting associated with anesthesia and surgery.

BENZTHIAZIDE
(Aquatag, Exna, Hydrex, Marazide, Proaqua)

Benzthiazide, a thiazide diuretic (50 to 200 mg p.o. daily), is indicated in the treatment of edema and hypertension (see also Table 25).

BENZTROPINE MESYLATE
(Cogentin)

Benztropine may be used in the management of Parkinson's disease (1 to 2 mg/day), neuroleptic-induced parkinsonism (1 to 4 mg once or twice/day), and neuroleptic-induced acute dystonic syndrome (1 to 2 mg IM or IV). In parkinsonian patients, the deficiency of dopamine causes the cholinergic receptors to be hyperactive. Therefore, anticholinergic drugs may be used to mitigate some of the symptoms. These agents include: trihexyphenidyl (Artane), cycrimine (Pagitane), procyclidine (Kemadrin), biperiden (Akineton), orphenadrine (Disipal), and benztropine (Cogentin).

Neuroleptics such as chlorpromazine or haloperidol may cause **parkinsonian** symptoms characterized by postural instability, stooped posture, shuffling and festinating gate, or rigidity, due to enhanced muscle tone, with, at times, "cogwheel" or "ratchet" resistance to passive movements in any direction. There is also tremor at rest with regular rhythmic oscillations of the extremities, especially the hands and fingers as well as akinesia (poverty of movement) or bradykinesia (slowness in initial volitional activities). These symptoms, which are due to blockade of dopaminergic receptor sites in the striatum, are lessened by reducing the dosage of neuroleptics and by the oral administration of anticholinergic compounds, such as **trihexyphenidyl hydrochloride** (Artane) or **benztropine mesylate** (Cogentin).

Neuroleptics such as chlorpromazine or haloperidol may cause acute dystonia which is characterized by an exaggerated posturing of the head, neck, or jaw; by spastic contraction of the muscles of the lips, tongue, face or throat, which makes drinking, eating, swallowing, and speech difficult; by torticollis, retrocollis, opisthotonus, distress, and ultimately anoxia. Neuroleptic-induced dystonia, which may occur in children treated actively with phenothiazine derivatives for their antiemetic properties, disappears in sleep and is treated effectively with **diphenhydramine hydrochloride** (Benadryl), which possesses both anticholinergic and antihistaminic properties. Benztropine is also effective. Contraindications to the use of benztropine are the same as those for atropine and other anticholinergic drugs and are: glaucoma, prostatic hypertrophy, myasthenia gravis, stenosing peptic ulcer, and duodenal or pyloric obstruction. Urinary retention and tachycardia should be heeded and regarded as signs of impending toxicity.

BEPRIDIL HYDROCHLORIDE
(Vascor)

Bepridil, a calcium channel blocker (200 mg p.o. daily), is indicated in the treatment of chronic stable angina (classic effort-associated angina) in patients who are unresponsive or inadequately responsive to other antianginals (see also Table 20).

BERACTANT
(Natural Lung Surfactant) (Survanta)

Beractant, a bovine lung extract (administered by intratracheal instillation), is indicated for prevention and treatment (rescue) of respiratory distress syndrome (hyaline membrane disease) in premature infants.

BETA-ADRENERGIC RECEPTOR BLOCKING AGENTS					
	α Blockade	β_1 Selectivity	MSA	ISA	Lipid-solubility
Acebutolol	0	+	+	+	Low
Atenolol	0	+	0	0	Low
Betaxolol	0	+	±	0	Low
Carteolol	0	0	0	+	Low
Labetalol	+	0	+	0	Moderate
Metoprolol	0	+	0	0	Moderate
Nadolol	0	0	0	0	Low
Penbutolol	0	0	0	+	High
Pindolol	0	0	+	+++	Moderate
Propranolol	0	0	+	0	High
Timolol	0	0	0	0	Low
MSA, membrane stabilizing activity; ISA, intrinsic sympathomimetic activity					

BETA-ARRESTIN

Two different kinases are involved in phosphorylating beta-adrenergic receptors. **Protein kinase A** is positively regulated by cyclic AMP and is stimulated by substances that activate adenylate cyclase. **Beta adrenergic receptor kinase (BARK)** is related functionally to rhodopsin kinase and may be important for regulating neural transmission (see Figure 42). A cytosolic protein, **beta-arrestin**, interacts with the BARK-phosphorylated receptors and disrupts the activation of G_S by the beta receptor.

BETAMETHASONE
(Celestone)

BETAMETHASONE (SYSTEMIC)
(Celestone)

BETAMETHASONE SODIUM PHOSPHATE
(BSP, Celestone Phosphate, Prelestone, Selestoject)

BETAMETHASONE SODIUM PHOSPHATE AND BETAMETHASONE ACETATE
(Celestone Soluspan)

Betamethasone, a glucocorticoid with antiinflammatory properties, is indicated in the treatment of adrenocortical insufficiency, severe inflammation, or immunosuppression (see also Tables 10 and 14, and Figure 16).

BETAMETHASONE BENZOATE
(Uticort)

BETAMETHASONE DIPROPIONATE
(Alphatrex, Diprolene AF, Diprolene, Diprosone, Maxivate)

BETAMETHASONE VALERATE
(Betatrex, Beta-Val, Valisone)

Betamethasone, a topical glucocorticoid with antiinflammatory properties (lotion, ointment 0.1%, cream 0.01%, 0.1%, aerosol solution 0.1%), is indicated in inflammation of corticosteroid-responsive dermatoses.

BETAMETHASONE BENZOATE
(Benisone; Uticort)

See **Corticosteroids**.

BETAMETHASONE DIPROPIONATE
(Diprosone)

See **Corticosteroids**.

BETAMETHASONE SODIUM PHOSPHATE
(Celestone Phosphate)

See **Corticosteroids**.

BETAMETHASONE SODIUM PHOSPHATE AND ACETATE
(Celestone Soluspan)

See **Corticosteroids**.

BETAMETHASONE VALERATE
(Beta-Val; Valisone)

See **Corticosteroids** (and Table 10).

BETAXOLOL HYDROCHLORIDE
(Betoptic)

Betaxolol (one drop in each eye b.i.d.), a cardioselective beta$_1$-adrenergic blocking agent, is used in chronic open-angle glaucoma and ocular hypertension. It reduces intraocular pressure by reducing the production of aqueous humor. Betaxolol is known to have caused brief discomfort, tearing, erythema, itching, photophobia, corneal sensitivity, corneal staining, keratitis, and anisocoria. Betaxolol should be used cautiously in patients with bronchial asthma, sinus bradycardia, second or third degree AV block, cardiac failure, and cardiogenic shock.

BETHANECHOL CHLORIDE
(Urecholine Chloride)

Bethanechol (5 mg sc) is indicated in acute postoperative and postpartum nonobstructive (functional) urinary retention and neurogenic atony of the urinary bladder with retention. The two currently used derivatives of acetylcholine are **bethanechol** and **carbachol** (Miostat). Unlike acetylcholine, both agents are resistant to hydrolysis by cholinesterase (see also Figure 18). The **cardiovascular actions** of acetylcholine are vasodilation and negative chronotropic and inotropic effects. The cardiovascular effects of **methacholine** are more pronounced than those of acetylcholine, which in turn are greater than those of carbachol or bethanechol. The **gastrointestinal effects** (increase in tone, amplitude of contractions, and peristalsis) of bethanechol and carbachol are equal but greater than those of acetylcholine. The effects of carbachol and bethanechol on the **urinary tract**, consisting of ureteral peristalsis, contraction of the detrusor muscle of the urinary bladder, and an increase in voluntary voiding pressure, are equivalent and exceed those produced by acetylcholine.

Higher than therapeutic doses of bethanechol may cause abdominal discomfort, colicky pain, belching, diarrhea, salivation, borborygmi, fall in blood pressure, with reflex tachycardia and bronchial constriction. Atropine (0.6 mg sc) is a specific antidote. The contraindication to larger than therapeutic doses of bethanechol are hyperthyroidism, peptic ulcer, latent or active asthma, pronounced bradycardia, atrioventricular conduction defects, vasomotor instability, coronary artery disease, epilepsy, parkinsonism, coronary occlusion, or hypotension. Bethanechol should not be used in bladder neck obstruction or mechanical obstruction of the gastrointestinal tract.

BETHANIDINE SULFATE

Bethanidine is being investigated as an orphan drug to be used in treatment of primary ventricular fibrillation and to treat or prevent the recurrence of primary ventricular fibrillation.

BEVANTOLOL

Bevantolol is a new adrenoreceptor blocking agent with a weak alpha$_1$-adrenoreceptor blocking activity which is indicated initially in hypertension and in angina pectoris. By virtue of its apparent lack of effect on serum lipids, decrease in peripheral vascular resistance, minimal or no effect on sexual function, low incidence of central nervous system side effects, and absence of effects on renal function, bevantolol may offer advantages over existing treatments for patients with hypertension and angina pectoris. Bevantolol is contraindicated for patients with sinus bradycardia, greater than first-degree conduction block, cardiogenic shock, or overt cardiac failure.

BIOAVAILABILITY OF DRUGS: FACTORS INFLUENCING	
Physicochemical Properties of the Drugs	
Solubility in aqueous and organic solvents pH-solubility profile Lipid-water partition coefficient pKa Particle size and size distribution	Crystalline and polymorphic forms Solvation and hydration Salt form Stability in solid state and solution Molecular weight
Physiologic Factors	
pH Temperature Surface area Surface tension	Volume and composition of biologic fluids Disease state Sex Age
Manufacturing Variables	**Environmental Factors**
Diluents Manufacturing factors Packaging	Humidity Temperature

BIPERIDEN

(Akineton)

Biperidine (2 mg t.i.d.) is indicated in the treatment of Parkinson's disease and drug-induced parkinsonism (2 mg t.i.d.). In parkinsonian patients, the deficiency of dopamine causes the cholinergic receptors to be hyperactive. Therefore, **anticholinergic drugs** may be used to mitigate some of the symptoms. These agents include: trihexyphenidyl (Artane), cycrimine (Pagitane), procyclidine (Kemadrin), biperiden (Akineton), orphenadrine (Disipal), and benztropine (Cogentin).

Contraindications to the use of anticholinergic drugs in treating parkinsonism are the same as those for atropine, and are: glaucoma, prostatic hypertrophy, myasthenia gravis, stenosing peptic ulcer, and duodenal or pyloric obstruction. Urinary retention and tachycardia should be heeded and regarded as signs of impending toxicity.

BISACODYL

(Biscolax, Carter's Little Pills, Dacodyl Tabs, Deficol, Dulcolax, Theralax Suppositories)

Bisacodyl, a stimulant laxative (10 to 15 mg p.o.), is indicated in the treatment of constipation; preparation for delivery, surgery, or rectal or bowel examination.

BISMUTH SUBGALLATE

(Devron)

BISMUTH SUBGALLATE

(Chewable Tablets)

BISMUTH SUBSALICYLATE

(Pepto-Bismol)

Bismuth salts, adsorbent with antidiarrheal properties, are indicated for prevention and treatment of traveler's diarrhea.

BISOPROLOL
(Zebeta)

Bisoprolol, a beta-adrenergic receptor blocking agent (5 mg p.o. once daily), is used in the treatment of hypertension (alone or in combination with other antihypertensives) (see also Figure 27).

BITOLTEROL MESYLATE
(Tornalate)

Bitolterol is indicated for the prophylaxis and treatment of bronchial asthma and reversible bronchospasm. It may be used with or without concurrent theophylline or steroid therapy. The selective beta$_2$-adrenergic stimulants cause bronchodilation without cardiac acceleration. **Metaproterenol** and **terbutaline** are available in tablet form, and terbutaline is also available for subcutaneous injection (see also Figure 86). Metaproterenol and albuterol are available in metered-dose inhalers.

Inhaled selective beta$_2$-adrenergic receptor agonists (**albuterol, terbutaline, fenoterol**, and **bitolterol**) have a rapid onset of action and are effective for 3 to 6 hours. **Formoterol** and **salmeterol** are longer-acting agents (12 hours) and may prove useful in treating nocturnal symptoms.

The **side effects** of beta-adrenergic receptor agonists are tremor, tachycardia, and palpitations.

BLACK WIDOW SPIDER (LATRODECTUS MACTANS) ANTIVENIN

Black widow spider antivenin, which provides immune globulins that specifically bind black widow spider venom, is used in black widow spider bites (see also Figure 18).

BLEOMYCIN
(Blenoxane)

Causes chain scission and fragmentation of DNA. With the exception of the skin and lungs, most tissues can enzymatically inactivate bleomycin. Bleomycin is used in the management of squamous cell carcinoma of the head, neck, and esophagus, and in the treatment of Hodgkin's disease and other lymphomas. Bleomycin causes stomatitis, ulceration, hyperpigmentation, erythema, and pulmonary fibrosis.

BORIC ACID
(Borofax, Ear-Dry, Neo-Flo, Ocu-Bath, Swim Ear, Ting)

BORIC ACID AND SODIUM BORATE
(Blinx, Collyrium)

Boric acid, a topical antiinfective agent (fill ear canal with solution and plug with cotton; repeat t.i.d. or q.i.d.), is used for the treatment of external ear canal infection. In addition, 5% ointment is used for the relief of abrasions, dry skin, minor burns, insect bites, and other skin irritations.

BOTULINUM TOXIN TYPE A
(Botox, Dysport)

Botulinum toxin Type A is used as an orphan drug or as an investigational drug in blepharospasm and strabismus associated with dystonia in adults; cervical dystonia; dynamic muscle contracture in pediatric cerebral palsy, and essential blepharospasm; and synkinetic closure of the eyelid associated with VIII cranial nerve aberrant regeneration. Botulinum toxin

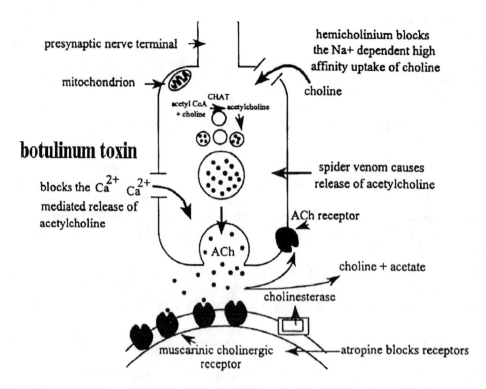

FIGURE 18 Botulinum toxin causes skeletal muscle paralysis by binding to acetylcholine receptors on the motor end plate. (Adapted from Ebadi, M., *Pharmacology, An Illustrated Review with Questions and Answers*, 3rd Edition, Lippincott-Raven Press, Philadelphia, 1996.)

produced by clostridium botulinum blocks neuromuscular conduction by binding to receptor pits on motor nerve terminals and preventing the release of acetylcholine (see Figure 18). The effect of botulinum toxin may be potentiated by aminoglycoside antibiotics or any other drug that interferes with neuromuscular transmission.

The integration of botulinum toxin into the orbicularis muscle can cause reduced blinking and lead to corneal exposure and ulceration.

BOTULINUM TOXIN A: USES OF			
Dystonia:	Blepharospasm Cervical dystonia Spasmodic dysphonia Oromandibular dystonia Focal hand dystonia Limb dystonia	Spasticity:	Multiple sclerosis Cerebral palsy Head injury Paraplegia Stroke
Muscle Spasms:	Hemifacial spasm Facial synkinesis Masticatory spasms	Tremor:	Dystonic tremor Essential tremor Vocal tremor Palatal tremor (myoclonus)
		Other:	Bruxism

Botulinum toxin acts selectively on cholinergic synapses to block Ca^{2+}-mediated release of acetylcholine. Unlike axotomy, botulinum toxin does not cause degeneration of the neuromuscular junction. Terminal motor axons are still capable of conducting impulses. An aqueous solution containing the botulinum toxin A, albumin and sodium chloride is injected intramuscularly into selected muscles to produce local neuromuscular blockade.

BRADYKININ AND KALLIDIN

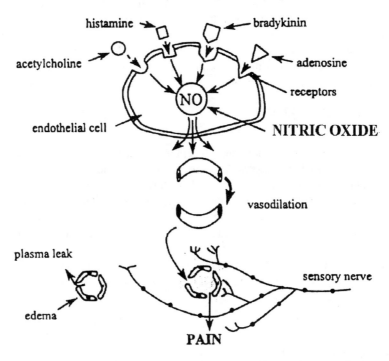

FIGURE 19   Bradykinin and kallidin increase vascular permeability, produce vasodilation, increase the synthesis of prostaglandins, and cause edema and pain. (Adapted from Ebadi, M., *Pharmacology, An Illustrated Review with Questions and Answers,* 3rd Edition, Lippincott-Raven Press, Philadelphia, 1996.)

BOTULINUM TOXIN TYPE A
(Oculinum)

Botulinum, a neurotoxin with muscle relaxant properties, is used in the treatment of strabismus (see also Figure 18).

BOTULISM ANTITOXIN, TRIVALENT (ABE) EQUINE

Botulism antitoxin, which binds and neutralizes toxin, is used in the treatment of botulism.

BRADYKININ

As autacoids, bradykinin and kallidin increase vascular permeability, produce vasodilation, increase the synthesis of prostaglandins, and cause edema and pain. Extensive evidence exists that bradykinin and other kallidin substances contribute to the pathogenesis of the inflammatory response that occurs in acute and chronic diseases including allergic reactions, arthritis, asthma, sepsis, viral rhinitis, and inflammatory bowel diseases (see Figure 19).

BRETYLIUM TOSYLATE
(Bretylol)

Bretylium is indicated in the treatment of life-threatening ventricular arrhythmias which have failed to respond to the first-line antiarrhythmic agents, such as lidocaine, and for prophylaxis and treatment of ventricular fibrillation. Bretylium initially and transiently releases norepinephrine, causing tachycardia and rise in blood pressure, but subsequently causes a chemical sympathectomy by inhibiting the release of catecholamine without reducing its concentration.

Bretylium reduces heterogeneity of repolarization times, an effect that is likely to suppress reentry, blocks K^+ channels, and has no effect on automaticity. A lag time of ~2 hours has been reported between peak plasma bretylium concentrations and peak prolongation of ventricular refractoriness after an intravenous dose. This lag time suggests that bretylium will be distributed to sites in peripheral tissues prior to exerting its pharmacological effect. Bretylium is excreted unchanged by the kidneys without undergoing significant hepatic metabolism. Reduction of a maintenance infusion rate has been recommended in patients with renal failure.

BROMOCRIPTINE MALEATE
(Parlodel)

Bromocriptine is an agonist for dopamine receptors and hence is used as an adjunct in the treatment of Parkinson's disease. As parkinsonism progresses, the activity of dopa-decarboxylase may become so reduced that it cannot adequately decarboxylate dopa to dopamine. In this case, it may be possible to stimulate the dopamine receptor sites located postsynaptically using compounds such as bromocriptine or pergolide. Bromocriptine is an ergot alkaloid that inhibits the secretion of **prolactin** by interfering with hypophyseal dopaminergic neurons, and has been used in the treatment of endocrine disorders such as **Chiari-Frommel syndrome** and **Forbes-Albright syndrome**. However, low-dose bromocriptine therapy is not effective in all patients. Bromocriptine has a longer duration of action than levodopa and is particularly useful in patients suffering from a high incidence of on-off phenomenon.

Bromocriptine is most effective when used with submaximal doses of levodopa. It should be regarded as an adjunct rather than as a substitute for levodopa. It is possible that more effective dopamine receptor agonists may replace bromocriptine in the future.

BROMPHENIRAMINE MALEATE
(Dimetane)

Brompheniramine is an alkylamine antihistaminic (H_1 receptor antagonist) agent used in allergic symptoms of rhinitis (4 to 8 mg p.o. t.i.d.). Brompheniramine is absorbed well from the gastrointestinal tract, exerts its effects in 15 to 30 minutes, and peak of action is seen in 2 to 5 hours. It is extensively (95%) metabolized in the liver, and 5% of it is excreted unchanged by the kidneys. Clinical manifestations of overdose may include either those of CNS depression (sedation, reduced mental alertness, apnea, and cardiovascular collapse) or of CNS stimulation (insomnia, hallucinations, tremors, or convulsions). Anticholinergic symptoms, such as dry mouth, flushed skin, fixed and dilated pupils, and GI symptoms, are common, especially in children. Monoamine oxidase inhibitors inhibit the metabolism of brompheniramine, prolonging its effects. Since brompheniramine has strong anticholinergic effects, it should be used cautiously in patients with narrow-angle glaucoma, or in those with pyloroduodenal obstruction or urinary bladder obstruction from prostatic hypertrophy or narrowing of the bladder neck.

BRONCHODILATORS: β-ADRENERGIC AGONISTS FOR THE TREATMENT OF ASTHMA			
Of the three classes of bronchodilators ($β_2$-adrenergic-receptor agonists, methylxanthines, and anticholinergic agents), the $β_2$-adrenergic-receptor agonists produce the greatest bronchodilation in patients with bronchial asthma. They are:			
Intermediate-acting (3-6 hr)			**Long-acting (>12 hr)**
Albuterol	Fenoterol	Pirbuterol	Formoterol
Bitolterol	Metaproterenol	Terbutaline	Salmeterol
$β_2$-Adrenergic agonists are generally preferred both for the relief of acute symptoms and for the prevention of exercise-induced bronchospasm. The introduction of long-acting inhaled $β_2$-adrenergic agonists have overcome the principal shortcoming of the previously available drugs of this class — their limited duration of action. However, the possibility of adverse effects with regular use of $β_2$-adrenergic agonists has been raised.			

BUCLIZINE HYDROCHOLORIDE
(Bucladin S)

Buclizine (50 mg p.o. 30 minutes prior to travel) is a centrally acting antiemetic agent used for the control of the nausea, vomiting, and dizziness of motion sickness. Buclizine depresses conduction in vestibular-cerebellar pathways and hence reduces labyrinth excitability (anti-vertigo action); and it inhibits the chemotrigger zone for emesis (antiemetic action) (see also Figure 73).

Similar to other antihistaminic agents, buclizine possesses anticholinergic properties and hence should be used cautiously in narrow-angle glaucoma, prostatic hypertrophy, and obstruction of the gastrointestinal and urinary tracts. Buclizine has additive CNS depressing effects with alcohol, barbiturates, anxiolytic agents, and many other medications. Buclizine should be used cautiously with ototoxic agents such as aminoglycosides, since the signs of ototoxicity may become masked with buclizine.

The manifestations with buclizine overdosage may include either those of CNS depression (sedation, reduced mental alertness, apnea, and cardiovascular collapse) or of CNS stimulation (insomnia, hallucinations, tremors, or convulsions). Anticholinergic symptoms, such as dry mouth, flushed skin, fixed and dilated pupils, and GI symptoms, are common, especially in children.

Buclizine contains **tartrazine** which may cause allergic reactions including asthma in susceptible individuals who also exhibit hypersensitivity to aspirin.

BUDESONIDE
(Rhinocort)

Budesonide, an antiinflammatory corticosteroid (32 mcg/actuation and 256 mcg/daily) is indicated in the management of seasonal or perennial allergic rhinitis in adults and children.

Corticosteroids do not inhibit the release of mediators from mast cells or block the early response to allergens, but they do block the late response and the subsequent bronchial hyperresponsiveness.

Steroids such as **beclomethasone dipropionate, budesonide, triamcinolone acetonide**, and **flunisolide** are active when given topically and can control asthma without causing the systemic effects or adrenal suppression. However, orally administered steroids such as **prednisone, prednisolone**, or **methylprednisolone** are still needed by some patients.

The **side effects** of high-dose inhalational steroids include oropharyngeal candidiasis and dysphonia. The orally administered steroids may produce osteoporosis, weight gain, hypertension, diabetes, myopathy, psychiatric disturbances, skin fragility, or cataracts (see also Table 10).

BUMETANIDE
(Bumex)

Bumetanide (0.5 to 2 mg/day p.o.), ethacrynic acid (Edecrin), furosemide (Lasix), and muzolimine are loop diuretics (see also Table 25 and Figure 4). These agents inhibit the active resorption of chloride (and sodium) in the thick, ascending medullary portion of the loop of Henle and also in the cortical portion of the loop or the distal tubule. The diuresis they produce, which is similar to that seen with the thiazides, predominantly causes a loss of chloride, sodium, and potassium, but HCO_3 excretion is not increased. Although large volumes of fluid can be excreted with the use of these agents, the ability of the kidney to produce either a dilute or concentrated urine is greatly diminished. These agents are the most efficacious of all the diuretics now on the market, usually producing about a 20% loss in the filtered load of sodium (**furosemide**, 15 to 30%; **ethacrynic acid**, 17 to 23%).

Loop diuretics are ordinarily taken orally but can be given intravenously if a very rapid onset of action is sought, as when used in combination with antihypertensive medications in the management of a **hypertensive crisis.** Furosemide and ethacrynic acid undergo some active renal tubular secretion as well as glomerular filtration. A minor portion is excreted by the liver.

Loop diuretics are used for treating the following conditions:

In the **edema** of cardiac, hepatic, or renal origin, including acute pulmonary edema and hypertensive crisis

In **acute renal failure**, to maintain urine flow, though an excessive loss of extracellular fluid volume can cause a decrease in the GFR

In **hypercalcemia,** excessive volume depletion, hyponatremia, and hyponatremia, and hypotension are major risks associated with the use of loop diuretics, and the side effects of **hypokalemia, hyperuricemia,** and **hyperglycemia** are always present. Loop diuretics should not be used concurrently with **ototoxic aminoglycoside antibiotics** (i.e., streptomycin, gentamicin, kanamycin, tobramycin).

BUPIVACAINE HYDROCHLORIDE

(Marcaine)

Bupivacaine, an amide local anesthetic, is indicated for the production of local or regional anesthesia or analgesia, for oral surgery, for surgery, for diagnostic procedures, or for obstetrical anesthesia.

When a local anesthetic is injected near a nerve, it blocks the flow of electrons along the axons and eliminates the pain without loss of consciousness (see Figure 20). These effects are reversible. When administering a local anesthetic, one must remember that the larger the diameter of the nerve fiber, the more anesthetic is needed to produce anesthesia.

Epinephrine is used in combination with a local anesthetic to reduce its uptake, prolong its duration of action, produce a bloodless field of operation, and protect against systemic effects (see Figure 72). Local anesthetic solutions containing epinephrine should not be used in areas supplied by end-arteries such as in the digits, ear, nose, and penis, because of the threat of ischemia and subsequential gangrene. Furthermore, under no circumstances should anesthetic solutions containing epinephrine be used intravenously in patients with cardiac arrhythmias. In general, solutions designed for multiple doses should not be used for spinal or epidural anesthesia.

Local anesthetics block the sodium channels, are cardiac depressants, and bring about a ventricular conduction defect and block that may progress to cardiac and ventilatory arrest if toxic doses are given. In addition, these agents produce arteriolar dilation. **Circulatory failure** may be treated with **vasopressors** such as ephedrine, metaraminol (Aramine), or mephentermine (Wyamine). Artificial respiration and cardiac massage may also become necessary. Among the local anesthetics, only cocaine blocks the uptake of norepinephrine, causes vasoconstriction, and may precipitate cardiac arrhythmias.

An overdosage of local anesthetics can produce dose-dependent CNS side effects such as insomnia, visual and auditory disturbances, nystagmus, shivering, tonic-clonic convulsions, and finally fatal CNS depression. The initial CNS excitation and convulsions may be brought under control by diazepam or thiopental.

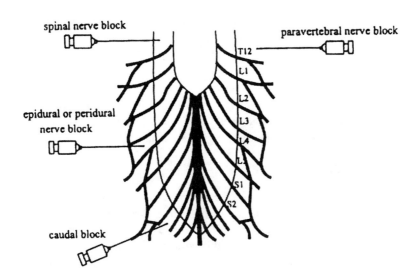

SITES OF INJECTION OF BUPIVACAINE

FIGURE 20   Bupivacaine, an amide local anesthetic, is sixteen times more potent than procaine and exhibits a long duration of action.

BUPRENORPHINE HYDROCHLORIDE

(Temgesic)

Buprinorphine is a semisynthetic opioid analgesic derived from thebaine. It binds readily to the opioid receptors in the CNS but dissociates from them slowly, which may be responsible for its long duration of action. Buprenorphine (0.3 mg IM) exerts its analgesic actions in 15 minutes and has a duration of action of 6 hours. It is bound to plasma proteins to the extent of 96%, is metabolized in the liver to a certain extent (N-dealkylmetabolite), and is excreted unchanged in the feces. Buprenorphine causes respiratory depression and elevates cerebrospinal pressure (contraindicated in head injury or conditions where intracranial pressure may be high).

Buprenorphine increases intracholedochal pressure to a similar degree as the other opiates. The adverse effects of buprenorphine are sedation, dizziness, vertigo, hypotension, hypoventilation, and miosis. Although **naloxone** is able to reverse several of the adverse effects of buprenorphine, it may not be as effective in reversing the respiratory depression requiring mechanical assistance of respiration.

BUPROPION HYDROCHLORIDE

(Wellbutrin)

Bupropion (100 mg p.o. b.i.d.) is indicated in the treatment of depression. It is reserved for patients who cannot tolerate or have not responded to other medications. Bupropion does not alter the uptake of serotonin, has an equivocal effect on the uptake of norepinephrine, but blocks the uptake of dopamine. Bupropion has no affinity for alpha 1 and 2 adrenergic receptors, H_1 histamine receptors, muscarinic cholinergic receptors, or D_2 dopaminergic receptors. It does not cause sedation or orthostatic hypotension. However, since it is structurally related to amphetamine, it may cause insomnia, agitation, and anxiety shortly after initiation of therapy. Bupropion lowers seizure threshold and hence is contraindicated in patients with a history of seizure disorder (see also Tables 3 through 5).

BURIMAMIDE

Histamine, as a normal constituent of the gastric mucosa, controls both **microcirculation** and **gastric secretion**. The gastric secretagogs are **acetylcholine, histamine**, and **gastrin**. The action of acetylcholine is blocked by atropine, and the action of **histamine** is blocked by **cimetidine, burimamide**, and **metiamide**. No specific antagonist is available for gastrin.

BUSPIRONE HYDROCHLORIDE
(BuSpar)

Buspirone (25 mg/day) is indicated in the management of anxiety disorders. The anxiolytic agents consist of **benzodiazepine** derivatives (see Table 8) and **azaspirodecanedione** derivatives, which include **buspirone, gepirone**, and **ipsapirone**. The introduction of novel anxiolytic agents such as buspirone, which interacts with the serotoninergic system, has suggested that serotoninergic fibers may be the final pathway through which anxiolytic effects are expressed.

Buspirone has a chemical structure that is distinct from that of the benzodiazepines. Without this structural homology, it is not surprising that buspirone does not interact with GABA receptors. Furthermore, the clinical profile of buspirone appears to be **anxioselective**, with a much reduced potential for abuse.

Several types of serotonin (5-HT) receptors exist in the mammalian brain, two of which are well characterized: 5-HT_3 and 5-HT_2 sites. The 5-HT_3 sites can be further subdivided into at least three distinct subsets, which differ in their regional distribution and functions and are currently termed 5-HT_{1A}, 5-HT_{1B}, and 5-HT_{1C} sites.

The 5-HT receptors in the hippocampus and other parts of the limbic system are primarily of the 5-HT_{1A} type. It is therefore tempting to speculate that drugs that display a high degree of selectivity for these receptor sites can selectively affect anxiety states. A breakthrough in that direction came with the discovery of **buspirone**, a drug with anxiolytic activity in humans that can help elucidate the role of 5-HT in anxiety. **Buspirone, gepirone**, and **ipsapirone may** therefore offer new therapeutic directions in the treatment of anxiety.

Buspirone is an anxiety agent but has no sedative, anticonvulsant, or muscle-relaxant properties. It binds selectively to the 5-HT_{1A} receptors, which are abundant in the hippocampus, a portion of the frontal cortex, and the dorsal raphe nucleus. The universal mechanism underlying its anxiolytic effects may be the inhibition of raphe cell firing. The most common side effects of buspirone are dizziness, headache, and nervousness.

The drug is rapidly absorbed after oral administration, and peak plasma concentrations occur about one hour later. Buspirone is extensively metabolized, with less than 1% of an administered dose excreted unchanged. Important routes of biotransformation are hydroxylation and oxidative dealkylation, the latter yielding 1-(2-pyrimidinyl) piperazines. This metabolite has been shown to concentrate in the brain and to have pharmacologic activity, though its capacity to interact with different brain receptors appears to differ from that of buspirone.

BUSULFAN
(Myleran)

Busulfan, an alkylsulfonate, is indicated in the palliative treatment of chronic myelogenous leukemia including myeloid, myelocytic, or granulocytic leukemia. Busulfan is of no value in chronic lymphocytic leukemia, acute leukemia, or in the "blastic crisis" of chronic myelogenous leukemia. Busulfan (4 to 8 mg/day) is a cell-cycle phase, nonspecific, polyfunctional alkylating agent which interacts with cellular thiol groups without crosslinking of nucleoproteins. In treating chronic granulocytic leukemia, the initial oral dose of busulfan varies with the total leukocyte count and the severity of the disease; daily doses from 2 to 8 mg are recommended to initiate therapy and are adjusted appropriately to subsequent hematological and clinical responses. Busulfan is well absorbed after oral administration, and it disappears from the blood with a half-life of 2 to 3 hours. Almost all of the drug is excreted in the urine as methanesulfonic acid (see also Figure 2).

The most frequent and serious side effects of busulfan is bone marrow failure. Therefore, the hemoglobin, hematocrit, white blood cells, platelets, and differential counts should be monitored weekly. A rare complication of busulfan therapy is the development of broncho-pulmonary dysplasia with pulmonary fibrosis. Busulfan is known to have caused cataract, hyperpigmentation of skin, adrenal insufficiency, gynecomastia, cholestatic jaundice, and myasthenia gravis.

BUTABARBITAL

(Barbased, Butalan, Buticaps, Butisol, Butartran, Sarisol No. 2)

Butabarbital, a barbiturate hypnotic sedative (15 to 30 mg p.o. t.i.d.), is indicated for causing sedation and preoperative sedation and treating insomnia.

BUTHIONINE SULFOXIMINE

One of the goals of cancer chemotherapy is to enhance the efficacy of antineoplastic agents and at the same time protect the nonmalignant tissues using chemoprotective agents. Buthionine sulfoximine is a chemoenhancing agent.

BUTOCONAZOLE NITRATE

(Femstat)

Butoconazole, a synthetic imidazole derivative with antifungal properties (2% vaginal cream with applicators to be used intravaginally at bedtime for three days), is indicated in the treatment of vulvovaginal candidiasis (moniliasis).

BUTORPHANOL TARTRATE

(Stadol)

Butorphanol is a narcotic agonist with analgesic action five times more potent than morphine; and a narcotic antagonist with antagonist action 1/40 that of naloxone. Butorphanol (2 to 3 mg IM) exerts its analgesic action in 10 to 15 minutes, with a peak of action in 30 to 60 minutes, and a duration of action of 3 to 4 hours. Butorphanol is metabolized in the liver to hydroxybutorphanol which is excreted mainly by the kidneys. Like pentazocine, butorphanol depresses respiration and increases pulmonary artery pressure, pulmonary wedge pressure, left ventricular end diastolic pressure, and systemic arterial pressure. Since it increases cardiac workload, it should be used cautiously in acute myocardial infarction, in ventricular dysfunction, or coronary insufficiency. Like morphine, butorphanol increases the cerebrospinal fluid pressure, and hence should be used cautiously in recent head injury. Naloxone is able to overcome the toxicity of butorphanol.

C

CAFFEINE

Oral caffeine (40 to 150 mg/5 oz. brewed coffee; 100 mg in **No-Doz**; 150 mg in **Quick Pep**; and 200 mg in **Caffedrine**) is used to remain mentally alert, and parenteral caffeine has been used as an analeptic to treat respiratory depression. Caffeine has been used as an orphan drug in neonatal apnea. Caffeine stimulates the CNS and produces cardiac stimulation, dilation of coronary and peripheral blood vessels, and constriction of cerebral blood vessels. It stimulates the skeletal muscles, enhances the secretion of gastric acid, and has diuretic properties. Caffeine exerts its various pharmacological effects by increasing calcium permeability in sarcoplasmic reticulum, by inhibiting phosphodiesterase, by raising the concentration of cyclic AMP, and by blocking adenosine receptors. Caffeine in adults is metabolized in the liver, but in neonates is excreted unchanged by the kidneys. The half-lives of caffeine in the newborn, three-month-old infant, and six-month-old infant are 70 hours, 15 hours, and 3 hours, respectively (see also Figure 10).

Overdosage of caffeine in a nontolerant individual causes insomnia, anxiety, diuresis, restlessness, excitement, nervousness, tinnitus, muscular tremor, headache, and scintillating scotoma.

CALCIFEDIOL

(Calderol)

Calcifediol, a vitamin D analog (300 to 350 mg p.o. weekly), is indicated in the treatment and management of metabolic bone disease associated with chronic renal failure (see also Figure 97).

CALCIPOTRIENE

(Dovonex)

Calcipotriene, vitamin D_3 analog (ointment 0.005%), is used topically in moderate plaque psoriasis. Calcipotriene is a synthetic vitamin D_3 analog that binds to vitamin D_3 receptors in skin cells (keratinocytes), regulating skin cell production and development (see also Figure 97).

CALCITONIN-HUMAN

(Cibacalcin – 0.5 mg SC; Calcitonin-Salmon, Calcimar, Miacalcin, 100 to 200 IUSC)

The **thyroid gland** synthesizes **thyroxine** (T_4) and **triiodothyronine** (T_3), and these hormones are involved in the regulation of growth and development, thermoregulation and calorigenesis, metabolism of carbohydrates, proteins, and lipids, and hypophyseal thyrotropin secretion (see Figure 56).

The thyroid gland also synthesizes **calcitonin**, which produces hypocalcemia by inhibiting bone resorption and by enhancing the urinary excretion of calcium and phosphate.

Calcitonin, a polypeptide consisting of 32 amino acids, is produced by parafollicular cells (C cells) of the thyroid gland. The secretion of calcitonin is stimulated by calcium, catecholamine and theophylline (increased cyclic adenosine monophosphate levels), glucagon, cholecysto-kinin, gastrin, and cerulean.

Calcitonin is indicated for patients with moderate to severe Paget's disease, characterized by abnormal and accelerated bone formation, and for patients with hypercalcemia associated with carcinoma multiple myeloma.

CALCITRIOL

(Rocaltrol)

Calcitriol, a vitamin D analog (0.25 mcg p.o. daily), is indicated in the management of hypocalcemia in patients undergoing chronic dialysis. In addition, calcitriol (0.5 mcg IV 3 times weekly), is used in the management of hypoparathyroidism and pseudohypoparathy-roidism (see Figure 97).

CALCIUM CHANNEL BLOCKERS

Many hormones, neurotransmitters, and autacoids exert their actions by altering phospho-inositide metabolism, increasing the concentration of ionized calcium in the cytosol of their target cells, and stimulating the turnover rate of phosphatidylinositol 4,5-biphosphate (PIP_2).

Under normal conditions, the extracellular concentration of calcium is in the millimolar range (10^{-3} M), whereas its intracellular concentration is less than 10^{-7} M. The cytoplasmic concentration of calcium is increased through the actions of **receptor-operated channels, voltage-activated channels**, or **ionic pumps**. In addition, calcium can be released from internal stores (see also Figures 76 and 95).

There are two types of voltage-activated channels:

1. **Low-voltage-activated channels** or low-threshold channels, which are also termed *T-type* channels.
2. **High-voltage-activated channels**, which are further subdivided into *L-type, N-type,* and *P-type* channels.

T-Type Channels

T-type calcium channels (with the *t* standing for "transient") require only a weak depolarization for activation and carry a transient current at negative membrane potentials that inactivates rapidly during a prolonged pulse. In neurons, the T-type channel is responsible for neuronal oscillatory activity and is thought to play a role in the regulation of wakefulness and motor coordination. The pyrazine diuretic, **amiloride**, inhibits the T-type calcium channel.

L-Type Channels

L-type calcium channels (with the *l* standing for "long lasting") exist in high numbers in the skeletal muscle and require a large depolarization for activation to take place. The channels are phosphorylated prior to opening. Each channel is composed of **five subunits**: $alpha_1$ (molecular weight [MW] = 175 kDa), $alpha_2$ (MW = 143 kDa), beta (MW = 54 kDa), gamma (MW = 30 kDa), and delta (MW = 27 kDa). The $alpha_1$ and beta subunits contain phospho-rylation sites for cyclic adenosine monophosphate (AMP)-dependent protein kinase. The $alpha_1$ subunit contains the **dihydropyridine**-binding sites. The L-type calcium channel is involved in the **generation of action potentials** and in **signal transduction** at the cell membrane.

N-Type Channels

The N-type channel (with the *n* standing for "neither T nor L or neuronal") appears to convey most of the whole-cell calcium current; it is insensitive to dihydropyridine and is blocked by

omega-conotoxin. The N-type channel is involved in the **release of transmitter** in some, but not all, tissues, with central nervous system (CNS) neurons being the exception.

P-Type Channels

The P-type channels were first observed in the Purkinje cells and are inhibited by a toxin derived from a funnel-web spider poison, but not by other calcium channel-blocking agents. P-type channels are widely distributed throughout the CNS and are thought to participate in the generation of **intrinsic activity** as well as serving as modulators of **neuronal integration** and **transmitter release**.

Calcium-activated potassium channels increase their **permeability to potassium ions** in response to increases in the intracellular calcium concentration. These potassium channels couple the membrane potential to the intracellular concentration of calcium, in that a rise in the intracellular calcium level leads to an efflux of potassium ions and hence hyperpolarization of the membrane.

The secretion of neurotransmitters and neurohormones is usually triggered by a rise in the intracellular calcium concentration. However, the release of **acetylcholine** from the Schwann cells and **renin** from the juxtaglomerular apparatus is triggered by a fall in the intracellular calcium level.

Unlike skeletal muscles, which contain endogenous stores of calcium ions, both cardiac muscle and vascular smooth muscle require extracellular calcium for contractile function. Therefore, cardiac muscle and vascular smooth muscle are subject to regulation by **calcium antagonists** or **calcium entry blockers** (Figures 76 and 95 and Table 20), which are used in the treatment of hypertension, Raynaud's disease, Prinzmetal's angina, and migraine syndromes.

Calcium enters the cell through voltage-dependent channels mainly during depolarization, and this process is regulated by the cyclic AMP level. Because the cellular content of cyclic AMP depends on a series of enzymatic steps initiated by receptor stimulation and ending with cyclic AMP degradation, an increase in cellular calcium uptake can be achieved by interventions that act at any of these stages. A major mechanism for calcium transport through the sarcolemma in both directions consists of **electrogenic sodium-calcium exchange**, which depends on the electrochemical gradient for sodium. A reduction in this gradient leads to increased calcium uptake by the exchanger. Therefore, a great variety of agents that promote an increase in the intracellular sodium level produce **positive inotropic effects**.

Calcium Entry Blockers

Calcium entry blockers include those agents that are **selective for slow calcium channels** in the myocardium (slow channel blockers), and consist of the following categories of substances:

Phenylalkylamines — verapamil, gallopamil, anipamil, desmethoxyverapamil, emopamil, falipamil, and ronipamil.

Dihydropyridines — nifedipine, nicardipine, niludipine, nimodipine, nisoldipine, nitrendipine, ryosidine, amlodipine, azodipine, dazodipine, felodipine, flordipine, iodipine, isradipine, mesudipine, oxodipine, and riodipine.

Benzothiazepines – diltiazem.

Agents that have no perceived action on the slow calcium inward current in the myocardium (voltage clamp) consist of the **diphenylpiperazines** and include cinnarizine and flunarizine.

There are also **nonselective calcium entry blockers** that act at similar concentrations on both calcium channels and fast sodium channels. These agents consist of: bencyclane, bepridil, caroverine, etafenone, fendiline, lidoflazine, perhexiline, prenylamine, proadifen, terodiline, and tiapamil.

Those agents that interact with calcium channels but have **another primary site of action** include: agents acting on **sodium channels** (local anesthetics and phenytoin), **catecholamine receptors** (benextramine, nicergoline, phenoxybenzamine, phenothiazines, pimozide, propranolol, and yohimbine derivatives), **benzodiazepine receptors** (diazepam and flurazepam), **opiate receptors** (loperamide and fluperamide), and **cyclic nucleotide phosphodiesterases** (amrinone, cromoglycate, and papaverine), as well as barbiturates, cyproheptadine, indomethacin, and reserpine.

Sodium-calcium exchange inhibitors include **amiloride** and its derivatives, specifically dantrolene, which acts on the sarcoplasmic reticulum, and ruthenium red, which acts on the mitochondria.

Calmodulin antagonists consist of the **phenothiazines** (trifluoperazine and chlorpromazine), **local anesthetics** (dibucaine), and **dopamine antagonists** (pimozide and haloperidol).

Calcium Entry Blockers and Their Use in Various Disorders

Hypertension
Verapamil, nifedipine, and **diltiazem** lower blood pressure with an efficacy comparable to that achieved by other commonly used agents. Their specific effects on the cardiovascular system are as follows:

Drugs	Heart Rate	Atrioventricular Nodal Conduction	Myocardial Contractility	Arteriolar Vasodilation
Verapamil	No change	Greatly decreased	Moderately decreased	Moderately increased
Nifedipine	Increased	—	No change	Greatly increased
Diltiazem	Decreased	Moderately decreased	Decreased	Increased

The intravenous administration of diltiazem or verapamil, or the oral or sublingual administration of nifedipine is effective in managing hypertensive emergencies.

Myocardial Infarction
Heart failure is associated with changes in the intracellular calcium levels. The rationale for using calcium entry blockers in preventing the secondary complications of myocardial infarction stems from the fact that these agents reduce systemic vascular resistance, afterload, myocardial contractility, blood pressure and oxygen consumption. However, despite these effects, the efficacy of calcium entry blockers in preventing the secondary complications of myocardial infarction or their usefulness in the context of cerebrovascular diseases such as aneurysmal subarachnoid hemorrhage needs to be established.

Angina
Beta-adrenergic blocking agents are effective for the prophylactic therapy of **exertional angina pectoris** by reducing heart rate and the force of myocardial contraction. However, verapamil, nifedipine, and diltiazem are also effective for the prophylactic treatment of stable exertional angina. The combination therapy with beta-blockers and calcium entry blockers is well tolerated, effective, and safe.

Psychiatric Disorders
Verapamil has also been used in the treatment of mania, depression, maintenance control of manic depression, and schizophrenia. In addition, it has been used in the management of premenstrual syndrome, stuttering, and intoxication with phencyclidine.

Cerebrovascular Disorders
Among the various types of calcium entry blockers, flunarizine has proved to be the most effective in the prophylaxis of **migraine**. It has also been shown to be beneficial in protecting

brain cells against hypoxia and in preventing the constriction of cerebrovascular smooth muscle cells. Moreover, it has been shown to be effective in the treatment of **epilepsy** and **hemiplegia**.

Parkinson's Disease
Calcium entry blockers may induce **extrapyramidal symptoms** and aggravate parkinsonism.

Drug Interactions and Calcium Entry Blockers
Following are some of the drug interactions seen with either specific calcium entry blockers or these agents in general:

- Verapamil inhibits several oxidative routes of hepatic metabolism.
- Verapamil and diltiazem decrease the clearance of **theophylline** and increase its half-life.
- Calcium channel blockers increase the toxicity of **lithium**, which has calcium antagonist effects itself.
- Calcium channel blockers potentiate the negative inotropic effects of type Ia anti-arrhythmic agents.
- Verapamil increases the plasma concentration of **digitoxin**.
- Calcium entry blockers potentiate the hypotensive effects of **prazocin**.
- Calcium entry blockers increase the plasma concentration of **carbamazepine**.
- Calcium entry blockers decrease the clearance of **cyclosporine**.
- Calcium entry blockers cause impaired myocardial conduction when given with **enflurane** and precipitate pronounced hypotension when given with **halothane**.

CALCIUM-CHANNEL BLOCKERS FOR THE TREATMENT OF HYPERTENSION		
Drugs		
Amlodipine	Isradipine	Nifedipine
Diltiazem	Lacidipine	Nitrendipine
Felodipine	Nicardipine	Verapamil
All calcium-channel blockers cause vasodilatation, but the cardiac response to the decrease in peripheral resistance is variable. An initial reflex increase in heart rate usually occurs with the dihydropyridines (nifedipine, nicardipine, isradipine, and felodipine); verapamil and diltiazem cause little or no change in heart rate. Verapamil and diltiazem can, however, slow atrioventricular (AV) conduction and should be used with caution in patients also taking a beta-blocker; dihydropyridines generally do not affect AV conduction and can be used with a beta-blocker, which decreases reflex tachycardia. All calcium-channel blockers should be used with caution in patients with heart failure.		

CALCIUM GLUCONATE

Calcium gluconate is indicated in hypocalcemia associated with neonatal tetany and tetany due to parathyroid difficulty, vitamin D deficiency, or alkalosis; in prevention of tetany during exchange transfusions; and in conditions related to malabsorption.

The concentration of calcium in extracellular fluids is $10^{-3} M$ and the concentration of cytoplasmic calcium is $10^{-6} M$. The **mitochondria** and **microsomes** contain 90 to 99% of the intracellular calcium, which is bound largely to organic and inorganic phosphates. The low cytoplasmic concentration of calcium is maintained by three **calcium pump-leak-transport systems**. Each pump is oriented in a direction of calcium egress from the cytosol (see also Figures 76 and 95).

Calcium functions at both extracellular and cellular sites. Its **extracellular functions** consist of the maintenance of normal ion products for mineralization, cofactor for prothrombin factors VII, IX, and X, and maintenance of plasma membrane stability and permeability.

Its **cellular functions** comprise skeletal and cardiac muscle contraction, cellular secretion, exocrine, endocrine, and neurotransmitters, neural excitation and light transmission, regulation of membrane ion transport, enzyme regulation (gluconeogenesis and glycogenolysis), and cell growth and division.

The symptoms of hypocalcemia are: tetany, paresthesias, laryngospasm, muscle spasms, seizures (usually grand mal), irritability, depression, psychosis, prolonged QT interval, intestinal cramps, and respiratory arrest.

Calcium salts are contraindicated in hypercalcemia, ventricular fibrillation, and in digitalized patients, which may be predisposed to arrhythmias. Inadvertent calcium overloading may be treated by IV infusion of sodium chloride which competes with calcium for reabsorption in the distal renal tubercle and by furosemide (see also Figure 4).

CALCIUM POLYCARBOPHIL
(Equalactin, Fiberall, FiberCon, Mitrolan)

Calcium polycarbophil, a hydrophilic agent which absorbs water (1 g p.o. q.i.d.), is used in the treatment of constipation.

CALCIUM PRODUCTS	
Preparation	mg Elemental Calcium/Tablet
Calcium Carbonate (40% elemental calcium)	
Cal-Sup	300
Caltrate	600
Os-Cal	500
Tums	200
Titralac	168
Generic Calcium Gluconate (9% elemental calcium)	58.5
Generic Calcium Lactate (13% elemental calcium)	84.5
Generic Dibasic Calcium Phosphate (23% elemental calcium)	115

CALCIUM SALTS

CALCIUM ACETATE
(Calcium Acetate Injection, Phos-Ex, Phoslo)

CALCIUM CARBONATE
(Alka-Mints, Amitone, Bio-Cal, Calcilac, Calglycine, Caltrate, Cal-Sup, Chooz, Dicarbosil, Equilet, Gustalac, Os-Cal 500, PAMA NO. 1, Suplical, Titracid, Titralac, Tums, Tums E-X)

CALCIUM CHLORIDE

CALCIUM CITRATE
(Citracel)

CALCIUM GLUBIONATE
(Neo-Calglucon)

CALCIUM GLUCEPTATE

CALCIUM GLUCONATE
(Kalcinate)

CALCIUM GLYCEROPHOSPHATE

CALCIUM LACTATE

CALCIUM PHOSPHATE, DIBASIC

CALCIUM PHOSPHATE, TRIBASIC
(Posture)

The calcium salts are used in the emergency treatment of hypocalcemia, in hyperkalemia, in hypermagnesemia, and in hyperphosphatemia in end-stage renal failure. In addition, they are used in prevention of osteoporosis (see also Figure 97).

CANNABINOID

Delta^9-Tetrahydrocannabinol (**delta^9-THC**) is considered to be the predominant compound in preparations of *Cannabis sativa* (marijuana, hashish, bhang) responsible for CNS effects in humans. The recognized CNS responses to these preparations include alterations in cognition and memory, euphoria, and sedation. Potential therapeutic applications of *Cannabis* preparations include analgesia, attenuation of the nausea and vomiting of cancer chemotherapy, appetite stimulation, decreased intestinal motility of diarrhea, decreased bronchial constriction of asthma, decreased intraocular pressure of glaucoma, antirheumatic and antipyretic actions, and treatment of convulsant disorders.

CANNABINOID

(Nabilone)

Nausea and vomiting are frequent side effects of radiotherapy and cancer chemotherapy. The incidence of this is relatively low for bleomycin, vincristine, and chlorambucil but is high for the remaining agents. In addition to prochlorperazine and metoclopramide (**dopamine-receptor-blocking agents**), nabilone (a **cannabinoid**), batanopride, granisetron, and ondansetron (all **serotonin-receptor-blocking agents**) have been shown to be effective in ameliorating these symptoms (see also Figures 64 and 73).

CANRENOATE POTASSIUM

(Soldactone S)

It is generally assumed that the intracellular content of sodium in vascular smooth muscle is increased in essential hypertension. Although the major role of aldosterone in the regulation of blood pressure is a renal one, it may also be involved in some extrarenal effects responsible for the regulation of body fluid and blood pressure. Recent studies have suggested that vascular walls specifically bind to aldosterone and that aldosterone has a direct vasoconstrictive effect on vascular smooth muscle *in vitro*. Indeed, **canrenoate potassium** (Soldactone S), an **aldosterone antagonist**, reduces blood pressure (Figure 21).

CANTHARIDIN
(Cantharone, Verr-Canth)

Cantharidin, a cantharide derivative with keratolytic properties (0.7% solution), is used for removal of ordinary and periungual warts.

CAPREOMYCIN SULFATE
(Capastat Sulfate)

Capreomycin, a polypeptide antibiotic (15 mg/kg up to 1 g IM daily for 60 to 120 days), is used as an adjunctive treatment in pulmonary tuberculosis.

CAPSAICIN
(Zostrix, Zostrix-HP)

Capsaicin, a naturally occurring nonenamide derived from plants of the solanacease family, with analgesic properties (creams 0.025% and 0.075% 3 to 4 times daily), is used topically in temporary pain relief from rheumatoid arthritis, osteoarthritis, and certain neuralgias, such as pain associated with shingles (herpes zoster) or diabetic neuropathy.

CAPTOPRIL
(Monopril)

Captopril, an angiotensin-converting enzyme inhibitor (ACE), is indicated in the management of hypertension by itself or in combination with other antihypertensive medications, in heart failure when the patients have not responded adequately to digitalis, after myocardial infarction associated with left ventricular dysfunction, and in diabetic nephropathy.

In studying the role of the renin-angiotensin system in the development of hypertension, it has become apparent that there are two systems: a **tissue** and a **circulating renin angiotensin**. The control of hypertension is focused primarily on the renin-angiotensin system in the cardiovascular center of the brain. **Angiotensin-converting enzyme** (ACE) is found in the lung, plasma, the brush borders of the proximal renal tubule, the endothelium of vascular beds, the brain, and the testis. Its two most important actions are the **inactivation of bradykinin** and the **conversion of angiotensin I to angiotensin II**.

Receptors for angiotensin II are found in the medulla oblongata in neurons involved in the regulation of **baroreceptor activity**. Because studies in hypertensive patients have indicated that **ACE inhibitors** reduce sympathetic activity and enhance baroreceptor sensitivity, it is possible that the primary hypotensive mechanism of these agents is mediated through the blockade of angiotensin II formation in the cardiovascular centers of the brain.

The relationship of the renin-angiotensin-aldosterone system to **bradykinin** and **prostaglandin** production is shown in Figure 21.

Captopril and other drugs in this class inhibit the converting enzyme peptidyl dipeptidase that hydrolyzes angiotensin I to angiotensin II and inactivates bradykinin, a potent vasodilator (see also Figure 19). Unlike **saralasin**, captopril has no pressor activity. Thus, the hypotensive activity of captopril probably results from an inhibitory action on the renin-angiotensin system and stimulating action on the kallikrein-kinin system.

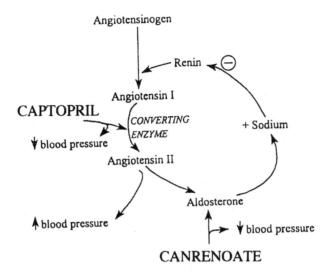

Angiotensinogen

Renin ⊖

Angiotensin I

CAPTOPRIL *CONVERTING ENZYME*   + Sodium

▼blood pressure

Angiotensin II

Aldosterone

▲blood pressure   ▼blood pressure

CANRENOATE

FIGURE 21 Captopril, an angiotensin-converting enzyme inhibitor, is used in hypertension and congestive heart failure.

Captopril is absorbed rapidly, partly metabolized to disulfide conjugate, and is excreted unchanged in the urine. With the exception of **fosinopril**, all ACE inhibitors are eliminated by the kidneys, and their doses should be reduced in renal insufficiency. Captopril, in high doses and in renal impairment, has caused neutropenia or proteinuria.

Alteration in taste occurs with captopril, but the incidence is less with enalapril and lisinopril.

Nonsteroidal antiinflammatory agents may impair the hypotensive effects of captopril by blocking bradykinin and prostaglandin mediated vasodilatation. triamterene-induced hyperkalemia is enhanced by captopril.

CARBACHOL

(Miostat)

Carbachol (1 to 2 drops into each eye t.i.d.) is indicated for lowering intraocular pressure in the treatment of glaucoma; and for causing miosis during surgery (0.5 ml of 0.01% into the anterior chamber causing miosis in 2 to 5 minutes).

Methacholine, carbachol, and bethanechol are all agents that mimic the effects of stimulation of cholinergic nerves (see also Figure 18).

The two currently used derivatives of acetylcholine are **bethanechol** (Urecholine chloride) and **carbachol** (Miostat). Unlike acetylcholine, both agents are resistant to hydrolysis by cholinesterase. Both agents are muscarinic agonists. The **nicotinic action** of carbachol is greater than that of acetylcholine, whereas bethanechol is devoid of nicotinic action. The **cardiovascular actions** of acetylcholine are vasodilation and negative chronotropic and inotropic effects. The cardiovascular effects of **methacholine** are more pronounced than those of acetylcholine, which in turn are greater than those of carbachol or bethanechol. The **gastrointestinal effects** (increase in tone, amplitude of contractions, and peristalsis) of bethanechol and carbachol are equal but greater than those of acetylcholine. The effects of carbachol and bethanechol on the **urinary tract**, consisting of ureteral peristalsis, contraction of the detrusor muscle of the urinary bladder, and an increase in voluntary voiding pressure, are equivalent and exceed those produced by acetylcholine.

The **miotic effects** of carbachol and bethanechol are greater than those of acetylcholine.

Atropine is able to antagonize all cholinergic (muscarinic) effects produced by acetylcholine, methacholine, carbachol, and bethanechol. However, this antagonist is least evident with carbachol (see also Figure 14).

CARBAMATES

The cholinesterase inhibitors are divided into two categories: **organophosphorous compounds** (such as parathion, malathion, and tetraethyl pyrophosphate [TEPP]) and the **carbamates** (such as naphthyl-N-methyl carbamate [carbaryl and Sevin]).

The clinical manifestations of acute and severe poisoning from the organophosphorous insecticides include **cholinergic crisis** (see also Figure 71), resulting from: the stimulation of muscarinic cholinergic receptors (bronchoconstriction, salivation, sweating, lacrimation, bradycardia, hypotension, and urinary and fecal incontinence); the stimulation of nicotinic cholinergic receptors (muscular fasciculation); and the CNS effects (with initial restlessness, tremors, ataxia, and convulsions, followed by CNS depression and respiratory and circulatory depression). The treatment of a cholinergic crisis caused by organophosphorous compounds includes the administration of a cholinesterase reactivator such as a pralidoxime (2-PAM) together with atropine (see Figure 71). The poisoning stemming from antidoting with 2-PAM can be avoided in the event of carbaryl toxicity, because this agent is a reversible cholinesterase inhibitor.

CARBAMAZEPINE

(Tegretol)

Carbamazepine is as effective as phenobarbital, phenytoin, and primidone in the prevention of **generalized tonic-clonic seizures**, but is significantly more effective than the others in the treatment of **complex partial seizures**. Carbamazepine is also used for the management of **trigeminal neuralgia** and **complex partial seizures with temporal lobe symptomatology**. Besides its antiepileptic effect, carbamazepine possesses sedative, anticholinergic, antidepressant, muscle relaxant, antiarrhythmic, antidiuretic, and neuromuscular transmission inhibitory actions. Therefore, carbamazepine has been used in the treatment of the childhood episodic behavior disorder, multiple sclerosis, central diabetes insipidus, and dystonia. Additional clinical trials should clarify the usefulness of carbamazepine in these conditions (see Figure 22).

Carbamazepine is structurally related to phenytoin and to the tricyclic antidepressant, imipramine. The oral bioavailability of carbamazepine, which may depend on a particular pharmaceutical preparation, is 75 to 85%. After absorption, it is bound to plasma proteins to the extent of 60 to 70%. Carbamazepine is metabolized to 10,11-epoxide and 10,11-dihydroxide derivatives of carbamazepine, some of which are excreted unchanged; the other portion is conjugated with glucuronic acid. The 10,11-epoxide derivatives are active anticonvulsants.

Phenobarbital has been shown to decrease serum carbamazepine half-life and plasma concentration levels when given in combination. Significant changes in carbamazepine serum concentrations were seen within 5 days after the addition of phenobarbital to the therapeutic regimen. Conversely, carbamazepine appears to have no effect on serum phenobarbital levels. Carbamazepine has been reported to lower serum concentrations of primidone, but the decrease does not appear to be clinically significant. Other barbiturates (e.g., amobarbital, butabarbital, secobarbital) may interact in a manner similar to phenobarbital because of pharmacologic similarity.

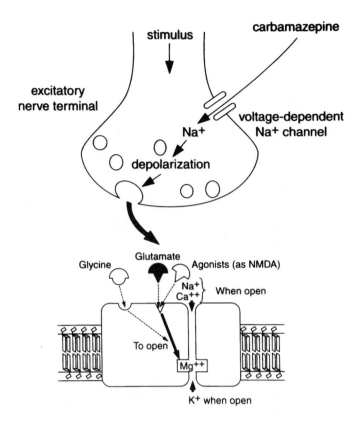

FIGURE 22 Carbamazepine inhibits seizure propagation by reduction of post-tetanic potentiation of synaptic transmission.

Phenobarbital is thought to induce the metabolism of carbamazepine to its epoxide metabolite. Accordingly, after phenobarbital administration, decreased serum carbamazepine concentrations were accompanied by increased epoxide levels.

The mode and mechanism of carbamazepine action are similar but not identical to those of phenytoin. In high but therapeutic doses, carbamazepine decreases sodium and potassium conductances and depresses post-tetanic potentiation. Furthermore, carbamazepine increases the taurine level, decreases the glutamic acid concentration, and enhances GABAergic transmission (see Figure 22).

The most frequent CNS adverse reactions of carbamazepine are dizziness, drowsiness, and unsteadiness. In addition, carbamazepine is known to have caused confusion, headache, fatigue, blurred vision, hallucinations, speech disturbances, abnormal involuntary movements, peripheral neuritis and paresthesias, depression with agitation, talkativeness, tinnitus, and hyperacusis (an abnormally acute sense of hearing or a painful sensitivity to sounds).

CARBENICILLIN INDANYL SODIUM

(Geocillin)

Carbenicillin is indicated for the treatment of acute and chronic infections of the upper and lower urinary tract and in asymptomatic bacteriuria due to susceptible strains of: *Escherichia coli, Proteus mirabilis, Morganella morganii, Providencia rettgeri, P. vulgaris, Pseudomonas, Enterobacter,* and enterococci. It is also indicated in the treatment of prostatitis due to susceptible strains of: *E. coli,* enterococcus (*S. faecalis*), *P. mirabilis,* and *Enterobacter* species.

Levodopa alone   Levodopa + Carbidopa

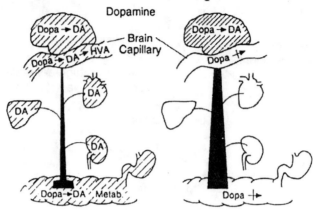

FIGURE 23   Carbidopa substantially decreases the formation of dopamine in the periphery and thus increases its formation in the brain. (Adapted from Ebadi, M., *Pharmacology, An Illustrated Review with Questions and Answers*, 3rd Edition, Lippincott-Raven Press, Philadelphia, 1996.)

Carbenicillin cures serious infections caused by *Pseudomonas* species and *Proteus* strains resistant to ampicillin. It is not absorbed from the gastrointestinal tract, and therefore must be administered intraperitoneally. **Carbenicillin indanyl** is acid stable and hence can be given orally. **Ticarcillin** is four times more potent than carbenicillin in treating a *Pseudomonas aeruginosa* infection, and **azlocillin** is ten times more potent than carbenicillin against *Pseudomonas*. **Mezlocillin** and **piperacillin** are more active against *Klebsiella* infection than is carbenicillin.

CARBIDOPA

(with Levodopa as Sinemet)

Carbidopa has no effect when given alone. It is used along with levodopa in the management of Parkinson's disease. When administered orally, levodopa is metabolized substantially in the gut and tissues, and very little penetrates into the brain to be converted to dopamine. The combined administration of levodopa with a peripheral dopa-decarboxylase inhibitor (**carbidopa**), substantially decreases the formation of dopamine in the periphery and thus increases its formation in the brain where it can work on the corpus striatum (Figure 23).

The **pharmacology** and **advantages** of the combined administration of a peripheral dopa-decarboxylase along with levodopa (e.g., Sinemet 10) are as follows:

The peripheral dopa-decarboxylase inhibitors such as carbidopa do not penetrate the blood-brain barrier, hence they do not affect the formation of dopamine in the brain. Because the metabolism of levodopa in the periphery is reduced, it can therefore be given in smaller doses and this lessens its peripheral side effects (hypotension and tachycardia). Once converted to dopamine, levodopa stimulates the chemoreceptor trigger zone for emesis located in the area postrema and causes nausea and vomiting. This side effect is reduced when levodopa is given with carbidopa. Peripheral dopa-decarboxylase inhibitors dramatically reduce the incidence of levodopa-induced tachycardia. In the presence of carbidopa, vitamin B_6 is not contraindicated. Adding vitamin B_6 may even enhance the formation of dopamine in the brain. Peripheral dopa-decarboxylase reduces the onset of the on-off phenomenon.

The appropriate starting dose for dopa-decarboxylase (Sinemet) varies among individuals. Many tolerate very well an initial dose of Sinemet 25/100, one tablet three times daily. However, older individuals, or those taking multiple medications, may tolerate only smaller initial doses, sometimes as low as one-half tablet daily. Because Sinemet 25/100 provides a higher ratio of carbidopa to levodopa and allows quicker attainment of the 75 to 100 mg of carbidopa necessary to sufficiently block the peripheral decarboxylation of levodopa to dopamine, it should be used instead of Sinemet 10/100 when initiating therapy. One can, however, later switch a patient to Sinemet 10/100 to take advantage of its lower cost. Sinemet 25/250 should not be used during the initiation of Sinemet therapy. **Sinemet CR 50/200**, the controlled-release form, can also be used in the initiation of therapy at an initial dose of one-half or one tablet twice daily.

CARBIMAZOLE

Propylthioural, methimazole, and **carbimazole** exert their effects by inhibiting **iodide organification**, and by inhibiting the **formation of DIT** (see also Figure 56).

These agents all possess a thiocarbamide moiety:

$$(-N-\overset{\overset{\displaystyle S}{\|}}{C}-R)$$

which is essential for their antithyroid actions. The onset of their beneficial effects is slow and takes 3 to 4 weeks.

CARBINOXAMINE MALEATE

(Clistin)

Carbinoxamine compound syrup (Pennex) containing 60 mg pseudoephedrine HCl, 4 mg carbinoxamine maleate, and 15 mg dextromethorphan HBr in 0.2% alcohol is indicated for relief of cough and upper respiratory systems including nasal congestion associated usually with allergy or common cold. Carbinoxamine possesses H_1 antihistaminic activity with mild anticholinergic-sedative properties. Carbinoxamine which is metabolized completely, has a serum half-life of 10 to 12 hours.

CARBONIC ANHYDRASE INHIBITORS

The carbonic anhydrase inhibitors consist of **acetazolamide** (Diamox), **ethoxzolamide** (Cardrase), and **dichlorphenamide** (Daranide). Acetazolamide is an old agent, whereas ethoxzolamide and dichlorphenamide are newer preparations. Dichlorphenamide is the most potent carbonic anhydrase inhibitor in use today. The presence of SO_2NH_2 (sulfonamide) causes such compounds to inhibit carbonic anhydrase (CA), which catalyzes the hydration of carbon dioxide as follows:

$$CO_2 + H_2O \xrightarrow{\text{CA}} H_2CO_3 \rightleftharpoons H^+ + HCO_3^-$$

These agents inhibit carbonic anhydrase in the renal tubular cells in both the proximal and distal tubules. When the rate of hydrogen generation is reduced, HCO_3^- is lost in urine and the patient tends to become acidotic. However, the plasma concentration of HCO_3^- is lowered and less is filtered, so the diuresis becomes less effective. In addition, the sodium output is increased because its resorption in exchange for hydrogen is limited by the decreased availability of hydrogen. With less hydrogen available, the exchange of sodium for potassium predominates, and this fosters the loss of potassium. Chloride excretion is not altered significantly. Because the aqueous humor has a high concentration of bicarbonate, carbonic anhydrase inhibitors are primarily used in the treatment of **glaucoma**. They are no longer used as diuretics or as antiepileptic agents (see also Figure 4).

CARBOPLATIN
(Paraplatin)

Carboplatin and cyclophosphamide are indicated in the treatment of advanced ovarian carcinoma. Cisplatin and carboplatin produce predominantly interstrand DNA crosslinks rather than DNA-protein crosslinks, and the effect is cell-cycle nonspecific. Carboplatin is not bound to plasma proteins, whereas platinum from carboplatin becomes bound to plasma protein and is eliminated slowly with a half-life of 5 days. The major route of elimination of carboplatin is the kidneys, and its doses should be reduced in renal impairment. Furthermore, the coadministration of aminoglycosides increases the chance of nephrotoxicity. Carboplatin causes anemia, neutropenia, leukopenia, and thrombocytopenia requiring transfusions. Cisplatin and, to a lesser extent, carboplatin cause emesis which requires treatment with antiemetic agents. Alopecia, pain, and asthenia do occur (see also Figure 2).

CARBOPROST TROMETHAMINE
(Hemabate)

Carboprost is used for abortion and in refractory postpartum uterine bleeding. Prostaglandins are mostly used as **abortifacients**. They may be administered by vaginal suppository (**Dinoprostone**), which contains prostaglandin E_2, by intramuscular injection (**carboprost and tromethamine**), which contains 15-methyl prostaglandin F_{2a}, or by intra-amnionic administration (**dinoprost and tromethamine**), which contains prostaglandin F_{2a}. Other possible uses of prostaglandins may include the treatment of ductus arteriosus (prostaglandin E_1) to maintain patency (see Figure 51), and as a vasodilator. High levels of prostaglandin F_{2a} may cause **dysmenorrhea**, and substances such as indomethacin and ibuprofen are effective in relieving these symptoms.

CARISOPRODOL
(SOMA)

Carisoprodol (350 mg p.o. t.i.d.) is indicated as an adjunct to physical therapy in acute painful musculoskeletal conditions. Carisoprodol causes muscular relaxation by blocking interneuronal activity in the descending reticular formation and spinal cord. Drowsiness, dizziness, vertigo, and tremor may be managed by dose reduction.

CARMUSTINE
(BCNU)

Carmustine is indicated in brain tumors such as glioblastoma, brainstem glioma, medulloblastoma, astrocytoma, ependymoma and metastatic brain tumors; in combination with prednisone in multiple myeloma; and as a secondary therapy in Hodgkin's disease and non-Hodgkin's lymphomas in patients who fail to respond to primary therapy. Carmustine, which does not exhibit cross resistance with other alkylating agents, exerts its antineoplastic effects by alkylating DNA and RNA and by carbamyolating amino acids and inhibiting enzymes. Carmustine crosses the blood-brain barrier readily and is excreted in the urine and in respiratory CO_2. High-dose carmustine causes myelosuppression, progressive azotema and renal failure, pulmonary infiltrates or fibrosis, and retinal hemorrhages. Cimetidine may enhance the carmustine-induced myelosuppression (see also Figure 2).

CAROTENOIDS

Carotenoids are a group of pigments that can be divided into two main classes: **carotenes** and **xanthophylls**. Carotenoids are introduced into the human body through dietary intake (mainly from fruits and vegetables and as food additives). Some are nutritionally active as precursors of vitamin A, but only approximately 10% of those identified in nature possess this property.

Aside from the nutritional context, the carotenoids have other important, well-defined functions, such as those related to their antioxidant properties (singlet oxygen quenching and scavenging oxyradicals) and their photoprotective activities, aspects which are now being considered to be of some significance in disease prevention.

CARTEOLOL HYDROCHLORIDE

(Cartrol)

Carteolol, a beta-adrenergic receptor blocking agent (2 to 5 mg as a single daily dose), is used to treat hypertension.

CARVEDILOL

Carvedilol (25 to 50 mg b.i.d.) is indicated in the treatment of hypertension. Carvedilol is a nonselective competitive $beta_1$ and $beta_2$ adrenergic blocking agent, with no intrinsic sympathomimetic activity, but with a membrane-stabilizing action. Carvedilol lowers blood pressure by diversified mechanisms which include beta-blockade, $alpha_1$-blockade, calcium channel blockade, and direct vasodilating effects resembling those produced by nitrates or prostaglandins. Carvedilol is a lipid-soluble substance, crosses the blood-brain barrier, and produces some of the side effects seen with other beta-adrenergic receptor blocking agents.

CASCARA SAGRADA

CASCARA SAGRADA AROMATIC FLUID EXTRACT

CASCARA SAGRADA FLUID EXTRACT

Cascara sagrada, an anthraquinone glycoside mixture (325 mg p.o. h.s., 1 ml fluid extract daily; or 5 ml aromatic fluid extract daily), is used in acute constipation and preparation for bowel or rectal examination.

CASTOR OIL

(Alphamul, Emulsoil, Neoloid, Purge)

Castor oil, a glyceride *Ricinus communis* derivative with stimulant laxative properties (15 to 60 ml p.o.), is used for preparation for rectal or bowel examination or surgery.

CASTOR OIL

(Apothecon, Purepac)

Irritant agents used in the treatment of constipation include cascara sagrada, castor oil, senna, rhubarb, phenolphthalein, and acetphenolisatin. Phenolphthalein is a constituent of many over-the-counter preparations, including Ex-Lax and Feen-A-Mint. Most of these agents, with the exception of castor oil, are slow in their onset of action (24 hours).

Phenolphthalein is thought to exert its effect by inhibiting the movement of water from the colon into the blood and by stimulating mucous secretion. If misused on a prolonged basis, a consequential loss of mucus may lower the plasma protein level. **Castor oil** is hydrolyzed to **ricinoleic acid**, the active cathartic. It has an onset of action of 2 to 6 hours.

The **misuse** of any of these agents has been shown to cause hypokalemia, dehydration, and a cathartic colon (resembling ulcerative colitis). Phenolphthalein-containing products may color alkaline urine red.

CATECHOLAMINE

Dopamine, norepinephrine, and epinephrine are classified as **catecholamines** and are synthesized according to the scheme depicted in Figure 27.

Tyrosine is converted to dopa by the rate-limiting enzyme, **tyrosine hydroxylase**, which requires tetrahydrobiopterin, and is inhibited by alpha-methyltyrosine. Dopa is decarboxylated to dopamine by L-**aromatic amino acid decarboxylase**, which requires pyridoxal phosphate (vitamin B$_6$) as a coenzyme. **Carbidopa**, which is used with L-dopa in the treatment of parkinsonism, inhibits this enzyme (see Figure 23). Dopamine is converted to norepinephrine by **dopamine beta-hydroxylase**, which requires ascorbic acid (vitamin C), and is inhibited by diethyldithiocarbamate. Norepinephrine is converted to epinephrine by **phenylethanolamine N-methyltransferase (PNMT)**, requiring S-adenosyl-methionine. The activity of PNMT is stimulated by corticosteroids.

The **catecholamine-synthesizing enzymes** are not only able to synthesize dopamine and norepinephrine from a physiologically occurring substrate such as L-dopa, but also from exogenous substrates such as **alpha-methyldopa**, which is converted to alpha-methyldopamine and in turn to alpha-methylnorepinephrine. Alpha-methyldopamine and alpha-methyl-norepinephrine are called *false transmitters* and, in general (except for alpha-methylnorepi-nephrine), are weaker agonists. Alpha-methyldopa is used in the management of hypertension.

In addition to being synthesized in the peripheral nervous system, dopamine is also synthesized in the corpus striatum and in the mesocortical, mesolimbic, and tuberoinfundibular systems. Norepinephrine is synthesized and stored primarily in sympathetic noradrenergic nerve terminals, as well as in the brain and the adrenal medulla. Epinephrine is synthesized and stored primarily in the adrenal medulla, and, to a certain extent, in the hypothalamic nuclei.

In sympathetic nerve terminals, as well as the brain, the adrenal medulla, and sympathetic postganglionic terminals, there are osmophilic granules (synaptic vesicles) that are capable of storing high concentrations of catecholamine (a complex with adenosine triphosphate [ATP] and protein). The stored amines are not metabolized by the intersynaptosomal mito-chondrial enzyme (monoamine oxidase).

Besides releasing norepinephrine (through exocytosis), the stimulation of sympathetic neurons also releases ATP, storage protein, and dopamine beta-hydroxylase. The released norepineph-rine interacts with receptor sites located postsynaptically (alpha$_1$) to produce the desired effects.

The action of norepinephrine is terminated by reuptake mechanisms, two of which have been identified: **Uptake 1** is located in the presynaptic membrane, requires energy for the transport, is sodium and temperature dependent, and is inhibited by **ouabain** (a cardiac glycoside), **cocaine** (a local anesthetic), and **imipramine** (an antidepressant). **Uptake 2** is located extra-neuronally in various smooth muscles and glands, requires energy, and is temperature dependent.

Approximately 20% of the amine is either taken up by the Uptake 2 mechanism or is metabolized. There are two enzymes capable of metabolizing catecholamines. The first is **monoamine oxidase** (MAO), a mitochondrial enzyme that oxidatively deaminates catecholamines, tyramine, serotonin, and histamine. MAO is further subclassified as either **monoamine oxidase A,** which metabolizes norepinephrine and is inhibited by **tranylcypromine**, and **monoamine oxidase B,** which metabolizes dopamine and is inhibited by L-deprenyl (selegiline, see Figure 79). **Catechol-O-methyltransferase** (COMT), a soluble enzyme present mainly in the liver and kidney, is also found in postsynaptic neuronal elements. About 15% of norepinephrine is metabolized postsynaptically by COMT (see also Figure 27).

CATHARTICS

Constipation may be defined as the passage of excessively dry stools, infrequent stools, or stools of insufficient size. Constipation is a symptom and not a disease. It may be of brief duration (e.g., when one's living habits or diet changes abruptly) or it may be a life-long problem, as occurs in congenital aganglionosis of the colon (Hirschsprung's disease). The causes of constipation are multiple and include the following:

Functional causes
    Fiber-deficient diets
    Variants of irritable bowel syndrome
    Debilitation and extreme old age
Colonic diseases
    Chronic obstructive lesions (e.g., tumors or strictures)
    Ulcerative colitis
    Collagen vascular diseases
Rectal diseases
    Stricture (e.g., ulcerative colitis)
    Painful conditions (fissure or abcess)
Neurologic diseases
    Hirschsprung's disease
    Spinal cord injuries and disease
    Parkinson's disease
    Cerebral tumors and cerebrovascular disease
Metabolic diseases
    Porphyria
    Hypothyroidism
    Hypercalcemia
    Pheochromocytoma
    Uremia

Use of the following drugs may also lead to constipation.

Anticholinergic drugs contained in many over-the-counter medications.
Antiparkinsonian drugs possessing anticholinergic properties (e.g., trihexyphenidyl and ethopropazine).
Antihistaminic drugs with anticholinergic properties (e.g., diphenhydramine).
Neuroleptics with anticholinergic properties (e.g., thioridazine).
Antidepressants with anticholinergic properties (e.g., amitriptyline).
Anticonvulsants with anticholinergic properties (e.g., carbamazepine).
Analgesics (e.g., morphine, codeine, and diphenoxylate).
Ganglionic blocking agents (e.g., mecamylamine hydrochloride and pempidine).
Antacids (calcium- or aluminum-containing compounds).

Laxatives and Cathartics

Although used interchangeably, the terms **laxative** and **cathartic** do have slightly different meanings. A **laxative effect** refers to the excretion of a soft, formed stool; **catharsis** implies a more fluid and complete evacuation.

Irritants

Irritant agents used in the treatment of constipation include cascara sagrada, castor oil, senna, rhubarb, phenolphthalein, and acetphenolisatin. Phenolphthalein is a constituent of many over-the-counter preparations, including Ex-Lax and Feen-A-Mint. Most of these agents, with the exception of castor oil, are slow in their onset of action (24 hours).

Phenolphthalein is thought to exert its effect by inhibiting the movement of water and sodium from the colon into the blood and by stimulating mucus secretion. If misused on a prolonged basis, a consequential loss of mucus may lower the plasma protein level. **Castor oil** is hydrolyzed to **ricinoleic acid**, the active cathartic. It has an onset of action of 2 to 6 hours.

The **misuse** of any of these agents has been shown to cause hypokalemia, dehydration, and a cathartic colon (resembling ulcerative colitis). Phenolphthalein-containing products may color alkaline urine red.

Bulk Saline Laxatives

Bulk saline laxatives fall into two categories: **inorganic salts** (magnesium sulfate, magnesium citrate, milk of magnesia, sodium sulfate, and sodium phosphate), and **organic hydrophilic colloids** (methylcellulose, carboxymethylcellulose [Metamucil], plantago seed, agar, psyllium, bran, and fruits). They exert their effects by absorbing and retaining water, increasing bulk, stimulating colonic peristaltic movements, and lubricating and hydrating the desiccated fecal materials.

These agents are more effective when administered with water. The onset of action of organic salts is relatively fast (2 to 6 hours) and that of colloids is relatively slow (1 to 3 days). These agents, which are very effective and safe, should not be used when the intestinal lumen has been narrowed. The prolonged use of saline cathartics may create problems for certain individuals. For example, magnesium salts have been known to cause hypermagnesemia, coma, and death in patients with renal insufficiency. Sodium salts may also be responsible for causing congestive heart failure.

Lubricants

The lubricants consist of mineral oil and dioctyl sodium sulfonsuccinate (Colace). Colace is used in the pharmaceutical industry as an emulsifying and dispersing substance. Both agents are taken orally. These agents, which do not influence peristalsis, soften desiccated stools or delay the desiccation of fecal materials. They are especially useful in patients with painful bowel movements resulting from inspissated stools or inflammation of the anal sphincter such as occurs with hemorrhoids or anal fissures. Colace is also useful for patients in whom the consequences of "straining at stool" may be harmful.

When used for a long time, mineral oil may come to interfere with the absorption of fat-soluble vitamins and other essential nutrients. Lipid pneumonitis may evolve if mineral oil is used as a vehicle for drugs that are taken nasally.

Other Uses of Laxatives

In Poisoning

Laxatives are used to hasten the elimination and reduce the absorption of a poison that has been taken.

Antihelmintics

Laxatives are used before and after treatment with antihelmintic drugs.

Radiology

Laxatives are used to clean the gastrointestinal tract before radiographic techniques are performed.

CEFACLOR

(Ceclor)

Cefaclor, a second-generation cephalosporin antibiotic (250 to 500 mg p.o. q. 8 hours), is indicated in the treatment of infections of respiratory or urinary tracts, skin, and soft tissue; and in otitis media caused by susceptible organisms.

CEFADROXIL MONOHYDRATE

(Duricef, Ultracef)

Cefadroxil, a first-generation cephalosporin antibiotic (500 to 2 g p.o. daily), is indicated in urinary tract, skin, and soft-tissue infections caused by susceptible organisms.

CEFAMANDOLE NAFATE

(Mandol)

Cefamandole, a second-generation cephalosporin antibiotic (500 mg to 1 g q. 4 to 8 hours), is indicated in the treatment of serious respiratory, genitourinary, skin and soft-tissue, and bone and joint infections; in septicemia; and in peritonitis from susceptible organisms.

CEFAZOLIN SODIUM

(Ancef, Ketzol, Zolicef)

Cefazolin, a first-generation cephalosporin antibiotic (250 mg IM or IV q. 8 hours), is indicated in the treatment of serious respiratory, genitourinary, skin and soft-tissue, and bone and joint infections; septicemia and endocarditis from susceptible organisms.

CEFDITOREN

Cefditoren is a new cephalosporin available for oral administration as the pivaloyloxy methyl ester which is known to possess a broad spectrum of antibacterial activity.

CEFEPINE

Cefepine, the last generation of the first enhanced-potency broad-spectrum cephalosporins, possesses enhanced activity compared with other cephalosporins, and this may result from its improved penetration into the Gram-negative cell and the lower affinity of beta-lactamase for the drug.

CEFIXIME

(Suprax)

Cefixime, a third-generation cephalosporin antibiotic (400 mg p.o. daily in 1 to 2 doses), is indicated in the treatment of otitis media, acute bronchitis, acute exacerbations of chronic bronchitis, pharyngitis, and tonsillitis.

CEFMETAZOLE SODIUM

(Zefazone)

Cefmetazole, a second-generation cephalosporin antibiotic (1 to 8 g IV total dose divided q. 6 to 12 hours), is indicated in the treatment of serious respiratory, urinary, skin and soft-tissue, abdominal, and pelvic infections caused by susceptible organisms. It is also used as surgical prophylaxis.

CEFONICID SODIUM
(Monocid)

Cefonicid, a second-generation cephalosporin antibiotic (1 gm IV or IM q. 24 hours), is indicated in the treatment of serious lower respiratory, urinary tract, skin, and skin-structure infections; in septicemia; and in bone and joint infections from susceptible organisms.

CEFOPERAZONE SODIUM
(Cefobid)

Cefoperazone, a third-generation cephalosporin antibiotic (1 to 2 g q. 12 hours IM or IV), is indicated in the treatment of serious respiratory tract, intra-abdominal, gynecologic, and skin infections; in bacteremia; and in septicemia caused by susceptible organisms.

CEFOTAXIME SODIUM
(Claforan)

Cefotaxime, a third-generation cephalosporin antibiotic (1 g IV or IM q. 6 to 8 hours), is indicated in the treatment of serious lower respiratory, urinary, CNS, gynecologic, and skin infections; in bacteremia; and in septicemia caused by susceptible organisms.

CEFOTETAN DISODIUM
(Cefotan)

Cefotetan, a second-generation cephalosporin antibiotic (1 to 2 g IV or IM q. 12 hours), is indicated in the treatment of serious urinary, lower respiratory, gynecologic, skin, intra-abdominal, and bone and joint infections caused by susceptible organisms.

CEFOXITIN SODIUM
(Mefoxin)

Cefoxitin, a second-generation cephalosporin antibiotic (1 to 2 g q. 6 to 8 hours), is indicated in the treatment of serious respiratory, genitourinary, skin, soft-tissue, bone and joint, blood, and intra-abdominal infections caused by susceptible organisms.

CEFPODOXIME PROXETIL
(Vantin)

Cefpodoxime, a second-generation cephalosporin antibiotic (100 to 400 mg p.o. q. 12 hours for 7 to 14 days depending on infections), is used in the treatment of acute, community-acquired pneumonia caused by non-beta-lactamase-producing strains of *Haemophilus influenzae* or *Streptococcus pneumoniae*; in acute bacterial exacerbations of chronic bronchitis caused by non-beta-lactamase-producing strains of *Haemophilus influenzae, Streptococcus pneumoniae,* or *Moraxella catarrhalis*; in uncomplicated gonorrhea in men and women; rectal gonococcal infections in women; uncomplicated skin and skin-structure infections caused by *Staphylococcus aureus* or *Streptococcus pyogenes*; in acute otitis media caused by *S. pneumoniae, H. influenzae,* or *M. catarrhalis*; pharyngitis or tonsillitis caused by *S. pyogenes*; and in uncomplicated urinary tract infections caused by *Escherichia coli, Klebsiella pneumoniae, Proteus mirabilis,* or *Staphylococcus saprophyticus.*

CEFPROZIL
(Cefzil)

Cefprozil, a second-generation cephalosporin antibiotic, is indicated in the treatment of pharyngitis or tonsillitis caused by *Streptococcus pyrogenes*; otitis media caused by *S. pneumoniae, Haemophilus influenzae,* and *Moraxella (Branhamella) catarrhalis;* in secondary bacterial infections of acute bronchitis and acute bacterial exacerbation of chronic bronchitis caused by *S. pneumoniae, H. influenzae,* and *M. (B.) catarrhalis*; and in uncomplicated skin and skin-structure infections caused by *Staphylococcus aureus* and *Streptococcus pyrogenes.*

CEFTAZIDIME
(Fortaz, Tazicef, Tazidime)

Ceftazidime, a third-generation cephalosporin antibiotic (1 g IV or IM q. 8 to 12 hours), is indicated in the treatment of bacteremia, septicemia, and serious respiratory, urinary, gynecologic, intra-abdominal, CNS, and skin infections from susceptible organisms.

CEFTIZOXIME SODIUM
(Cetizox)

Ceftizoxime, a third-generation cephalosporin antibiotic (1 to 2 g IV or IM q. 8 to 12 hours), is indicated in the treatment of bacteremia, septicemia, meningitis, and serious respiratory, urinary, gynecologic, intra-abdominal, bone and joint, and skin infections from susceptible organisms.

CEFTRIAXONE SODIUM
(Rocephin)

Ceftriaxone, a third-generation cephalosporin antibiotic (1 to 2 g IM or IV once daily), is indicated in the treatment of bacteremia, septicemia, and serious respiratory, urinary, gynecologic, intra-abdominal, and skin infections from susceptible organisms.

CEFUROXIME AXETIL
(Ceftin)

CEFUROXIME SODIUM
(Kefurox, Zinacef)

Cefuroxime, a second-generation cephalosporin antibiotic (750 mg to 1.5 g IM or IV q. 8 hours), is indicated in the treatment of serious lower respiratory, urinary tract, skin and skin-structure infections; in septicemia; and in meningitis caused by susceptible organisms.

CELIPROLOL

Celiprolol is a potent beta$_1$ adrenergic receptor antagonist. It has intrinsic sympathomimetic action, possesses some alpha$_2$-adrenoreceptor antagonistic properties, is a direct vasodilator and a direct bronchodilator. Celiprolol is incompletely and variably absorbed, eliminated both in bile and urine, and has a half-life of 4 to 5 hours. Celiprolol (200 to 400 mg/day) has efficacy similar to atenolol or propranolol in reducing blood pressure and is useful in hypertensive patients with asthma or bronchitis. Furthermore, celiprolol is as effective as atenolol in treating patients with stable angina.

CEPHALEXIN HYDROCHLORIDE
(Keftab)

CEPHALEXIN MONOHYDRATE
(Keflet, Keflex)

Cephalexin, a first-generation cephalosporin antibiotic (250 mg to 1 g p.o. q. 6 hours), is indicated in the treatment of respiratory, genitourinary, skin and soft-tissue, or bone and joint infections, and in otitis media caused by susceptible organisms.

CEPHALOSPORINS

Cephalosporins are structurally related to the penicillins. The nucleus of the cephalosporin, **7-aminocephalosporanic acid**, resembles the nucleus of penicillin, 6-aminopenicillanic acid. Cephalosporins have a broad spectrum of antimicrobial activity and are effective against a variety of Gram-positive and some strains of Gram-negative bacteria, such as *E. coli* and *Klebsiella* and *Proteus* species. In addition, cephalosporins are effective against some strains of *Enterobacter, Serratia,* and *Pseudomonas*. Among the Gram-positive bacteria, the enterococci, penicillin-resistant pneumococci, and methicillin-resistant staphylococci are also resistant to cephalosporins. However, the second-generation and newer cephalosporins, such as cefamandole, cefoxitin, cefuroxime, and moxalactam, offer an even greater spectrum of activity and are more active than the first-generation cephalosporins, such as cephalothin, against Gram-negative microorganisms.

Like the penicillins, cephalosporins exert their effects by inhibiting the formation of cell walls in the bacteria (see Figure 67). Clinical resistance to some of the second- and third-generation cephalosporins has been reported. These agents are resistant to **penicillinase-producing organisms** (see also Table 22).

Cephalexin, cefaclor, cefadroxil, and cephradine are absorbed well from the gastrointestinal tract and thus are given orally. Cephaloridine, cephalothin, cephapirin, cefoxitin, cefotaxime, cefamandole, and cefazolin are poorly absorbed from the gastrointestinal tract and must be given parenterally. Because the cephalosporins have short half-lives, they must be administered frequently. First- and second-generation (but not third-generation) cephalosporins do not readily penetrate the central nervous system and, therefore, are not effective for the treatment of meningitis. The cephalosporins are eliminated by **glomerular filtration** and **active tubular secretion**, which are blocked by probenecid. The acetylated derivatives of cephalosporins, such as cephalothin and cephapirin, are metabolized in the liver to inactive metabolites.

The **first-generation cephalosporins** consist of:

Cephalothin (Keflin) Cephalothin is not absorbed orally.
Cephapirin (Cefadyl)
Cefazolin (Ancef, Kefzol, and others)
Cephalexin (Keflet and Keflex)
Cefadroxil (Duricef and Ultracef)
Cephradine (Anspor and Velocef)

The **second-generation** cephalosporins are:

Cefamandole (Mandol)
Cefoxitin (Mefoxin)
Cefaclor (Ceclor)

Cefuroxime (Kefurox and Zinacef)
Cefuroxime axetil (Ceftin)
Cefonicid (Monocid)
Cefotetan (Cefotan)
Ceforanide (Precef)

These are more active than the first-generation cephalosporins against certain Gram-negative organisms, including *Haemophilus influenzae, Enterobacter* species, indole-positive *Proteus* species, *E. coli,* and *Klebsiella* species.

The **third-generation** cephalosporins are:

Cefotaxime (Claforan)
Ceftizoxime (Cefizox)
Ceftriaxone (Rocephin)
Cefoperazone (Cefobid)
Ceftazidime (Fortaz and others)

The pharmacologic features of the third-generation cephalosporins vary widely for each drug. They are effective in treating infections caused by aerobic Gram-negative organisms.

Decreased renal function affects the elimination of most third-generation cephalosporins, whereas the presence of hepatic disease does not require dose adjustment.

The cephalosporins, often in combination with aminoglycoside antibiotics, are used in suspected cases of bacteremia due to *Staphylococcus, Klebsiella*, coliform bacteria, *Proteus*, or *Pseudomonas* infection.

Cephalosporins may be used as alternative agents to penicillin G for the treatment of streptococcal and pneumococcal infections. The third-generation cephalosporins are the drugs of choice in Gram-negative bacillary meningitis. Cephalosporins are used on a very limited basis as prophylaxis prior to and following some surgical procedures that carry high risks for infections.

The adverse reactions caused by cephalosporins resemble those to be named for penicillin, and include injection-site complications, phlebitis following intravenous administration, hypersensitivity reactions, and rare anaphylactoid shock. Infrequently, nephrotoxicity does occur with some cephalosporins.

CEPHALOSPORINS		
First-Generation Cephalosporins	Cefazolin	Parenteral use only
	Cephalexin	Parenteral use only
	Cephalothin	Oral or parenteral administration
	Cephradine	Oral administration
Second-Generation Cephalosporins	Cefaclor	
	Cefamandole	
	Cefonicid	
	Cefotetan	
	Cefoxitin	
	Cefuroxime	
Third-Generation Cephalosporins	Cefoperazone	
	Cefotaxime	
	Ceftazidime	
	Ceftizoxime	
	Ceftriaxone	

CEPHALOTHIN SODIUM
(Keflin, Seffin)

Cephalothin, a first-generation cephalosporin antibiotic (500 mg to 1 g IM or IV q. 4 to 6 hours), is indicated in the treatment of serious respiratory, genitourinary, GI, skin and soft-tissue, bone and joint infections; in septicemia; and in endocarditis and meningitis.

CEPHAPIRIN SODIUM
(Cefadyl)

Cephapirin, a first-generation cephalosporin antibiotic (500 mg to 1 g IV of IM q. 4 to 6 hours), is indicated in the treatment of serious respiratory, genitourinary, GI, skin and soft-tissue, bone and joint infections (including osteomyelitis); in septicemia; and in endocarditis.

CEPHRADINE
(Anspor, Velosef)

Cephradine, a first-generation cephalosporin antibiotic (500 mg to 1 g IM or IV b.i.d.), is indicated in the treatment of serious respiratory, genitourinary, GI, skin and soft-tissue, bone and joint infections; and septicemia, endocarditis, and otitis media.

CEREBROACTIVE MEDICATIONS	
Bamethan	Naftidrofuryl
Bencyclane	Nicergoline
Bethahistine	Nicotinic acid derivatives
Cinnarizine	Nylidrin
Citicoline	Pentoxifylline
Cyclandelate	Papaverine
Dihydroergocristine	Pinacidil
Dihydroergotoxine	Piracetam
Ebunamonine	Piribedil
Flunarizine	Raubasine
Ginkgo-biloba extracts	Suloctidil
Isoxsuprine	Vincamine

These allegedly cerebroactive and vasodilating medications have been tried in vascular disorders. Their pharmacological properties are complex and their values remain to be established. For example, as a vasodilator pinacidil is three- and tenfold more potent than hydralazine and minoxidil, respectively. It does not interact with alpha, beta, cholinergic, or histaminergic receptors, and also does not produce vasodilation via an indirect effect that is mediated by adenosine, prostaglandin, or endothelial-derived relaxant factor. Its vasodilating activity does not resemble that brought about by the conventional calcium-channel antagonists. Thus, pinacidil-induced vascular relaxation is a direct effect mediated by a novel mechanism.

CETIRIZINE
(Reactine)

Cetirizine is indicated in the treatment of pollen-associated asthma in individuals with angioedema, atopic dermatitis, and certain types of physical urticaria such as delayed pressure urticaria, dermatographia and cold urticaria. **Terfenadine, astemizole, loratadine**, and **cetirizine** are **second-generation** antihistaminic agents that are relatively **nonsedating**. Cetirizine is a carboxylated metabolite of hydroxyzine (Vistaril), a piperazine derivative H_1 receptor antagonist. Cetirizine inhibits both histamine release and eosinophil chemotaxis during the secondary phase of the allergic response. It reduces inflammatory cell infiltration (i.e., eosinophils, neutrophils, basophils) by 75% during the late-phase response.

Cetirizine 10 mg is more potent than terfenadine 60 mg, loratadine (Claritin) 10 mg, and chlorpheniramine (e.g., Chlor-Trimeton) 6 mg, and equal in potency to diphenhydramine (e.g., Benadryl) 50 mg, hydroxyzine 25 mg, and terfenadine 180 mg. Cetirizine is absorbed well when given orally, is bound to plasma protein to the extent of 93%, does not cross the blood-brain barrier, has an elimination half-life of 7 to 10 hours, and is excreted mostly unchanged in the urine. The half-life of cetirizine is increased in renal impairment, requiring smaller dosage.

CHEMOPROTECTANTS

(e.g., Amifostine, Dexrazoxane)

One of the goals of cancer chemotherapy is to enhance the efficacy of antineoplastic agents and at the same time protect the nonmalignant tissues using chemoprotective agents. A few of the chemoenhancers and chemoprotectors are listed below:

Chemoenhancers	Chemoprotectors
Calcium channel blockers	Amifostine
Phenothiazines	Thiosulfate
Cyclosporine	Diethyldithiocarbamate
Buthionine suloximime	Diuretics, phorbol esters
Tamoxifen	Bismuth salts
Triparanol	Oxothiazolidine-4-carboxylate
Acridines	Glutathione esters
Amiodarone	Steroids
Phorbol esters	Metallothionein
Streptozocin	Dexrazoxane
Progesterone	
Ethacrynic acid	

Anthyracycline antibiotics (e.g., doxorubicin) causes unique cardiomyopathies. An acute form is characterized by abnormal electrocardiographic changes, including ST-T wave alterations and arrhthymias. This is brief and rarely a serious problem. Cineangiographic studies have shown an acute, reversible reduction in ejection fraction 24 hours after a single dose. An exaggerated manifestation of acute myocardial damage, the **"pericarditis-myocarditis syndrome,"** may be characterized by severe disturbances in impulse conduction and frank congestive heart failure, often associated with pericardial effusion. Chronic, cumulative dose-related toxicity is manifested by congestive heart failure that is unresponsive to digitalis.

Cardiac irradiation or administration of high doses of cyclophosphamide or another anthracycline may increase the risk of cardiotoxicity. There is evidence that cardiac damage is reduced by the concomitant administration of the iron chelator dexrazoxane (ADR-529) or by amifostine (WR-2721) or its active metabolite (WR-1065).

CHENODIOL

(Chenix)

Chenodiol, a bile acid with cholelitholytic properties (250 mg b.i.d. for two weeks), is indicated in dissolution of radiolucent cholesterol stones (gallstones) when systemic disease or age precludes surgery; and to increase bile flow in patients with bile duct prostheses or stents.

CHLAMYDIAL INFECTIONS: TREATMENT OF	
Infections	**Medications**
Uncomplicated urethral, endocervical, or rectal infection in adults	Doxycycline 100 mg p.o. two times daily for 7 days **or** Tetracycline 500 mg p.o. four times daily for 7 days
Urogenital infections during pregnancy	Erythromycin base 500 mg p.o. four times daily for 7 days **or** Erythromycin ethyl succinate 800 mg p.o. four times daily for 7 days (or 400 mg p.o. four times daily for 14 days)
Conjunctivitis of the newborn	Erythromycin suspension 50 mg/kg/d p.o. in four divided doses for 14 days)
Pneumonia in infants	Erythromycin suspension 50 mg/kg/d p.o. in four divided doses for 14 days
Acute epididymo-orchitis	Amoxicillin 3.0 g p.o., or ampicillin 3.5 g p.o., or aqueous procaine penicillin G 4.8 million units IM at two sites (each along with probenecid 1.0 g p.o.), or spectinomycin 2.0 g IM or ceftriaxone 250 mg IM followed by tetracycline 500 p.o. four times daily for 10 days **or** Doxycycline 100 mg p.o. two times daily for 10 days

CHLORAL HYDRATE

(Noctec, Somnos)

Chloral hydrate (500 to 1000 mg taken 15 to 30 minutes before bedtime) is indicated for nocturnal sedation in patients intolerant to barbiturates or benzodiazepine derivatives. It may be used in candidates for surgery to alleviate anxiety and induce sleep without depressing respiration or cough reflex. Chloral hydrate rectal suppositories are available. The CNS depressant effects of chloral hydrate are believed to be due to **trichlorethanol**, its metabolite. Chloral hydrate has additive CNS depressing effects when taken with alcohol. Chloral hydrate, when used on a chronic basis, is known to be habit forming. The toxic dose of chloral hydrate is 10 grams producing hypothermia, hypotension, slow- or rapid shallow breathing, pinpoint pupils, and comatose state. In surviving individuals, hepatic and renal impairments may result.

CHLORAMBUCIL

(Leukeran)

Chlorambucil (0.1 to 0.2 mg/kg/day for 3 to 6 weeks) will provide palliation in chronic lymphocytic leukemia, malignant lymphomas including lymphosarcoma, giant follicular lymphoma, and Hodgkin's disease. In addition, it has been used in the treatment of uveitis and meningoencephalitis associated with Behcet's disease. Chlorambucil is absorbed orally, metabolized extensively, and the metabolite is excreted in the urine. Chlorambucil causes reversible bone marrow suppression, hepatotoxicity with jaundice, infertility, sterility, bronchopulmonary dysplasia, seizures in susceptible individuals, and gastrointestinal problems such as oral ulceration, nausea, vomiting, or diarrhea. Chlorambucil, which is carcinogenic, mutagenic, and teratogenic should be used cautiously in all subjects including patients with leukemia and malignant lymphomas. Radiation therapy will enhance chlorambucil-induced bone marrow depression.

CHLORAMPHENICOL

(Chloromycetin)

Chloramphenicol is indicated for infection caused by susceptible strains of *Salmonella* species; and *H. influenzae*, specifically, meningeal infections and rickettsiae; for the lymphogranuloma-psittacosis group and various Gram-negative bacteria causing bacteremia, meningitis, or other serious Gram-negative infections; for infections involving anaerobic organisms when *Bacteroides fragilis* is suspected; and for other susceptible organisms which have been demonstrated to be resistant to all other appropriate antimicrobial agents.

Chloramphenicol has a broad spectrum of bacteriostatic activity for many bacteria, including *Rickettsia*. It is the preferred drug in the treatment of *Salmonella* infection (e.g., typhoid fever); *Haemophilus influenzae*, meningitis, laryngotracheitis, or pneumonia not responding to ampicillin; in *Bacteroides* infections and meningococcal infections in patients allergic to penicillin, and in *Rickettsia* infections (see also Figure 80).

Chloramphenicol exerts its effects by binding to 50S ribosomal subunits and thus inhibiting bacterial protein synthesis by preventing peptide-bond formation and by inhibiting the synthesis of mitochondrial proteins in the host. The resistance of chloramphenicol stems from the production of chloramphenicol acetyltransferase by microorganisms, which metabolizes the drug.

Chloramphenicol is completely absorbed from the gastrointestinal tract and is distributed widely throughout the body, including the cerebrospinal fluid. It is metabolized in the liver by glucuronyl transferase, and the metabolites are excreted by the kidneys. Newborn infants cannot metabolize chloramphenicol readily.

Chloramphenicol causes both dose-dependent and dose-independent hematologic reactions. Fatal **aplastic anemia** occurs in genetically susceptible patients taking chloramphenicol on a long-term basis. Reversible and dose-dependent disturbances of **hemopoiesis** can also arise, and are characterized by the altered maturation of red blood cells, vacuolated nucleated red blood cells in the marrow, and reticulocytopenia.

Newborn infants are deficient in **glucuronyl transferase**. Thus, when treating newborns, doses of chloramphenicol should not exceed 50 mg/kg per day. Large doses will precipitate **gray baby syndrome**, characterized by vomiting, hypothermia, gray skin tone, and shock.

CHLORAZEPATE DIPOTASSIUM
(Tranxene)

Chlorazepate, which enhances GABAergic transmission (see Figure 40), is indicated in acute alcohol withdrawal, in anxiety disorders, and as an adjunct in seizure management. Chlorazepate is hydrolyzed in the stomach to desmethyldiazepam, which is then absorbed completely, and bound to plasma proteins to the extent of 80 to 95%. Desmethyldiazepam is then metabolized to oxazepam, whose inactive metabolite conjugated to glucuronic acid is excreted in the urine.

Chlorazepate potentiates the CNS depressant effects of phenothiazines, narcotics, barbiturates, alcohol, antihistamines, monoamine oxidase inhibitors, general anesthetics, and antidepressants. Concomitant use with cimetidine and possibly disulfiram causes diminished hepatic metabolism of chlorazepate, which increases its plasma concentration.

Clinical manifestations of overdose with chlorazepate include somnolence, confusion, coma, hypoactive reflexes, dyspnea, labored breathing, hypotension, bradycardia, slurred speech, and unsteady gait or impaired coordination.

CHLORCYCLIZINE
(Mantadil)

Noscapine (Nectadon) is a naturally occurring opium alkaloid with a structure and function similar to papaverine's. It is antitussive and has no analgesic or additive properties.

Diphenhydramine and **chlorcyclizine** are antihistaminic agents that also have antitussive properties. **Dimethoxanate** (Cothera) and **pipazethate** (Theratuss) are phenothiazine derivatives without analgesic but with weak antitussive and local anesthetic properties.

CHLORDIAZEPOXIDE
(Librium)

Chlordiazepoxide is indicated for the management of anxiety disorders, for the short-term relief of symptoms of anxiety, for symptoms of acute alcohol withdrawal; and for preoperative apprehension and anxiety.

Chlordiazepoxide, a weakly basic substance, is unstable both in solution and when exposed to ultraviolet light. Thus, oral preparations are protected with opaque capsules, and solutions for parenteral injection must be prepared fresh and used immediately. The absorption of chlordiazepoxide from intramuscular sites is erratic and unpredictable. Thus, the oral and intravenous routes are used when reliable or rapid effects are desired. Chlordiazepoxide disappears from the plasma rapidly, but its metabolites, desmethylchlordiazepoxide, demoxepam, and desmethyldiazepam, are eliminated more slowly.

Chlordiazepoxide is about 94 to 97% bound to plasma proteins and has a **distribution volume** of 0.3 to 0.4 L/kg in males and a somewhat larger volume in females.

The **rate of elimination** of chlordiazepoxide is prolonged in the elderly, the clearance in those over 60 years of age being about half that of young adults. The elderly are also more "sensitive" to the CNS effects of chlordiazepoxide; thus, they should be given smaller doses. Clearance of chlordiazepoxide is also reduced in patients with cirrhosis, as are the rate and extent of formation of desmethylchlordiazepoxide. **Disulfiram** inhibits the metabolism of chlordiazepoxide (see also Figure 40 and Table 8).

CHLORGYLINE

Monoamine oxidase inhibitors are classified into A and B types. **Monoamine oxidase A** preferentially uses serotonin and norepinephrine as substrates and is inhibited by **chlorgyline** and harmaline. **Monoamine oxidase B** preferentially uses dopamine and is inhibited by **selegiline** (see also Figures 23 and 27).

CHLOROPROCAINE
(Nesacaine)

Chloroprocaine (1 to 2% injection with methylparaben as a preservative) is indicated for the production of local anesthesia by infiltration and peripheral nerve block. Chloroprocaine without methylparaben is indicated for peripheral and central nerve block, including lumbar and caudal epidural blocks. Chloroprocaine has an onset of action of 6 to 12 minutes.

Chloroprocaine, like other local anesthetics, blocks the generation and the conduction of nerve impulses, presumably by increasing the threshold for electrical excitation in the nerve by slowing the propagation of the nerve impulse and by reducing the rate of rise of the action potential. In general, the progression of anesthesia is related to the diameter, myelination, and conduction velocity of affected nerve fibers. Clinically, the order of loss of nerve function is as follows: pain, temperature, touch, proprioception, and skeletal muscle tone.

The adverse reactions of chloroprocaine, which are dose-dependent and may result from rapid absorption from injection site or unintentional intravascular injection, are central nervous system reactions (restlessness, anxiety, dizziness, tinnitus, blurred vision, tremor, and even convulsions) and cardiovascular reactions (depression of myocardium, bradycardia, hypotension, arrhythmias, and even cardiac arrest) (see also Figure 20).

CHLOROQUINE PHOSPHATE
(Aralen)

Chloroquine is indicated for prophylaxis and treatment of acute attacks of malaria due to *P. vivax, P. malariae, P. ovale,* and susceptible strains of *P. falcinarum.* It is also used for treatment of extraintestinal amebiasis. Chloroquine destroys schizonts in erythrocytes by interfering with DNA synthesis. The phosphate salts are active orally, whereas the hydrochloride salt is used for intravenous purposes. It accumulates in normal and parasitized erythrocytes. Overdosage has caused reversible corneal damage and permanent retinal damage. In toxic doses, chloroquine causes visual disturbances, hyperexcitability, convulsions, and heart block. It is an antimalarial of choice in all cases except chloroquine-resistant *Plasmodium falciparum.* In addition, it has a certain degree of effectiveness in amebiasis and in the late stages of rheumatoid arthritis. **Amodiaquine** (Camoquin) may be used as an alternate drug.

CHLOROTHIAZIDE
(Diuril)

Thiazides and related diuretics (see Table 25) are used in edema associated with congestive heart failure, hepatic cirrhosis, nephrotic syndrome, acute glomerulonephritis, or chronic renal failure. Thiazides are used as sole therapeutic agents, or in combination with other drugs in the management of hypertension. Thiazides in combination with amiloride or allopurinol have been used to prevent formation and recurrence of calcium nephrolithiasis in hypercalciuric and normal calciuric patients. Thiazide in combination with calcium and estrogen may be helpful in postmenopausal osteoporosis. Thiazide is useful in treating nephrogenic diabetes insipidus (see also Figure 4 and Table 25).

The thiazide diuretics, also called **sulfonamide** or **benzothiazide diuretics**, vary in their actions. For instance, the potency of **hydrochlorothiazide** (Hydro-Diuril and Esidrix) is ten times greater than that of **chlorothiazide** (Diuril), but the two drugs have equal efficacy. The duration of action of hydrochlorothiazide, which is 6 to 12 hours, is equal to that of chlorothiazide. On the other hand, **chlorthalidone** (Hygroton) has a duration of action lasting 48 hours. Some thiazide derivatives inhibit carbonic anhydrase, which is unrelated to their diuretic activity. Those that are active in this respect, may at sufficient dose, have the same effect on bicarbonate excretion as does acetazolamide. They cause a moderate loss of sodium (5 to 10% of the filtered load), chloride, and water, and the clearance of free water is impaired. They may cause **metabolic alkalosis** (resorption of bicarbonate and loss of hydrogen ions), **hyperuricemia** (enhanced resorption of uric acid), or **hyperglycemia** (inhibiting insulin release directly and due to **hypokalemia**).

Thiazide diuretics are used in the treatment of edema of cardiac and gastrointestinal origin and bring about a state of intravascular volume depletion. Because this depleted intravascular volume is replenished from the interstitial (edematous) sites, the thiazide diuretics should not be administered too frequently. For example, hydrochlorothiazide is given every other day and chlorthalidone is given once every 2 to 3 days. In small doses, thiazide diuretics are extremely effective in controlling essential hypertension. They exert their effects initially by bringing about volume depletion, then reduce the peripheral resistance and sensitivity of vascular receptor sites to catecholamine. Thiazide diuretics are also used in conjunction with antihypertensive medications.

The thiazides decrease the urinary calcium concentration by diminishing glomerular filtration and also enhance the urinary magnesium level. The thiazide diuretics can reduce free water formation in patients with diabetes insipidus, in whom large amounts of free water are eliminated. The loss of potassium can produce **hypokalemia**, which is particularly dangerous in patients receiving **digitalis** because it increases the risk of **arrhythmias**. Hypokalemia can be offset either by giving a potassium supplement (potassium chloride), or by the concurrent use of a potassium-sparing diuretic. However, not both measures should be adopted because **hyperkalemia** will result. **Hyperglycemia** is a potential hazard for patients with **diabetes mellitus. Hyperuricemia** can precipitate an acute attack of gout, but usually only in those patients who either have already had gout or have a propensity toward it. Since thiazides can cause a decrease in the GFR, they should not be used in patients whose renal function is less than one third of normal. The risk of thiazide-induced **hypercalcemia** should be kept in mind in patients with conditions such as **malignancies** or **hyperparathyroidism** that are associated with hypercalcemia.

CHLOROTRIANISENE

(Tace)

Chlorotrianisene is a nonsteroidal synthetic estrogen which is used in postpartum breast engorgement (12 mg 4 times/day for 7 days), vasomotor symptoms associated with menopause (12 mg/day cyclically for 30 days), atrophic vaginitis and *Kraurosis vulvae* (12 mg/day cyclically for 60 days), female hypogonadism (12 mg/day cyclically for 21 days), and inoperable prostate carcinoma (12 mg/day given chronically) (see also Figures 26 and 38).

CHLORPHENESINE CARBAMATE

(Maolate)

Chlorphenesine (400 to 800 mg t.i.d.) is indicated as an adjunct to rest and physical therapy for the relief of discomfort associated with acute and painful musculoskeletal conditions. Chlorphenesine-induced muscular relaxation may be related to its sedative properties, since it does not exert its effects either directly on skeletal muscles or myoneural junctions.

CHLORPHENIRAMINE MALEATE

(Chlor-Trimeton)

Chlorpheniramine (4 mg q. 4 to 6 hours) is an alkylamine derivative H_1 antihistaminic agent which is indicated in perennial and seasonal allergic rhinitis, vasomotor rhinitis, allergic conjunctivitis due to inhalant allergens and foods, mild, uncomplicated allergic skin manifestations of urticaria and angioedema, amelioration of allergic reactions to blood or plasma, demographism, or as therapy for anaphylactic reactions adjunctive to epinephrine and other standard measures after the acute manifestations have been controlled.

Chlorpheniramine has anticholinergic properties and hence is contraindicated in narrow-angle glaucoma, prostatic hypertrophy, stenosing peptic ulcer, pyloroduodenal obstruction, and bladder neck obstruction. In addition, it has sedative properties, and the drug may impair alertness needed to complete hazardous tasks. Chlorpheniramine maleate (2 mg)/codeine phosphate (10 mg)/guaifenesin (100 mg) is indicated for its antiallergic, antitussive, expectorant, and mucolytic properties and is marketed as **Tussar**. Chlorpheniramine maleate/codeine phosphate/phenylephrine hydrochloride/potassium iodide (**Demi-Cof**) is marketed for its antiallergic, antitussive, expectorant, and mucolytic properties to be used in common cold associated with bronchitis. Many other preparations containing chlorpheniramine sold as

Novahistine-Dh, Chem-Tuss, Anaplex-Hd, D-Allergy, Ru-Tuss, and **Lantussforte** are indicated for their antitussive properties associated with allergies and common cold.

CHLORPROMAZINE
(Thorazine)

Chlorpromazine is indicated for the management of manifestations of psychotic disorders, to control nausea and vomiting (see Figure 73), for relief of restlessness and apprehension before surgery, for acute intermittent porphyria, as an adjunct in the treatment of tetanus, to control the manifestations of the manic type of manic-depressive illness, for relief of intractable **hiccups**, for the treatment of severe behavioral problems in children marked by combativeness and/or explosive hyperexcitable behavior, and in the short-term treatment of hyperactive children who show excessive motor activity with accompanying conduct disorders consisting of some or all of the following symptoms: impulsivity, difficulty sustaining attention, aggressiveness, mood lability, and poor frustration tolerance.

Chlorpromazine is well absorbed mainly from the jejunum. It is extensively metabolized in the liver, which produces several active metabolites. When given intramuscularly, the phenothiazine neuroleptics avoid metabolic degradation (first-pass metabolism), making them more beneficial as long-acting depot antipsychotics (see Table 23).

Chlorpromazine produces a **tranquility** characterized by a detached serenity without depression of mental faculties or clouding of consciousness. It depresses the central nervous system (CNS) selectively by reducing input directed to the reticular formation through collaterals arriving from the sensory pathways. Chlorpromazine-induced sedation differs from that caused by barbiturates in that the patient can be easily aroused. In practice, the more sedative neuroleptics are often prescribed for agitated, overactive patients, and the less sedative agents are used for apathetic, withdrawn patients. However, **sedation** is not necessary for its antipsychotic property for two reasons: (1) tolerance develops to the sedative effects, and (2) **fluphenazine, prochlorperazine**, and **trifluoperazine** are excellent neuroleptics that lack pronounced sedative effects.

In general, chlorpromazine and other neuroleptics **reduce spontaneous motor activity** in proportion to their dosages.

The nausea and vomiting associated with circulating physical agents (radiation therapy and virus particles) or chemical agents (toxins and cancer chemotherapeutic agents) that stimulate the **chemoreceptor trigger zone for emesis** are treated with the phenothiazine derivatives such as chlorpromazine, perphenazine, promethazine, triethylperazine, and triflupromazine. With the exception of thioridazine (Mellaril), all have antiemetic effects because they depress the chemoreceptor zone for emesis. Larger than therapeutic doses inhibit the vomiting center (see Figure 73).

The phenothiazine derivatives are hypothermic, and the extent of hypothermia depends on the dosage and the environmental temperature. Substances that reduce the concentrations of norepinephrine (reserpine) or block its receptor site (chlorpromazine) are hypothermic, whereas substances that increase the release of norepinephrine (amphetamine) are hyperthermic.

Phenothiazine derivatives cause postural or orthostatic hypotension. This may be more pronounced in patients with reduced vascular volume resulting from acute hemorrhage or dehydration, and when used with diuretic agents. Hypotension is more frequent with phenothiazine derivatives having either an **aliphatic substitution** on N_{10} (e.g., chlorpromazine) or a **piperidine substitution** on N_{10} (e.g., mesoridazine or thioridazine). It occurs less frequently with compounds containing a piperazine substitution (e.g., trifluoperazine). The hypotension is due to direct vasodilation and an alpha-adrenergic receptor-blocking effect. The pressor effects of epinephrine can be reduced, blocked, or reversed by appropriate doses of chlorpromazine.

Surgical patients who are premedicated with chlorpromazine respond poorly to pressor drugs, requiring larger than anticipated doses. The **inotropic** effects of epinephrine (increase in the strength of muscular contraction) are reduced by chlorpromazine. The **chronotropic** effects of epinephrine (increase in the rate of contraction) are increased as the result of chlorpromazine's anticholinergic properties. The local vasoconstrictor action of epinephrine (as used with a local anesthetic) is blocked by chlorpromazine, but its hyperglycemic effect is not. The lethal effect of toxic doses of epinephrine or norepinephrine can be reversed by chlorpromazine.

Most phenothiazine neuroleptics (see Table 23) have weak anticholinergic properties. However, the anticholinergic effects of **thioridazine** or **ethaproprazine** are pronounced, and all the cautions cited for atropine apply to these agents as well. Indeed, fatal **tachyarrhythmias** and other electrocardiographic changes such as blunting and notching of T waves, prolongation of the QT interval, increased convexity of the ST segment, and appearance of V waves have been caused through the injudicious use of thioridazine (1500 to 3600 mg/day), especially in elderly patients.

Nausea, which may be patient related, occurs frequently with psychotropic drugs, but the incidence is also high in schizophrenic patients who are receiving placebo. Furthermore, the incidence of vomiting with thioridazine, which has no antiemetic effect, is high. Dry mouth, constipation, paralytic ileus, and decreased gastric secretion, which are all due to its **anticholinergic effects**, may occur.

Phenothiazine derivatives have been observed to cause jaundice in 5% of the patients. The jaundice is accompanied by intense pruritus, fever, chills, nausea, epigastric or right upper quadrant abdominal pain, and malaise. The jaundice is not dose dependent and develops after a typical delay of 2 to 3 weeks. With discontinuation of medication, the prognosis has been excellent.

Phenothiazine derivatives (thioridazine, trifluoperazine, prochlorperazine, and fluphenazine) have been known to cause reversible **galactorrhea**. This commonly occurs with large doses and long-term treatment. It arises because dopamine normally inhibits the release of **prolactin**, but, by blocking dopamine receptor sites, neuroleptics nullify this action. Thioridazine causes a reversible ejaculation disorder, in that erection and orgasm occurs without ejaculation. **Bromocriptine mesylate** (Parlodel), a dopaminergic agonist used in the treatment of parkinsonism, has been shown to be effective in **preventing postpartum lactation**. Chlorpromazine, by preventing the release of insulin, may cause diabetes mellitus in a borderline individual or unstabilize a diabetic patient.

Chlorpromazine and other phenothiazine derivatives (perphenazine, prochlorperazine, thioridazine, and triflupromazine) may cause **agranulocytosis**. The incidence of these side effects is higher among female and elderly patients whose bone marrow has lower proliferative potential. These agents inhibit DNA polymerase, thymidylate kinase, and the incorporation of ^{3}H-thymidine into DNA. Because the phenothiazine-induced agranulocytosis is a toxic reaction, it may be prevented by carefully monitoring the status of peripheral blood.

The dermatologic reactions following the use of phenothiazine derivatives can be divided into three categories: solar sensitivity, allergic dermatitis, and pigment retinopathy.

Solar sensitivity, which occurs only in sun-exposed areas of the body such as the hands and face, can be prevented by having patients avoid exposure to the sun.

Allergic dermatitis, which may be maculopapular, urticarial, or pruritic, should be regarded as a hypersensitivity reaction. Medication should be discontinued and other supportive therapy initiated.

Pigment retinopathy is manifested by the deposition of dotlike particles in the anterior capsular and subcapsular portion of the lens, pupillary area, cornea, conjunctiva, and retina. It is thought that, in the presence of ultraviolet light, the highly reactive metabolites of phenothiazine form free radicals that undergo covalent linkage with melanin. The synthesis of melanocyte-stimulating hormone, like that of prolactin, is stimulated following treatment with phenothiazine derivatives. These side effects may be prevented by using the lowest possible maintenance doses of neuroleptics, and by observing **"drug-free holidays"** to reduce the endogenous concentrations of neuroleptics which have long and protracted half-lives.

A variety of neurologic syndromes, involving particularly the extrapyramidal system, occur following short- or long-term use of neuroleptic (antipsychotic) drugs. These include **akathisia, dystonia, neuroleptic malignant syndrome, parkinsonism**, and **tardive dyskinesia**.

Akathisia is characterized by an inability to sit still, by shifting of the legs and tapping of feet while sitting, and by rocking and shifting of the weight while standing. This "motoric restlessness" is not caused by agitation or anxiety, occurs more frequently among female and elderly patients, is stopped volitionally, returns spontaneously when it is not controlled consciously, and is aggravated by physical inactivity. Reducing the total dosage of neuroleptic medications and the addition of either an anticholinergic drug, one of the benzodiazepine derivatives, or propranolol have been shown to reduce the severity of akathisia. **Restless legs syndrome** is characterized by a creeping or crawling sensation that most frequently affects movements in sleep; it is also called **nocturnal myoclonus** and causes intense and repetitive muscle jerking during sleep. Treatment with 100 to 200 mg of levodopa, levodopa plus **benserazide, bromocriptine**, or **piribedil** has been reported to be beneficial in managing both movement disorders.

Dystonia is characterized by an exaggerated posturing of the head, neck, or jaw; by spastic contraction of the muscles of the lips, tongue, face, or throat, which makes drinking, eating, swallowing, and speech difficult; by torticollis, retrocollis, opisthotonus, distress, and ultimately anoxia. Neuroleptic-induced dystonia, which may occur in children treated actively with phenothiazine derivatives for their antiemetic properties, disappears in sleep and is treated effectively with **diphenhydramine hydrochloride** (Benadryl), which possesses both anticholinergic and antihistaminic properties.

Parkinsonian symptoms may be characterized by postural instability, stooped posture, shuffling and festinating gate, or rigidity, due to enhanced muscle tone, with, at times, "cogwheel" or "ratchet" resistance to passive movements in any direction. There is also tremor at rest with regular rhythmic oscillations of the extremities, especially in the hands and fingers as well as akinesia (poverty of movement) or bradykinesia (slowness in initiating volitional activities). These symptoms, which are due to blockade of dopaminergic receptor sites in the striatum, are lessened by reducing the dosage of neuroleptics and by the oral administration of anticholinergic compounds, such as **trihexyphenidyl hydrochloride** (Artane) or **benztropine mesylate** (Cogentin).

Tardive dyskinesia, which was initially called *persistent dyskinesia* or *reversible drug-related dyskinesia,* is characterized by abnormal involuntary movements frequently involving the facial, buccal, and masticatory muscles and often extending to the upper and lower extremities, including the neck, trunk, fingers, and toes. For example, the typical abnormal facial movements include opening, protrusion, and retrieval of the tongue then closing of the mouth, chewing, licking, sucking, puckering, smacking, panting, and grimacing. Abnormal movements associated with the disorder, which may involve any part of the body, may be ballistic, athetotic, myoclonic, dyskinetic, or choreiform. The neuroleptic-induced dyskinesias, which have been reported and studied extensively in adult patients, also occur in children. It is generally believed that the **pathogenesis** of tardive dyskinesia relates closely to the ongoing **blockade of dopamine receptor sites**, which is the opposite of receptor desensitization. With continuous blockade, the dopaminergic receptors in the striatum up-regulate. Following the discontinued use of neuroleptics or a reduction in dosage, the dyskinesia becomes apparent. In the therapeutic management of neuroleptic-induced tardive dyskinesia, reserpine, lithium, diazepam, baclofen (see Figure 17), and gamma-vinyl-gamma-aminobutyric acid (vigabatrin) (see Figure 96) have all been used with unsatisfactory results. Therefore, in the absence of an effective treatment, the best prevention of tardive dyskinesia is to prescribe the neuroleptics at their lowest possible doses, have patients observe drug-free holidays, and avoid prescribing anticholinergic agents solely to prevent parkinsonism.

Neuroleptic Malignant Syndrome
Among the complications of neuroleptic chemotherapy, the most serious and potentially fatal complication is **malignant syndrome**, which is characterized by extreme hyperthermia; "lead pipe" skeletal muscle rigidity that causes dyspnea, dysphagia, and rhabdomyolysis; autonomic instability; fluctuating consciousness; leukeocytosis; and elevated creatine phosphokinase levels.

The treatment of neuroleptic malignant syndrome consists of immediately discontinuing the neuroleptic agent and administering **dantrolene sodium** and dopamine function-enhancing substances such as **levodopa-carbidopa, bromocriptine,** or **amantadine**.

Phenothiazine derivatives potentiate the CNS-depressing effects of alcohol and barbiturates and shorten the onset of action of anesthetics.

CHLORPROPAMIDE
(Diabinese)

Chlorpropamide (250 mg/day), an oral hypoglycemic agent, is indicated in the treatment of diabetic patients (see Table 1 and Figure 44). Oral hypoglycemic agents have advantages over insulin, because, by releasing insulin and by decreasing the release of glucagon, they mimic physiologic processes and cause fewer allergic reactions. Furthermore, they are effective in an oral form, thus eliminating the need for daily injections. The properties of chlorpropamide are compared in Table 1 with other orally administered hypoglycemic agents. The mechanisms that underlie the hypoglycemic actions of **sulfonylureas** are:

Pancreatic
    Improved insulin secretion
    Reduced glucagon secretion
Extrapancreatic
    Improved tissue sensitivity to insulin
Direct
    Increased receptor binding
    Improved post-binding action
Indirect
    Reduced hyperglycemia
    Decreased plasma free fatty-acid concentrations
    Reduced hepatic insulin extraction

Sulfonylurea oral hypoglycemic agents bind to sulfonylurea receptors located on the surface of beta cells and trigger insulin releases at nanomolar concentrations (Figure 44). Sulfonylureas bind to ATP-sensitive potassium channels and inhibit potassium efflux through these channels. The inhibition of ATP-sensitive potassium channels then leads to depolarization of the beta cell; this opens voltage-dependent calcium channels and allows the entry of extracellular calcium. The rising level of cytosolic free calcium next triggers the release of insulin. An increase in the cyclic adenosine monophosphate levels in the cells can also open the voltage-dependent calcium channels, thus increasing calcium influx into the cells.

CHLORPROTHIXENE

(Taractan)

Chlorprothixene (25 to 50 mg p.o. t.i.d.) is indicated for the management of manifestations of psychotic disorders. Chlorprothixene is absorbed rapidly, distributed throughout the body, is bound to plasma protein to the extent of 90 to 95%, and is excreted mostly unchanged via the biliary tract in feces. It exerts its antipsychotic effects in part by blocking dopamine receptors in the mesolimbic and mesocortical systems; and like chlorpromazine, it produces movement disorders such as parkinsonism (see also Table 23).

CHLORTETRACYCLINE HYDROCHLORIDE

(Aureomycin)

Chlortetracycline (see **Tetracycline**) is an antibiotic available for eye, ear, nose, and throat preparation. For example, it is available as 1% ointment to treat conjunctivitis and blepharitis. Chlortetracycline, like other tetracyclines, possesses a wide range of antimicrobial activity against aerobic and anaerobic Gram-positive and Gram-negative bacteria, which overlaps that of many other antimicrobial drugs. They also are effective against some microorganisms that are resistant to cell-wall-active antimicrobial agents, such as *Rickettsia, Coxiella burnetii, Mycoplasma pneumoniae, Chlamydia spp., Legionella spp., Ureaplasma*, some atypical mycobacteria, and *Plasmodium spp.*

Tetracyclines are thought to inhibit bacterial protein synthesis by binding to the 30S bacterial ribosome and preventing access of aminoacryl tRNA to the acceptor site on the mRNA-ribosome complex (see also Figures 80 and 88).

CHLORTHALIDONE

(Hygroton)

Chlorthalidone in a dose of 50 to 100 mg daily is indicated in edema and a dose of 25 mg/day is used in hypertension. The thiazide diuretics, also called *sulfonamide* or *benzothiadiazide diuretics*, vary in their actions. For instance, the potency of **hydrochlorothiazide** (Hydro-Diuril and Esidrix) is ten times greater than that of **chlorothiazide** (Diuril), but the two drugs have equal efficacy. The duration of action of hydrochlorothiazide, which is 6 to 12 hours, is equal to that of chlorothiazide. On the other hand, **chlorthalidone** has a duration of action lasting 48 hours. Some thiazide derivatives inhibit carbonic anhydrase, which is unrelated to their diuretic activity. Those that are active in this respect, may at sufficient dose have the same effect on bicarbonate excretion as does acetazolamide. They cause a moderate loss of sodium (5 to 10% of the filtered load), chloride, and water, and the clearance of free water is impaired. The loss of potassium can produce **hypokalemia**, which is particularly dangerous in patients receiving **digitalis** because it increases the risk of **arrhythmias**. Hypokalemia can be offset either by giving a potassium supplement (potassium chloride), or by the concurrent use of a potassium-sparing diuretic. However, not both measures should be adopted because **hyperkalemia** will result. **Hyperglycemia** is a potential hazard for patients with **diabetes mellitus. Hyperuricemia** can precipitate an acute attack of gout, but usually only in those patients who either have already had gout or have a propensity toward it. Since thiazides can cause a decrease in the GFR, they should not be used in patients whose renal function is less than one third of normal. The risk of thiazide-induced **hypercalcemia** should be kept in mind in patients with conditions such as **malignancies** or **hyperparathyroidism** that are associated with hypercalcemia (see also Table 25).

CHLORZOXAZONE
(Paraflex, Parafon Forte DSC)

Chlorzoxazone, a benzoxazole derivative with skeletal muscle relaxant properties (250 to 750 mg p.o. t.i.d.), is used as an adjunct medication in the treatment of acute and painful musculoskeletal conditions.

CHOLERA VACCINE

Cholera vaccine is a suspension of killed *Vibrio cholerae* (each millimeter contains 8 units of Inaba and Ogawa serotypes) which is used for primary immunization.

CHOLESTYRAMINE
(Questran)

Cholestyramine is indicated as adjunctive therapy to diet for the reduction of elevated serum cholesterol in patients with primary hypercholesterolemia (elevated low density lipoprotein (LDL) cholesterol) who do not respond adequately to diet. Similarly, cholestyramine is indicated for the relief of pruritus associated with partial biliary obstruction. Cholestyramine is not absorbed but binds to bile acids in the intestine, whereupon it is eliminated. To replenish the lost bile acid, cholesterol is then converted to bile acid and this lowers the level of cholesterol (see Figure 25). Cholestyramine has also been used in the treatment of **cholestasis** to control the intense pruritis. Cholestyramine reduces the LDL level in 4 to 7 days, and the maximum effect is seen in 14 days.

Besides binding to bile acid, cholestyramine binds to numerous other drugs used in the management of cardiovascular diseases, and which may be taken along with cholestyramine. These include chlorothiazide, phenylbutazone, phenobarbital, anticoagulants, digitalis, and fat-soluble vitamins (A, D, E, and K). Consequently, these and similar agents should be taken 1 hour before or 4 hours after the administration of cholestyramine. Cholestyramine, which is given in large doses of 16 to 30 g per day, causes severe constipation.

CHOLINE MAGNESIUM TRISALICYLATE
(Tricosal, Trilsate)

CHOLINE SALICYLATE
(Arthropan)

Choline salicylate, a non-narcotic analgesic, antipyretic, and antiinflammatory agent, is indicated in mild to moderate pain and fever, in arthritis, and in rheumatoid arthritis and osteoarthritis (see also Table 2).

CHOLINERGIC DRUGS: USES IN MEDICINE	
Cholinomimetics **Glaucoma** Carbachol Pilocarpine **Urinary retention** Bethanechol	**Cardiac/Pulmonary Disorders** Atropine sulfate Ipratropium bromide
Muscarinic Cholinergic Receptor Blocking Agents **Antispasmodics** Atropine sulfate Clidinium bromide Glycopyrrolate Isopropamide iodide *l*-hyoscyamine sulfate Methantheline bromide Methscopolamine bromide Propantheline bromide Scopolamine hydrobromide	**Mydriatic and Cycloplegic** Atropine sulfate Cyclopentolate hydrochloride Eucatropine hydrochloride Homatropine hydrobromide Scopolamine hydrobromide Tropicamide **Motion Sickness** Scopolamine hydrobromide **Anesthetic Premedication** Atropine sulfate Glycopyrrolate Scopolamine hydrobromide

Parkinson's Disease and Drug-induced Parkinsonism
Benztropine mesylate   Biperiden lactate   Procyclodine hydrochloride   Trihexyphenidyl hydrochloride

Cholinesterase Inhibitors	
Myasthenia gravis Edrophonium chloride Neostigmine bromide Pyridostigmine bromide	**Glaucoma** Demecarium bromide Echothiophate iodide Isoflurophate Physostigmine sulfate

Autonomic drugs have extensive clinical applications. They are used in the treatment of wide-angle glaucoma, in the diagnosis of myasthenia gravis, as a gastrointestinal and urinary tract stimulant in postoperative abdominal distention and urinary retention, as antidotes to poisoning from curare and the tricyclic antidepressants, as preanesthetic medications, as mydriatics, as cycloplegics, in peptic acid over-secretion to diminish the vagally-mediated secretion of gastric juices, in slowing of gastric emptying, in vestibular disorders, in parkinsonism, in conjugation with local anesthetics, in hypotension and shock, in heart block to improve atrioventricular conduction and stimulate ventricular automaticity, in bronchial asthma, as a nasal decongestant, in narcolepsy, in attention deficit hyperactivity disorders, in the diagnosis and treatment of pheochromocytoma, in cardiac arrhythmias, in angina pectoris, in hypertension, in thyrotoxicosis, and in tremor. In addition, numerous drugs such as neuroleptics and antidepressants produce side effects by modifying the function of the autonomic nervous system.

CHOLINERGIC RECEPTOR BLOCKING AGENTS: USES OF	
Tertiary Amines	
Adiphenine hydrobromide	Pyloric and biliary spasm, dysmenorrhea
Atropine sulfate	Preoperative medication; treatment of anticholinesterase poisoning
Benztropine methanesulfonate	Antagonizes extrapyramidal symptoms of the antipsychotics
Cyclopentolate	Mydriatic, cycloplegic
Dicyclomine	Alleviates gastrointestinal spasm, dysmenorrhea: pylorospasm, and biliary distention

Tertiary Amines	
Homatropine hydrobromide	Mydriatic and cycloplegic; anterior uveitis
Oxyphencyclimine	Antisecretory compound in peptic ulcer
Scopolamine hydrobromide	Preoperative medication
Trihexyphenidyl	Similar uses as benztropine methanesulfonate
Tropicamide	Mydriatic, cycloplegic

Quaternary Amines	
Atropine methylbromide (and methylnitrate)	Mydriatic, cycloplegic, antispasmodic in pyloric stenosis
Clidinium bromide	Spasmolytic in ulcer
Glycopyrrolate	Spasmolytic for ulcer therapy; preoperative medication
Homatropine methylbromide	In gastric acidity and spasm
Ipratropium	Chronic emphysema
Isopropamide iodine	In Zollinger-Ellison syndrome
Methantheline bromide	Spasmolytic to treat peptic ulcer
Methscopolamine bromide	Decreases gastric hyperacidity and hypermotility
Propantheline bromide	Spasmolytic in peptic ulcer
Tridihexethyl chloride	Antispasmodic, preoperative medication

CHOLINESTERASE INHIBITORS

Acetylcholine, an ester of choline and acetic acid, is synthesized in cholinergic neurons according to the following scheme:

$$\text{Acetyl CoA + choline} \xrightarrow{\text{Choline acetyltransferase}} \text{acetylcholine}$$

The acetylcholine, in turn, is hydrolyzed by both **acetylcholinesterase** and plasma butyrylcholinesterase. **Choline** is actively transported into nerve terminals (synaptosomes) by a high affinity uptake mechanism. Furthermore, the availability of choline regulates the synthesis of acetylcholine (see Figure 18).

Hemicholinium blocks the transport of choline into synaptosome, whereas **botulinum toxin** blocks the calcium-mediated release of acetylcholine. The released acetylcholine is hydrolyzed rapidly by acetylcholinesterase to choline and acetate. The cholinesterase inhibitors are divided into two categories: **organophosphorous compounds**, such as parathion, malathion, and tetraethyl pyrophosphate (TEPP), and the **carbamates**, such as naphthyl-N-methyl carbamate (carbaryl and Sevin).

The clinical manifestations of acute and severe poisoning from the organophosphorous insecticides include **cholinergic crisis**, resulting from the stimulation of muscarinic cholinergic receptors (bronchoconstriction, salivation, sweating, lacrimation, bradycardia, hypotension, and urinary and fecal incontinence); the stimulation of nicotinic cholinergic receptors (bronchoconstriction, salivation, sweating, lacrimation, bradycardia, hypotension, and urinary and fecal incontinence); the stimulation of nicotinic cholinergic receptors (muscular fasciculation); and the CNS effects (with initial restlessness, tremors, ataxia, and convulsions, followed by CNS depression and respiratory and circulatory depression). The treatment of a cholinergic crisis caused by organophosphorous compounds includes the administration of a cholinesterase reactivator such as **pralidoxime** (2-PAM) together with **atropine**. The poisoning stemming from antidoting with 2-PAM can be avoided in the event of carbaryl toxicity, because this agent is a reversible cholinesterase inhibitor (see Figure 71).

CHORIONIC GONADOTROPIN, HUMAN

(HCG) (A.P.L., Chorex 5, Chorex 10, Chorigon, Choron 10, Corgonject 5, Follutein Gonic, Pregnyl, Profasi HP)

Chorionic gonadotropin, a gonadotropin with ovulation and spermatogenesis stimulating properties (5,000 to 10,000 USP units IM), is indicated in the treatment of hypogonadotropic hypogonadism.

CHYMOPAPAIN

(Chymodiactin)

Chymopapain is a **proteolytic** enzyme with **chemonucleolytic** properties (2,000 to 4,000 pKat units per disk injected intradiskally). Maximum dose in a patient with multiple disk herniation is 8,000 pKat units. The drug is indicated in the treatment of herniated lumbar intervertebral disk.

CICLOPIROX OLAMINE

(Loprox)

Ciclopirox olamine is indicated for the treatment of tinea pedis (athlete's foot), tinea cruris (jock itch), and tinea corporis (ringworm) due to *T. rubrum, T. mentagrophytes, E. floccosum, and M. canis;* for candidiasis (moniliasis) due to *C. albicans*; and for tinea (pityriasis) versicolor due to *M. fufur.* Loprox is available as 1% cream (water-miscible base, 1% benzyl alcohol mineral oil in 15, 30, and 90 g, and 1% lotion (water-miscible base, 1% benzyl alcohol, mineral oil, in 30 ml).

CIMETIDINE

(Tagamet)

Cimetidine is indicated in treating duodenal ulcer, benign gastric ulcer, gastrointestinal reflux disease, pathological hypersecretory conditions, and in preventing upper GI bleeding in critically ill patients (Figure 24 and Table 9). There are two types of histamine receptors: **H_1 receptors**, which are blocked by agents such as diphenhydramine and other antiallergic compounds, and **H_2 receptors**, which are blocked by cimetidine, ranitidine (Zantac), famotidine (Pepcid), and nizatidine (Axid). Cimetidine has no effect on most H_1 receptor-mediated symptoms, such as bronchoconstriction.

The clinical use of **H_2-receptor** antagonists stems from their capacity to inhibit gastric acid secretion, especially in patients with peptic ulceration. **Cimetidine**, which is far more efficacious than anticholinergic drugs, is used in the treatment of duodenal ulcers and gastrinoma, and in patients suffering from gastroesophageal reflux disorders. It is absorbed orally, has a plasma half-life of 2 hours, and is excreted mainly unchanged by the kidney. Doses of cimetidine must be reduced in the presence of impaired renal function. The few and infrequent **adverse effects** of cimetidine use include gynecomastia (may bind to androgen receptor sites), galactorrhea (especially in patients with gastrinoma), granulocytopenia, agranulocytosis (very rare), mental confusion (especially in the elderly), restlessness, seizures, and reduced sperm count. **Ranitidine** is more effective than cimetidine and allegedly has fewer side effects.

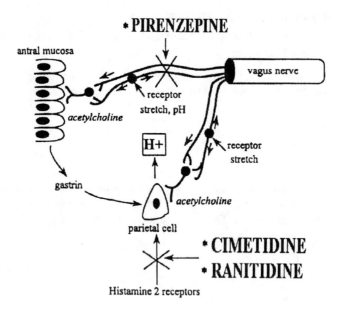

FIGURE 24   Cimetidine, a histamine$_2$ receptor antagonist, inhibits basal and nocturnal gastric acid secretion.

TABLE 9
Comparison of H$_2$-Receptor Antagonists

Actions	Cimetidine	Ranitidine	Famotidine
Ability to inhibit acid production	+++	+++	+++
Ability to inhibit pepsin	+++	+++	+++
Relative potency (in comparison to cimetidine)	1	5	32
Neuropsychiatric side effects	+	—	—
Pituitary stimulation	+	—	—
Antiandrogen effect	+	—	—
Inhibition of drug metabolism	++	+	—
Inhibition of cation transport	+	—	—
Frequency recommended for drug administration (doses per day)	4	2	1

CINOXACIN

(Cinobac)

Cinoxacin, a quinolone antibiotic (1 g daily in 2 to 4 divided doses for 7 to 14 days), is indicated in initial and recurrent urinary tract infections caused by susceptible organisms (see also Figure 77).

The quinolones include: **nalidixic acid** (NegGram), **cinoxacin, norfloxacin** (Noroxin), and **ciprofloxacin** (Cipro). Other members of the quinolone family are **pefloxacin, ofloxacin, enoxacin,** and **fleroxacin**. The bacterial **DNA gyrase** is responsible for the continuous introduction of negative supercoils into DNA, and the quinolones inhibit this gyrase-mediated DNA supercoiling (see Figure 77).

Nalidixic acid and **cinoxacin** are bactericidal Gram-negative organisms that cause urinary tract infections. The **fluoroquinolones** are bactericidal and considerably more potent against

Escherichia coli and various species of *Salmonella, Shigella, Enterobacter, Campylobacter,* and *Neisseria.* **Ciprofloxacin** also has good activity against staphylococci, including methicillin-resistant strains. The quinolones and fluoroquinolones may produce arthropathy, and hence should not be used in prepubertal children or pregnant women.

Nalidixic acid and **cinoxacin** are useful only for treating urinary tract infections. **Ciprofloxacin** is useful for both urinary tract infections and prostatitis.

CIPROFLOXACIN

Lower respiratory tract infections account for a large proportion of prescribed antibiotics and, with emerging resistance to standard agents, the introduction of the fluoroquinolones, in particular ciprofloxacin, has provided a further component in the armamentarium. Ciprofloxacin is able to eradicate *Streptococcus pneumoniae, Haemophilus influenzae,* and *Moraxella catarrhalis* readily. These findings suggest that the high respiratory tissue penetration of ciprofloxacin and the achievable minimum inhibitory concentrations lead to acceptable clinical outcomes in lower respiratory tract infections.

CIPROFLOXACIN

(Cipro)

The quinolones include: **nalidixic acid** (NegGram), **cinoxacin, norfloxacin** (Noroxin), and **ciprofloxacin** (Cipro). Other members of the quinolone family are **pefloxacin, ofloxacin, enoxacin,** and **fleroxacin.** The bacterial **DNA gyrase** is responsible for the continuous introduction of negative supercoils into DNA, and the quinolones inhibit this gyrase-mediated DNA supercoiling (see Figure 77).

Nalidixic acid and **cinoxacin** are bactericidal Gram-negative organisms that cause urinary tract infections. The **fluoroquinolones** are bactericidal and considerably more potent against *Escherichia coli* and various species of *Salmonella, Shigella, Enterobacter, Campylobacter,* and *Neisseria.* **Ciprofloxacin** also has good activity against staphylococci, including methicillin-resistant strains. The quinolones and fluoroquinolones may produce arthropathy, and hence should not be used in prepubertal children or pregnant women.

Nalidixic acid and **cinoxacin** are useful only for treating urinary tract infections. **Ciprofloxacin** is useful for both urinary tract infections and prostatitis.

CIPROFLOXACIN HYDROCHLORIDE

(Ophthalmic) (Ciloxan)

Ciprofloxacin, a fluoroquinolone antibacterial agent (2 drops in the affected eye q. 15 minutes for the first six hours, then 2 drops q. 30 minutes for the remainder of the first day), is indicated for corneal ulcers caused by *Pseudomonas aeruginosa, Staphylococcus aureus, S. epidermidis, Streptococcus pneumoniae,* and possibly *Serratia marcescens* and *Streptococcus viridans*; and for bacterial conjunctivitis caused by *Staphylococcus aureus* and *S. epidermidis* and possibly *Streptococcus pneumoniae.*

CIRRHOSIS: TREATMENT OF
Hepatic cirrhosis may be associated with portal hypertension, ascites, encephalopathy, spontaneous bacterial peritonitis, and hepatocellular carcinoma. Portal hypertension is directly responsible for the formation of esophageal varices, which may give rise to massive upper gastrointestinal bleeding. Therapy is aimed at correcting hypovolemic shock and at achieving hemostasis at the bleeding site.

Drug therapy is based on the use of agents that may decrease pressure and blood flow at the esophageal varices. This can be achieved either by the use of splanchnic vasoconstrictors (vasopressin, glypressin, or somatostatin) which decrease portal-collateral blood flow, or by drugs which decrease the vascular resistance at the intrahepatic and portal collateral circulation (nitroglycerine), or by combination therapy. Terlipressin or glypressin is a synthetic vasopressin derivative with prolonged biological activity, which allows its administration as IV injections of 2 mg/4 hr until achieving a bleeding-free period of 24 to 48 hours.

Treatment of ascites is directed toward eliminating the intra-abdominal fluid by increasing urinary excretion of water and sodium with diuretics and through paracentesis and/or peritonea-venous shunt. The therapeutic approach to chronic hepatic encephalopathy is based on dietary protein restriction and the use of nonabsorbable disaccharides. Since spontaneous bacterial peritonitis may precipitate numerous potentially lethal complications (septic shock, progressive circulatory and renal impairment, liver failure), antibiotic administration must be started as soon as the diagnosis is established. The combination of an aminoglycoside, gentamicin or tobramycin, plus a β-lactam antibiotic, ampicillin or cefalotin, has been the most frequently used empiric antibiotic regimen in cirrhotic patients.

Hepatocellular carcinoma constitutes a frequent clinical program during the follow-up of cirrhotic patients requiring surgical treatment by liver transplantation, radiotherapy, or immunotherapy.

CISAPRIDE
(Propulsid)

Cisapride, a serotonin$_4$ receptor agonist (10 mg p.o. q.i.d.) with gastrointestinal prokinetic properties, is indicated in the symptomatic treatment of nocturnal heartburn due to gastro-esophageal reflux disease.

CISPLATIN (CIS-PLATINUM)
(Platinol, Platinol AQ)

Cisplatin, an alkylating agent, is indicated as an adjunctive therapy in metastatic testicular cancer; adjunctive therapy in metastatic ovarian cancer, head and neck cancers, lung cancer, and esophageal cancer, and in the treatment of advanced bladder cancer (see also Figure 2).

CITALOPRAM

Citalopram, a new serotonin uptake inhibitor (20 to 60 mg) is an effective antidepressant.

Citalopram together with fluoxetine, fluvoxamine, paroxetine, and sertraline belong to the group of selective serotonin reuptake inhibiting (SSRI) antidepressants (see also Tables 3 through 5 and Figure 78).

CLADRIBINE
(Leustatin)

Cladribine, a purine nucleoside analog, with antineoplastic properties (0.09 mg/kg daily by continuous IV infusion for 7 days), is indicated in the treatment of active hairy cell leukemia. In addition, it has been used in advanced cutaneous T-cell lymphomas, chronic lymphocytic leukemia, non-Hodgkin's lymphomas, acute myeloid leukemias, autoimmune hemolytic anemia, mycosis fungoides, or Sezary syndrome (see also Figure 2).

Cladribine has been designed to stimulate the immunodeficiency state of hereditary adenosine deaminase by causing the accumulation of deoxynucleotides in lymphocytes. Cladribine, an immunosuppressive drug, stabilizes the condition of patients with chronic progressive multiple sclerosis.

CLARITHROMYCIN

(Biaxin Filmtabs)

Clarithromycin, a macrolide antibiotic, is indicated in the treatment of pharyngitis or tonsillitis caused by *Streptococcus pyogenes,* acute maxillary sinusitis caused by *S. pneumoniae,* acute exacerbations of chronic bronchitis caused by *Moraxella (Branhamella) catarrhalis* or *S. pneumoniae,* pneumonia caused by *S. pneumoniae* or *Mycoplasma pneumoniae,* acute exacerbations of chronic bronchitis caused by *Haemophilus influenzae,* and uncomplicated skin and skin-structure infections caused by *Staphylococcus aureus, Streptococcus aureus,* or *Streptococcus pyogenes.*

CLEMASTINE FUMARATE

(Tavist, Tavist-1)

Clemastine, an ethanolamine derivative antihistamine, is indicated in the treatment of rhinitis and allergy symptoms, and the allergic skin manifestation of urticaria and angioedema (see also Figure 49).

CLIDINIUM BROMIDE

(Quarzan)

Clidinium, an anticholinergic agent with gastrointestinal, antispasmodic properties (2.5 to 5.0 mg p.o. t.i.d.), is indicated as an adjunctive therapy for peptic ulcers (see also Figure 24).

CLINDAMYCIN PHOSPHATE

(Cleocin)

Clindamycin, an aminoglycoside, is indicated in serious respiratory tract infections such as empyema, anaerobic pneumonitis, and lung abscess; serious skin and soft-tissue infections; septicemia; intra-abdominal infections such as peritonitis and intra-abdominal abscess; infections of the female pelvis and genital tract such as endometriosis, nongonococcal tubo-ovarian abscess, pelvic cellulitis, and postsurgical vaginal cuff infection.

Aminoglycosides are bactericidal and **inhibit protein synthesis** in susceptible microorganisms (see Figure 80). They exert this effect by (1) interfering with the initiation complex of peptide formation, (2) inducing the misreading of the code on the messenger RNA template, which causes the incorporation of inappropriate amino acids into peptides, and (3) rupturing the polysomes into monosomes, which become nonfunctional (see Figure 80). Resistance to aminoglycosides may be due to one or a combination of the following mechanisms:

Interference with the transport of aminoglycosides into bacterial cells
Deletion of receptors on the 30S ribosomal subunit; thus preventing the functioning of aminoglycosides
The bacterial biotransformation of aminoglycosides to inactive forms.

In addition, because the initial transport of aminoglycosides into bacterial cells is an **oxygen-dependent process,** microorganisms that are able to grow under **anaerobic conditions** show or develop resistance. The aminoglycosides are poorly absorbed from the gastrointestinal tract, and, for this reason, they are administered intramuscularly. Furthermore, since they do not penetrate the central nervous system, they may have to be given intrathecally or intraventricularly in the treatment of meningitis. Aminoglycosides are excreted by glomerular filtration, which is greatly reduced in the presence of renal impairment, thus leading to toxic blood levels.

The most serious reactions following aminoglycoside therapy are cochlear damage and vestibular impairment, which lead to vertigo and disturb the ability to maintain postural equilibrium. Aminoglycosides given during pregnancy cause deafness in the newborn. Nephrotoxicity and reversible neuromuscular blockade causing respiratory paralysis have also been seen following the use of high doses.

The neuromuscular blocking effects of depolarizing and nondepolarizing agents are enhanced by aminoglycosides, and prolonged respiratory depression may occur.

CLINDAMYCIN HYDROCHLORIDE
(Cleocin HCL)

CLINDAMYCIN PALMITATE HYDROCHLORIDE
(Cleocin Pediatric)

CLINDAMYCIN PHOSPHATE
(Cleocin Phosphate, Cleocin T)

Clindamycin, a lincomycin derivative (150 to 450 mg p.o. q. 6 hours), is indicated in infections caused by sensitive organisms.

CLOBAZAM

Clobazam, a 1,5 benzodiazepine derivative, is indicated in the management of ambulant patients with anxiety. Clobazam lacks sedative and amnestic effects and does not cause impairment of psychomotor skills (see also Table 8).

CLOBETASOL PROPIONATE
(Temovate)

Clobetasol, a topical adrenocorticoid with antiinflammatory properties (0.05% cream, lotion, or ointment), is indicated in inflammation of corticosteroid-responsive dermatoses.

CLOFAZIMINE
(Lamprene)

Clofazimine, a substituted aminophenazine dye, with leprostatic properties (50 to 100 mg p.o. once daily), is indicated in the treatment of dapsone-resistant leprosy and erythema nodosum leprosum.

CLOFIBRATE
(Atromid S)

Clofibrate is indicated for the treatment of primary dysbetalipoproteinemia (type III hyperlipidemia) not responding to diet. Clofibrate (Atromid S) reduces VLDL, triglyceride, and cholesterol levels (Figure 25). Clofibrate does not inhibit cholesterol synthesis. Its primary mechanism of action is activation of lipoprotein lipase. Clofibrate is also considered effective in patients with elevated VLDL levels, especially those who do not respond to dietary restrictions. Because clofibrate displaces coumarin and phenytoin from binding sites, the **prothrombin time** should be checked on a regular basis in patients who are taking both agents. A flu-like syndrome, characterized by muscular cramps, tenderness, stiffness, and weakness, may occur in some patients.

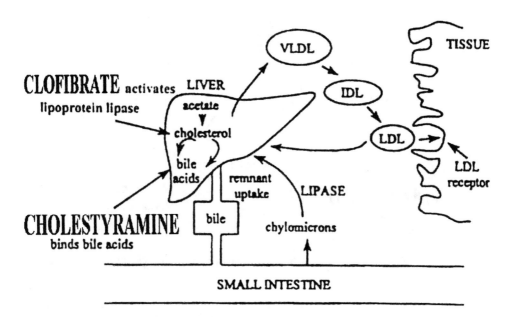

FIGURE 25   Clofibrate lowers serum triglyceride levels by accelerating catabolism of very low density lipoproteins. (Adapted from Ebadi, M., *Pharmacology, An Illustrated Review with Questions and Answers,* 3rd Edition, Lippincott-Raven Press, Philadelphia, 1996.)

CLOMIPHENE CITRATE

(Clomid)

Clomiphene citrate is indicated for the treatment of ovulatory failure. **Clomiphene** and **tamoxifen** (Nolvadex) modify or inhibit the actions of estrogens. They accomplish this by binding to the cytoplasmic estrogen receptors that are then translocated to the nucleus. By diminishing the number of estrogen-binding sites, they interfere with the physiologic actions of estrogens. Furthermore, by interfering with the normal hypothalamic and hypophyseal feedback inhibition of estrogen synthesis, these agents cause an increased stimulation of luteinizing hormone-releasing hormone, follicle-stimulating hormone-releasing hormone, and gonadotropins. This leads to ovarian stimulation and ovulation. Clomiphene has been used successfully in some cases of infertility but causes multiple births. Antiestrogens are able to arrest the growth of estrogen-dependent malignant mammary cells. Clomiphene has been used in certain cases of disseminated breast cancer (see Figure 26).

CLOMIPRAMINE HYDROCHLORIDE

(Anafranil)

Clomipramine is indicated for the treatment of obsessive-compulsive disorder. It mildly blocks the uptake of norepinephrine, but strongly blocks the uptake of serotonin. In addition, clomipramine blocks alpha$_1$-adrenergic, H$_1$-histamine, and muscarinic cholinergic receptors. Clomipramine lowers the seizure threshold and should be used cautiously in seizure disorders (see also Tables 3 through 5).

CLONAZEPAM

(Clonopin)

Clonazepam (1.5 mg/day in three divided doses) is used alone or as adjunctive treatment of Lennox-Gastaut syndrome (petit mal variance) and akinetic and myoclonic seizures. It may

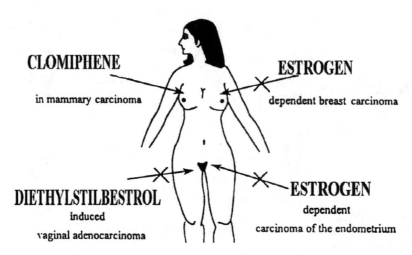

FIGURE 26 Clomiphene, an ovulation stimulant, is a partial estrogen receptor agonist.

be used in patients with petit mal (absence) seizures who have failed to respond to succinamides. Clonazepam is actually a broad-spectrum anticonvulsant, since it is also effective in tonic-clonic (grand mal) and complex partial (psychomotor-temporal lobe) seizures. Clonazepam causes drowsiness (increased by barbiturate administration) and a dose-dependent ataxia. In addition, behavioral abnormalities such as hypersensitivity, irritability, and aggression may occur, but these are mostly seen in children (see also Figure 40).

CLONIDINE HYDROCHLORIDE
(Catapress)

Clonidine stimulates alpha$_2$-adrenoreceptors in the brain stem, resulting in a reduced sympathetic outflow and a decrease in peripheral resistance (see Figure 27). Although clonidine is indicated in hypertension, it is being used and/or investigated for alcohol withdrawal, Gille de la Tourette syndrome, methadone/opiate detoxification, neuralgia, and smoking cessation. Clonidine (0.1 mg b.i.d.) reduces blood pressure within 30 to 60 minutes, has a half-life of 12 to 16 hours, is metabolized partly in the liver, is excreted (50%) unchanged, and its half-life is increased to 30 to 40 hours in renal impairment. Treatment with clonidine should not be stopped abruptly since rebound hypertension occurs, and this effect may be greater in patients receiving beta-adrenergic blocking agents.

Tricyclic antidepressants, which block the uptake sites for biogenic amines, may block the antihypertensive effects of clonidine.

Overdosage with clonidine causes bradycardia, hypotension, CNS depression, respiratory depression, hypothermia, apnea, and hypoventilation. Atropine sulfate is able to reverse bradycardia, and epinephrine, dopamine, or tolazine are effective in combating hypotension.

CLORAZEPATE DIPOTASSIUM
(Tranxene-SD Half Strength)

Clorazepate, a benzodiazepine derivative with antianxiety, anticonvulsant, and sedative hypnotic properties (30 mg p.o. initially), is indicated in acute alcohol withdrawal and is used as an adjunct in epilepsy (see also Table 8).

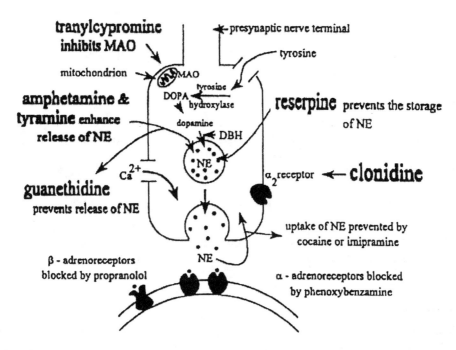

FIGURE 27 Clonidine, a centrally acting antiadrenergic agent, is used in treating hypertension. (Adapted from Ebadi, M., *Pharmacology, An Illustrated Review with Questions and Answers*, 3rd Edition, Lippincott-Raven Press, Philadelphia, 1996.)

CLOTRIMAZOLE
(Gyne-Lotrimin)

Clotrimazole, an antifungal agent, is used only topically and is available as a 1% cream, lotion, or solution (Lotrimin and Mycelex), as a 1% vaginal cream, as 100 mg or 500 mg vaginal tablets (Gyne-Lotrimin, Mycelex-G), and as 10 mg troches (Mycelex).

CLOXACILLIN SODIUM
(Tegopen)

Cloxacillin (500 mg every 4 to 6 hours for at least five days) is indicated for the treatment of infections due to penicillinase-producing staphylococci. Cloxacillin sodium is an acid-stable and penicillinase-resistant penicillin, absorbed orally rapidly but incompletely. It binds to albumin to the extent of 95% and is excreted unchanged in the urine.

Penicillinase-resistant penicillins should be administered cautiously to persons with a history of sensitivity to any penicillins. Tetracycline, a bacteriostatic antibiotic, may antagonize the bactericidal effects of penicillin (see also Table 22).

CLOZAPINE
(Clozaril)

Clozapine, which is associated with higher risk of agranulocytosis and seizures, is indicated (25 mg once or twice daily) only for the management of schizophrenic patients who fail to respond adequately to standard antipsychotic drug treatment. Clozapine, on the other hand, is relatively free from extrapyramidal side effects such as parkinsonism. Approximately 50%

of the administered dose is excreted in the urine and 30% in the feces as inactive demethylated, hydroxylated, and N-oxide derivatives. Clozapine has anticholinergic properties and causes tachycardia and hence poses a serious risk for a patient with compromised cardiovascular function (see also Table 23).

CLUSTERIN

Clusterin is a heterodimeric glycoprotein produced by a wide array of tissues and found in most biological fluids. The proposed physiologic functions of clusterin include complement regulation, lipid transport, sperm maturation, initiation of apoptosis, endocrine secretion, membrane protection, and promotion of cell interactions.

COCCIDIOIDIN
(Spherulin)

Coccidioidin, a *Coccidioides immitis* antigen, is used as a diagnostic aid in coccidioidomycosis and to assess cell-mediated immunity (see also Figure 16).

CODEINE
(Methylmorphine)

Codeine, which is an analgesic and antitussive, is methylmorphine and pharmacologically resembles morphine, with the following exceptions. The **analgesic potency** of codeine is approximately one sixth that of morphine. Codeine raises the pain threshold without altering the patient's reaction to pain and produces very little euphoria. Therefore, 10 mg of morphine is far superior for alleviating pain than is 60 mg of codeine.

Unlike morphine, codeine is **absorbed orally**. The side effects are the same as morphine's but are milder and far less frequent. Codeine produces miosis, respiratory depression, urinary retention, and constipation, but these are not of clinical or toxicological significance (see also Figure 58).

Tolerance to codeine develops very slowly and the **addiction liability** is far less than that observed for morphine. Most narcotics such as **morphine, codeine, dihydrocodeine, methadone,** and **levorphanol** have antitussive properties. Codeine is used primarily because its addictive liability is low and it is effective orally. The antitussive doses of narcotics are lower than the doses used for analgesic purposes.

COLCHICINE

Colchicine, an alkaloid obtained from meadow saffron or autumn crocus, may be used both diagnostically to ascertain the presence of gout and prophylactically to prevent its further occurrence. Usually 0.5 mg oral doses of colchicine are given hourly until either the therapeutic effects appear or the side effects develop. In addition to colchicine, phenylbutazone, indomethacin, ACT, and steroid antiinflammatory agents may be used to treat the acute attack of gout.

Colchicine is tolerated well in moderate doses. Nausea, vomiting, diarrhea, and abdominal pain are the most common and earliest untoward effects of overdosage.

In the event of acute poisoning with colchicine, there is hemorrhagic gastroenteritis, extensive vascular damage, nephrotoxicity, muscular depression, and an ascending paralysis of the central nervous system.

Colchicine produces a leukopenia that is soon replaced by a leukocytosis. The long-term administration of colchicine may lead to myopathy, neuropathy, agranulocytosis, aplastic anemia, alopecia, and azoospermia (see also Figure 11).

COLESTIPOL HYDROCHLORIDE
(Colested)

Colestipol (5 to 30 g/day given once or in divided doses) is indicated as adjunctive therapy to diet for the reduction of elevated serum total and low-density lipoprotein (LDL) and cholesterol in patients with primary hypocholesterolemia who do not respond adequately to diet.

Colestipol and cholestyramine are very large polymeric cationic exchange resins that are insoluble in water. They bind bile acids in the intestinal lumen and prevent their reabsorption (see Figure 25). Chloride is released from cationic quaternary ammonium binding sites in exchange for bile acids, but the resin itself is not absorbed.

Colestipol causes constipation and a bloating sensation. The absorption of fat soluble vitamins and certain drugs such as digitalis, thiazides, tetracycline, and phenylbutazone may be altered. Therefore, medications are given either one hour before or two hours after colestipol.

CONGESTIVE HEART FAILURE: TREATMENT OF
Overt congestive heart failure (CHF) has a prevalence of 1% of the population. The predominant symptoms of patients with CHF are **fatigue and dyspnea**. Fatigue is thought to result from changes in peripheral muscle metabolism secondary to decreased vasodilative capacity and physical inactivity. An increase of peripheral perfusion by vasodilator therapy and physical activity are therefore recommended. Beside overt decompensation, where dyspnea results from acute pulmonary congestion due to backward failure, increased physiological dead space ventilation caused by pulmonary ventilation/perfusion mismatch accounts, to a large degree, for dyspnea, and can be improved by **vasodilator therapy**.
According to the pathophysiology of CHF, normalization of loading conditions and myocardial inotropy are the parameters addressed by various pharmacological agents in order to alleviate symptoms and slow progression of the disease. **Diuretics** are rapid-acting and effective agents to improve congestion and decrease filling pressures. **Digitalis** improves hemodynamics and symptomatology by increasing inotropy and slowing resting heart rate in atrial fibrillation; however, prognostic effects have yet to be proved. The introduction of **vasodilators** has significantly improved the prognosis of the disease, and the administration of **ACE inhibitors** in particular has been shown to slow progression of CHF. This results in a substantial decrease in morbidity and mortality.

CONSTIPATION: DRUG-INDUCED
Antacids Containing Calcium Carbonate or Aluminum Hydroxide
Barium sulfate
Clonidine
Diuretics (non-potassium-sparing)
Drugs Possessing Anticholinergic Properties
Antihistamines
Antiparkinsonian agents (e.g., benztropine or trihexyphenidyl)
Phenothiazines
Tricyclic antidepressants
Ganglionic Blocking Agents
Inhibitors of prostaglandin synthesis
Iron preparations
Narcotic Analgesics (opiates)
Polystyrene sodium sulfonate
Skeletal Muscle Blocking Agents
d-Tubocurarine
Succinylcholine

COLLAGENASE

(Santyl)

Collagenase, an enzyme concentrate derived from *Clostridium histolytica,* is used to promote debridement of necrotic tissue in dermal ulcers and severe burns.

CORTICOSTEROIDS

Corticosteroids (Table 10) are synthetic adrenocortical steroids with antiinflammatory actions and effects and are used in numerous disorders including bronchial asthma. For example, beclomethasone dipropionate (Beclovent, 85 mcg 3 to 4 times daily), dexamethasone sodium phosphate (Decadron phosphate), and triamcinolone acetonide (Azmacort), which are not bronchodilators and are not indicated for rapid relief of acute asthma, are used in broncho-spastic states intractable to adequate trial of conventional therapy.

CORTICOSTEROIDS: USES FOR (see also Table 10)		
Replacement Therapy Congenital adrenal hyperplasia Primary adrenal insufficiency Secondary adrenal insufficiency Selective aldosterone deficiency	**Hematologic and Neoplastic Diseases** Aplastic anemias (some forms) Complications of malignancy Hypercalcemia Hematologic malignancies	**Gastrointestinal Diseases** Chronic active hepatitis Crohn's disease Nontropical sprue Ulcerative colitis

Musculoskeletal Diseases
Mixed connective tissue syndromes
Polymyalgia rheumatica
Polymyositis
Rheumatoid arthritis
Systemic lupus erythematosus
	Acute lymphoblastic leukemia
	  Lymphomas
	  Multiple myeloma
	Immune hemolytic anemia
	Immune thrombocytopenia
	Inflammatory bowel disease
	Transfusion reactions
		Neurologic Conditions
		Acute cerebral edema
		Multiple sclerosis
		Myasthenia gravis
		
		Eye Diseases
		Allergic conjunctivitis

Pulmonary Diseases
Aspiration pneumonitis
Bronchoconstrictive diseases
  Acute asthma
  Chronic asthmatic bronchitis
Interstitial diseases
  Hypersensitivity pneumonitis
  Idiopathic pulmonary fibrosis
  Sarcoidosis
Pulmonary vasculitides
	Allergic and Immune Diseases
	Acute hypersensitivity reactions
	Allergic rhinitis
	Anaphylaxis
	Angioedema and urticaria
	Insect venom allergy
	Serum sickness
	Some drug allergies
	Transplantation rejection
		Exophthalmos
		Optic neuritis
		Scleritis
		Uveitis
		
		Skin Diseases
		Atopic dermatitis
		Contact dermatitis
		Erythema multiform
		Mycosis fungoides
		Pemphigus
		Seborrheic dermatitis

	Cardiovascular Diseases Giant cell arteritis Myocarditis Pericarditis Temporal arteritis	

CORTICOTROPIN

(Adrenocorticotropic Hormone, ACTH, Acthar, ACTHGel, Cortigel-40, Cortigel 80, Cortrophin Gel, Cortrophin-Zinc, HP Acthar Gel)

Corticotropin, an anterior pituitary hormone, is indicated as a diagnostic test of adrenocortical function, as a replacement hormone, in the treatment of multiple sclerosis, in the treatment of severe allergic reactions, collagen disorders, dermatologic disorders, inflammation, and of infantile spasm.

TABLE 10
Preparations of Adrenocortical Steroids and Their Synthetic Analogs

Nonproprietary and Proprietary Names	Oral Forms	Injectable Forms
Fludrocortisone acetate (Florinef Acetate)	0.1 mg	—
Cortisol (hydrocortisone) (Cortef, Hydrocortone, others)	5–20 mg	25, 50 mg/ml (susp.)
Beclomethasone dipropionate (Beclovent, Vanceril, others)	Inhalation aerosol	—
Betamethasone (Celestone)	0.6 mg 0.6 mg/5 ml syrup	— —
Betamethasone benzoate (Benisone, Uticort)	Topical	—
Betamethasone dipropionate (Diprosone, others)	Topical	—
Betamethasone sodium phosphate (Celestone Phosphate, others)	—	4 mg/ml
Betamethasone sodium phosphate & acetate (Celestone Soluspan)	—	6 mg/ml (susp.)
Betamethasone valerate (Beta-Val, Valisone, others)	Topical	—
Cortisone acetate (Cortone Acetate)	5–25 mg	25, 50 mg/ml (susp.)
Dexamethasone (Decadron, others)	0.25–6.0 mg 0.5 mg/5 ml (elixir, soln.) 0.5 mg/0.5 ml (soln.)	—
Dexamethasone acetate (Decadron-LA, others)	—	8, 16 mg/ml (susp.)
Dexamethasone sodium phosphate (Decadron Phosphate, Hexadrol Phosphate, others)	—	4–24 mg/ml
Methylprednisolone (Medrol)	2–32 mg	—
Methylprednisolone acetate (Depo-Medrol, Medrol Acetate, others)	—	20–80 mg/ml (susp.)
Paramethasone acetate (Haldrone)	1.2 mg	—
Prednisolone (Delta-Cortef)	5 mg 3 mg/ml (syrup)	— —
Prednisolone acetate (Econopred, others)	—	25–100 mg/ml (susp.)
Prednisolone tebutate (Hᴜᴅᴇʟᴛʀᴀ-T.B.A., others)	1 mg/ml (liquid)	—
Prednisone (Deltasone, others)	1–50 mg 1 mg/ml (syrup) 1, 5 mg/ml (soln.)	— — —
Triamcinolone (Aristocort, Kenacort)	1–8 mg	—
Triamcinolone acetonide (Kenalog, others)	—	3,10,40 mg/ml (susp.)
Triamcinolone diacetate (Aristocort, Kenacort Diacetate, others)	2,4 mg/5 ml (syrup)	25,40 mg/ml (susp.)
Triamcinolone hexacetonide (Aristospan)	—	5, 20 mg/ml (susp.)

susp. = suspension; soln. = solution

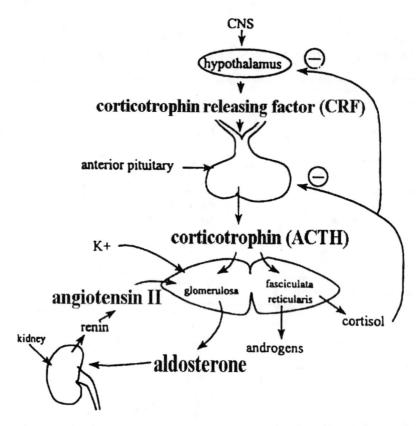

FIGURE 28 Corticotropin (adrenocorticotropic hormone), originating from anterior pituitary gland, has been used in the treatment of multiple sclerosis and nonsuppurative thyroiditis. (Adapted from Ebadi, M., *Pharmacology, An Illustrated Review with Questions and Answers*, 3rd Edition, Lippincott-Raven Press, Philadelphia, 1996.)

CORTICOTROPIN-RELEASING FACTOR

Corticotropin-releasing factor and **arginine vasopressin**, which are released predominantly by the paraventricular nucleus of the hypothalamus, are important regulators of corticotropin (ACTH) release, which in turn triggers the release of cortisol and other steroids by the adrenal gland. Both the administration of certain psychoactive agents and emotional arousal originating from the limbic system are able to modify the functions of the pituitary-adrenal axis and to stimulate the synthesis of cortisol. ACTH elicits the following effects. It enhances the synthesis of pregnenolone, activates adenylate cyclase and elevates the cyclic adenosine monophosphate level, enhances the level of adrenal steroids, especially cortisol, and reduces the level of ascorbic acid.

The level of cortisol is thought to directly control the secretion of ACTH through a negative feedback mechanism that may be directed at both the hypothalamus and the anterior pituitary gland. Conversely, a reduced concentration of cortisol or cortisol-like substances eliminates the negative effect and enhances the release of ACTH (see Figure 28).

The **metyrapone test** may be used diagnostically to evaluate the proper functioning of the anterior pituitary gland. When administered orally, metyrapone inhibits the activity of 11-beta-hydroxylase, which is necessary for the synthesis of cortisol, corticosterone, and aldosterone, promotes the release of corticotropin, which in turn increases production of the precursors

(11-deoxycortisol and 11-deoxycorticosterone), and enhances the appearance of 17-hydroxy-corticosteroids and 17-ketogenic steroids.

In the event that the pituitary gland is nonfunctional, and therefore cannot stimulate ACTH secretion, the levels of these urinary metabolites will not increase.

CORTISONE

Cortisone (25 to 300 mg/day) is insoluble in water. Cortisone acetate (Bioline) is available in 25 mg tablet. Hydrocortisone (Cortisol, 20 to 240 mg/day) exists in suspension and is insoluble in water. Hydrocortisone cypionate (Cortef, 20 to 240 mg/day) is available in oral suspension. Hydrocortisone sodium phosphate, a water-soluble salt with a rapid onset but short duration of action, is available for IV, IM, or SC injection. Hydrocortisone sodium succinate (Solu-Cortef) in an initial dose of 100 to 500 mg may be administered IV or IM. The antiinflammatory effect of cortisol is relatively weak (Table 14).

CORTISONE ACETATE

(Cortone)

Cortisone, a substance with glucocorticoid and mineralocorticoid properties (25 to 300 mg p.o. or IM daily on an alternate-day schedule), is indicated in the treatment of adrenal insufficiency, allergy, and inflammation.

COSYNTROPIN

(Cortrosyn)

Cosyntropin, an anterior pituitary hormone (0.25 to 1 mg IM or IV), is used as a diagnostic test of adrenocortical function.

CO-TRIMOXAZOLE

(Trimethoprim-Sulfamethoxazole) (Bactrim, Bactrim DS, Bactrim I.V. Infusion, Cotrim, Septra, Septra DS, Septra IV Infusion, SMZ-TMP, Sulfatrim, UroPlus SS, UroPlus OS)

Co-trimoxazole, a sulfonamide and folate antagonist agent with antibiotic properties, is used in urinary tract infections and shigellosis, in otitis media, in *Pneumocystis carinii* pneumonitis, in chronic bronchitis, and in traveler's diarrhea (see Figure 82).

COUMARIN ANTICOAGULANTS

The **coumarin anticoagulants**, which are orally active, include dicumarol, warfarin sodium (coumadin sodium), warfarin potassium (Athrombokin-K), acenocoumarol (Sintrom), and phenopromcouman (Liquamar).

CROHN'S DISEASE: TREATMENT OF
Crohn's disease is an indolent, chronic inflammatory disorder capable of involving the entire alimentary tract from mouth to anus. The etiology and pathogenesis remain unknown, and Crohn's disease might represent more than one etiologically distinct entity. The term "Crohn's disease" is preferable to "granulomatous enteritis" because granulomas are not required for diagnosis and because other inflammatory disorders can affect "regions" of the bowel. Inflammation extends through all layers of the gut wall and involves the adjacent mesentery and lymph nodes. Distal ileum and colon are the most common sites, and the inflammatory process is characteristically discontinuous. The disease is characterized by its prolonged and variable course, by its diversity of clinical manifestation, by its perianal and systemic complications, and by its remarkable tendency to recur after surgical resection of involved gut.

Development of specific therapies for Crohn's disease has been hampered by the incomplete understanding of the underlying etiology and pathogenesis of this disease. In addition, the great variability in its location, extent, and behavior, as well as the imperfect correlation between clinical status and findings on endoscopy and histology, has made the design and interpretation of clinical trials difficult. Considering the dramatically variable natural history of the disease and frequent spontaneous improvement seen in patients on no therapy, the frequent reporting of uncontrolled trials only adds to the confusion.

Traditional medical therapies for Crohn's disease include **sulfasalazine** and **corticosteroids**. These are pluripotent, reducing the production of inflammatory mediators and cytokines, although the complex and multiple mechanisms remain incompletely understood. Novel therapies related to newer aminosalicylate preparations such as **balsalazide** (colazide) or **olsalazine** (dipentum); newer corticosteroids such as **budesonide**; immunomodulators such as **azathioprine, 6-mercaptopurine,** or **methotrexate**; and antibiotics such as **metronidazole** are aimed at more specific delivery of active compounds to the site of disease, reduction of systemic absorption and side effects, and modulation of more focal targets within the immune response and the action of specific proinflammatory cytokines.

CROMOLYN SODIUM
(Disodium Cromoglycate)

Cromolyn sodium (inhalation 20 mg/2 ml), **Intal** in capsules (20 mg for inhalation only), solution (20 mg per amp for nebulizer only), and aerosol spray (delivers 800 mcg), **Nasalcrom** (nasal solution in 40 mg/ml), and **Gastrocom** (100 mg capsule for oral administration) are used for prophylactic management of severe bronchial asthma. As an antiasthmatic, antiallergic, and mast cell stabilizer, cromolyn has no bronchodilating, antiinflammatory, anticholinergic, or vasoconstricting properties.

Cromolyn sodium is given by inhalation as an aerosol powder four times a day only as a prophylactic medication (see also Figure 29). Since it is not a bronchodilator, it is not used in the management of status asthmaticus. Because it can inhibit the immediate response to allergen or exercise, it is thought that it suppresses the release of the mediator from mast cells. Cromolyn also prevents the late response and the subsequent hypersecretion, and this suggests it acts on other inflammatory cells such as macrophages or eosinophils. Cromolyn is not effective in all patients. It is the preferred antiinflammatory agent for use in children. The drug is well tolerated and, with the exception of causing minor throat irritation, has no side effects. Nedocromil sodium has biologic and chemical properties similar to those of cromolyn sodium (Figure 29).

CROTALINE (CROTALIDAE) ANTIVENIN, POLYVALENT

Crotaline, a snake antivenin, is indicated in the treatment of crotalid (pit viper) bites, including those from rattlesnakes, copperheads, and cottonmouth moccasins.

CROTAMITON
(Eurax)

Crotamiton, a synthetic chloroformate salt possessing scabicide and antipruritic properties (10% cream or lotion), is used for its antipruritic efficacy.

CYANOCOBALAMIN (VITAMIN B_{12})

(Berubigen, Betalin 12, Cabadon-M, Cobex, Crystimin-1000, Cyanoject, Cyomin, Kaybovite-1000, Redisol, Rubesol-1000, Rubramin PC, Sytobex)

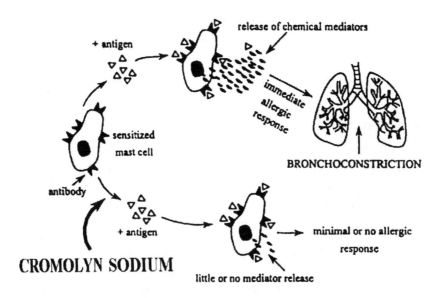

FIGURE 29 Cromolyn sodium, an antiasthmatic preparation, prevents the release of the mediators of Type I allergic reactions. (Adapted from Ebadi, M., *Pharmacology, An Illustrated Review with Questions and Answers*, 3rd Edition, Lippincott-Raven Press, Philadelphia, 1996.)

HYDROXOCOBALAMIN (VITAMIN B$_{12A}$)

(Alphamin, AlphaRedisol, Codroxomin, Droxomin, Hybalamin, Hydrobexan, Hydro-Cobex, Hydroxo-12, LA-12)

Cyanocobalamin, a water-soluble vitamin (25 mcg p.o. daily as a dietary supplement), is indicated in vitamin B$_{12}$ deficiency resulting from any cause except malabsorption related to pernicious anemia or other GI disease (see Figure 98).

CYCLIZINE HYDROCHLORIDE

(Marezine)

Cyclizine (50 mg taken one-half hour before departure and then every 4 to 6 hours as needed) has antihistaminic, anticholinergic, and antiemetic properties, and is used in the prevention and treatment of nausea, vomiting, and dizziness associated with motion sickness. The side effects of cyclizine are drowsiness, dry nose and throat, urinary retention, tachycardia, and constipation.

CYCLOBENZAPRINE HYDROCHLORIDE

(Flexeril)

Cyclobenzaprine (10 mg t.i.d.) is a centrally acting skeletal muscle relaxant and is indicated as an adjunct to rest and physical therapy for relief of muscular spasm associated with injury-related to painful musculoskeletal conditions. However, cyclobenzaprine is not effective in spasticity associated with cerebral or spinal cord injury. Cyclobenzaprine is structurally related to tricyclic antidepressants possessing sedative and anticholinergic properties. Therefore, cyclobenzaprine should be used cautiously in individuals with angle-closure glaucoma and urinary retention due to obstruction or prostatic hypertrophy. Since it causes drowsiness and blurred vision, it should be used carefully when alertness is required.

CYCLOPENTOLATE HYDROCHLORIDE

(AK-Pentolate, Cyclogyl, I-Pentolate, Pentolair)

Cyclopentolate, an anticholinergic agent with mydriatic and cycloplegic properties (2 drops of 0.5% solution), is used in diagnostic procedures requiring mydriasis and cycloplegia (see also Figure 69).

CYCLOPHOSPHAMIDE

(Cytoxan, Endoxan)

Cyclophosphamide, which is chemically related to nitrogen-mustard, is indicated for multiple myeloma including malignant lymphomas, Hodgkin's disease, lymphocytic lymphoma, mixed-cell type lymphoma, histiocytic lymphoma, Burkitt's lymphoma, and for leukemia including chronic lymphocytic leukemia, chronic granulocytic leukemia, acute myelogenous and monocytic leukemia, and acute lymphoblastic leukemia in children, and in mycosis fungoides, neuroblastoma, carcinoma of the ovary, retinoblastoma, and carcinoma of the breast.

Cyclophosphamide is hydroxylated to 4-hydroxycyclophosphamide and aldophosphamide, which in turn are oxidized to the active antineoplastic alkylating agents, non-nitrogen mustard, and phosphoramide mustard. These agents crosslink cell DNA interfering with the growth of rapidly dividing normal and neoplastic cells (see Figure 16). Cyclophosphamide interferes with normal wound healing and impairs oogenesis and spermatogenesis and hence may cause sterility and infertility.

Cyclophosphamide causes immunosuppression and may cause secondary neoplasm especially when taken with radiation therapy. The side effects of cyclophosphamide are anorexia, nausea, vomiting, diarrhea, stomatitis, and alopecia. Leukopenia, interstitial pulmonary fibrosis, and hemorrhagic cardiac necrosis occur with large doses.

CYCLOPROPANE

Cyclopropane, an inflammable gas capable of explosion when improperly mixed with oxygen, is a general anesthetic which is rarely used.

Cyclopropane increases the irritability of the heart by acting on its autonomic tissue and has a tendency to induce irregularities which may terminate in fatal fibrillation. The use of epinephrine is contraindicated in cyclopropane anesthesia since this drug tends to induce ventricular fibrillation (see Table 15).

The advantages of cyclopropane are that it is nonirritating, not unpleasant to the patient, and has little effect on the respiration. It differs from the other gaseous anesthetics in that a high concentration of oxygen (85%) is used in conjunction with a relatively low concentration (15%) of cyclopropane, thus providing an adequate supply of oxygen. There is also less pulmonary irritation than with ether (except in asthma, where it is poorly tolerated) and less excitement during induction. Its disadvantages are explosiveness, lack of respiratory stimulation, difficulty in detecting the planes of anesthesia, and the tendency to produce cardiac arrhythmias and postanesthetic headache.

CYCLOSERINE

(Seromycin)

Cycloserine, an isoxizolidone, d-alanine analog (250 mg p.o. q. 12 hours), is indicated as an adjunctive treatment in pulmonary or extra-pulmonary tuberculosis.

CYCLOSPORIN
(Cyclosporin A)

Cyclosporin (Sandimmune) is an immunosuppressant which, in combination with cortico-steroids, is indicated in prophylaxis of organ rejection in kidney, liver, and heart allogenic transplants. Cyclosporin exerts its effects by inhibition of immunocompetent lymphocytes in the G_0 or G_1-phase of the cell cycle, T-lymphocytes are preferentially inhibited. The T-helper cell is the main target, but the T-suppressor cell may also be suppressed. Cyclosporin also inhibits lymphokine production and release including interleukin-2 or T-cell growth factor (TCGF). It does not cause bone marrow suppression. Cyclosporin has caused nephrotoxicity, hepatotoxicity, thrombocytopenia, microangiopathic hemolytic anemia syndrome, hyperkale-mia, hyperuricemia, and hypertensive and convulsion seizures. Cyclosporin should not be used with potassium-sparing diuretics. Since hypertension is a common side effect, cyclosporin should be used along with an antihypertensive medication.

CYCRIMINE
(Pagitane)

In parkinsonian patients, the deficiency of dopamine causes the cholinergic receptors to be hyperactive. Therefore, **anticholinergic drugs** may be used to mitigate some of the symptoms. These agents include trihexyphenidyl (Artane), cycrimine (Pagitane), procyclidine (Kemadrin), biperiden (Akineton), orphenadrine (Disipal), and benztropine (Cogentin).

Contraindications to the use of anticholinergic drugs in treating parkinsonism are the same as those for atropine: glaucoma, prostatic hypertrophy, myasthenia gravis, stenosing peptic ulcer, and duodenal or pyloric obstruction. Urinary retention and tachycardia should be heeded and regarded as signs of impending toxicity.

CYPROHEPTADINE
(Periactin)

Cyproheptadine, a serotonin and histamine$_1$ receptor- and muscarinic cholinergic receptor-blocking agent, has been used in the treatment of the postgastrectomy dumping syndrome and the intestinal hypermotility seen with carcinoids.

CYPROTERONE ACETATE
(Androcur)

Cyproterone, a substance with antiandrogenic properties, is being investigated for the treatment of severe hirsutism (see Figure 87).

CYTARABINE
(Cytarabine, Cytosar, ARAC)

Cytarabine is an analog of deoxycytidine, differing only in its substitution of sugar arabinose for deoxyribose. It is converted to Ara-CTP, and thereby inhibits DNA-polymerase according to the following reactions:

$$\text{Ara-C} \xrightarrow{\text{Deoxycytidine kinase}} \text{Ara-CMP} \xrightarrow{\text{dCMP kinase}} \text{Ara-CDP}$$

$$\text{Ara-CDP} \xrightarrow{\text{NDP kinase}} \text{Ara-CTP}$$

$$\text{Deoxynucleotides} \xrightarrow[\text{DNA-polymerase}]{\quad/\quad/\quad} \text{DNA}$$

Cytosine arabinoside is used in the treatment of **acute granulocytic leukemia**. Doxorubicin, daunorubicin and cytarabine, cytarabine and thioguanine, or cytarabine, vincristine, and prednisone are the combinations of agents employed. Resistance to cytosine arabinoside may stem from the deletion of deoxycytidine kinase, an increased intracellular pool of dCTP, a nucleotide that competes with ARA-CTP, or increased cytidine deaminase activity, converting Ara-C to inactive Ara-U.

The **toxic effects** of cytosine arabinoside are myelosuppression and injury to the gastrointestinal epithelium, which cause nausea, vomiting, and diarrhea.

CYTOKINES

Cellular diversity in the nervous system evolves from the concerted processes of cell proliferation, differentiation, migration, survival, and synapse formation. Neural adhesion and extracellular matrix molecules have been shown to play crucial roles in axonal migration, guidance, and growth cone targeting.

Cytokines are a heterogeneous group of polypeptide mediators that have been associated with activation of numerous functions, including the immune system and inflammatory responses. The cytokine families include, but are not limited to, interleukins (IL_1-alpha, IL_1-beta, ILIra, and IL-2–IL-15), chemokines (IL-8/NAP-1, NAP-2, MIP_1-alpha and beta, MCAF/MCP-1, MGSA, and RANTES), tumor necrosis factors (TNF-alpha and TNF-beta), interferons (IFN-alpha, beta, and gamma), colony stimulating factors (G-CSF, M-CSF, GM-CSF, IL-3, and some of the other ILs), growth factors (EGF, FGF, PDGF, TFG-alpha, TGF-beta, and ECGF), neuropoietins (LIF, CNTF, OM, and IL-6), and neurotrophins (BDNF, NGF, NT-3–NT-6, and GDNF).

The neurotrophins represent a family of survival and differentiation factors that exert profound effects on the central and peripheral nervous system. The neurotrophins are currently under investigation as therapeutic agents for the treatment of neurodegenerative disorders and nerve injury either individually or in combination with other trophic factors such as ciliary neurotrophic factor or fibroblast growth factor. Responsiveness of neurons to a given neurotrophin is governed by the expression of two classes of cell surface receptors. For NGF, these are $p75^{NTR}$ (p75) and $p140^{trk}$ (referred to as trk or trk-A) which binds both BDNF and NT-4/5, and trk C receptor which binds only NT-3. After binding ligand, the neurotrophin-receptor complex is internalized and retrogradely transported in the axon to the soma. Both receptors undergo ligand-induced dimerization that activates multiple signal transduction pathways. These include the ras-dependent pathway utilized by trk to mediate neurotrophin effects such as survival and differentiation.

Nerve growth factor and brain-derived neurotrophic factor are important neurotrophic factors that are essential for the differentiation and survival of some neural tissues, especially sympathetic neurons. Proinflammatory cytokines, released by activated macrophages and monocytes during infection, can act on neural targets that control thermogenesis, behavior, and mood. In addition to induction of fever, cytokines induce other biologic functions associated with the acute phase response, including hypophagia and sleep. Cytokine production has been detected within the CNS as a result of brain injury, following stab wounds to the brain, during viral and bacterial infections (AIDS and meningitis), and in neurodegenerative processes (multiple sclerosis and Alzheimer's disease). Novel cytokine therapies, such as anticytokine antibodies or specific receptor antagonists acting on the cytokine network, may provide an optimistic feature for treatment of multiple sclerosis and other diseases in which cytokines have been implicated (see also Figure 53).

CYTOKINES: THEIR ACTIONS		
Cytokine	Select Sources	Select Actions
IL-1	Macrophages	Immunoaugmentation
IL-2	T lymphocytes and LGL	T and B cell growth factor
IL-3	T lymphocytes	Hematopoietic growth factor
IL-4	TH cells	T and B cell growth factor; promotes IgE reactions
IL-5	TH cells	Stimulates B cells and eosinophils
IL-6	Fibroblasts	Hybridoma growth factor; augments inflammation
IL-7	Stromal cells	Lymphopoietin
IL-8	Macrophages	Chemoattracts neutrophils and T lymphocytes
G-CSF	Monocytes	Myeloid growth factor
M-CSF	Monocytes	Macrophage growth factor
GM-CSF	T cells	Monomyelocytic growth factor
IFN-α	Leukocytes	Antiviral, antiproliferative, and immunomodulating
IFN-β	Fibroblasts	Induce cell membrane antigens (e.g., MHC)
IFN-γ	T lymphocytes and NK cells	Vascular thromboses and tumor necrosis
TNFα	Macrophages	Inflammatory, immunoenhancing, and tumoricidal
LT = TNFβ TGFβ	T lymphocytes Platelets and bone	Fibroplasia and immunosuppression

CYTOMEGALOVIRUS IMMUNE GLOBULIN

(CMV-IGIV, Cytomegalovirus Immune Serum Intravenous [HUMAN], Cytomune-IV) (Cytogam)

Cytomegalovirus immune globulin (150 mg/kg IV within 75 hours of transplant, and then in reduced dosage 2 to 16 weeks post transplant), is used to attenuate cytomegalovirus (CMV) disease in seronegative kidney transplant recipients who receive a kidney from a CMV seropositive donor.

D

DACARBAZINE
(DTIC-Dome)

Dacarbazine, a cell cycle phase nonspecific antineoplastic agent (see Figure 2), is indicated for treatment of metastatic malignant melanoma (3 mg/kg/day for 10 days) and second-line therapy for Hodgkin's disease. Dacarbazine is thought to exert its effects by alkylation of a carbonium ion, inhibition of DNA synthesis by acting as a purine analog, and interaction with sulfhydryl groups in proteins. It is metabolized partly to 5-aminomidazole-4-carboxamide (AIC) and partly is excreted unchanged by active tubular secretion. The half-life of carboxamide is altered in hepatic and renal impairment. Dacarbazine causes nausea, vomiting, flu-like syndrome with fever and myalgia, leukopenia, and thrombocytopenia.

DACTINOMYCIN
(Actinomycin D; ACT; Cosmegen)

Dactinomycin (0.5 mg/day IV for 5 days) in combination with vincristine, radiotherapy, and surgery it is used in Wilm's tumor; in conjunction with vincristine, cyclophosphamide, and doxorubicin it is used in choriocarcinoma; in combination with methotrexate it is used in testicular carcinoma; and in combination with cyclophosphamide and radiotherapy it is used in Ewing's sarcoma. Dactinomycin inhibits messenger RNA synthesis by anchoring to a purine–pyrimidine (DNA) base pair by intercalation (see Figure 2). The toxicity of dactinomycin increases when combined with radiation therapy.

Adverse effects of dactinomycin, which begin 3 to 4 days after initiation of therapy, include cheilitis, dysphagia, esophagitis, ulcerative stomatitis, pharyngitis, anorexia, abdominal pain, diarrhea, GI ulceration, proctitis, hepatic toxicity, anemia, leukopenia, thrombocytopenia, alopecia, erythema, fatigue, malaise, and lethargy. Many of these adverse effects will continue after cessation of therapy.

DANTROLENE SODIUM
(Dantrium)

Dantrolene, which has a high risk for causing hepatic toxicity, is indicated for the management of spasticity resulting from upper motor neuron disorders such as spinal cord injury, stroke, cerebral palsy, or multiple sclerosis. In addition, it is used in malignant hyperthermia, neuroleptic malignant syndrome, and heat stroke causing painful muscular contraction and rigidity. Dantrolene does not influence myoneural function but exerts its effects directly on the muscle by interfering with the release of Ca^{++} from sarcoplasmic reticulum and dissociating the excitation–contraction coupling (see Figure 30).

The reported side effects of dantrolene are drowsiness, dizziness, weakness, hepatitis, constipation, increased urinary frequency, crystalluria, seizures, visual disturbances, pruritis, urticaria, acne, and skin eruption.

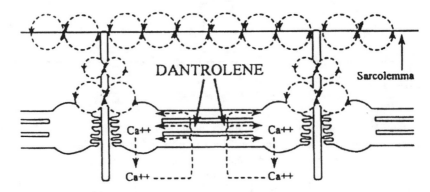

FIGURE 30   Dantrolene, a skeletal muscle relaxant, interferes with the release of calcium ion from the sarcoplasmic reticulum, resulting in decreased muscle contraction.

DAPSONE
(DDS)

Leprosy (Hansen's disease) is a chronic granulomatous disease that attacks superficial tissues such as the skin, nasal mucosa, and peripheral nerves. There are two types of leprosy: **lepromatous** and **tuberculoid**. The **sulfones**, which are derivatives of 4,4′-diaminodiphenyl-sulfone, are bacteriostatic. **Dapsone** (DDS) and **sulfoxone sodium** are the most useful and effective agents currently available. They should be given in low doses initially, and then the dosage should be gradually increased until a full dose of 300 to 400 mg per week is reached. During this period, the patient must be monitored carefully. With adequate precautions and appropriate doses, sulfones may be used safely for years. Nevertheless, side effects such as anorexia, nervousness, insomnia, blurred vision, paresthesia, and peripheral neuropathy do occur. **Hemolysis** is common, especially in patients with glucose 6-phosphate dehydrogenase deficiency. A fatal exacerbation of lepromatous leprosy and an infectious mononucleosis-like syndrome rarely occur. **Clofazimine** (Lamprene) may be effective in patients who show resistance to the sulfones and may also dramatically reduce an exacerbation of leprosy. Red discoloration of the skin and eosinophilic enteritis have occurred following clofazimine therapy.

Not all mycobacterial infections are caused by *Mycobacterium tuberculosis* or *Mycobacterium leprae*. These atypical mycobacteria require treatment with secondary medications as well as other chemotherapeutic agents. For example, *Mycobacterium marinum* causes skin granulomas, and effective drugs in the treatment of infection are **rifampin** or **minocycline**. *Mycobacterium fortuitum* causes skin ulcers, and the medications recommended for treatment are **ethambutol, cycloserine**, and **rifampin** in combination with **amikacin**.

DAUNORUBICIN
(Cerubidine, Daunomycin)

Daunorubicin and doxorubicin (Adriamycin) bind to and cause the intercalation of the DNA molecule, thereby inhibiting DNA template function. They also provoke DNA chain scission and chromosomal damage.

Daunorubicin is useful in treating patients with acute lymphocytic or acute granulocytic leukemia. Adriamycin is useful in cases of solid tumors such as sarcoma, metastatic breast cancer, and thyroid cancer. These agents cause stomatitis, alopecia, myelosuppression, and cardiac abnormalities ranging from arrhythmias to cardiomyopathy (see also Figure 2).

DEBRISOQUIN

Debrisoquin is an antihypertensive medication. **Bethanidine** is a short-acting adrenergic neuron blocker; **debrisoquin** and **guanadrel** are medium-acting adrenergic neuron blockers; whereas **guanethidine** is a long-acting adrenergic neuron blocker and also depletes axonal stores of norepinephrine. Debrisoquin causes postural hypotension, fluid retention, failure of ejaculation, and depression. Debrisoquin should be avoided with tyramine-containing substances such as cheese. Debrisoquin and other adrenergic neuron-blocking drugs may interact with amphetamines, ephedrine, phenylephrine, tricyclic antidepressants, and chlorpromazine.

DECAMETHONIUM

Acetylcholine receptors are classified as either **muscarinic** or **nicotinic**. The alkaloid **muscarine** mimics the effects produced by stimulation of the parasympathetic system. These effects are postganglionic and are exerted on exocrine glands, cardiac muscle, and smooth muscle. The alkaloid **nicotine** mimics the actions of acetylcholine, which include stimulation of all autonomic ganglia, stimulation of the adrenal medulla, and contraction of skeletal muscle (see Figure 18).

Dimethylphenylpiperazinium stimulates the autonomic ganglia; tetraethylammonium and **hexamethonium** block the autonomic ganglia; phenyltrimethylammonium stimulates skeletal motor muscle end plates, decamethonium produces neuromuscular blockade; and d-tubocurarine blocks both the autonomic ganglia and the motor fiber end plates.

Among the agents cited, only d-tubocurarine (see Figure 92) is useful as a drug (skeletal muscle relaxant); the rest are useful only as research tools.

DEFEROXAMINE
(Desferal)

A lethal dose of iron consists of 12 g of an iron preparation containing 1 or 2 g of elemental iron. Therefore, iron toxicity rarely occurs in adults but is frequently seen in children. The mortality rate among untreated children is high (45%). The initial signs and symptoms of iron poisoning are gastrointestinal and usually consist of nausea, vomiting, and diarrhea. If untreated, acidosis, cyanosis, and circulatory collapse may ensue. If the patient survives, there may be gastric scarring and pyloric stenosis resulting from the corrosive action of the iron preparation. Treatment should include induced vomiting and lavage if the poisoning is discovered early, catharsis to hasten evacuation, sodium bicarbonate therapy to combat the acidosis, and the administration of **deferoxamine**, a specific iron-chelating agent.

One hundred milligrams of deferoxamine is able to bind 8.5 mg of iron. The chelating effects of deferoxamine are maximum at an acidic pH; therefore, when given orally, deferoxamine must be administered before the sodium bicarbonate. In the event of iron poisoning; deferoxamine may also be administered intramuscularly. Besides its usefulness in counteracting the effects of iron poisoning, deferoxamine has been used in disorders that involve **iron overload** such as ocular hemosiderosis or hemochromatosis.

DEMECLOCYCLINE HYDROCHLORIDE
(Declomycin, Ledermycin)

Demeclocycline, a tetracycline antibiotic (600 mg p.o. q. 6 hours), is indicated in the treatment of infections caused by susceptible organisms, gonorrhea, and uncomplicated urethral, endocervical, or rectal infection (see also Figure 88).

DEOXYNIVALENOL

Deoxynivalenol, also called **vomitoxin**, is a naturally occurring trichotecene mycotoxin produced by several species of *Fusarium fungi* on a variety of cereal grains. Reports of contaminated grain are not uncommon. Feed refusal and emesis are the major symptoms in individuals fed diets containing deoxynivalenol. Deoxynivalenol delays gastric emptying through serotonin 3-receptors ($5HT_3$) (see also Figure 64).

DERMATAN SULFATE

(DS)

Dermatan sulfate (DS) is a member of a family of structurally complex, sulfated, linear polysaccharides called **glycosaminoglycans**. The other members of this family of molecules are heparin, heparin sulfate, chondroitin sulfates, and hyaluronic acid. DS and chondroitin sulfates are structurally similar and make up a subfamily of glycosaminoglycans called galactosaminoglycans. Glycosaminoglycans are often found attached to a protein core, resulting in a macromolcule called a proteoglycan. These proteoglycans localize on cell surfaces and in the extracellular matrix. There, they function in the important role of cell–cell interaction, binding a variety of biologically important proteins and localizing these at the cell surface. Glycosaminoglycan DS has been used as an experimental therapeutic agent to modulate a variety of these biological processes.

DERMATOLOGICAL DISORDERS: TREATMENT WITH RETINOIDS	
Acne	
Cystic acne	Hidradenitis suppurativa
Gram-negative folliculitis	Papular acne
Cutaneous Aging	
Disorders of Keratinization	
Darier's disease	Pityriasis rubra pilaris
Erythrokeratoderma variabilis	The ichthyoses
Precancerous Conditions	
Actinic keratosis	
Dysplastic nevus	
Leukoplakia	
Skin Cancer	
Basal cell cancer	Keratoacanthoma
Cutaneous T-cell lymphoma	Squamous cell cancer
Psoriasis	
Erythrodermic psoriasis	Pustular psoriasis
Psoriasis vulgaris	Pustular psoriasis, palms and soles
Psoriatic arthritis	

DESFLURANE

(Suprane)

Desflurane, a tetrafluorethyl difluoromethyl ether, is used to induce and maintain anesthesia.

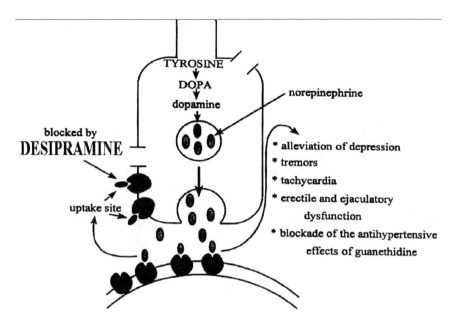

FIGURE 31 Desipramine, a tricyclic antidepressant, causes a strong blockade of serotonin uptake mechanism. It causes a mild degree of sedation and orthostatic hypotension and has a weak anticholinergic property. (Adapted from Ebadi, M., *Pharmacology, An Illustrated Review with Questions and Answers*, 3rd Edition, Lippincott-Raven Press, Philadelphia, 1996.)

DESIPRAMINE

(Norpramin)

Desipramine (75 to 150 mg p.o./day in divided doses) is indicated in endogenous depression; major depression with melancholia or psychotic symptoms; depression associated with organic brain disease, alcoholism, schizophrenia, or mental retardation; and depressive phase of manic-depressive disorder. Desipramine is absorbed rapidly from the GI tract, distributed widely in the body, and appears also in breast milk. It is bound to plasma proteins to the extent of 90%, undergoes extensive first-pass metabolism, and its metabolites are excreted in the urine. Desipramine strongly blocks the norepinephrine uptake mechanism and has no effect on the uptake of serotonin. Desipramine has weak alpha$_1$ adrenergic and muscarinic cholinergic receptor blocking effects (see also Tables 3 through 5). The concomitant use of desipramine with sympathomimetic amines may cause elevated blood pressure. On the other hand, desipramine, by blocking the uptake sites for norepinephrine may attenuate the antihypertensive effects of guanethidine, guanabenz, guanadrel, clonidine, methyldopa, and reserpine (see Figure 31).

DESLANOSIDE

Among the useful available cardiac glycosides are the following:

Digitalis purpurea	Digitalis lanata	Strophanthus gratus
Digitoxin	Digoxin	Ouabain
Digoxin	Lanatoside C	
Digitalis leaf	Deslanoside	

Of these, only digoxin and digitoxin and, to a certain extent, ouabain are used extensively.

The structures of the cardiac glycosides, including digoxin, have three common components: a steroid nucleus (aglycones or genins), a series of sugar residues in the C_3 position, and a five- or six-membered lactone ring in the C_{17} position.

DESMOPRESSIN ACETATE
(1-Deamino-8-D-Arginine Vasopressin)

Desmopressin, a synthetic analog of arginine vasopressin, is indicated for nocturnal enuresis; for neurogenic diabetes insipidus; for polyuria following surgery or trauma in the pituitary region; in combination with factor VIII in the treatment of hemophilia A; and in combination with factor VIII in the treatment of Von Willebrand's disease. Since desmopressin may be used intranasally, changes in nasal mucosa including scarring, edema, discharge, blockage, congestion, and atrophic rhinitis may occur.

Many agents alter the secretion or action of vasopressin, and these are cited in Figure 94.

DESONIDE
(DesOwen, Tridesilon)

Desonide, a topical adrenocorticoid with antiinflammatory properties (0.05% cream, lotion, and ointment), is used as an adjunctive therapy for inflammation in acute and chronic corticosteroid-responsive dermatoses (see also Table 10).

DEXAMETHASONE (OPHTHALMIC SUSPENSION)
(Maxidex)

DEXAMETHASONE SODIUM PHOSPHATE
(AK-Dex, Decadron, Dexair, 1-Methasone, Maxidex, Ocu-Dex)

Dexamethasone, a corticosteroid with ophthalmic antiinflammatory properties (0.1% solution), is used in the treatment of uveitis; iridocyclitis; inflammation of eyelids, conjunctiva, cornea, anterior segment of globe; and corneal injury from burns or penetration by foreign bodies (see also Table 10).

DEXAMETHASONE SODIUM PHOSPHATE
(Decadron Phosphate, Hexadrol Phosphate)

Dexamethasone sodium phosphate, an antiinflammatory corticosteroid, is available as a nasal aerosol (84 mcg/metered spray) and is used in the management of perennial or seasonal rhinitis and prevention of recurrence of nasal polyps after surgical removal. It is also used as an oral inhalant to treat bronchial asthma in patients who require corticosteroids to control symptoms. The nasal inhalations may cause itchy nose, dryness, burning, irritation, sneezing, epistaxis, and bloody mucus; oral inhalation may cause flushing, rash, dry mouth, hoarseness, irritation of the tongue or throat, and impaired sense of taste. Prolonged and inappropriate usage of dexamethasone in higher than therapeutic dosage may result in suppression of immune mechanism and fungal overgrowth (see Table 10).

DEXAMETHASONE (SYSTEMIC)
(Decadron, Dexone, Hexadrol, SK-Dexamethasone)

DEXAMETHASONE ACETATE

(Dalalone D.P., Decadron L.A., Decaject L.A., Decameth L.A., Dexacen, Dexasone L.A., Dexone L.A., Solurex L.A.)

DEXAMETHASONE SODIUM PHOSPHATE

(AK-Dex, Dalalone, Decadrol, Decadron, Decaject, Decameth, Dexacen, Dexasone, Dexon, Dexone, Hexadrol Phosphate, Solurex)

Systemic dexamethasone is used in shock (other than adrenal crisis), dexamethasone suppression test, and adrenal insufficiency.

DEXAMETHASONE (TOPICAL)

(Aeroseb-Dex, Decaderm, Decaspray)

DEXAMETHASONE SODIUM PHOSPHATE

(Decadron Cream)

Topical dexamethasone (gel and cream 0.1%) is indicated in inflammation of corticosteroid-responsive dermatoses.

DEXAMETHASONE SODIUM PHOSPHATE

(Inhalant)

Dexamethasone (100 mcg/metered spray) is indicated in the control of bronchial asthma in patients with steroid-dependent asthma, and relief of symptoms of perennial or seasonal rhinitis; and in prevention of recurrence of nasal polyps after surgical removal.

DEXFENFLURAMINE

Dexfenfluramine, the dextroisomer of fenfluramine, altering serotoninergic transmission, (15 mg b.i.d.) causes weight loss and enhances adherence to weight-lowering programs such as counseling, following dietary advice, behavioral modification, and physical exercise.

DEXTRAN

(Dextran 40 & 70)

Dextran, a branched polysaccharide plasma volume expander, may be used as a supportive measure to treat shock resulting from hemorrhage, burns, surgery, or other trauma. Low-molecular-weight dextran (Dextran 40) has an average molecular weight of 40,000, and its 2.5% solution is equivalent in colloid osmotic pressure to normal plasma. High-molecular-weight dextran (Dextran 70) has an average molecular weight of 70,000. Dextran is excreted gradually by the kidneys, 50% of it within 3 hours, 60% of it within 6 hours, and 75% of it within 24 hours. Dextran is used as a prophylaxis against venous thrombosis and thromboembolism in that it inhibits vascular stasis, platelet adhesion, and fibrous clot formation. Dextrans are antigenic, and those with the smallest molecular weights are least antigenic.

DEXTRIFERRON

The parenteral iron medications available include **iron-dextran** (ferric hydroxide and high-molecular-weight dextran) for intramuscular use, **dextriferron** (a complex of ferric hydroxide and partially hydrolyzed dextran) for intravenous use, and **saccharated iron oxide** (a complex of ferric hydroxide and sucrose) for intravenous use. These preparations are reserved for those cases in which oral preparations are not tolerated, absorbed, or rapid enough in their onset of action, or are otherwise not suitable for noncompliant patients.

DEXTROAMPHETAMINE
(Dexedrine)

Dextroamphetamine is a sympathomimetic amine which is used in narcolepsy and in attention deficit disorder in children. Dextroamphetamine releases norepinephrine and, in high doses, also dopamine. It is absorbed from the gastrointestinal tract, metabolized in the liver, and is excreted unchanged in the urine. Acidification of urine shortens amphetamine's half-life, whereas alkalinization of urine prolongs it. The accumulation of hydroxy metabolite of amphetamine has been thought to cause amphetamine-induced psychosis. Therapeutic doses of amphetamine may cause insomnia, tremor, and restlessness; and toxic doses of amphetamine may cause mydriasis, hypertension, and arrhythmia. **Chlorpromazine** is an excellent antidote in amphetamine toxicity. The continuous use of amphetamine causes tolerance, requiring higher doses, and hence there exists a high potential for its abuse. Amphetamine should not be used with a monoamine oxidase A inhibitor such as tranylcypromine, since the chance of inducing hypertension becomes magnified.

Similar caution should be exercised with biogenic amine uptake blockers such as tricyclic antidepressant. Amphetamine is contraindicated in advanced arteriosclerosis; symptomatic cardiovascular disease; moderate to severe hypertension; hyperthyroidism; hypersensitivity or idiosyncrasy to the sympathomimetic amines; glaucoma, agitated states; history of drug abuse; during or within 14 days following administration of monoamine oxidase (MAO) inhibitors.

DEXTROMETHORPHAN
(Romilar)

Dextromethorphan (Romilar) is the dextroisomer of the methyl ether of **levorphanol**. Unlike its levorotatory congener, it possesses no significant analgesic property, exerts no depressant effects on respiration, and lacks addiction liability. It is an antitussive agent with a potency approximately one half that of codeine.

Therapeutic doses of dextromethorphan (15 to 30 mg) produce few or no side effects, whereas excessively high doses (300 to 1500 mg) have been reported to produce a state resembling intoxication accompanied by euphoria.

Besides its antitussive property, recent studies have shown that dextromethorphan has anticonvulsant and **neuroprotective properties**. Because dextromethorphan interacts with NMDA or sigma receptors, it may become important in ameliorating the cerebrovascular and functional consequences of **global cerebral ischemia**.

DEXTROPROPOXYPHENE
(Darvon)

Propoxyphene is structurally very similar to methadone and possesses four stereoisomers. Dextropropoxyphene is an analgesic with a potency two thirds that of codeine. Levopropoxyphene is an antitussive, but lacks analgesic properties.

Adverse reactions to dextropropoxyphene include nausea, vomiting, sedation, dizziness, constipation, and skin rash, with a frequency of incidence somewhat less than that seen with codeine use. Although respiratory depression is a cardinal sign of acute dextropropoxyphene poisoning, the drug apparently does not affect respiration in the usual therapeutic doses of 32 to 65 mg.

DEXTROSE
(D-Glucose)

Dextrose, a carbohydrate, is used in fluid replacement and caloric supplementation in patients who cannot maintain adequate oral intake or who are restricted from doing so.

DEXTROTHYROXINE SODIUM
(Choloxin)

Dextrothyroxine, a thyroid hormone with antilipemic effect (1 to 2 mg daily), is used primarily in type II hyperlipoproteinemia.

DEZOCINE
(Dalgan)

Dezocine, an opiate receptor agonist–antagonist, possessing analgesic property (5 to 20 mg IM q. 3 to 6 hours), is used in the management of moderate to severe pain.

DIABETES MELLITUS: TREATMENT FOR NON-INSULIN-DEPENDENT CASES	
Drugs for NIDDM	**Usual Daily Dosage**
Sulfonylureas	
First Generation	
Acetohexamide	500 to 750 mg once or divided
Chlorpropamide	250 to 375 mg once
Tolazamide	250 to 500 mg once or divided
Tolbutamide	1000 to 2000 mg once or divided
Second Generation	
Glimepiride	4 mg once
Glipizide	10 to 20 mg once or divided
Glucotrol	
Glucotrol XL sustained-release tablets	5 to 10 mg once
Glyburide	5 to 10 mg once or divided
DiaBeta	
Micronase	
Glynase micronized tablets	3 to 12 mg once or divided
Biguanide	
Metformin	850 mg b.i.d.
Alpha-glucosidase inhibitor	
Acarbose	50 to 100 mg t.i.d.

DIACETYLMORPHINE
(Heroin)

Heroin, a synthetic alkaloid formed from morphine by substituting acetyl for its two hydroxyl groups, resembles morphine in its general effects but acts more strongly on both cerebrum and medulla than does morphine, and is therefore more poisonous, the usual dose being about one fourth that of morphine (see Figure 58). Heroin is a highly addictive substance, and the social danger from it, moreover, seems to be greater than with morphine in that it produces a change in the personality as shown by an utter disregard for the conventions and morals of civilization. Degenerative changes in the individual progress faster than with any of the other narcotic drugs, and all the higher faculties of the mind, such as judgment, self-control, and attention, are weakened, and the addict rapidly becomes a mental and moral degenerate. The heroin habit is most difficult to cure, not only in the active withdrawal period but also in the convalescent stage, and relapse is frequent. Habitues take it either by snuffing or by hypodermic injection. Because of its marked tendency to addiction and its minor therapeutic value, the manufacture and importation of heroin has been outlawed in the United States.

DIAMIDINES

(Pentamidine)

Trypanosomiasis is produced by protozoa of the genus *Trypanosoma* and leads to Gambian or mid-African sleeping sickness (*T. gambiense*), Rhodesian or East African sleeping sickness (*T. rhodesiense*), and Chagas' disease, which is seen in the populations of Central and South America (*T. cruzi*).

Agents effective in the treatment of trypanosomiasis are the **aromatic diamidines** (pentamidine, stilbamidine, and propamidine). **Pentamidine** is the preferred drug for the prevention and early treatment of *T. gambiense* infections; however, it cannot penetrate the central nervous system. **Melarsoprol** is the drug recommended for *T. gambiense* infections that do not respond to pentamidine or for managing the late meningoencephalitic stages of infection. It does reach the central nervous system. **Nifurtimox** (Lampit) is the drug of choice for treating the acute form of Chagas' disease. **Suramin** (Naphuride) is effective only as therapy for African sleeping sickness.

DIARRHEA: DRUG-INDUCED	
Antacids (magnesium-containing agents)	
Antibiotics	
Any broad-spectrum antibiotic	Sulfonamides
Clindamycin	Tetracyclines
Antihypertensives	
Guanabenz	Methyldopa
Guanadrel	Reserpine
Guanethidine	
Cholinesterase Inhibitors	
Metaclopramide	
Cholinomimetics	
Bethanechol	
Cardiac Agents	
Digitalis	
Digoxin	
Quinidine	

DIAZEPAM

(Valium)

Diazepam is a lipid-soluble but water-insoluble substance. The solvent for parenteral diazepam consists of 40% propylene glycol, 10% ethyl alcohol, 5% sodium benzoate, and 1.5% benzyl alcohol. Injection site complications such as phlebitis may result from the injudicious administration of these compounds. Like chlordiazepoxide, diazepam should be given either orally or intravenously. The peak plasma concentration of orally administered diazepam is reached in two hours. The short duration of action of diazepam when given intravenously is caused by its tissue redistribution and not by metabolism. In this case, diazepam behaves identically to the ultra-short-acting barbiturates such as **thiopental**. As a matter of fact, diazepam is metabolized slowly, with the reported half-life varying from 50 to 75 hours. Because some of the metabolites are also active pharmacologically, steady-state concentrations develop slowly, usually 7 to 10 days after the initiation of oral therapy.

When compared to **oxazepam**, diazepam is absorbed more rapidly and produces discernible sedative effects. Such rapid absorption (peak levels attained in one hour) could account for its vast popularity, but could also predispose patients to abuse it. When alcohol in small concentration (10% by volume) is taken at the same time as an oral dose of diazepam, the rate of absorption is decreased, but not the amount absorbed; a higher concentration of alcohol (50% by volume) may increase diazepam absorption (see also Table 8).

As with chlordiazepoxide, the dosage of diazepam should be lower in the elderly (initial dose, about half the usual), not only because of the pharmacokinetic differences but also because accumulation of the parent drug and active metabolites is more likely to lead to confusion and muscle weakness in the elderly. Furthermore, the elderly seem to be more sensitive to the depressant effects of diazepam than are younger patients.

The plasma protein binding of diazepam is about 97 to 99% in adults, regardless of age, but the distribution volume of around 1 liter per kilogram is higher in the elderly and females. Hypoalbuminemia leads to an increase in the fraction of unbound drug in plasma and a faster rate of elimination, since more drug is available for metabolism.

Diazepam readily crosses the placenta, particularly in the later stages of pregnancy and during labor; its pathways of metabolism are altered in the fetus and newborn and this prolongs the elimination of both diazepam and desmethyldiazepam. Diazepam must therefore be used judiciously in patients who are pregnant and in labor. Diazepam and desmethyldiazepam appear in breast milk and in the plasma of breast-fed infants (see also Figure 40).

DIAZOXIDE

(Hyperstat)

Diazoxide, which is administered intravenously, is used exclusively in the management of **malignant hypertension** or a hypertensive crisis. It brings about reflex cardiac acceleration and increased cardiac output. However, it can cause hyperglycemia due to its inhibition of insulin release from the beta cells. Because diazoxide also produces sodium and water retention, it should be given with a diuretic such as **furosemide** or **ethacrynic acid**.

DIBENZAPINE DERIVATIVES

Antidepressants are divided into the following classes: The **dibenzapine derivatives** are called **tricyclic antidepressants** and include **imipramine** (Tofranil), **desipramine** (Norpramin), **amitriptyline** (Elavil), **nortriptyline** (Aventyl), **protriptyline** (Vivactil), and **doxepin** (Adapin). The **monoamine oxidase inhibitors** are used occasionally to treat depression. The **hydrazine** derivatives consist of **isocarboxazid** (Marplan) and **phenelzine sulfate** (Nardil). The **nonhydrazine** derivatives include **tranylcypromine** (Parnate). **L-Tryptophan** is the only member of the **monoamine precursors** used to treat depression. The newer and second-generation antidepressants include **amoxapine, doxepin, fluoxetine, maprotiline, trazodone, mianserin, alprazolam,** and **bupropion** (see also Tables 3 through 5).

DIBUCAINE
(Nupercainal)

Dibucaine, an amine local anesthetic (1% ointment; 0.5% cream), is used topically for temporary relief of pain and itching associated with abrasions, sunburn, minor burns, hemorrhoids, and other minor skin conditions (see also Figure 20).

DICHLORPHENAMIDE
(Daranide)

The carbonic anhydrase inhibitors consist of **acetazolamide** (Diamox), **ethoxzolamide** (Cardrase), and **dichlorphenamide** (Daranide). Acetazolamide is an old agent, whereas ethoxzolamide and dichlorphenamide are newer preparations. Dichlorphenamide is the most potent carbonic anhydrase inhibitor in use today. The presence of SO_2NH_2 (sulfonamide) causes such compounds to inhibit carbonic anhydrase (CA), which catalyzes the hydration of carbon dioxide as follows:

$$CO_2 + H_2O \xrightarrow{\ CA\ } H_2CO_3 \rightleftharpoons H^+ + HCO_3^-$$

These agents inhibit carbonic anhydrase in the renal tubular cells in both the proximal and distal tubules. When the rate of hydrogen generation is reduced, HCO_3^- is lost in urine and the patient tends to become acidotic. However, the plasma concentration of HCO_3^- is lowered and less is filtered, so the diuresis becomes less effective. In addition, the sodium output is increased because its resorption in exchange for hydrogen is limited by the decreased availability of hydrogen. With less hydrogen available, the exchange of sodium for potassium predominates, and this fosters the loss of potassium. Chloride excretion is not altered significantly. Because the aqueous humor has a high concentration of bicarbonate, carbonic anhydrase inhibitors are primarily used in the treatment of **glaucoma**. They are no longer used as diuretics or as antiepileptic agents.

DICLOFENAC SODIUM
(Voltaren)

Diclofenac has analgesic and antiinflammatory properties and in the dose of 150 to 250 mg/day is indicated in acute and chronic treatment of the signs and symptoms of rheumatoid arthritis, osteoarthritis, and ankylosing spondylitis. In addition, it is effective in a dose of 50 mg t.i.d. in the management of pain primarily associated with dysmenorrhea (see also Table 2).

DICLOXACILLIN SODIUM
(Pathocil)

Dicloxacillin is indicated in the treatment of infections resulting from penicillinase-producing staphylococci. Penicillins, which are the safest of the antibiotics, produce few direct toxic reactions, and most of the serious side effects are **hypersensitivity reactions**. Penicillins and their by-products, penicilloic acid and penicilloylpolylysine, are antigenic in susceptible individuals who develop immunoglobulin G antibodies to them. Furthermore, all penicillins cross-sensitize and cross-react. Allergic reactions, including **anaphylactoid shock**, occur in sensitized patients following the repeated administration of penicillin. Anaphylactoid reactions, which are more common following the parenteral administration of penicillin, may be reversed by the administration of corticosteroids (see Figure 65).

The direct toxicity of penicillin following the administration of large doses may include **phlebitis** if it is given intravenously, **injection site inflammatory reactions** when given intramuscularly, **degeneration of nerve tissue** if injected into a nerve, and **central nervous system excitability** if given intrathecally.

The **broad-spectrum penicillins**, such as **ampicillin** and **amoxicillin**, may cause gastrointestinal irritation. Occasionally, the overgrowth of *Staphylococci, Pseudomonas, Proteus,* or yeasts may be responsible for causing **enteritis**. Methicillin and nafcillin may precipitate **granulocytopenia,** and methicillin has been known to cause **nephritis**. Carbenicillin may cause **hypokalemic alkalosis**. The properties of the various penicillins are shown in Table 22.

DICUMAROL

The **coumarin anticoagulants** include dicumarol, warfarin sodium (coumadin sodium), warfarin potassium (Athrombin-K), acenocoumarol (Sintrom), and phenprocouman (Liquamar).

Phytonadisone (vitamin K_1; phylloquinone) is identical to naturally occurring vitamin K_1, which is required for the synthesis of blood coagulation factors such as prothrombin (II), proconvertin (VII), Christmas factor or plasma thromboplastin component (IX), and Stuart-Prower factor (X) in the liver. Dicumarol and ethylbiscoumacetate act as competitive antagonists of vitamin K and interfere with the synthesis of these factors in the liver. Similarly, hypoprothrombinemic-induced bleeding can be rectified by the administration of vitamin K.

DICYCLOMINE HYDROCHLORIDE

(Bentyl)

Dicyclomine (80 to 160 mg in four equally divided doses) is indicated in the treatment of irritable colon, spastic colon, and mucous colitis. Dicyclomine is an antispasmodic-anticholinergic agent which relieves smooth muscle spasm of the gastrointestinal tract. Dicyclomine is contraindicated in obstructive uropathy, obstructive disease of the gastrointestinal tract, severe ulcerative colitis, reflux esophagitis, unstable cardiovascular status in acute hemorrhage, glaucoma, and myasthenia gravis. The side effects of dicyclomine include dry mouth, dizziness, and blurred vision.

DIDANOSIDE

(ddl) (Videx)

Didanoside, a purine analog with antiviral effects (75 mg/kg p.o. q. 12 hours), is used in advanced human immunodeficiency virus (HIV) infection in patients who cannot tolerate or no longer respond to zidovudine therapy (see also Figure 99).

DIENESTROL

(Estraguard)

Dienestrol cream is indicated in the treatment of atrophic vaginitis and kraurosis vulvae. Like all estrogens, dienestrol is contraindicated in known or suspected cancer of the breast, known or suspected estrogen-dependent neoplasia, undiagnosed abnormal genital bleeding, active thrombophlebitis or thromboembolic disorders, and a history of thrombophlebitis, thrombosis, or thromboembolic disorders associated with previous estrogen use (see also Figure 26).

DIETHYLDITHIOCARBAMATE

(Imuthiol)

Diethyldithiocarbamate is under investigation for its possible effectiveness in the treatment of **acquired immunodeficiency syndrome** (AIDS) which is caused by the human immuno-deficiency virus (HIV), which impairs both cellular and humoral immune functions, and this results in increased susceptibility to opportunistic infection and certain malignancies.

DIETHYLPROPION HYDROCHLORIDE

(Nobesine, Nu-Dispoz, Regibon, Ro-Diet, Tenuate, Tepanil)

Diethylpropion, a sympathomimetic agent resembling amphetamine (25 mg p.o. t.i.d.), is used for a short period of time in the treatment of obesity.

DIETHYLSTILBESTROL

(Stilbestrol)

Diethylstilbestrol is indicated in female hypogonadism, ovariectomy, or primary ovarian failure (0.2 to 0.5 mg p.o. daily in cycles of three weeks on and one week off); moderate to severe vasomotor symptoms of menopause, atrophic vaginitis or kraurosis vulvae (0.2 to 2 mg p.o. daily in cycles of three weeks on and one week off); in postcoital contraception as morning-after pill (25 mg p.o. b.i.d. for five days); for prostatic cancer (1 to 3 mg p.o. daily); and for breast cancer in postmenopausal women (15 mg daily p.o.). Diethylstilbestrol mimics the action of estrogen in treating female hypogonadism, menopausal symptoms, and atrophic vaginitis. Diethylstilbestrol inhibits the growth of hormone sensitive tissues in advanced inoperable prostatic cancer. Diethylstilbestrol is contraindicated in patients with thrombophlebitis, thromboembolism or history of thromboembolism associated with estrogen use, estrogen-responsive carcinoma, or undiagnosed abnormal genital bleeding, and in preg-nant and breast-feeding women. Diethylstilbestrol, when it was given to pregnant women, occasionally caused immediate nausea and vomiting. The slow toxicity included fluid reten-tion and uterine bleeding. The delayed toxicities, which appear many years later in the female offspring when they reach puberty, are vaginal adenosis and clear-cell vaginal adenocarcinoma (see also Figure 26).

DIFENOXIN HYDROCHLORIDE

(with Atropine Sulfate) (Motofen)

Difenoxin, an opiate receptor agonist with antidiarrheal properties (2 mg p.o.), is indicated as an adjunctive treatment of acute nonspecific exacerbations of chronic functional diarrhea.

DIFLORASONE DIACETATE

(Florone, Florone E, Maxiflor, Psorcon)

Diflorasone, a topical adrenocorticoid with antiinflammatory properties (0.05% cream or ointment), is used in inflammation of corticosteroid-responsive dermatoses (see also Table 10).

DIFLUNISAL

(Dolobid)

Diflunisal (initially 1 g followed by 500 mg every 8 to 12 hours) is indicated for acute or long-term symptomatic treatment of mild to moderate pain associated with rheumatoid arthritis and osteoarthritis. Similar to aspirin, diflunisal inhibits prostaglandin synthetase and platelet functions (see Figures 11 and 12). Diflunisal is eliminated primarily by the kidneys, and its plasma half-life of 8 to 12 hours is lengthened in renal impairment. Diflunisal increases the plasma level of acetaminophen; displaces coumarins from protein binding sites, and enhances the hypoprothrombinemic effects of anticoagulant; and as a uricosuric agent, antagonizes the hyperuricemic effects of hydrochlorothiazide (see also Table 2).

DIGITALIS

(Cardiac Glycosides)

In congestive heart failure, the patient's cardiac compensatory mechanism becomes fully activated. This consists of **cardiac dilatation** and hypertrophy — taking advantage of the Frank–Starling relationship to utilize more contractile elements; **sympathetic stimulation** — increasing the heart rate to maintain contractility and cardiac output, **increasing oxygen consumption** through the arterial venous oxygen difference-increasing extraction of oxygen from limited blood flow; and **production of aldosterone** — increasing sodium and fluid retention, which may not be advantageous to the organism (see Figure 32). Agents with **positive inotropic actions** that may be used in the management of congestive heart failure include the **cardiac glycosides** (e.g., digoxin and digitoxin), **dopaminergic analogs** (e.g., dobutamine), **phosphodiesterase inhibitors** (e.g., amrinone and milrinone), **angiotensin antagonists** (e.g., captopril, enalapril, and lisinopril), and **vasodilators** (nitrates and hydralazine).

The most important and often-used drugs in the treatment of congestive heart failure are the cardiac glycosides, which may exist and occur naturally in the body. Unfortunately, the **margin of safety** for these drugs is very narrow (therapeutic index, 3.0). **Toxicity** can develop readily, and careful attention to pharmacokinetic principles is absolutely crucial (see Table 11).

Cardiac glycosides (digitalis) potentiate the coupling of electrical excitation with mechanical contraction, and, by augmenting the myoplasmic concentration of calcium, they provoke a more forceful contraction. It is thought that digitalis inhibits sodium-calcium exchanges by inhibiting $Na^+K^+ATPase$. This results in an enhanced intracellular concentration of sodium, which in turn leads to greater sodium influx that then elicits stronger systolic contraction.

The cardiac glycosides increase **cardiac output** through their positive inotropic effect. They slow **heart rate** by relieving the sympathetic tone and through their vagotonic effects. They reduce the **heart size** by relieving the Frank–Starling relationship. They increase **cardiac efficiency** by increasing cardiac output and decreasing oxygen consumption (decreased heart size and rate).

Blood pressure remains unchanged following the administration of cardiac glycosides. In **congestive heart failure**, the cardiac output is reduced but the total peripheral resistance is increased, and these effects are reversed by cardiac glycosides.

Cardiac glycosides bring about **diuresis** by increasing both cardiac output and renal blood flow; the latter in turn reverses the **renal compensatory mechanism** activated in congestive heart failure. Consequently, the production of **aldosterone** is reduced, sodium retention is reversed, and the excretion of edematous fluid is enhanced (see Figure 32).

Cardiac glycosides have a vagotonic effect and may decrease impulse formation in the sinoatrial node. Although **automaticity** is not directly influenced by digitalis, **conduction velocity** is decreased. This effect of digitalis on the atrioventricular node is more prominent in the context of congestive heart failure, where the vagal tone is low and the adrenergic tone is high. Digitalis shortens the refractory period, in part due to enhanced intracellular calcium

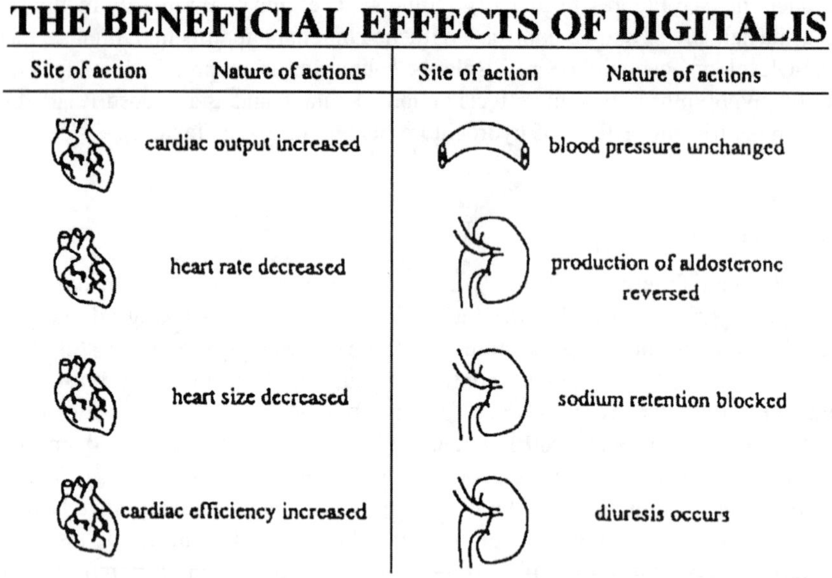

THE BENEFICIAL EFFECTS OF DIGITALIS

Site of action	Nature of actions	Site of action	Nature of actions
	cardiac output increased		blood pressure unchanged
	heart rate decreased		production of aldosterone reversed
	heart size decreased		sodium retention blocked
	cardiac efficiency increased		diuresis occurs

FIGURE 32   The mode of action of digitalis.

levels, decreasing membrane resistance, and increasing membrane potassium conductance, which lead to shortening of the action potential and contribute to shortening of atrial and ventricular refractoriness. The electrophysiologic properties of digitalis make it a useful compound in the treatment of **atrial arrhythmias** (for its vagotonic effect), **atrial flutter** (for its depressant effect on atrioventricular conduction), and **atrial fibrillation** (also for its vagotonic effect).

The toxic effects of digitalis are frequent and may be fatal. Toxicity may result from **overdosage, decreased metabolism and excretion,** and **hypokalemia** stemming from the use of thiazide diuretics, diarrhea, and vomiting. Digitalis toxicity has several manifestations and includes any arrhythmia occurring *de novo*, renal insufficiency, electrolyte disturbances, hypothyroidism, visual symptoms, headache, psychotic symptoms, pulmonary disease, and anorexia.

Digitalis toxicity should also be closely watched in **elderly** patients and those who have had a **recent myocardial infarction**, as these predispose to toxic reactions. The most commonly reported signs of toxicity are **dysrhythmia** such as ventricular ectopic depolarization, second- and third-degree heart block, junctional tachycardia, atrial tachycardia with block, ventricular tachycardia, sinoatrial block, and sinus arrest. Anorexia is seen as a gastrointestinal complication of cardiac glycoside use, and is followed by nausea and vomiting. The most common visual side effects are blurring, dimness of vision, flickering or flashing lights, color vision (yellow, green, red, and white), cycloplegia, and diplopia. A few of the neuropsychiatric symptoms that have been reported in conjunction with cardiac glycoside use are agitation, apathy, aphasia, ataxia, belligerence, changes in affect or personality, confusion, delirium, delusions, depression, disorientation, dizziness, drowsiness, euphoria, excitement, fatigue, hallucinations, headache, insomnia, irritability, mania, muscle pain, nervousness, neuralgias, nightmares, paresthesia, vertigo, violence, and weakness. Once digitalis toxicity is diagnosed, digitalis and diuretic use should be stopped. Furthermore, the patient should be monitored closely for any alteration in the pharmacokinetic profile of the cardiac glycoside being used. Treatment with **potassium** and magnesium may be indicated. Potassium is recommended for patients with digitalis-induced ectopic beat or tachycardia, provided the patient is neither hyperkalemic, uremic, or oliguric. It is the drug of choice if the patient is hypokalemic. To manage digitalis-induced arrhythmia, **lidocaine**, with its fast onset and short duration of action, is the drug of choice. Because lidocaine is metabolized, it should be used cautiously in patients with liver disease. **Phenytoin** may be used if potassium or lidocaine prove ineffective. **Propranolol** is effective in treating ventricular tachycardia. **Atropine** is effective if digitalis-induced conduction delay is at the atrioventricular node and is mediated via the vagus. Calcium-channel blocking agents such as **verapamil** are effective if the arrhythmia is due to reentry, increased diastolic depolarization in the Purkinje fibers, or oscillatory after-potential. In addition to these drugs, a temporary pacemaker may be indicated. The following interventions are contraindicated: **quinidine** should not be used because it displaces digoxin from binding sites, and **bretylium** should not be used because it releases norepinephrine. **Carotid sinus stimulation** should be discouraged, as it may precipitate ventricular fibrillation. The antidigitoxin or the antidigoxin antibodies (**Digibind**) have been used to control digitalis intoxication. The antibody mobilizes depot digoxin and is excreted by the kidney as an antibody-digoxin complex.

DIGITOXIN

(Crystodigin)

DIGOXIN

(Lanoxin)

The structures of the cardiac glycosides, including digoxin and digitoxin have three common components, which include a steroid nucleus (aglycones or genins), a series of sugar residues in the C_3 position, and a five- or six-membered lactone ring in the C_{17} position.

The **sugar residue** in digoxin and digitoxin is -O-digitoxose-digitoxose-digitoxose. Digoxin varies from digitoxin in having a hydroxy group at C_{12}. Glycosides possess both lipophilic residues (a steroid nucleus) and hydrophilic residues (a lactone ring and OH group). These residues and other factors strongly influence the pharmacokinetic profiles of these cardiac glycosides. **Digitoxin** is more lipid soluble than digoxin, is absorbed better when given orally, has a longer half-life, depicts a higher protein binding, and is more extensively metabolized by the liver. **Digoxin** is excreted primarily unchanged by the kidney. Renal insufficiency alters its half-life and safety. An elevated blood urea nitrogen (BUN) level signals the diminished capacity to eliminate digoxin. A direct relationship exists between the clearance of digoxin and that of creatine, which, in addition to BUN, may be used to assess a patient's ability to excrete digoxin. Table 11 compares the pharmacokinetic profiles of digoxin and digitoxin. Because a drug may require four to five half-lives before attaining a steady-state (maintenance) level, it is logical to assume that it will take digoxin approximately one week and digitoxin four weeks to reach their maintenance levels (see **Digitalis**).

DIGOXIN IMMUNE FAB

(Ovine) (Digibind)

Digoxin immune fab, an antibody fragment, is used in potentially life-threatening digoxin or digitoxin intoxication.

DIHYDRALAZINE

Hydralazine and nitrates have been used in patients with congestive heart failure. An **angiotensin-converting enzyme** inhibitor such as **lisinopril** increases the left ventricular ejection fraction in patients with congestive heart failure, and the drug's effectiveness is not diminished in the presence of impaired renal function. In addition, a **vasodilator** in combination with

TABLE 11
Comparison of the Pharmacokinetic Profiles of Digoxin and Digitoxin

Properties	Digoxin	Digitoxin
Lipid solubility	Low	High
Gastrointestinal absorption	Good	Excellent
Protein binding	Low (25%)	High (90%)
Half-life	Short (1–2 days)	Long (6–9 days)
Enterohepatic recycling	Minimal	High
Liver metabolism	Low	High
Excretion	Active drug	Inactive metabolites
Onset of action after intravenous administration	Fast (5–30 min)	Slow (4–8 hours)

an angiotensin-converting enzyme inhibitor has been used in congestive heart failure. The vasodilators may be classified as **venodilators, arterial dilators,** or **balanced-type vasodilators** (see Table 26). The rationale for vasodilation in the management of congestive heart failure is based on the increased arteriolar vasotone that occurs. This initiates a vicious circle in which cardiac function is further depressed by an increase in afterload and in resistance to ejection.

DIHYDROCODEINONE

Most narcotics such as **morphine, codeine, dihydrocodeinone, methadone,** and **levorphanol** have antitussive properties. Codeine is used primarily because its addictive liability is low and it is effective orally. The antitussive doses of narcotics are lower than the doses used for analgesic purposes.

DIHYDROCYCLOSPORIN C

This group consists of cyclosporin A and dihydrocyclosporin C. Cyclosporin A, a fungal metabolite, is a cyclic polypeptide that consists of 11 amino acids. It has a biologic half-life of 4 to 6 hours and displays a preferential T-cell cytotoxic property, in that it inhibits the factors that stimulate T-lymphocyte proliferation. Cyclosporin A has been used as the sole immunosuppressant (without prednisone or other drugs) for cadaveric transplants of the kidney, pancreas, and liver. Cyclosporin A has been observed to cause reversible hepatic toxicity and nephrotoxicity. Another fungal metabolite, dihydrocyclosporin C is even more selective than cyclosporin A, in that it suppresses T-lymphocyte production with only marginal effects on the antibody response.

DIHYDROEMETINE

Dehydroemetine is given for 5 days and effects rapid relief of the symptoms of acute amebic dysentery. The patient is then switched to **metronidazole**. If the response to metronidazole is not satisfactory, dihydroemetine plus **tetracycline** or dihydroemetine plus **paromomycin** are given along with the metronidazole.

DIHYDROERGOTAMINE MESYLATE
(DHE 45)

Dihydroergotamine, an ergot alkaloid with vasoconstricting properties (1 mg IM or IV), is used to prevent or abort vascular headaches, including migraine and cluster headaches (see also Figure 85).

DIHYDROMORPHINONE

(Numorphan)

Dihydromorphinone (1 mg IM SC) is a semisynthetic narcotic analgesic which is far more potent than morphine and has a duration of action of 4 to 6 hours.

DIHYDROMORPHINONE HYDROCHLORIDE

(Dilaudid)

Dilaudid is 5 to 10 times as potent and more toxic than morphine, but its duration of action is shorter, and its effects on the gastrointestinal tract are less. Chemically, it differs from morphine in that the alcoholic hydroxyl group of that alkaloid is replaced by ketonic oxygen and the adjacent double bond is removed by hydrogenation. Dihydromorphinone produces analgesia and narcosis and acts upon the respiration in a manner similar to morphine, with the difference that it is effective in about one quarter of the dosage. Dihydromorphinone is powerfully analgesic and also markedly depressing to the respiration, while nausea, vomiting, and constipation are not so marked as with morphine. Tolerance and addition occur readily and the same care should be exercised in prescribing it as is used in the case of the natural opium alkaloids.

Dihydromorphinone is used in the same manner as morphine for the relief of pain but in much smaller doses — usually 1 to 2 mg. For cough, a dose about half that size is used. Administered orally, dihydromorphinone is more effective than morphine, and it may also be administered in a rectal suppository. Its principal indication is for acute pain of short duration (see also Figure 58).

DIHYDROPYRIDINE

When calcium homeostasis fails, as occurs in the presence of **anoxia**, cell viability is threatened by the uncontrolled influx of calcium through the plasma membrane or by the massive release of calcium from intracellular binding and sequestration sites. Agents that affect calcium movements consist of **calcium entry blockers** and **calcium antagonists** (see Table 20 and Figures 76 and 95).

Calcium entry blockers include those agents that are **selective for slow calcium channels** in the myocardium (slow channel blockers) and consist of the following categories of substances benzothiazepines — diltiazem, dihydropyridines — nifedipine, nicardipine, niludipine, nimodipine, nisoldipine, nitrendipine, ryosidine, amlodipine, azodipine, dazodipine, felodipine, flordipine, iodipine, isradipine, mesudipine, oxodipine, and riodipine; and, phenylalkylamines — verapamil, gallopamil, anipamil, desmethoxyverapamil, emopamil, falipamil, and ronipamil.

DIHYDROTACHYSTEROL

(DHT, DHT Intensol, Hytakerol)

Dihydrotachysterol, a vitamin D analog with antihypocalcemic property, is indicated in the treatment of familial hypophosphatemia; hypocalcemia associated with hypoparathyroidism and pseudohypoparathyroidism; or renal osteodystrophy in chronic uremia (see also Figure 66).

DIIODOTYROSINE

(DIT)

The steps involved in the synthesis of thyroid hormones are depicted in Figure 56. First the ingested iodide (100 to 150 microgram/day) is actively transported (**iodide trapping**) and then accumulated in the thyroid gland. Following this, the trapped iodide is oxidized by a peroxidase system to active iodine, which iodinates the tyrosine residue of glycoprotein to yield **monoiodotyrosine (MIT) and diiodotyrosine (DIT)**. This process is called **iodide organification**. The MIT and DIT combine to form T_3, whereas two molecules of DIT combine to form T_4. T_3 and T_4 are released from thyroglobulin through the actions of pinocytosis and the proteolysis of thyroglobulin by lysosomal enzymes. In the circulation, 75% of T_4 is bound to **thyroxine-binding globulin** (TBG), and the remainder is bound mostly to **thyroxine-binding prealbumin** (TBPA). Approximately 0.05% of T_4 remains free. T_3 is similarly bound to TBG, allowing only 0.5% of it to remain in the free form.

DILEVALOL

Dilevalol, a noncardioselective beta-adrenergic blocking agent, is an isomer of labetalol, has no alpha$_1$-adrenergic blocking action, but has a potent vasodilating effect, which appears to be mediated via its beta$_2$-agonist effect, and this effect is blocked by propranolol, but not metoprolol (see Figures 14 and 57). Dilevalol decreases peripheral vascular resistance without influencing cardiac output. Dilevalol in a daily dose of 100 to 800 mg is effective in the treatment of mild to moderate hypertension. The plasma concentration of dilevalol is not altered in renal impairment and only 3% of the drug is excreted unchanged.

DILTIAZEM HYDROCHLORIDE

(Cardizem)

Diltiazem, a calcium channel blocking agent, is indicated for angina pectoris due to coronary artery spasm, chronic stable angina, and essential hypertension (Cardizem CD sustained-release preparation). Diltiazem dilates systemic arteries, decreases total peripheral resistance and afterload. It also decreases myocardial oxygen demand and cardiac work by reducing heart rate, relieving coronary artery spasm and dilating peripheral vessels. Diltiazem is absorbed from the gastrointestinal tract rapidly, is subjected to massive first-pass effect in the liver, is bound to plasma proteins to the extent of 70 to 85%, is metabolized in the liver, and partly (35%) is excreted unchanged by the kidneys. Overdosage with diltiazem may cause heart block, asystole, and hypotension (see Table 20 and Figure 76).

DIMENHYDRINATE

(Dramamine)

Dimenhydrinate consists of diphenhydramine and chlorotheophylline. It is indicated (50 to 100 mg every 4 to 6 hours) in the prevention and treatment of nausea, vomiting, dizziness, or vertigo of motion sickness. Dimenhydrinate, possessing anticholinergic action, should be used cautiously in prostatic hypertrophy, stenosing peptic ulcer, pyloroduodenal obstruction, bladder neck obstruction, narrow angle glaucoma, bronchial asthma, cardiac arrhythmias, and any other conditions in which atropine-like compounds are contraindicated. Dimenhydrinate may mask the ototoxic symptoms of aminoglycosides, when used concomitantly. The side effects of dimenhydrinate are drowsiness, diplopia, tachycardia, thickening of bronchial secretions, and dryness of mouth, nose, and throat.

DIMERCAPROL

(BAL in Oil)

Dimercaprol, a metal chelating agent (30 mg/kg IM), is used to treat severe **arsenic** or **gold** poisoning.

DIMETHOXANATE
(Cothera)

Noscapine (Nectadon) is a naturally occurring opium alkaloid with a structure and function similar to papaverine's. It is antitussive and has no analgesic or addictive properties. **Diphenhydramine** and **chlorcyclizine** are antihistaminic agents that also have antitussive properties. **Dimethoxanate** and **pipazethate** (Theratuss) are phenothiazine derivatives without analgesic but with weak antitussive and local anesthetic properties.

DINOPROST TROMETHAMINE
(Prostin F2S)

Prostaglandins are mostly used as **abortifacients**. They may be administered by vaginal suppository (**Dinoprostone**), which contains prostaglandin E_2, by intramuscular injection (**carboprost** and **tromethamine**), which contains 15-methyl prostaglandin F_{2a}, or by intraamnionic administration (dinoprost and **tromethamine**), which contains prostaglandin F_{2a}. Other possible uses of prostaglandins may include the treatment of **ductus arteriosus** (prostaglandin E_1), in the management of peripheral vascular diseases (see also Figure 51). High levels of prostaglandin F_{2a} may cause **dysmenorrhea**, and substances such as indomethacin and ibuprofen are effective in relieving these symptoms.

DINOPROSTONE
(Prostin E_2)

Dinoprostone is used to "ripen" an unfavorable cervix in pregnant woman near term. Dinoprostone is the naturally occurring form of prostaglandin E_2 (PGE_2). When administered endocervically, it will stimulate the gravid uterus to contract. In addition to its oxytoxic effect, dinoprostone has a local effect in softening and dilating the cervix. Dinoprostone is contraindicated in fetal distress where delivery is not imminent or where vaginal delivery should not take place, such as in cases of active herpes genitalia. Dinoprostone is metabolized in the lung, liver, and kidney, and the metabolite is eliminated by the kidneys, and hence it should be used cautiously in renal and hepatic dysfunction.

DIPHENADIONE
(Dipaxin)

The **coumarin anticoagulants** include dicumarol, warfarin sodium (coumadin sodium), warfarin potassium (Athrombin-K), acenocoumarol (Sintrom), and phenprocouman (Liquamar). The **inanedione derivatives** are **phenidione** (Hedulin), **diphenadione** (Dipaxin), and **anisindione** (Miradon). The pharmacologic properties of oral anticoagulants are identical qualitatively, but their pharmacokinetic parameters and their toxicities vary. **Racemic warfarin sodium** is the most widely used anticoagulant (see Tables 16 and 17).

DIPHENHYDRAMINE HYDROCHLORIDE
(Benadryl)

Diphenhydramine is an H_1-antihistaminic agent with anticholinergic and sedative properties. Diphenhydramine (25 to 50 mg t.i.d.) is indicated for allergic conjunctivitis, urticaria, and angioedema resulting from food, blood, or plasma; in combination with epinephrine in anaphylactic reactions; for active and prophylactic treatment of motion sickness; and for neuroleptic-induced dystonic reactions. Diphenhydramine has potent anticholinergic effects, and hence should be used cautiously in prostatic hypertrophy, stenosing peptic ulcer, pyloroduodenal obstruction, bladder neck obstruction, narrow angle glaucoma, bronchial asthma, or cardiac arrhythmias. The sedative properties of diphenhydramine become potentiated by alcohol, sedative-hypnotic, neuroleptics, and tricyclic antidepressants. Monoamine oxidase inhibitors prolong and intensify the anticholinergic effects of diphenhydramine. Overdosage with diphenhydramine may cause profound CNS depression in adults or CNS excitation in children (see also Figures 24 and 49).

DIPHENIDOL
(Vontrol)

Diphenidol (25 mg every four hours as needed) is indicated in vertigo and associated nausea and vomiting seen in labyrinthitis and Meniere's disease, and in controlling nausea and vomiting due to malignant neoplasms. Diphenidol may cause auditory and visual hallucination, disorientation, or confusion and hence should be used under careful supervision. Since 90% of diphenidol is excreted in the urine, it should be used cautiously in renal impairment. The antiemetic effects of diphenidol may mask the nausea and vomiting associated with a toxic dosage of digitalis (see also Figure 73).

DIPHENOXYLATE HYDROCHLORIDE WITH ATROPINE SULFATE
(Lomotil)

Diphenoxylate is an opiate (schedule V) with antidiarrheal properties. Diphenoxylate is usually dispensed with **atropine** and sold as Lomotil. The atropine is added to discourage the abuse of diphenoxylate by narcotic addicts who are tolerant to massive doses of narcotic but not to the CNS stimulant effects of atropine. Diphenoxylate should be used cautiously in patients with obstructive jaundice because of potential for hepatic coma, and in patients with diarrhea caused by pseudomembranous colitis because of potential for toxic megacolon. In addition, it should be used cautiously in the treatment of diarrhea caused by poisoning or by infection by *Shigella, Salmonella,* and some strains of *Escherichia coli* because expulsion of intestinal contents may be a protective mechanism. Diphenoxylate should be used with extreme caution in patients with impaired hepatic function, cirrhosis, advanced hepatorenal disease, or abnormal liver function test results, because the drug may precipitate hepatic coma. Since diphenoxylate is structurally related to meperidine, it may cause hypertension when combined with monoamine oxidase inhibitors. As a narcotic, it will augment the CNS depressant effects of alcohol, hypnotic-sedative, and numerous other drugs, such as neuroleptics or antidepressants which cause sedation.

DIPHTHERIA AND TETANUS TOXOIDS, ABSORBED, COMBINED
(TD)

Diphtheria, a diphtheria and tetanus prophylaxis agent, is used for primary immunization.

DIPHTHERIA AND TETANUS TOXOIDS AND PERTUSSIS VACCINE, ABSORBED
(DTP) (Tri-Immunol)

This combination, toxoid and vaccine, is used for primary immunization and booster immunization.

DIPHTHERIA ANTITOXIN, EQUINE

This diphtheria antitoxin is used to prevent or treat diphtheria.

DIPHTHERIA TOXOID, ABSORBED

(for pediatric use)

This diphtheria prophylaxis agent is used in diphtheria immunization.

DIPYRIDAMOLE

(Persantine)

Dipyridamole is indicated as an adjunct to therapy with coumarin anticoagulant in the prevention of postoperative thromboembolic complications of cardiac valve replacement; as an alternative to exercise in thallium myocardial perfusion imaging for the evaluation of coronary artery disease in patients who are unable to exercise; and for long-term therapy of angina pectoris. Dipyridamole inhibits platelet adhesion and is a coronary vasodilator. Inappropriate use of dipyridamole has caused myocardial infarction, ventricular fibrillation, tachycardia, bronchospasm, and transient cerebral ischemia (see also Figures 12 and 84).

DIPYRONE

Dipyrone is a water-soluble pyrazolone derivative available in oral, rectal, and injectable forms. It has been recognized as an effective analgesic, antipyretic, and antispasmodic drug. Some antiinflammatory properties have also been recognized in pharmacological models, although whether this is of any clinical relevance is still questionable. It is indicated for severe pain and, particularly, for pain associated with smooth muscle spasm or colic affecting the gastrointestinal, biliary, or urinary tracts. It is also useful for fever that is refractory to other treatment.

DISOPYRAMIDE PHOSPHATE

(Norpace)

Disopyramide, a type 1 antiarrhythmic agent, in a dose of 100 mg every six hours, is indicated in the treatment of life-threatening ventricular arrhythmias. Disopyramide depresses automaticity primarily in the **ventricular conducting system**. It depresses conduction velocity throughout the heart, but has less effect at the AV node than either **quinidine** or **procainamide**. It does not have a vagolytic effect in the heart. Disopyramide terminates reentry by producing **bidirectional block**. It does not greatly depress blood pressure. Contractility and cardiac output are mildly depressed with its use, but, because the compound is not a vasodilator, a reflex increase in peripheral resistance tends to offset the decline in cardiac output. Like quinidine and procainamide, it is excreted 50% unmetabolized in the urine. Disopyramide's side effects are primarily gastrointestinal in nature, due to its peripheral anticholinergic action that causes dry mouth and urinary hesitancy. Disopyramide's major therapeutic use is for treating premature ventricular contractions and ventricular tachycardia. It does not appear to be particularly useful in controlling atrial arrhythmias (see also Figure 76).

DISULFIRAM

(Anabuse)

Disulfiram, an inhibitor of aldehyde dehydrogenase (500 mg/day for 5 to 10 days), is used as an adjunct regimen in the management of chronic alcoholism.

DIURETICS		
Carbonic Anhydrase Inhibitor Acetazolamide		
Osmotic Agent Mannitol		
Loop Diuretics		
Azosemide	Furosemide	Torsemide
Bumetanide	Muzolimine	Tripamide
Ethacrynic acid	Piretanide	
Thiazide Diuretics		
Bendroflumethiazide	Cyclothiazide	Metolazone
Benzthiazide	Hydrochlorothiazide	Polythiazide
Chlorothiazide	Hydroflumethiazide	Quinethazone
Chlorthalidone	Indapamide	Trichlormethiazide
Clopamide	Methyclothiazide	
Potassium-Retaining Diuretics		
Amiloride		
Spironolactone		
Triamterene		

DOBUTAMINE HYDROCHLORIDE
(Dobutrex)

Dobutamine (infusion of 2.5 to 10 mcg/kg/min) is indicated in the short-term treatment of adults with cardiac decompensation due to decreased contractility, resulting from either organic heart disease or surgical procedures involving the heart. Often digitalis is used prior to infusing dobutamine in patients with atrial fibrillation. The actions of dobutamine on various adrenergic and dopaminergic receptors are summarized in Table 12. In patients with depressed cardiac output, dobutamine increases cardiac output without increasing cardiac rate, and is contraindicated in patients with idiopathic hypertrophic subaortic stenosis. Dobutamine exerts its effects within 1 to 2 minutes, has a half-life of two minutes, is metabolized to 3-0 methyldobutamine, which is then excreted in the urine (see also Figure 39).

DOCETAXEL
(Taxotere)

Docetaxel is the second representative of the new entity of drugs that have a unique taxane ring in common, such as the one seen in **paclitaxel**. Docetaxel, being more efficacious than paclitaxel, is used in ovarian cancer. Paclitaxel and docetaxel inhibit microtubule depolymerization, thereby reducing the formation of stable microtubule bundles (see also Figure 26).

DOCUSATE CALCIUM
(D-C-S, PRO-CAL-SOF, SURFAK)

DOCUSATE POTASSIUM
(Dialose, Diocto-K, Kasof)

DOCUSATE SODIUM
(Colace, Diocto, Dioeze, Diosuccin, Disonate, Di-Sosul, DOS, Doxinate, D.S.S., Duosol, Modane Soft, Pro-Sof, Regulax SS, Regutol, Theravac-SB)

Docusate salts (50 to 300 mg p.o. daily) are used as stool softeners.

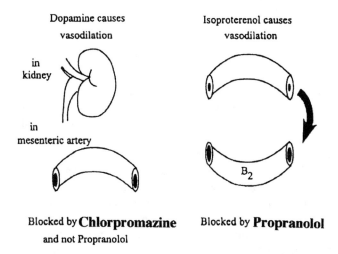

Dopamine causes vasodilation

in kidney

in mesenteric artery

Isoproterenol causes vasodilation

B₂

Blocked by **Chlorpromazine** and not Propranolol

Blocked by **Propranolol**

FIGURE 33 Stimulation of the **dopamine receptors** in renal and mesenteric arteries causes vasodilation, which is not blocked by propranolol (beta antagonist) but is blocked by a dopamine receptor-blocking agent such as **chlorpromazine**.

DOMPERIDONE

Domperidone (100 mg p.o.) is an antiemetic agent which blocks selectively peripheral dopamine receptors in the chemoreceptor trigger zone for emesis as well as those in the gastrointestinal tract. Unlike **metoclopramide**, domperidone does not pass across the blood-brain barrier, and hence it is thought to be devoid of any extrapyramidal side effects. The clinical evidence indicates that domperidone, by blocking dopamine receptors in the wall of the gastrointestinal tract, enhances normal synchronized GI peristalsis and motility in the proximal portion of the GI tract (see also Figure 73).

DOPAMINE HYDROCHLORIDE
(Intropin)

Peripheral dopaminergic receptor agents are useful in the treatment of congestive heart failure. Two distinct subtypes of dopamine receptors have been identified. The **dopamine₂** (DA₂) receptors are located at various sites within the sympathetic nervous system, and their activation results in inhibition of the sympathetic nervous system. In contrast, activation of the postsynaptic **dopamine₁** (DA₁) receptors, which are located on vascular smooth muscles, causes vasodilation in the renal, mesentery, cerebral, and coronary vascular beds. Thus, the pharmacologic response to activation of the DA₂ and DA₁ receptors is hypotension, bradycardia, diuresis, and natriuresis (see Figure 33 and Table 12). **Dopamine** stimulates dopamine, alpha-, and beta-adrenergic receptors. The use of dopamine in congestive heart failure is limited because it causes nausea and vomiting, becomes inactive when given orally, increases afterload (alpha-adrenergic receptor-mediated peripheral vasoconstriction), and enhances oxygen demand on the left ventricle (see also Figures 39 and 75).

DORNASE ALFA RECOMBINANT
(Pulmozyme)

Dornase alpha, a recombinant human deoxyribonuclease I, a mucolytic enzyme with respiratory stimulant properties, is used to improve pulmonary function and reduce the frequency of moderate to severe respiratory infections in patients with cystic fibrosis.

DOXACURIUM
(Nuromax)

Doxacurium is indicated as an adjunct to general anesthesia in order to produce skeletal muscle relaxation; and to facilitate endotracheal intubation. Doxacurium is a long-acting nondepolarizing skeletal muscle relaxant which binds to cholinergic receptors on the motor end plate, and its action is antagonized by neostigmine, an inhibitor of acetylcholinesterase. Doxacurium, which is 3 and 10 times more potent than pancuronium and metocurine, respectively, does not alter heart or blood pressure in therapeutic doses. Doxacurium should be used cautiously in patients with neuromuscular diseases such as myasthenia gravis and the myasthenic syndrome. The action of doxacurium, like other skeletal muscle relaxing agents, is altered in conditions where electrolytes and/or acid-base balance have been disturbed. For example, the action of doxacurium is altered by magnesium salts used in the management of eclampsia or preclampsia. Carbamazepine delays the onset of action and shortness of action of doxacurium. Isoflurane, enflurane, and halothane decrease the ED_{50} and prolong the duration of neuromuscular blockade (see also Figure 92).

DOXAPRAM HYDROCHLORIDE
(Dopram)

Doxapram (0.5 to 1 mg/kg) is used as a postanesthesia respiratory stimulation, in drug-induced CNS depression, and in acute hypercapnia associated with chronic obstructive pulmonary disease.

DOXAZOSIN MESYLATE
(Cardura)

Doxazosin, an alpha adrenergic blocking agent (1 mg p.o. daily), is used in the treatment of essential hypertension.

DOXEPIN HYDROCHLORIDE
(Adapin)

Doxepin (75 mg p.o. daily) is indicated in psychoneurotic patients with depression or anxiety; depression and/or anxiety of chronic alcoholism; depression and/or anxiety associated with organic disease; and in manic-depressive disorders. Doxepin blocks the uptake sites for norepinephrine and to a lesser extent that of serotonin. Doxepin blocks $alpha_1$-adrenergic receptors, H_1 histaminergic receptors, and muscarinic cholinergic receptors. It causes heavy sedation and marked orthostatic hypotension. Because of its anticholinergic properties, it should be used cautiously in prostatic hypertrophy, stenosing peptic ulcer, pyloroduodenal obstruction, bladder neck obstruction, narrow angle glaucoma, bronchial asthma, and cardiac arrhythmias (see Tables 3 through 5).

DOXORUBICIN
(Adriamycin)

Daunorubicin (daunomycin and cerubidine) and doxorubicin bind to and cause the intercalation of the DNA molecule, thereby inhibiting DNA template function. They also provoke DNA chain scission and chromosomal damage. Daunorubicin is useful in treating patients with acute lymphocytic or acute granulocytic leukemia. **Adriamycin** is useful in cases of solid tumors such as sarcoma, metastatic breast cancer, and thyroid cancer. These agents cause stomatitis, alopecia, myelosuppression, and cardiac abnormalities ranging from arrhythmias to cardiomyopathy (see also Figure 2).

DOXYCYCLINE HYCLATE

(Vibramycin)

Doxycycline is indicated for gonorrhea in patients allergic to penicillin; in primary or secondary syphilis in patients allergic to penicillin; Chlamydia trachomatis, nongonococcal urethritis, and uncomplicated urethral, endocervical, or rectal infections and prophylaxis for rape victims; and to prevent "traveler's diarrhea," commonly caused by enterotoxigenic *Escherichia coli*. Doxycycline, which is absorbed well (90 to 100%), has the least affinity for calcium, and hence its absorption is not altered by milk products. Doxycycline is excreted primarily unchanged by the kidneys, and its half-life is prolonged in renal impairment. Doxycycline is contraindicated in pregnancy and young children since it discolors teeth permanently. When doxycycline is used with digoxin or oral anticoagulant, the dosage for digoxin and anticoagulant should be reduced (see also Table 22 and Figures 80 and 88).

DROLOXIFENE

The new antiestrogen droloxifene has a 10- to 60-fold higher binding affinity to the estrogen receptor compared to the related compound **tamoxifen**. A similar relationship was found in growth inhibition studies which showed that droloxifene inhibited human breast cancer cells more effectively than tamoxifen, predominantly in drug concentrations which are found in humans during therapy. Therefore, it can be assumed that droloxifene may represent an important step forward in the treatment of mammary carcinomas in women through its better tolerability and increased efficacy compared with tamoxifen. For long-term adjuvant or preventative treatment of breast cancer, droloxifene may well be the safer choice (see also Figure 26).

DRONABINOL

(Marinol) (THC)

Dronabinol is a cannabinoid with antiemetic effects and is used in a dosage of 5 mg/m^2 p.o. 1 to 3 hours prior to administration of antineoplastic agents. Dronabinol is excreted primarily in feces via the biliary tract. Dronabinol may cause euphoria, drowsiness, altered thinking, hallucination, confusion, and impaired coordination (see also Figures 64 and 73). In addition, dronabinol is used to stimulate appetite in anorexia associated with AIDS-related weight loss.

DROPERIDOL

(Inapsine)

Droperidol is used as an adjunct for induction and maintenance of general anesthesia and as an anesthetic in diagnostic procedures. Droperidol, which has antiemetic properties, causes marked sedation and potentiates the CNS depressant effects of alcohol, hypnotic-sedatives, and numerous psychoactive agents. Droperidol is absorbed well through an IM injection — sedation begins in 3 minutes, peaks at 30 minutes, and lasts for 2 to 4 hours. Droperidol is metabolized by the liver to p-fluoro-phenylacetic acid and p-hydroxypiperidine, and its metabolites are excreted in urine and feces.

DUODENAL ULCERS: TREATMENT OF	
Histamine$_2$ (H$_2$) Receptor Antagonists	
Cimetidine	Nizatidine
Famotidine	Ranitidine
Proton Pump Inhibitors	
Omeprazole	

Aluminum Hydroxide Complex of Sucrose-Enhancing Mucosal Defense Mechanism Sucralfate
Prostaglandin Analog Misoprostol
Antacids Aluminum hydroxide Magnesium hydroxide Simethicone antacids

DYCLONINE HYDROCHLORIDE
(Dyclone, Sucrets)

Dyclonine, a topical local anesthetic, is indicated for relief of pain and itching from minor burns, insect bites, or irritations, or episiotomy or anogenital lesion; and to anesthetize mucous membranes before endoscopic procedures such as laryngoscopy, bronchoscopy, or endotracheal procedures. For example, for bronchoscopy, dyclonine (1% solution) is sprayed into the larynx and trachea every five minutes until laryngeal reflex is abolished. Dyclonine blocks conduction of nerve impulses at the sensory nerve endings by altering cell membrane permeability to ionic transfer.

DYPHYLLINE
(Dylline)

Dyphylline (200 to 800 mg p.o. every 6 hours) is indicated for relief of acute and chronic bronchial asthma and reversible bronchospasm associated with chronic bronchitis and emphysema. Dyphylline should be used cautiously in patients with compromised cardiac or circulatory function, diabetes, glaucoma, hypertension, hyperthyroidism, peptic ulcer, or gastroesophageal reflux, because the drug may worsen these symptoms or conditions. Sympathomimetic agents act synergistically with dyphylline, and probenecid enhances the half-life of dyphylline by blocking its renal tubular secretion (see also Figure 86).

E

EBASTINE

Histamine$_1$ (H$_1$) receptors mediate such actions as bronchoconstriction and the contraction of smooth muscles in the gastrointestinal tract. Ebastine is a histamine$_1$ receptor blocker. **Terfenadine, astemizole, loratadine,** and **certirizine** are **second-generation** antihistamine agents that are relatively **nonsedating**. Other H$_1$-receptor antagonists currently undergoing clinical trials are **azelastine, ebastine,** and **levocabastine** (see also Figure 49).

ECHOTHIOPHATE IODIDE

(Phospholine Iodide)

Echothiophate, a cholinesterase inhibitor with miotic properties (1 drop of 0.03 to 0.125% solution into conjunctival sac daily), is used in open-angle glaucoma or conditions obstructing aqueous outflow (see also Figure 18).

ECONAZOLE NITRATE

(Spectazole)

Econazole, which is applied topically and daily, is indicated in the treatment of tinea pedis (athlete's foot), tinea cruris (jock itch), and tinea corporis (ringworm) caused by *T. rubrum, T. mentagrophytes, T. tonsurans, M. canis, M. audouini, M. gypseum,* and *E. floccosum*; and as therapy for cutaneous candidiasis and tinea versicolor.

EDETATE CALCIUM DISODIUM

(Calcium EDTA) (Calcium Disodium Versenate)

Edetate calcium disodium, a metal chelating agent, is indicated in the treatment of symptomatic lead poisoning without encephalopathy and blood lead concentrations less than 100 mcg/dl, or in the treatment of severe lead poisoning with symptoms of encephalopathy and/or blood lead concentrations greater than 100 mcg/dl.

EDETATE DISODIUM

(EDTA) (Chealamide, Disotate, Endrate)

Edetate disodium, heavy metal antagonist, is indicated in hypercalcemia (500 mg/kg daily by slow IV infusion) and in digitalis-induced cardiac arrhythmias (15 mg/kg/hour by IV infusion). EDTA will lower serum levels of calcium, magnesium, and zinc. EDTA should not be used in anuria, and renal excretory functions (BUN and creatinine) should be monitored carefully. EDTA should be used cautiously in hypokalemia and in patients with limited cardiac reserve.

EDROPHONIUM CHLORIDE

(Enlon, Tensilon)

Edrophonium chloride, a cholinesterase inhibitor (10 mg IV given over 30 to 45 seconds), may be used as a curare antagonist (to reverse neuromuscular blocking action), and for reversal of nondepolarizing muscle relaxants (see also Figures 18 and 92).

EFLORNITHINE HYDROCHLORIDE
(DFM0) (Ornidyl)

Eflornithine, an ornithine decarboxylase inhibitor with antiprotozoal activity (100 mg/kg q. 6 hours), is used in the treatment of the meningoencephalitic stage of *Trypanosoma brucei gambiense* infection (sleeping sickness) and in treatment of *Pneumocystis carinii* pneumonia in acquired immunodeficiency syndrome patients.

ELECTROLYTES AND SKELETAL MUSCLE RELAXANTS

The generation of **action potentials** by muscle and nerve result from changes in the conductance of their membranes to **sodium** and **potassium**, and normal neuromuscular function depends on the maintenance of the correct ratio between intracellular and extracellular ionic concentrations. An acute decrease in the extracellular **potassium** concentration tends to elevate the **end plate transmembrane potential**, causing hyperpolarization together with a greater sensitivity to the nondepolarizing muscle relaxants. Conversely, an increased extracellular potassium concentration lowers the resting end plate transmembrane potential and thereby partially depolarizes the membrane, which should augment the effects of the depolarizing agents and oppose the action of the nondepolarizing drugs. Diuretic-induced chronic hypokalemia reduces the pancuronium requirements for neuromuscular blockade and thus more neostigmine is required to achieve antagonism. The release of **acetylcholine** from the **motor nerve terminal** is also affected by calcium and magnesium ion concentrations, which have opposing effects. **Calcium** increases the quantal release of the postjunctional membrane to transmitter and enhances the excitation-contraction coupling mechanisms of muscle. In contrast, **magnesium** decreases acetylcholine release and reduces the sensitivity of the postjunctional membrane to acetylcholine. Consequently, the action of the nondepolarizing muscle relaxants can be accentuated by low calcium and high magnesium levels. In addition, magnesium augments the block produced by depolarizing relaxants. Therefore, the dose of a muscle relaxant should be reduced in patients who have **toxemia** associated with **pregnancy** and are undergoing magnesium replacement therapy (see also Figures 30 and 92).

EMEDASTINE

The most common symptoms of allergic conjunctivitis treated by ophthalmologists include ocular pruritis, erythema, edema, and tearing. The traditional drugs of choice to treat these symptoms of allergic conjunctivitis have been antihistamines alone or in combination with vasoconstrictors. Antihistamines currently employed in this area as topical solutions include **pheniramine, antazoline, pyrilamine**, and **levocabastine**. However, these drugs have some disadvantages such as low potency (antazoline), slow onset of action (levocabastine), short duration of action (antazoline, pyrilamine, pheniramine), discomfort/tolerance (**ketotifen**, levocabastine), and significant side effects (e.g., they can raise intraocular pressure and cause mydriasis and ocular dryness) due to other receptor binding activities. Emedastine is a novel antihistaminic/antiallergic drug that potentially inhibits histamine-induced vascular permeability in the conjunctiva and blocks the allergic response in a model of passive conjunctival anaphylaxis. In addition, emedastine potently inhibits histamine-induced airway resistance and skin vascular permeability (see also Figure 49).

EMETICS

Ipecac is a mixture of the alcohol-soluble alkaloid which is obtained from the South American plant *Cephaelis ipecacuanha* and is used solely in the form of **syrup of ipecac. Apomorphine hydrochloride** and **copper sulfate** are also emetics. Syrup of ipecac and copper sulfate cause emesis by locally irritating the stomach, whereas apomorphine stimulates the **chemoreceptor**

trigger zone for emesis located in the caudal portion of the fourth ventricle (area postrema), which in turn stimulates the vomiting center in the lateral reticular formation of the medulla (see also Figure 73).

EMLA
(Astra)

Emla is a topical anesthetic ointment containing a mixture of lidocaine (2 to 5%) and prilocaine (2 to 5%) which is useful in reducing the pain associated with venipuncture.

ENALAPRIL MALEATE
(Vasotec)

Enalapril is indicated in the treatment of hypertension either by itself or in combination with thiazide like diuretics; and in the symptomatic treatment of congestive heart failure, usually in combination with a diuretic and digitalis. Enalapril becomes hydrolyzed to enalaprilat, which in turn inhibits angiotensin-converting enzyme (ACE). The beneficial effects of enalapril in hypertension or heart failure appear to result primarily from suppression of the renin angiotensin-aldosterone system. The lower plasma level of angiotensin II leads to decreased vasopressor activity and to decreased aldosterone secretion. Since enalapril lowers blood pressure in low renin hypertension, it may exert its effects also by increasing the level of bradykinin. Enalapril is known to have caused angioedema of the face, extremities, lips, tongue, glottis, and/or larynx. Antihistaminics are effective in relieving the symptoms (see also Figure 21).

ENCAINIDE HYDROCHLORIDE

Encainide, a class IC antiarrhythmic agent, is available on a limited basis only to patients with life-threatening ventricular arrhythmias. Encainide slows conduction velocity, inhibits automaticity, and increases the ratio of the effective refractory period to action potential duration. It blocks the sodium channel of Purkinje fibers and the myocardium. Encainide is absorbed well, reaches peak plasma level in 30 to 90 minutes, becomes metabolized to 0-demethyl encainide (ODE) and 3-methoxy-0-demethyl encainide (MODE), which are active antiarrhythmic agents, and the metabolites are excreted by the kidneys. In renal impairment, the clearance of ODE and MODE is decreased, and hence the dosage should be reduced. Encainide may either worsen or create new arrhythmias, especially in electrolyte-imbalanced patients. Encainide is known to have caused sinus bradycardia, sinus pause, or sinus arrest (see also Figure 76).

ENDORPHINS

For many years, pharmacologists considered the possibility that opioids mimic a naturally ongoing process. Investigations isolated opiate-like peptides from the brain that consisted of two similar pentapeptides with the following sequences:

    Try-Gly-Gly-Phe-Met (met-enkephalin)
    Try-Gly-Gly-Phe-Leu (leu-enkephalin)

Both peptides behave as agonists and inhibit opiate receptor binding, with affinities comparable to the affinity of morphine. The effects of met-enkephalin and leu-enkephalin are reversed by **naloxone**. Three distinct families of peptides have been identified thus far: the **enkephalins**, the **endorphins**, and the **dynorphins**.

ENDOTHELINS

Endothelial cells synthesize and release substances that cause vasoconstriction or vasorelaxation. **Endothelin** is a potent, slow-acting, and long-lasting vasoconstrictor peptide that exerts

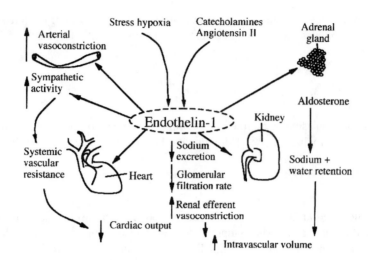

FIGURE 34   Endothelial cells synthesize and release substances that cause vasoconstriction or vasore-laxation. **Endothelin** is a potent, slow-acting and long-lasting vasoconstrictor peptide that exerts a wide variety of effects.

a wide variety of effects, which include constriction of airway, intestinal, and uterine smooth muscle, positive inotropic and chronotropic actions plus stimulation of atrial natriuretic peptide release, inhibition of renin release from isolated glomeruli, and inhibition of ouabain-sensitive $Na^+K^+ATPase$ in the inner medullary collecting duct cells. It also blocks the antidiuretic effect of vasopressin *in vivo*, modulates catecholamine release from the sympathetic termini and adrenomedullary chromaffin cells, stimulates aldosterone release in adrenocortical glomerular cells, and stimulates CNS effects, including a potent pressor action that is mediated by increased sympathetic outflow and the stimulation of substance P release from the spinal cord (see Figure 34).

The currently available data suggest that the **signal transduction** at the endothelium receptor in vascular smooth muscle may be similar to that of **angiotensin II** and **vasopressin**.

ENFLURANE

(Enthrane)

Enflurane is indicated to provide analgesia for vaginal delivery, and in combination with other anesthetic agents, it is used for delivery by cesarean section. It does provide adequate muscular relaxation. Enflurane, an inhalation anesthetic produces rapid induction and recovery. It obtunds pharyngeal and laryngeal reflexes and causes salivary secretion. Since it releases fluoride ion, it may cause renal failure in susceptible individuals (see also Table 15).

ENKEPHALINS

For many years, pharmacologists considered the possibility that opioids mimic a naturally ongoing process. Investigations isolated opiate-like peptides from the brain that consisted of two similar pentapeptides with the following sequences:

   Try-Gly-Gly-Phe-Met (met-enkephalin)
   Try-Gly-Gly-Phe-Leu (leu-enkephalin)

Both peptides behave as agonists and inhibit opiate receptor binding, with affinities comparable to the affinity of morphine. The effects of met-enkephalin and leu-enkephalin are reversed by **naloxone**. Three distinct families of peptides have been identified thus far: the **enkephalins**, the **endorphins**, and the **dynorphins**.

ENOXACIN
(Penetrex)

Enoxacin (single dose of 400 mg) is indicated in the treatment of uncomplicated urethral or cervical gonorrhea due to *Neisseria gonorrhoeae*; or uncomplicated cystitis (200 mg q. 12 hr/7 days) due to *Escherichia coli, Staphylococcus epidermidis,* or *S. saprophyticus*; complicated due to *E. coli, Klebsiella pneumoniae, Proteus mirabilis, Pseudomonas aeruginosa, S. epidermidis,* or *Enterobacter cloacae*. Enoxacin diffuses into cervix, fallopian tube, and myometrium at levels approximately 1 to 2 times those achieved in plasma, and into kidney and prostate at levels approximately 2 to 4 times those achieved in plasma. Enoxacin becomes bound to the extent of 40%, and this is decreased to 15% in patients with renal impairment requiring a reduction in total dosage. Bismuth subsalicylate decreases the availability of enoxacin. The activity of cytochrome P450 isoenzyme responsible for metabolism of methylxanthines (caffeine, theophylline, and theobromine) is inhibited by enoxacin prolonging their actions. Quinolones, including enoxacin reduce the clearance of warfarin. The side effects of enoxacin may include headache, dizziness, somnolence, gastrointestinal pain, skin rash, and vaginal moniliasis. The quinolones and fluoroquinolones may produce arthropathy, and hence should not be used in pregnant women (see also Figure 77).

ENOXAPRIN SODIUM
(Lovenox)

Enoxaprin (30 mg b.i.d. SC) is indicated for the prevention of deep vein thrombosis, which may lead to pulmonary embolism, following hip replacement surgery. Enoxaprin is a low-molecular-weight heparin which has antithrombotic properties. It is contraindicated in a patient with active major bleeding or with thrombocytopenia. Furthermore, enoxaprin should be used cautiously in conditions with increased risk of hemorrhage such as bacterial endocarditis, congenital or acquired bleeding disorders, active ulceration, hemorrhagic stroke, or shortly after brain, spinal, or ophthalmological surgery. Protamine sulfate (1% solution) is able to antidote the overdosage of enoxaprin (see also Figure 35 and Tables 16 and 17).

ENOXIMONE

Amrinone, milrinone, and **enoximone** differ from aminophylline in that they exhibit a certain degree of selectivity for peak III phosphodiesterase (Figure 10), which is found predominantly in myocardial and vascular tissues. These agents exert both positive inotropic and direct vasodilating actions. Circulating catecholamines released from adrenergic nerve terminals, and exogenous sympathomimetic drugs act on beta-adrenergic and alpha-adrenergic receptors, respectively. Simulation of beta-adrenergic receptors activates adenylate cyclase, resulting in increased cyclic adenosine monophosphate (cyclic AMP) production, which in turn augments calcium influx through the slow calcium channels, presumably due to the activation of protein kinases that phosphorylate the slow calcium channel (see Figure 76). The mechanism by which the stimulation of alpha-adrenergic receptors increases myocardial contractility is not fully understood, but it may also involve an action on the slow calcium channel. **Tyramine** acts on adrenergic nerve terminals to release catecholamines, which then act on adrenergic receptors. **Calcium channel agonists** act directly on the calcium channel to increase calcium influx, intracellular cyclic AMP is degraded by phosphodiesterase, and the subsequent inhibition of cardiac phosphodiesterases results in increased intracellular cyclic AMP levels. This mechanism appears to be largely responsible for the actions of several of the newer positive inotropic agents. The cyclic AMP concentration can also be increased independently of beta-adrenergic receptors through the direct stimulation of adenylate cyclase with **forskolin** (see also Figure 42).

ENPROFYLLINE

Enprofylline is a methylxanthine bronchodilator which may be used in the treatment of bronchial asthma. The methylxanthines consist of **aminophylline, dyphylline, enprofylline,** and **pentoxifylline**. Aminophylline (theophylline ethylenediamine) is the most widely used of the soluble theophyllines. Its main therapeutic effect is bronchodilation. In addition, it causes central nervous system stimulation, cardiac acceleration, diuresis, and gastric secretion. Aminophylline is available in an oral, rectal (pediatric), or intravenous solution, which is used in the treatment of status asthmaticus. Although aminophylline is a less effective bronchodilator than beta-adrenergic agonists, it is particularly useful in preventing nocturnal asthma (see also Figure 86).

ENTACAPONE

Entacapone, a peripherally acting inhibitor of catechol-o-methyltransferase, is a valuable adjunct to levodopa in parkinsonian patients.

ENZYMES AND HORMONES OF GASTROINTESTINAL TRACT: ACTIONS OF		
Enzymes/Hormones	**Sites of Secretion**	**Main Actions**
Amylase	Parotid and submandibular glands	Converts carbohydrates, starch, and glycogen to simple disaccharides
Cholecystokinin	Duodenum, jejunum	Stimulates pancreatic enzyme secretion and gallbladder contraction
Chymotrypsinogen	Pancreas	Breaks down proteins into proteases and peptides
Enteroglucagon	Duodenum	Inhibits pancreatic enzyme secretion and bowel motility
Gastric inhibitory peptide	Small intestine	Decreases gastric motility and stimulates insulin secretion
Gastrin	Stomach, duodenum	Stimulates gastric acid secretion and mucosal growth
Glucagon	Pancreas	Stimulates hepatic glycogenolysis and inhibits motility
Lipase	Pancreas	Hydrolyzes short-chain and medium-chain triglycerides, involved in fat absorption
Pancreatic polypeptide	Pancreas	Inhibits gallbladder contraction and pancreatic and biliary secretion
Pepsinogen	Stomach	Converts large proteins into polypeptides
Secretin	Small intestine	Stimulates hepatic and pancreatic water and bicarbonate secretion
Trypsinogen	Pancreas	Breaks down proteins into proteases and peptides
Vasoactive inhibitory peptide	Small intestine, pancreas	Vasodilator; stimulates water and bicarbonate secretion, release of insulin and glucagon, and production of small intestinal juice

EPHEDRINE
(Bofedrol)

EPHEDRINE HYDROCHLORIDE
(Efedron)

EPHEDRINE SULFATE
(Ectasule Minus, Ephed II, Slo-Fedrin, Vicks Va-tro-nol)

Ephedrine, a sympathomimetic amine, is used to correct hypotensive states (25 to 50 mg IM or SC), to treat orthostatic hypotension (25 mg p.o. once daily to q.i.d.), and as a broncho-dilator or nasal congestant (see also Table 24).

Ephedrine (25 to 50 mg p.o. t.i.d.) is indicated in the treatment of allergic disorders, such as bronchial asthma; of nasal congestion in acute coryza; of vasomotor rhinitis, acute sinusitis, and hayfever. Ephedrine (25 to 30 mg slowly SC, IM, or IV) has been used to relieve acute bronchospasm, but epinephrine is more effective. Ephedrine is also used in shock. Ephedrine is a naturally occurring sympathomimetic agent which stimulates alpha and beta receptors and CNS. It is less potent than epinephrine but has a longer duration of action (see also Figure 27).

EPILEPTIC SEIZURES: TREATMENT OF		
Seizure Type	**Drug of Choice**	**Alternate**
Partial Seizures		
Simple partial	Carbamazepine, phenytoin, phenobarbital, primidone, valproate	Gabapentin, lamotrigine
Complex partial	Carbamazepine, phenobarbital, phenytoin, primidone, valproate	Gabapentin, lamotrigine
Partial with secondarily generalized tonic-clonic seizure	Carbamazepine, phenobarbital, phenytoin, primidone, valproate	Gabapentin, lamotrigine
Generalized Seizures		
Absence seizure	Clonazepam, ethosuximide, valproate	Lamotrigine
Myoclonic seizure	Valproate	
Tonic-clonic seizure	Carbamazepine, phenobarbital, phenytoin, primidone, valproate	

EPINEPHRINE
(Bronkaid Mist, EpiPen, EpiPen Jr, Primatene Mist Solution, Sus-Phrine)

EPINEPHRINE BITARTRATE
(AsthmaHaler, Bronitin Mist, Bronkaid Mist Suspension, Epitrate, Medihaler-Epi, Primatene Mist Suspension)

EPINEPHRINE HYDROCHLORIDE
(Adrenalin Chloride, AsthmaNefrin, Epifrin, Glaucon, microNefrin, S-2 Inhalant, Vaponefrin)

EPINEPHRYL BORATE
(Epinal, Eppy/N)

Epinephrine, a sympathomimetic amine, is used as a bronchodilator (one inhalation per metered aerosol); to restore cardiac rhythm in cardiac arrest (0.5 to 1 mg IV bolus); to treat open-angle glaucoma (1 to 2 drops of 1 to 2% solution), and to prolong the effect of local anesthetics. Epinephrine is a sympathomimetic drug that activates an adrenergic receptor mechanism on effector cells and initiates cell actions of the sympathetic nervous system except on the arteries of the face and sweat glands (see Figure 27). Epinephrine acts on both alpha and beta receptors, but the beta effect may predominate; norepinephrine acts on both alpha and beta receptors, but the alpha effects may predominate. The functions associated with **alpha receptors** are vasoconstriction, mydriasis, and intestinal relaxation. The functions associated with **beta receptors** are vasodilation, cardioacceleration, bronchial relaxation, positive inotropic effect, intestinal relaxation, and glycogenolysis and fatty acid release. The $beta_1$ receptors are responsible for cardiac stimulation and vasodepression. $Beta_2$ agonists are especially useful in the treatment of asthma because they produce bronchodilation without causing much cardiac acceleration.

The actions of norepinephrine and epinephrine on the cardiovascular system may be quite different when both drugs are administered in small doses (0.1 to 0.4 microgram/kg/min in a slow intravenous infusion), but are essentially the same when given in large doses. Following are the effects of **small doses of norepinephrine** in humans: systolic pressure — increased; diastolic pressure — increased; mean pressure — increased; heart rate — slightly decreased; cardiac output — slightly decreased; and peripheral resistance — increased.

The effects of **small doses of epinephrine** in humans are: systolic pressure — increased; diastolic pressure — decreased (increased by larger dose); mean pressure — unchanged; cardiac output — increased; and peripheral resistance — decreased. Epinephrine increases the heart rate, force of contraction, irritability, and coronary blood flow. The inherent **chronotropic effect of norepinephrine** is opposed by reflex slowing that is secondary to vasoconstriction and elevated blood pressure. Epinephrine is a dilator of bronchial smooth muscle ($beta_2$ receptor), whereas norepinephrine is a weak dilator. Isoproterenol is more active than epinephrine. Both epinephrine and isoproterenol elevate the blood glucose level by stimulating glycogenolysis and by inhibiting glucose utilization. The therapeutic uses of epinephrine and its related drugs are as a bronchodilator ($beta_2$ receptor activation in asthma), as a mydriatic (contracts radial muscle), in glaucoma (lowers intraocular pressure), for allergic reactions (prevents antigen-induced histamine releases), in hypotension (increases the mean pressure), as a nasal decongestant (**mephentermine**), as a local anesthesia (produces a bloodless field of operation, delays absorption and yields a longer duration of anesthetic action, and protects the brain and heart against the toxic effects of local anesthetics), and as cardiac stimulants (epinephrine or isoproterenol may be injected in heart block to improve atrioventricular conduction velocity and stimulate ventricular automaticity) (see also Figure 72).

EPIRUBICIN

Epirubicin is a new anthracycline that has activity similar to doxorubicin (Adriamycin) in a variety of solid neoplasms and hematologic malignancies. Importantly, epirubicin causes less cardiotoxicity than doxorubicin (see also Figure 2).

EPOETIN ALFA
(Erythropoietin) (Epogen, Procrit)

Epoetin alfa, a glycoprotein with antianemic effects (50 to 100 units/kg three times weekly), is used to treat anemia associated with chronic renal failure and anemia related to zidovudine therapy in patients infected with human immunodeficiency virus (HIV) (see Figures 36 and 37).

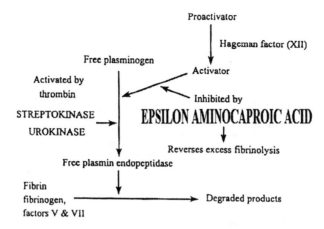

FIGURE 35   The effects of streptokinase or urokinase may be counteracted by **epsilon-aminocaproic acid**. (Adapted from Ebadi, M., *Pharmacology, An Illustrated Review with Questions and Answers*, 3rd Edition, Lippincott-Raven Press, Philadelphia, 1996.)

EPSILON-AMINOCAPROIC ACID

Fibrinolysis takes place according to the scheme depicted in Figure 35. Plasmin, an endopeptide that is converted from plasminogen by an activator, hydrolyzes fibrin, fibrinogen, factor V, and factor VIII to their inactive products. **Hageman factor** (factor XII) converts a proactivator to the active activator. Agents such as thrombin, streptokinase, and urokinase therefore enhance the formation of plasmin and hence have fibrinolytic properties. **Epsilon-aminocaproic acid** inhibits the activator-mediated formation of plasmin and hence may be used as an antidote to streptokinase-urokinase, or in a defibrination syndrome when bleeding from a mucous membrane occurs (Figure 35).

ERECTILE DYSFUNCTIONS: TREATMENT OF	
Impotence is usually defined as the inability to obtain or maintain a penile erection that is sufficient for vaginal penetration in 50% or more attempts during intercourse. There is no age after puberty at which intercourse is not physiologic, and, as such, the development of impotence represents a pathologic process. It is also evident that the frequency of erectile dysfunction is higher in men older than 60 compared with those younger than 40 (see also the section on Sexual Dysfunctions Caused by Drugs).	
Neurologic diseases causing erectile dysfunction are:	
Alzheimer's disease	Primary autonomic insufficiency
Amyloidosis	Primary and metastatic tumors
Cerebrovascular accidents	Spinal arachnoiditis
Cervical spondylosis	Spinal cord trauma
Multiple sclerosis	Syphilis
Parkinson's disease	Temporal lobe epilepsy
Pelvic trauma	
Surgical or traumatic causes of erectile dysfunctions are:	
Abdominoperineal resection	Penectomy
Aortoiliac surgery	Proctocolectomy
Bilateral orchiectomy	Prostate biopsy
Cystectomy	Prostatectomy; radical or simple
Genital trauma	Renal transplantation
Inguinoscrotal surgery	Retroperitoneal lymphadenectomy
Internal urethrotomy; sphincterotomy	Spinal cord injury
Pelvic fractures	Sympathectomy
Pelvic radiation therapy	

Pharmacological management of erectile dysfunction are:	
Drugs used for intracavernous vasoactive injection therapy	
Alprostadil (prostaglandin E₁)	Moxisylyte
Atropine	Multiple-drug mixtures
Calcitonin gene-related peptide	Papaverine
Linsidomine	Phentolamine
Oral pharmacological therapy	
Apomorphine	Pentoxifylline (oxpentifylline)
Arginine	Phentolamine
Bromocriptine	Testosterone replacement therapy
Fluoxetine	Trazodone
Naltrexone	Yohimbine
Topical pharmacological therapy	
Alprostadil and dinoprostone (prostaglandin E₂)	Nitroglycerin (glyceryl trinitrate)
Minoxidil	Papaverine

ERGOCALCIFEROL

(Vitamin D) (Calciferol, Deltalin, Gelseals, Drisdol, Vitamin D Capsules)

Ergocalciferol, a vitamin with antihypocalcemic properties, is indicated in nutritional rickets or osteomalacia (25 to 125 mcg p.o. daily), in familial hypophosphatemia (250 mcg to 1.5 mg p.o. daily), in vitamin D-dependent rickets (250 mcg to 1.5 mg p.o. daily), and in hypoparathyroidism (625 mcg to 5 mg p.o. daily) (see also Figure 97).

ERGONOVINE MALEATE

(Ergotrate)

Ergonovine (0.2 mg IM) is indicated for prevention and treatment of postpartum and post-abortal hemorrhage. It exerts its effects by acting as a partial agonist or antagonist at alpha adrenergic, dopaminergic, or tryptaminergic receptors. The onset of action of ergonovine is 40 seconds, and 7 to 8 minutes when given intravenously or intramuscularly. Inappropriate uses of ergonovine in higher than therapeutic concentrations may cause impairment of the uteroplacental blood flow, uterine rupture, cervical and perineal laceration, and trauma to the infant.

ERGOT ALKALOIDS	
Bromocriptine, used in Parkinson's disease	Methylergonovine
Dihydroergotamine	Methysergide, used in headaches
Ergotamine	
Ergot alkaloids have complex and diverse actions. For example, the marked effects of ergotamine on the cardiovascular system are due to vasoconstriction, depression of vasomotor centers, and peripheral adrenergic blockade.	

ERGOTAMINE TARTRATE

(Ergomar, Ergostat, Medihaler-Ergotamine, Wigrettes)

Ergotamine, an ergot alkaloid (2 mg sublingually), is used to prevent or abort vascular headache, including migraine and cluster headaches (see also Figure 85).

ERYTHRITYL TETRANITRATE

(Cardilate)

Erythrityl tetranitrate (5 to 10 mg sublingually) is used for prophylaxis and long-term treatment of frequent or recurrent angina pain and in reduced exercise tolerance associated with angina pectoris (see **Nitroglycerin**) (see Figures 59 and 60).

ERYTHROMYCIN

(Erythocin)

Erythromycin, as a penicillin alternative, is a medium- to broad-spectrum antibiotic. It possesses both bactericidal and bacteriostatic properties, depending on the concentration of the drug being used and the microorganisms being treated. Erythromycin is effective against Gram-positive organisms such as *Streptococcus pyogenes* and *pneumoniae*. In larger doses, erythromycin is effective against *Staphylococcus epidermidis* and *aureus*. In addition, Gram-positive bacilli such as *Clostridium perfringens, Corynebacterium diphtheriae,* and *Listeria monocytogenes* are also susceptible to erythromycin. Erythromycin is also effective against *Mycoplasma pneumoniae* and *Legionella pneumophilia*, which causes legionnaires' disease. Erythromycin exerts its effect by binding to a 23S ribosomal RNA on the 50S ribosomal subunit, and this inhibits protein synthesis. Aminoacyl translocation reactions and elongation of the peptide chain are then blocked (see Figure 80). Resistance occurs from the methylation of ribosomal RNA receptors, preventing the attachment of erythomycin to 50S ribosomes. Erythromycin, which is destroyed by gastric secretions, is supplied as enteric-coated tablets, which are absorbed well from the upper part of the small intestine. Erythromycin stearate is acid resistant. Erythromycin is largely excreted in the bile and the urinary excretion is negligible. Erythromycin, and especially erythromycin estolate, can cause **cholestatic hepatitis**.

ERYTHROMYCIN BASE

(E-Mycin, ERYC, Eryfed, Ethril 500, Erythrocin, Erythromycin Base Filmtabs, Robimycin)

ERYTHROMYCIN ESTOLATE

(Ilosone)

ERYTHROMYCIN ETHYLSUCCINATE

(E.E.S., E-Mycin E, EryPed, Pediamycin, Pediazole, Wyamycin E)

ERYTHROMYCIN STEARATE

(Erypar Filmseal, Erythrocin Stearate, Ethril, Wyamycin S)

ERYTHROMYCIN (TOPICAL)

(Akne-Mycin, A/T/S/, EryDerm, Erymax, Eryvette, Staticin, T-Stat)

Erythromycin, an antibiotic, is indicated in acute pelvic inflammatory disease caused by *Neisseria gonorrhoeae*, in endocarditis prophylaxis for dental procedures in patients allergic to penicillin, erythromycin base, estolate, or stearate; and in the treatment of intestinal amebiasis in patients who cannot receive metronidazole, erythromycin base, estolate, or stearate. It is used as treatment for mild to moderate severe respiratory tract, skin, and soft-tissue infections caused by susceptible organisms, as well as for syphilis, Legionnaires' disease, uncomplicated urethral, endocervical, or rectal infections when tetracyclines are

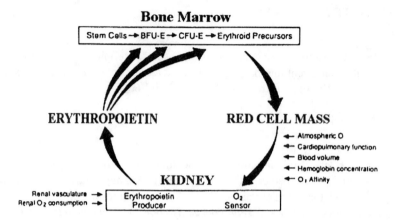

FIGURE 36 Erythropoietin is produced primarily by **peritubular cells** in the proximal tubule of the kidney. These cells not only produce erythropoietin but also the **oxygen sensor** that stimulates erythropoietin production. (Adapted from Ebadi, M., *Pharmacology, An Illustrated Review with Questions and Answers*, 3rd Edition, Lippincott-Raven Press, Philadelphia, 1996.)

contraindicated, urogenital *Chlamydia trachomatis* infections during pregnancy, conjunctivitis caused by *Chlamydia trachomatis* in neonates, pneumonia of infancy caused by *Chlamydia trachomatis*, and topical treatment of acne vulgaris.

ERYTHROPOIETIN

(Procrit)

Hematopoietic stem cells and progenitor cells undergo extensive proliferation and differentiation *in vitro* under the influence of at least eleven **hematopoietic growth factors**. These include interleukin-1, -3, and -6; interferon alpha, beta, and gamma; and erythropoietin.

Erythropoietin is produced primarily by **peritubular cells** in the proximal tubule of the kidney (Figure 36). These cells not only produce erythropoietin but also the oxygen sensor that stimulates erythropoietin production. Erythropoietin, which consists of 193 amino acid residues, has a molecular weight of 34,000 and is glycosylated. Its synthesis increases in the presence of **anemia** and **hypoxia** (Figure 36).

Erythropoietin is effective for the treatment of anemia associated with **chronic renal failure**. It is also effective in managing the anemia seen in patients with acquired immunodeficiency syndrome (AIDS) who are being treated with zidovudine (AZT) and the anemia associated with cancer chemotherapy. Patients who are to undergo elective surgery may receive erythropoietin preoperatively to increase red cell production, thus permitting the storage of large volumes of blood for autologous transfusion (see Figure 37).

ESMOLOL

(Brevibloc)

Esmolol is an ultra short-acting intravenous cardioselective beta-adrenergic receptor antagonist with a short elimination half-life of nine minutes. Esmolol is used in situations where a brief duration of adrenergic block is required, such as tracheal intubation and stressful surgical stimuli. Esmolol causes hypotension which is accompanied by diaphoresis (see also Figures 33, 57, 61, and 75). Esmolol, a beta$_1$-adrenergic blocking agent with antiarrhythmic properties (50 to 200 mcg/kg/min), is indicated in the treatment of intraoperative tachycardia and/or hypertension.

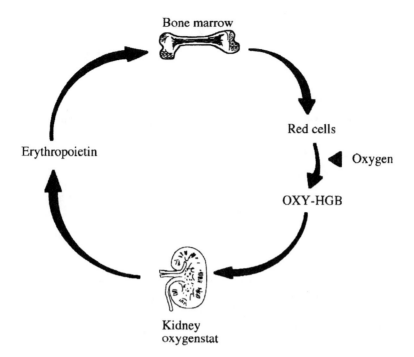

FIGURE 37   Erythropoietin is effective for the treatment of anemia associated with **chronic renal failure**.

ESMOLOL HYDROCHLORIDE

(Brevibloc)

Esmolol is a class II antiarrhythmic agent with ultra short-acting beta-adrenergic blocking activity which is used (50 to 200 mcg/kg/min) to treat supraventricular tachycardia such as atrial fibrillation or atrial flutter. Esmolol is rapidly metabolized by erythrocyte esterases via hydrolysis of the methyl ester. Unlike succinylcholine, esmolol is not metabolized by plasma cholinesterase (see also Figures 57 and 76).

ESTAZOLAM

(Prosom)

Estazolam (1 mg at bedtime) is indicated for the short-term management of insomnia characterized by difficulty in falling asleep, frequent nocturnal awakening, or early morning awakenings. Estazolam may cause fetal damage and hence is contraindicated in pregnancy. It causes CNS depression and potentiates the CNS depressant effects of alcohol, and other CNS drugs should be used cautiously whenever alertness and vigilance are required (see also Table 8).

ESTERIFIED ESTROGENS

(Estratab, Menest)

Esterified estrogen is used in prostatic cancer (1.25 to 2.5 mg p.o. t.i.d.); and in female hypogonadism, ovariectomy, and primary ovarian failure (2.5 mg daily p.o. in a cycle of three weeks on medication and one week medication-free); and in menopausal symptoms (Figure 38).

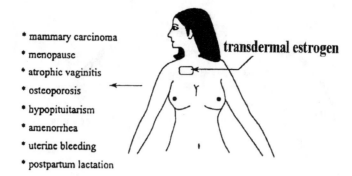

* mammary carcinoma
* menopause
* atrophic vaginitis
* osteoporosis
* hypopituitarism
* amenorrhea
* uterine bleeding
* postpartum lactation

transdermal estrogen

FIGURE 38   The therapeutic uses of estrogen.

ESTRADIOL

(Estraderm)

Estradiol transdermal system is indicated in the treatment of vasomotor symptoms associated with menopause. It is also used to treat female hypogonadism, primary ovarian failure, atrophic conditions (atrophic vaginitis or kraurosis vulvae), and in the prevention of osteoporosis (see **Estrogen** and Figure 38).

ESTRADIOL

(Estrace, Estrace Vaginal Cream, Estraderm)

ESTRADIOL CYPIONATE

(Depestro, DepGynogen, Depo-Estradiol Cypionate, Depogen, Dura-Estrin, Estra-D, Estro-cyp, Estrofem, Estroject-L.A., Estronol-L.A., Hormogen Depot)

ESTRADIOL VALERATE

(Dioval, Dioval XX, Dioval 40, Duragen, Estradiol L.A., Estradiol L.A. 20, Estradiol L.A. 40, Estraval Gynogen L.A. 10, Gynogen L.A. 20, L.A.E. 20, Valergen-10, Valergen-20, Valergen-40)

POLYESTRADIOL PHOSPHATE

(Estradurin)

These various estradiol preparations, available in oral, injectable, and cream forms, are used in atrophic vaginitis, atrophic dystrophy of the vulva, menopausal symptoms, hypogonadism, ovariectomy, primary ovarian failure; postpartum breast engorgement; female hypogonadism; inoperable breast cancer; inoperable prostatic cancer; and in advancing prostatic carcinoma deemed inoperable (see also Figure 38).

ESTRAMUSTINE PHOSPHATE SODIUM

(EMCYT)

Estramustine (10 to 16 mg/kg p.o. in 3 to 4 divided doses), is used as a palliative treatment of metastatic or progressive cancer of the prostate.

ESTROGEN AND PROGESTIN

(Brevicon 21-Day, Brevicon 28-Day, Demulen 1/35-21, Demulen 1/35-28, Enovid 5 mg, Enovid E-21, Loestrin 21 1/20, Loestrin 21 1.5/30, Loestrin Fe 1/20, Loestrin Fe 1.5/30,

Lo/Ovral, Lo/Orval-28, Modicon 21, Modicon 28, Nordette-21, Nordette-28, Norinyl 1+35 21Day, Norinyl 1+50 28-Day, Norinyl 1+80 21-Day, Norinyl 1+80 28-Day, Norinyl 2 mg, Norlestrin 21 1/50, Norlestrin 21 2.5/50, Norlestrin 28 1/50, Norlestrin Fe 1/50, Norlestrin Fe 2.5/50, Ortho-Novum 1/35 21, Ortho-Novum 1/35 28, Ortho Novum 1/50 21, Ortho-Novum 1/50 28, Ortho-Novum 1/80 21, Ortho-Novum 1/80 28, Ortho Novum 2 mg 21, Ortho-Novum 7/7/7-21, Ortho-Novum 7/7/7-28, Ortho-Novum 10/11-21, Ortho-Novum 10/11-28, Ovcon-35, Ovcon-50, Ovral, Ovral-28, Ovulen-21, Ovulen-28, Tri-Norinyl-21, Tri-Norinyl-28, Triphasil-21, Triphasil-28)

Estrogen and progestin hormonal combination is used as oral contraceptive medication.

ESTROGENIC PREPARATIONS	
Estrone	
Injectable	Estrone aqueous suspension and estrogenic substance or estrogens aqueous suspension (primarily estrone)
Oral	Conjugated estrogens (50-65% sodium estrone sulfate and 20-35% sodium equilin sulfate) Esterified estrogens (75-85% estrone sulfate and 6-15% sodium equilin)
Vaginal creams	Estropiate Conjugated estrogens
Estradiol	
Injectable	Estradiol valerate (in oil) Estradiol cypionate (in oil)
Oral	Micronized estradiol
Vaginal creams	Micronized estradiol
Transdermal	Estradiol
Others	
Oral	Ethinyl estradiol Quinestrol Chlorotrianisene
Vaginal creams	Dienestrol

ESTROGENIC SUBSTANCES, CONJUGATED

(Estracon, Premarin, Progen Tabs)

Estrogen, possessing antineoplastic and antiosteoporotic properties, is indicated in abnormal uterine bleeding (hormonal imbalance), in castration, primary ovarian failure, and osteoporosis, in female hypogonadism, in menopausal symptoms, atrophic vaginitis, or kraurosis vulvae, in prostatic cancer, and in breast cancer (see also Figure 38).

ESTROGENS

Estrogens are synthesized mainly in the ovaries, the placenta, and the adrenal glands. A minute amount of estradiol is synthesized in the testes. Estrogens are synthesized according to the following scheme.

Cholesterol → pregnenolone → progesterone → androstenedione

→ estradiol 17 beta → estrone → estriol

Estrogen dramatically influences the growth and development of the **female reproductive organs**. The uterus and vagina are sensitive to the biochemical actions of estrogens, which are as follows: Early events — release of histamine, synthesis of cyclic adenosine monophosphate (cyclic AMP), stimulation of RNA polymerase, and increased excitability of the myometrium. Intermediate events — synthesis of RNA and DNA, inhibition of water, and stimulation of certain enzymes. Late events — increased secretory activity, morphologic changes, increased protein synthesis, stimulation of lipid and carbohydrate metabolism, and increased gravimetric responses.

Estrogens are used extensively in the treatment of endocrine and non-endocrine disease, a few of which are cited: menopause — as a replacement therapy; atrophic vaginitis — to thicken epithelial cells and to cause mucosal cells to proliferate; hypopituitarism — to correct vaginal mucosal atrophy, maintain breast development, and minimize calcium loss from bone; cancer — used in postmenopausal mammary carcinoma; primary hypogonadism — to correct ovarian failure; osteoporosis — estrogen by itself or with a hypercalcemic steroid is used in the treatment of osteoporosis; primary amenorrhea — to cause endometrium to proliferate; uterine bleeding — to reverse estrogen deficiency (in this case, oral contraceptives containing 80 to 100 micrograms of estrogen are recommended); postpartum lactation — to relieve postpartum painful breast engorgement and prevent postpartum lactation; bromocriptine is also effective; control of height — to cause closure of the epiphyses in unusually tall young girls; and dermatologic problems — used with some success in the treatment of acne. Low-dose estrogens are safe only when taken for a limited period. The most often reported side effects are breakthrough bleeding, breast tenderness, and very infrequently gastrointestinal upsets. When estrogens are used in large doses or injudiciously, they may cause thromboembolic disorders, hypertension in susceptible individuals, and cholestasis. Estrogens are contraindicated in patients with estrogen-dependent neoplasms such as carcinoma of the breast or endometrium. Vaginal adenocarcinoma has been reported in young women whose mothers were treated with **diethylstilbestrol** in an effort to prevent miscarriage (see also Figure 26).

ESTRONE

(Bestrone, Estrone-A, Estronol, Kestrone-5, Theelin Aqueous)

ESTROPIPATE

(Ogen)

Estrone or estropipate is used in the treatment of atrophic vaginitis and menopausal symptoms, female hypogonadism, primary ovarian failure, after castration, or in prostatic cancer (see also Figure 26).

ETHACRYNIC ACID

(Edecrin)

The major loop diuretics are **furosemide** (Lasix) and **ethacrynic acid**. Furosemide is chemically related to the thiazide diuretics, but ethacrynic acid is not. These agents inhibit the active resorption of chloride (and sodium) in the thick, ascending medullary portion of the loop of Henle and also in the cortical portion of the loop or the distal tubule. The diuresis they produce, which is similar to that seen with the thiazides, predominantly causes a loss of chloride, sodium, and potassium, but HCO_3 excretion is not increased. Although large volumes of fluid can be excreted with the use of these agents, the ability of the kidney to produce either a dilute or concentrated urine is greatly diminished. These agents are most efficacious with about a 20% loss in the filtered load of sodium (furosemide, 15 to 30%; ethacrynic acid, 17 to 23%). Loop diuretics are ordinarily taken orally, but can be given intravenously if a rapid onset of action is sought, as when used in combination with antihypertensive medications in the management of hypertensive crisis. Furosemide and ethacrynic acid undergo some active renal tubular secretion as well as glomerular filtration. A minor portion is excreted by the liver. Loop diuretics are used for treating the following conditions: in **edema** of cardiac, hepatic, or renal origin, including acute pulmonary edema and hypertensive crisis; in **acute renal failure**, to maintain urine flow, though an excessive loss of extracellular fluid volume can cause a decrease in the GFR; and in **hyperkalemia** (see Figure 4).

Excessive volume depletion, hyponatremia, and hypotension are major risks associated with the use of loop diuretics, and the side effects of **hypokalemia, hyperuricemia**, and **hyperglycemia** are always present. Loop diuretics should not be used concurrently with **ototoxic aminoglycoside antibiotics** (i.e., streptomycin, gentamicin, kanamycin, tobramycin) (see also Table 25).

ETHAMBUTOL HYDROCHLORIDE
(Myambutol)

Ethambutol (15 to 25 mg/kg/day) is used in conjunction with other antituberculosis drugs in pulmonary tuberculosis. It is effective against strains of *Mycobacterium tuberculosis* but does not seem to be active against fungi, viruses, or other bacteria. Ethambutol is metabolized in the liver (20%), and a significant portion of it (50%) is excreted unchanged in the urine, and hence the dosage should be reduced in renal impairment. Ethambutol may cause retrobulbar neuritis, and patients treated for a prolonged period of time should have vision examination including visual fields. Most visual effects are reversible following discontinuation of the drug. In addition, ethambutol has caused dermatitis, pruritis, anorexia, headache, dizziness, vomiting, fever, and joint pain. Aluminum salts delays and reduces the absorption of ethambutol.

ETHANOLAMINE OLEATE
(Ethamolin)

Ethanolamine, a sclerosing agent, is indicated in the treatment of patients with esophageal varices that have recently bled, with the intention of preventing rebleeding. When injected IV, it acts primarily by irritation of the intimal endothelium of the vein and produces a sterile dose-related inflammatory response. This results in fibrosis and occlusion of the vein. The adverse reactions following ethanolamine include pleural effusion, infiltration, esophageal ulcer, esophageal stricture, pneumonia, pyrexia, and retrosternal pain.

ETHAPROPRAZINE HYDROCHLORIDE
(Parsidol)

Ethaproprazine is used as an adjunct in the treatment of Parkinson's disease or in neuroleptic-induced parkinsonism. Most phenothiazine neuroleptics have weak anticholinergic properties. However, the anticholinergic effects of **thioridazine** or **ethaproprazine** are pronounced, and all the cautions cited for atropine apply to these agents as well. Indeed, fatal **tachyarrhythmias** and other electrocardiographic changes, such as blunting and notching of T waves, prolongation of the QT interval, increased convexity of the ST segment, and appearance of V waves have been caused through the injudicious use of thioridazine (1500 to 3600 mg/day), especially in elderly patients.

ETHAVERINE HYDROCHLORIDE
(Circubid, Ethaquin, Ethatab, Ethavex-100, Isovex, Pavaspan)

Ethaverine, an isoquinoline derivative with peripheral vasodilating properties (100 to 200 mg p.o. t.i.d. q. 12 hours), is indicated in peripheral and cerebrovascular insufficiency associated with arterial spasm and in spastic conditions of the gastrointestinal and genitourinary tracts.

ETHCHLORVYNOL
(PLACIDYL)

Ethchlorvynol (500 mg at bedtime), which has sedative-hypnotic, anticonvulsant, and muscle relaxant properties, is indicated in the management of insomnia. The onset and duration of action are 15 minutes and 6 hours, respectively. Ethchlorvynol, which should not be used more than one week, causes psychological and physical dependence when used for a prolonged period of time, and its sudden discontinuation will produce abstinence syndromes characterized by convulsions, delirium, schizoid reaction, perceptual distortions, memory loss, ataxia, insomnia, slurring of speech, unusual anxiety, irritability, agitation, tremors, anorexia, nausea, vomiting, weakness, dizziness, sweating, muscle twitching, or weight loss.

Ethchlorvynol or phenobarbital may be used in the management of withdrawal symptoms. The CNS depressant effects of ethchlorvynol will be enhanced by alcohol, barbiturates, narcotics, and numerous other drugs. Ethchlorvynol will reduce the hypoprothrombinemic effects of anticoagulants requiring dose adjustment of the anticoagulant.

ETHER

The pharmacology of nitrous oxide, cyclopropane, halothane, and ether is summarized in Table 15. Ether and cyclopropane are seldom used in anesthesiology.

ETHINYL ESTRADIOL
(Estinyl)

Ethinyl tablets are indicated in the treatment of vasomotor symptoms associated with the menopause; in female hypogonadism; in prostatic carcinoma; and in breast cancer. For additional information, see **Estrogen** and Figure 38.

ETHINYL ESTRADIOL-ETHYNODIOL DIACETATE
(Demulen)

Demulen contains 1 mg of ethynodiol diacetate and 35 mcg of ethinyl estradiol. Demulen 1/35 and Demulen 1/50 are indicated for prevention of pregnancy and are used as oral contraceptive medications (see Figure 46). They act by suppression of gonadotropins. Oral contraceptive medications should be used cautiously in thrombophlebitis, thromboembolic disorders, cerebral vascular disease, myocardial infarction, coronary artery disease, carcinoma of the breast, carcinoma of any section of the reproductive tract, abnormal genital bleeding, suspected pregnancy, and history of cholestatic jaundice. Ethinyl estradiol-levonorgestrel (**Nordette**), ethinyl estradiol-norethindrone (**Ortho-Novum**), ethinyl estradiol-norethindrone acetate-ferrous fumarate (**Loestrin Fe**), and ethinyl estradiol-norgestrel (**Lo/Ovral**) are all oral contraceptive medications with the same indication or contraindications as cited for Demulen.

ETHIONAMIDE
(Trecator-SC)

Ethionamide, which has bacteriostatic actions against mycobacterium tuberculosis, (0.5 to 1 g/day in divided doses) is indicated in the treatment of tuberculosis where first-line drugs such as **isoniazid** and **rifampin** have failed. The side effects of ethionamide may include nausea and vomiting, diarrhea, metallic taste, hepatitis, jaundice, stomatitis, depression, drowsiness, asthenia, peripheral neuritis, olfactory disturbances, diplopia, blurred vision, optic neuritis, convulsions, postural hypotension, thrombocytopenia, gynecomastia, impotence, menorrhagia, or diabetes mellitus.

ETHOSUXIMIDE
(Zarotin)

Ethosuximide, methsuximide (Celontin), and **phensuximide** (Milontin) are indicated for control of absence (petit mal) seizures. These agents suppress the paroxysmal three cycle per second spike and wave activity associated with lapses of consciousness common in absence seizures. Ethosuximide is extensively metabolized in the liver to inactive metabolites, and 20% of it is excreted unchanged by the kidneys. Ethosuximide is not effective in grand mal seizures and may increase their frequency. Ethosuximide is known to have caused systemic lupus erythematosus, blood dyscrasias, and impairment of hepatic and renal function. The most frequent side effects of ethosuximide are nausea, vomiting, gastric upset, cramps, anorexia, diarrhea, weight loss, epigastric and abdominal pain, and constipation.

ETHOTOIN
(Peganone)

Ethotoin (250 mg p.o. q.i.d.) is indicated in the management of generalized tonic-clonic (grand mal) or complex partial (psychomotor) seizures. Similar to phenytoin, ethotoin stabilizes neuronal membrane, increases the efflux of sodium, and prevents the spread of the seizure process. Unlike phenytoin, ethotoin has no antiarrhythmic activity. The side effects of ethotoin may include fatigue, insomnia, dizziness, headache, numbness, chest pain, rash, diplopia, nystagmus, gingival hyperplasia, and blood dyscrasias (see also Figure 68).

ETHOXZOLAMIDE
(Cadrase, Ethamide)

The carbonic anhydrase inhibitors consist of **acetazolamide** (Diamox), **ethoxzolamide**, and **dichlorphenamide** (Daranide). Acetazolamide is an old agent, whereas ethoxzolamide and dichlorphenamide are newer preparations. Dichlorphenamide is the most potent carbonic anhydrase inhibitor in use today. The presence of SO_2NH_2 (sulfonamide) causes such compounds to inhibit carbonic anhydrase (CA), which catalyzes the hydration of carbon dioxide as follows:

$$CO_2 + H_2O \xrightarrow{\quad CA \quad} H_2CO_3 \rightleftharpoons H^+ + HCO_3^-$$

These agents inhibit carbonic anhydrase in the renal tubular cells in both the proximal and distal tubules. When the rate of hydrogen generation is reduced, HCO_3^- is lost in urine and the patients tends to become acidotic. However, the plasma concentration of HCO_3^- is lowered and less is filtered, so the diuresis becomes less effective. In addition, the sodium output is increased because its resorption in exchange for hydrogen is limited by the decreased availability of hydrogen. With less hydrogen available, the exchange of sodium for potassium predominates, and this fosters the loss of potassium. Chloride excretion is not altered significantly. Because the aqueous humor has a high concentration of bicarbonate, carbonic anhydrase inhibitors are primarily used in the treatment of **glaucoma**. They are no longer used as diuretics or as antiepileptic agents.

ETHYL ALCOHOL

As a CNS depressant, ethyl alcohol (**ethanol**) obeys the law of descending depression, in that it first inhibits the cerebral cortex, then the cerebellum, spinal cord, and medullary center. Taken in small quantities, alcohol brings about a feeling of well-being. When consumed in large quantities, alcohol produces more boisterous behavior. Self-control is lost and judgment is impaired. Alcohol works by depressing the **inhibitory control mechanism** and the **reticular activating system**. If a large amount of alcohol is consumed within a short time, unconsciousness and general anesthesia ensue. **Death** is due to respiratory and cardiac failure. Because numerous drugs in toxic doses can produce ataxia and slurred speech (e.g., **phenytoin**), for medico-legal purposes, the only acceptable means of proving intoxication is by determining the level of alcohol in any biologic fluid or in expired air. Alcohol produces dilation of the skin vessels, flushing, and a sensation of warmth. Alcohol also interferes with the normal cutaneous vasoconstriction in response to cold. The body heat is therefore lost very rapidly and the internal temperature consequently falls. At toxic alcohol levels, the hypothalamic temperature-regulating mechanism becomes depressed, and the fall in body temperature becomes pronounced. For these reasons, consuming alcoholic beverages for the purpose of keeping warm in cold weather is obviously irrational. As a **gastric secretagogue**, alcohol stimulates the secretion of gastric juice, which is rich in acid and pepsin. Therefore, the consumption of alcohol is contraindicated in subjects with untreated **acid-pepsin disease.** In addition, alcohol releases histamine, which in turn releases gastric juice. This effect is not blocked by atropine. In toxic doses (20%), gastric secretion is inhibited and peptic activity is depressed. From this, it is easy to deduce that small amounts of alcohol stimulate appetite and aid digestion, but large amounts may produce indigestion. Alcohol is also a **carminative** substance in that it facilitates the expulsion of gas from the stomach. Alcohol enhances the accumulation of fat in the liver. In alcoholics, this fat accumulation continues, and cirrhosis of the liver may ensue; however, the two phenomena are not related. Alcohol may release epinephrine, which leads to transient hyperglycemia and hyperlipemia. Therefore, alcohol consumption is contraindicated in diabetics. Alcohol causes diuresis by increasing fluid intake and by inhibiting the secretion of **antidiuretic hormone** elaborated by the posterior pituitary gland. Alcohol has **teratogenic effects** that are manifested by CNS dysfunction (such as low IQ and microencephaly), slow growth, a characteristic cluster of facial abnormalities (such as short palpebral fissures, hypoplastic upper lip, and short nose), and a variable set of major and minor malformations. Alcohol is absorbed from the stomach and very rapidly from the small intestine. Patients who have undergone gastrectomy may therefore become intoxicated relatively quickly. The absorption that takes place through unbroken skin is negligible. As a water-soluble substance with a low molecular weight, alcohol is distributed uniformly throughout all tissues and tissue fluids. It passes across the placental barrier, is found in spinal fluid, and accumulates in the brain. Consequently, any physiologic fluids (urine, blood, spinal fluid, breast milk, or saliva) are suitable for determining the concentration of alcohol. The metabolism of ethanol, which shows genetic polymorphism, is catalyzed primarily by **alcohol dehydrogenase** with **zero-order kinetics**, according to the following scheme.

$$\text{Ethanol} \xrightarrow[\text{NAD}^+ \quad \text{NADH}]{\text{Alcohol dehydrogenase}} \text{acetaldehyde} \xrightarrow[\text{NAD}^+ \quad \text{NADH}]{\text{Acetaldehyde dehydrogenase}} \text{acetic acid}$$

The rate-limiting factor in the metabolism of ethanol is the availability of NAD^+.

Ethanol is not metabolized by cytochrome P-450 enzymes (microsomal drug-metabolizing systems [MEDS]). However, it is metabolized to a certain extent by the microsomal ethanol-oxidizing system (MEDS).

Although ethanol is not metabolized by the microsomal drug-metabolizing system, it inhibits it and increases the rate of its synthesis. This effect may create a significant alcohol-drug interaction in both nonalcoholics and alcoholics who are taking medications.

Poisoning may be characterized by inebriation, muscular incoordination, blurred vision, impaired reaction time, excitement due to loss of inhibitions, impairment of consciousness, coma, tachycardia, and slow respiration. A blood alcohol level of 80 mg/dl can produce recognizable features of drunkenness; a level above 300 mg/dl is life-threatening. In children, severe hypoglycemia and convulsions may also occur.

Acute poisoning is treated with gastric aspiration and lavage combined with intensive supportive therapy, including thorough assessment of the patient plus measures to prevent respiratory failure. In cases of very severe poisoning, peritoneal dialysis or hemodialysis may be necessary.

Chronic alcoholism produces pathologic changes such as chronic gastritis, cirrhosis of the liver, alcoholic cardiomyopathy, **Korsakoff's syndrome**, bloatedness, flabby muscles, fine tremors, impaired physical capacity and stamina, diminished will power, and impaired memory. Accompanying malnutrition may contribute to alcohol-induced tissue injury.

Delirium tremens usually arises in a chronic alcoholic. The clinical features may include hallucinations, intense fear, sleeplessness, restlessness, agitation, delirium, and sometimes grand mal convulsions. In addition, tachycardia, hypotension, and clover-shaped ST changes in the electrocardiogram are evident.

The treatment of patients during a delirium tremens episode includes the intravenous administration of another CNS depressant (usually diazepam) during the acute phase, followed by the oral administration of chlordiazepoxide or oxazepam. In addition, other medications plus dietary management may become essential.

ETHYL CHLORIDE
(Chloroethane) (Ethyl Chloride Spray)

Ethyl chloride, a halogenated hydrocarbon with local anesthetic and counterirritant properties, is used as a local anesthetic in minor operative procedures and to relieve pain caused by insect stings and burns; and as a counterirritant to relieve myofascial and visceral pain syndromes.

ETHYLENEDIAMINETETRAACETIC ACID
(EDTA)

Ethylenediaminetetraacetic acid, by chelating calcium ions, is a direct anticoagulant in an *in vitro* system. EDTA is poorly administered from the gastrointestinal tract. The rapid intravenous administration of sodium EDTA causes **hypocalcemic tetany**. In addition, ethylene glycolbis (beta-aminoethyl ether)-N, N, N', N'-tetraacetic acid (EGTA), potassium fluoride, and potassium citrate are calcium-binding agents. Fluoride poisoning causes gastrointestinal disturbances, clonic convulsions, and hypotension, as well as respiratory and cardiac failure.

ETHYLESTRENOL
(Maxibolin)

Ethylestrenol (4 mg p.o. daily) is an anabolic steroid which is used to promote weight gain; to combat tissue depletion, anemia; and to overcome the catabolic effects of corticosteroids, osteoporosis, immobilization, and debilitation. Ethylestrenol enhances the production of erythropoietin by the kidneys and hence increases the red blood cell mass and volume (see Figure 37). Ethylestrenol may retain electrolytes and fluid and hence may become detrimental in patients with severe cardiac and renal diseases. Ethylestrenol is contraindicated in prostatic hypertrophy with obstruction and severe types of cancer (see also Table 6).

ETIDOCAINE HYDROCHLORIDE
(Duranest)

Etidocaine is a long-acting derivative of lidocaine but is far more potent. It is effective for filtration anesthesia, peripheral nerve block, and epidural and caudal blockade (see also Figure 20).

ETINTIDINE

Stimulation of the H_2 receptors elicits a variety of responses, the most widely studied of which is **gastric acid secretion** from the parietal cells of the gastric glands. However, many other effects mediated by H_2 receptors are manifested in peripheral tissues. These include the positive chronotropic action in the auricular muscle, the inotropic action in the ventricular muscle, and the lipolytic effect in fat cells. In addition, the extensive use of **cimetidine** has led to the synthesis and marketing of more specific and efficacious analogs (see also Figure 24).

Examples of the various H_2 receptor blocking agents are:

Imidazole derivatives
   Cimetidine and etintidine
Furan derivatives
   Ranitidine and nizatidine
Guanidinothiazole derivatives
   Famotidine
Piperidinomethylphenoxy derivatives
   Roxatidine acetate and roxatidine

The pharmacological properties of cimetidine, ranitidine, and famotidine are outlined in Table 9.

ETODOLAC
(Lodine)

Etodolac, which inhibits prostaglandin biosynthesis (see Figure 11), is indicated for acute and long-term use in the management of the signs and symptoms of osteoarthritis. Etodolac is a nonsteroidal antiinflammatory agent that possesses analgesic, antipyretic, and antiinflammatory properties. The most common side effects of etodolac are dyspepsia, abdominal pain, diarrhea, flatulence, nausea, vomiting, gastritis, or constipation (see also Table 2).

ETOMIDATE
(Amidate)

Etomidate is a nonbarbiturate hypnotic without analgesic activity and is used for induction of general anesthesia, for supplementing subpotent anesthetics such as nitrous oxide in oxygen, and for maintenance of anesthesia for short operative procedures. Etomidate lowers cerebral blood flow, and similar to ketamine, methohexital, or thiopental also reduces cerebral oxygen consumption (see also Table 15).

The onset of action of etomidate when given intravenously (0.2 to 0.6 mg/kg) is 1 minute, and duration of its action is 3 to 6 minutes. The addition of 0.1 mg of IV **fentanyl** will hasten recovery, in part because less etomidate will be required to induce anesthesia.

ETOPOSIDE

(Vepesid)

Etoposide (70 mg/m²/day p.o.) is an antineoplastic agent, which is indicated in small cell carcinoma of the lung and testicular carcinoma. Etoposide exerts its cytotoxic action by arresting cells in the metaphase portion of cell division. The drug also inhibits cells from entering mitosis and depresses DNA and RNA synthesis (see also Figure 2).

Etoposide is mostly excreted unchanged by the kidneys. The adverse effects of etoposide include nausea and vomiting, headache, weakness, paresthesia, hypotension, palpitation, tachycardia, bone marrow depression, leukopenia, thrombocytopenia, and reversible alopecia.

EUCATROPINE

Eucatropine is a synthetic muscarinic cholinergic receptor antagonist. The various applications of synthetic muscarinic receptor antagonists are listed below:

Ophthalmology:
> Homatropine
>> Produces mydriasis and cycloplegia
> Eucatropine
>> Produces only mydriasis

Preoperative uses:
> Atropine
>> To prevent excess salivation and bradycardia
> Scopolamine
>> In obstetrics, to produce sedation and amnesia

Cardiac uses:
> Atropine
>> To reduce severe bradycardia in hyperactive carotid sinus reflex
>> Diagnostically in Wolff-Parkinson-White syndrome to restore the PRS complex to normal duration

Gastrointestinal disorders:
> In peptic ulcer
>> To diminish vagally mediated secretion of gastric juices and slow gastric emptying (**propantheline, oxyphenonium, pirenzepine**)
> In diarrhea associated with dysenteries and diverticulitis
> In excess salivation associated with heavy metal poisoning or in parkinsonism

Neurologic diseases:
> In parkinsonism (trihexyphenidyl or benztropine)
> In drug-induced pseudoparkinsonism (trihexyphenidyl or benztropine)
> In vestibular disorders such as motion sickness (scopolamine)

Methantheline and propantheline are synthetic derivatives that, besides their antimuscarinic effects, are ganglionic blocking agents and block the skeletal neuromuscular junction. **Propantheline** and **oxyphenonium** reduce gastric secretion, while **pirenzepine**, in addition to reducing gastric secretion, also reduces gastric motility (see Figure 24).

EXPECTORANTS: DRUGS THAT INCREASE RESPIRATORY TRACT FLUID		
Classes of Expectorant	**Examples**	**Mechanism of Action**
Mucolytics Compounds with free thiol group	N-acetylcysteine Ethylcysteine Mercaptoethane sodium sulfonate Mecysteine	Destroy disulfide bonds of proteins and glycoproteins
Proteolytic enzymes	Trypsin, chymotrypsin	Hydrolyze peptide bonds of proteins or glycoproteins
Deoxyribonuclease	Deoxyribonuclease	Destroys deoxyribonucleic acid fibers
Mucoregulators	Bromhexine Ambroxol Carbocysteine	Alter the secretory activity of the bronchial mucosa Activate sialomucin synthesis
"Hydrating" agents	Sodium chloride Sodium bicarbonate, water	Correct water and electrolyte disorders in secretions
Tensio-Active agents	Tyloxapol	Make secretions less adhesive
Other compounds	Eprazinone	Modify fibrillate structures

Expectorants may have a demulcent (soothing and irritation-allaying) effect on the cells of the respiratory tract and assist in repelling invasion through providing a medium for the upward propulsion of foreign particles by ciliary action.

F

FACTOR IX COMPLEX

(AlphaNine SD, Bebulin VH Immuno Konyne 80, Monanine, Profilinine Heat-Treated, Proplex SX-T, Proplex T)

Factor IX complex, a blood derivative with hemostatic properties, is used in factor IX deficiency (hemophilia B or Christmas disease), in patients with Factor VIII inhibition, in Factor VII deficiency, and in overdosage with anticoagulant (see also Tables 16 and 17 and Figure 35).

FAMCICLOVIR

(Famvir)

Famciclovir, the oral formulation of penciclovir, is a new antiherpes agent which is well absorbed following oral administration with little intersubject variability and is rapidly converted to penciclovir with a bioavailability of 77%. Furthermore, while the activities of penciclovir and acyclovir against varicella-zoster virus (VZV) in infected cell lines appear to be comparable, penciclovir-triphosphate persists in virus-infected cells far longer than acyclovir-triphosphate, resulting in more prolonged antiviral activity. The intracellular half-life of penciclovir-triphosphate in VZV-infected cells is reported to be 9 h, while that of acyclovir-triphosphate is 0.8 h. These findings indicate that famciclovir has the potential to be administered without compromising therapeutic efficacy (see also Figure 3).

FAMOTIDINE

(Pepcid)

Famotidine (40 mg once a day at bed time) is indicated for the short-term (4 weeks) treatment of active duodenal ulcer; maintenance therapy for duodenal ulcer at reduced dosage after healing has taken place; for short-term treatment of gastroesophageal reflux disease; and in the treatment of hypersecretory conditions such as **Zollinger-Ellison syndrome,** or multiple endocrine adenoma. Famotidine, which is a competitive inhibitor of H_2 receptors, inhibits gastric secretion. It is absorbed incompletely (40 to 50%), metabolized partly to an S-oxide metabolite, and partly is excreted unchanged in the urine (see also Table 9 and Figure 24).

FASUDIL HYDROCHLORIDE

Fasudil, a novel intracellular calcium antagonist, dilates the spastic cerebral arteries in the chronic stage of an experimental model of subarachnoid hemorrhage. Fasudil increases cerebral blood flow and does not change systemic blood pressure (see also Table 20 and Figure 76).

FAT EMULSIONS

(Intralipid 10%, Intralipid 20%, Liposyn 10%, Liposyn 20%, Liposyn II 10%, Liposyn II 20%, Liposyn III 10% and 20%, Nutrilipid 10% and 20%, Soyacal 10%, Soyacal 20%, Travamulsion 10%, Travamulsion 20%)

Fat emulsions are used as a source of calories adjunctive to total parenteral nutrition.

FAZADINIUM

Fazadinium, similar to *d*-tubocurarine chloride, is a nondepolarizing or competitive blocking skeletal muscle relaxant. Fazadium, which is slightly less potent than *d*-tubocurarine, has a rapid onset and a long duration of action. It has anticholinergic properties and raises heart rate and cardiac output (see also Figure 92).

FELBAMATE
(Felbatol)

Felbamate (1200 mg/day) is indicated in partial seizures and in **Lennox-Gastaut syndrome**. Felbamate increases the seizure threshold and prevents the spread of the seizure process. It is absorbed well, becomes bound to plasma proteins to the extent of 90%, is metabolized to parahydroxyfelbamate, and 2-hydroxyfelbamate, and 30 to 40% of the dosage is excreted unchanged in the urine. Felbamate causes aplastic anemia and hence should be used cautiously. It increases the level of phenytoin and valproic acid, and decreases the level of carbamazepine (see also Figure 22).

FELODIPINE
(Plendil)

Felodipine, a calcium channel antagonist, is indicated in the treatment of hypertension. Following administration of felodipine, a reduction in blood pressure occurs within two hours, the heart rate increases during the first week, and the renal vascular resistance is decreased while the glomerular filtration rate remains unchanged. The reported adverse effects in descending order of occurrence are: peripheral edema (20%), headache, flushing, dizziness, upper respiratory infection, asthenia, cough, paraesthesia, dyspepsia, chest pain, nausea, muscle cramps, palpitation, abdominal pain, constipation, diarrhea, pharyngitis, rhinorrhea, back pain, and rash (2%) (see also Table 20 and Figure 76).

FENFLURAMINE HYDROCHLORIDE
(Pondimin)

Fenfluramine (20 mg t.i.d. before meals), an amphetamine-like drug, is an anorexic drug. The antiappetite effect of fenfluramine is blocked by agents which lower the level of serotonin receptor in the brain. Fenfluramine also enhances the utilization of glucose. Fenfluramine is deethylated to norfenfluramine which is subsequently oxidized to M-trifluoromethylhippuric acid. Fenfluramine and norfenfluramine are also excreted unchanged in the urine. A greater amount of fenfluramine is excreted when urine is acidic. The half-lives of amphetamine and fenfluramine are 5 and 20 hours, respectively. Fenfluramine is contraindicated in glaucoma or psychosis; and should not be coadministered with a monoamine oxidase inhibitor (see also Figure 27).

FENOLDOPAM

Peripheral dopaminergic receptor agents are useful in the treatment of congestive heart failure. Two distinct subtypes of dopamine receptors have been identified. The **dopamine** (DA_1) receptors, which are located on vascular smooth muscles, cause vasodilation in the renal, mesentery, cerebral, and coronary vascular beds (see Figure 39). Thus, the pharmacologic response to activation of the DA_2 and DA_1-receptor receptors is hypotension, bradycardia, diuresis, and natriuresis. **Fenoldopam** is an orally active DA_1-receptor agonist. It is more potent than dopamine in causing renal vasodilation without having adrenergic, cholinergic, or histaminergic properties. The comparative actions of **norepinephrine, dopamine, dobutamine, ibopamine, propylbutyldopamine**, and **fenoldopam** are shown in Table 12.

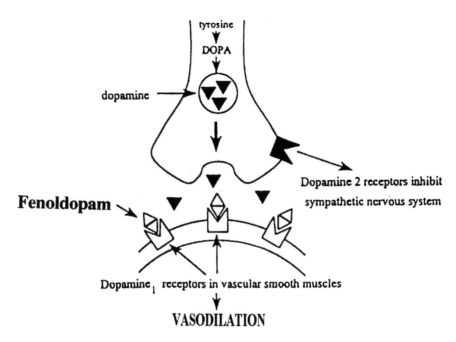

tyrosine

DOPA

dopamine

Fenoldopam

Dopamine 2 receptors inhibit
sympathetic nervous system

Dopamine$_1$ receptors in vascular smooth muscles

VASODILATION

FIGURE 39 Fenoldopam, an oral drug, is more potent than dopamine in causing renal vasodilation without having adrenergic, cholinergic, or histaminergic properties. (Adapted from Ebadi, M., *Pharmacology, An Illustrated Review with Questions and Answers*, 3rd Edition, Lippincott-Raven Press, Philadelphia, 1996.)

FENOPROFEN CALCIUM

(Ansaid)

Fenoprofen (200 to 300 mg in divided doses b.i.d. or t.i.d.) is indicated for acute or long-term treatment of the signs and symptoms of rheumatoid arthritis and osteoarthritis. Fenoprofen is a propionic acid derivative and, similar to ibuprofen, naproxen, flurbiprofen, or ketoprofen, has analgesic, antipyretic, and antiinflammatory properties (see also Table 2).

FENOTEROL HYDROBROMIDE

Fenoterol (200 to 400 mcg by inhalation), a beta$_2$-adrenergic receptor agonist, is being used in patients with moderate to severe asthma, with chronic obstructive pulmonary disease, in protection against exercise-induced asthma, and for acute treatment of asthma attack. However, no apparent advantage of fenoterol over equipotent doses of albuterol or terbutaline has been demonstrated in clinical trials (see also Figure 86).

FENTANYL

(Sublimaze)

Fentanyl (0.05 to 0.1 mg IM) is an opioid analgesic, which is used as an analgesic of short duration during anesthesia; is used in combination with a neuroleptic such as droperidol to produce **dissociative anesthesia**; and as an anesthetic agent in combination with oxygen in high-risk surgery such as open heart surgery. Fentanyl interacts predominantly with the opioid mu receptors which are distributed in the spinal cord and brain. Fentanyl produces analgesia, miosis, sedation, and respiratory depression which lasts longer than its analgesic effects. Like morphine, fentanyl raises the pain threshold and alters the patient's reactions to pain (see also Figure 58). Fentanyl increases the tone and decreases the propulsive contractions of the

TABLE 12
Actions of Adrenergic and Dopaminergic Agents on Their Receptor

Sympathetic Amines Prolactin	Beta$_1$ Positive Inotropy Positive Chronotropy Positive Dromotropy	Beta$_2$ Vasodilation	Alpha$_1$ Vasoconstriction	Alpha$_2$ Vasoconstriction	DA$_1$ Vasodilation	DA$_2$ Vasodilation Emesis
Norepinephrine	+++	–	+++	+++	–	–
Dopamine	+++	±	++	++	±	±
Dobutamine	+++	+	+	–	–	–
Ibopamine	++	+	–	–	–	+
Propylbutyldopamine	–	–	+	+	+	+++
Fenoldopam	–	–	–	–	+++	–

DA = dopamine receptor; +++ = major action; ++ = moderate action; + = minimal action; – = actions absent smooth muscles in the gastrointestinal tract and hence causes constipation. **Duragesic** is a transdermal system providing continuous system delivery of fentanyl for 72 hours. Duragesic, which causes life-threatening hypoventilation, is contraindicated in the management of acute or postoperative pain.

FEPRADINOL

Fepradinol is an antiinflammatory agent which possesses inhibitory activity on acute inflammation, and this effect does not seem to be related to an inhibitory effect on prostaglandin biosynthesis. Therefore, the mechanism of antiinflammatory effects of fepradinol are different from those of indomethacin or piroxicam (see also Table 2 and Figure 11).

FERROUS SALTS

Ferrous sulfate (20% elemental iron) and ferrous gluconate (11.6% elemental iron) are used in iron deficiency anemia. Extensive numbers of oral preparations are available for the treatment of iron deficiency. In general, the **ferrous salts** (ferrous sulfate, ferrous gluconate, and ferrous fumerate) are better absorbed than the **ferric salts** (ferric sulfate). Ferrous calcium citrate is mostly used in patients during pregnancy to provide iron as well as calcium. The parenteral iron medications available include **iron-dextran** (ferric hydroxide and high-molecular-weight dextran) for intramuscular use, **dextriferron** (a complex of ferric hydroxide and partially hydrolyzed dextran) for intravenous use, and **saccharated iron oxide** (a complex of ferric hydroxide and sucrose) for intravenous use. These preparations are reserved for those cases in which oral preparations are not tolerated, absorbed, or rapid enough in their onset of action, or are otherwise not suitable for noncompliant patients. A lethal dose of iron consists of 12 g of an iron preparation containing 1 or 2 g of elemental iron. Therefore, iron toxicity rarely occurs in adults but is frequently seen in children. The mortality rate among untreated children is high (45%). The initial signs and symptoms of iron poisoning are gastrointestinal and usually consist of nausea, vomiting, and diarrhea. If untreated, acidosis, cyanosis, and circulatory collapse may ensue. If the patient survives, there may be gastric scarring and pyloric stenosis resulting from the corrosive action of the iron preparation. Treatment should include induced vomiting and lavage if the poisoning is discovered early, catharsis to hasten evacuation, sodium bicarbonate therapy to combat the acidosis, and the administration of **deferoxamine** (Desferal), a specific iron-chelating agent. One hundred milligrams of deferoxamine is able to bind 8.5 mg of iron. The chelating effects of deferoxamine are maximum at an acidic pH; therefore, when given orally, deferoxamine must be administered before the sodium bicarbonate. In the event of iron poisoning, deferoxamine may also be administered intramuscularly. Besides its usefulness in counteracting the effects of iron poisoning, deferoxamine has been used in disorders that involve **iron overload** such as ocular **hemosiderosis** or **hemochromatosis**.

FIBRINOLYSIN AND DEOXYRIBONUCLEASE, COMBINED (BOVINE)
(Elase)

Fibrinolysin and deoxyribonuclease, a proteolytic enzyme and a topical debriding agent, are used as a topical debridement of inflamed or infected skin lesions and wounds.

FILGRASTIM
(Granulocyte Colony Stimulating Factor, G-CSF) (Neupogen)

Filgrastim, a colony stimulating factor (5 mcg/kg SC or IV), is used to decrease incidence of infection after cancer chemotherapy for nonmyeloid malignancies (see also **Cytokines** and Figure 53).

FINASTERIDE

Finasteride is a potent 5 alpha-reductase inhibitor that has shown limited success in men treated for benign prostatic hyperplasia. 5 Alpha-reductase is necessary for the prostatic conversion of testosterone to dihydrotestosterone (DHT), the specific steroid that stimulates prostate transitional zone growth. Finasteride reduces the size of the prostate gland by 20%, but this does not correlate well with improvement in symptoms (see also Figure 87).

FLAVOXATE HYDROCHLORIDE

(Uripas)

Flavoxate, a flavone derivative and urinary tract spasmolytic (100 to 200 mg p.o. t.i.d.), is used in the symptomatic relief of dysuria, frequency, urgency, nocturia, incontinence, and suprapubic pain associated with urologic disorders.

FLECAINIDE ACETATE

(Tambocor)

Flecainide, is an antiarrhythmic agent which is indicated for prevention of paroxysmal supraventricular tachycardia including atrioventricular nodal reentrant tachycardia, atrioventricular reentrant tachycardia, and paroxysmal atrial fibrillation and flutter (see also Figure 76).

Flecainide, one of a classic membrane-stabilizing group of antiarrhythmic agents, decreases intracardiac conduction in all parts of the heart with the greatest effects being noted in the His-Purkinje system. Effects upon atrioventricular (AV) nodal conduction time and intra-atrial conduction time, although present, are less pronounced than those on the ventricular conduction system.

Flecainide is absorbed well, has a long half-life of 3 to 5 days, is metabolized to –O dealkylated flecainide (active antiarrhythmic agent with less potency than flecainide) and to –O dealkylated lactam of flecainide, which is an inactive metabolite. A portion of flecainide is excreted unchanged. Flecainide, like other antiarrhythmic agents, can cause new or worsen supraventricular or ventricular arrhythmias. Ventricular proarrhythmic effects range from an increase in frequency of PVCs to the development of more severe ventricular tachycardia, e.g., tachycardia that is more sustained or more resistant to conversion to sinus rhythm, with potentially fatal consequences.

The noncardiac side effects of flecainide in descending order of occurrence are: dizziness (20%), visual disturbances, dyspnea, headache, nausea, fatigue, palpitation, chest pain, asthenia, tremor, constipation, edema, and abdominal pain (2%).

FLEROXACIN

(Megalone)

The quinolones include: **nalidixic acid** (NegGram), **cinoxacin** (Cinobac), **norfloxacin** (Noroxin), and **ciprofloxacin** (Cipro). Other members of the quinolone family are **pefloxacin, ofloxacin, enoxacin,** and **fleroxacin**. The bacterial enzyme **DNA gyrase** is responsible for the continuous introduction of negative supercoils into DNA, and the quinolones inhibit this gyrase-mediated DNA supercoiling. **Nalidixic acid** and **cinoxacin** are bactericidal against Gram-negative organisms that cause urinary tract infections. The **fluoroquinolones** are bactericidal and considerably more potent against *Escherichia coli* and various species of *Salmonella, Shigella, Enterobacter, Campylobacter*, and *Neisseria*. **Ciprofloxacin** also has good activity against staphylococci, including methicillin-resistant strains. The quinolones and fluoroquinolones may produce arthropathy, and hence should not be used in prepubertal children or pregnant women. **Nalidixic acid** and **cinoxacin** are useful only for treating urinary tract infections. **Ciprofloxacin** is useful for both urinary tract infections and prostatitis (see also Figure 77).

FLESTOLOL

Flestolol is a nonselective, ultra short-acting beta adrenergic receptor blocking agent. It is 50 times more potent than esmolol, is given by intravenous infusion, and has a half-life of 7.2 minutes. Flestolol contains an ester group (Figure 57) and hence is rapidly metabolized by tissue esterases to inactive metabolites. Flestolol has no intrinsic sympathomimetic activity or alpha adrenergic receptor blocking effects, and possesses a weak membrane stabilizing property. Flestolol is able to control heart rate in patients with atrial flutter or fibrillation, improve the hemodynamic status of patients with ischemic heart disease, and relieve chest pain in patients with unstable angina.

FLOSEQUINAN

Flosequinan is a vasodilator. **Vasodilators** in combination with an angiotensin-converting enzyme inhibitor have been used in congestive heart failure. The vasodilators may be classified as **venodilators, arterial dilators**, or **balanced-type vasodilators** (Table 26). The rationale for vasodilation in the management of congestive heart failure is based on the increased arteriolar vasotone that occurs. This initiates a vicious circle in which cardiac function is further depressed by an increase in afterload and in resistance to ejection.

FLOXURIDINE
(FUDR)

Floxuridine, an antimetabolite and antineoplastic agent (0.1 to 0.6 mg/kg daily by intra-arterial infusion), is used to treat brain, breast, head, neck, liver, gall bladder, and bile duct cancer (see also Figure 2).

FLUCONAZOLE
(Diflucan)

Fluconazole (50 to 400 mg given daily) is indicated in the treatment of oropharyngeal and esophageal candidiasis. It is employed in the treatment of candidal urinary tract infections, peritonitis, and systemic candidal infections (including candidemia, disseminated candidiasis and pneumonia), as a prophylactic measure to reduce the incidence of candidiasis in patients undergoing bone marrow transplantation who receive cytotoxic chemotherapy or radiation therapy, and in the treatment of cryptococcal meningitis. Fluconazole, a synthetic broad-spectrum antifungal agent, inhibits fungal cytochrome P450 and sterol C-14 alpha demethyl-ation. The steady-state concentration of fluconazole is reached in 5 to 10 days, the concentration in cerebrospinal fluid approaches 80% of the corresponding plasma concentration, and 80% of the administered dose is excreted unchanged in the urine. Hence, the dosage in renal impairment should be adjusted downward. Fluconazole is excreted in breast milk, and its use in nursing mothers is discouraged. Most fungi show a higher sensitivity to fluconazole *in vivo* than *in vitro*. Fluconazole interacts with numerous drugs, some of which will be cited here. **Cimetidine** reduces the plasma level of fluconazole; **hydrochlorothiazide** enhances the plasma level of fluconazole; **rifampin** reduces the half-life of fluconazole; fluconazole increases the plasma level of **cyclosporin**; fluconazole enhances the hypoprothrombinemic effects of **warfarin**; and fluconazole increases the hypoglycemic effects of the sulfonylureas **tolbutamide, glyburide**, and **glipizide**. The reported side effects of fluconazole are dizziness, headache, itching, rash, nausea, vomiting, abdominal pain, diarrhea, thrombocytopenia, elevated transaminase levels, and hypokalemia (see also Figure 54).

FLUCYTOSINE

(Ancobon)

Flucytosine (5 FC, 5-fluorocytosine) is indicated in the treatment of septicemia, endocarditis, and urinary tract infection (candida), and in meningitis and pulmonary infections (cryptococcus). Flucytosine, which usually is used in combination with amphotericin B, has activity against candida and cryptococcus in both *in vivo* and *in vitro* systems. Flucytosine is absorbed well, distributed throughout the body, exhibits low binding to plasma proteins, and 80 to 90% of the administered dosage is excreted unchanged in the urine. Flucytosine should be used cautiously in patients with a history of bone marrow depression or hematologic disease, and in patients receiving radiation therapy along with drugs known to cause bone marrow depression. The antifungal action of flucytosine may be reduced by cytosine. Flucytosine has caused emesis; abdominal pain; diarrhea; anorexia; dry mouth; duodenal ulcer; GI hemorrhage; hepatic dysfunction; jaundice; ulcerative colitis, bilirubin elevation; elevation of hepatic enzymes; azotemia; creatinine and BUN elevation; crystalluria; renal failure; anemia; agranulocytosis; aplastic anemia; eosinophilia; leukopenia; pancytopenia; thrombocytopenia; ataxia; hearing loss; headache; paresthesia; parkinsonism; peripheral neuropathy; pyrexia; vertigo; sedation; confusion; hallucinations; and psychosis. The side effects and toxicity occur at blood levels greater than 100 mcg/ml.

FLUDARABINE PHOSPHATE

(Fludara)

Fludarabine, an antimetabolite with antineoplastic properties, is indicated in the treatment of B-cell chronic lymphocytic leukemia (CLL) in patients who have not responded or responded inadequately to at least one standard alkylating regimen. Fludarabine works primarily by inhibiting DNA synthesis. The compound also possesses lymphocytotoxic activity with preferential activity toward T-lymphocytes (see also Figure 2).

FLUDROCORTISONE ACETATE

(Florinef Acetate)

Fludrocortisone (0.1 mg/day) is indicated as a partial replacement therapy for primary and secondary adrenocortical insufficiency in Addison's disease and for the treatment of salt-losing adrenogenital syndrome. Fludrocortisone is an adrenal cortical steroid with both glucocorticoid and pronounced mineralocorticoid activities (Table 10), but it is used primarily for its mineralocorticoid effects. It acts on the renal distal tubules to enhance the reabsorption of sodium and increase the urinary excretion of both potassium and hydrogen ions. Fludrocortisone is readily absorbed from the GI tract, having a plasma half-life of 3.5 hours, and a biological half-life of 18 to 36 hours. The side effects of fludrocortisone, when it is given in larger than therapeutic doses and for a prolonged period of time, are hypokalemia, alkalosis, edema, hypertension, weight gain, enlarged heart, and congestive heart failure. High sodium diets will aggravate and accelerate the side effects. Patients with Addison's disease are more sensitive to the action of fludrocortisone and exhibit these side effects to an exaggerated degree (see also Figure 4).

FLUMAZENIL

(Romazicon)

Flumazenil (0.1 to 1.0 mg IV) is indicated for reversal of the sedative effects of benzodiazepine derivatives. Flumazenil is an antagonist at the benzodiazepine receptor in the benzodiazepine-GABA receptor chloride channel complex. Flumazenil does not antagonize the

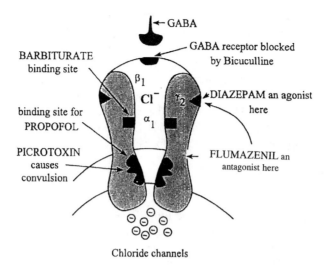

Chloride channels

FIGURE 40 Flumazenil, a benzodiazepine receptor antagonist, is used to reverse the sedative effects of benzodiazepines after anesthesia. (Adapted from Ebadi, M., *Pharmacology, An Illustrated Review with Questions and Answers*, 3rd Edition, Lippincott-Raven Press, Philadelphia, 1996.)

CNS depressant effects of ethanol, barbiturates, or general anesthetics, although these agents influence GABAergic transmission (see Figure 40).

The pharmacokinetics of flumazenil is not altered by age, gender, or renal failure. Flumazenil may precipitate benzodiazepine withdrawal syndrome (dizziness, mild confusion, emotional lability, agitation, anxiety) or convulsive seizures, especially in patients who have taken benzodiazepines in large doses and for a long period of time. Following administration of flumazenil, the patient's vital signs should be monitored carefully. Flumazenil does not consistently reverse amnesia.

FLUNARIZINE

Flunarizine, which interacts with serotonergic receptors (see Figures 64 and 78), is undergoing clinical investigation for its efficacy in migraine headache (see Figure 85). Extensive ligand-binding studies and molecular biologic examination of membrane preparations have revealed that there are at least 14 types of serotonin receptors, including: $5HT_{1A}$, $5HT_{1B}$, $5HT_{1D}$, $5HT_3$, and $5HT_4$. Serotonin possesses many actions. It:

Is involved in the neural network that regulates intestinal motility,
Is released by a carcinoid,
Is released by platelets (also ADP) during aggregation,
Causes vasoconstriction by stimulating $5HT_2$ receptors, and this effect is blocked by
   ketanserine,
Causes vasodilation by stimulating $5HT_1$ receptors,
Causes positive inotropic and chronotropic effects by interacting with both $5HT_1$ and
   $5HT_3$ receptors,
Increases the motility of the stomach as well as small and large intestines,
Causes uterine contractions,
Causes bronchial contractions.

Ketanserine, a $5HT_2$ and alpha$_1$-adrenergic receptor antagonist, lowers blood pressure. **Methysergide**, a $5HT_{1C}$ antagonist, has been used for the prophylactic treatment of migraine and other vascular headache, including Horton's syndrome. Calcium entry blockers such as **flunarizine** have been shown to be effective in treating migraine. **Cyproheptadine**, a serotonin and histamine$_1$ receptor-and muscarinic cholinergic receptor-blocking agent, has been used in the treatment of the postgastrectomy dumping syndrome and the intestinal hypermotility seen with carcinoid. **Sumatriptan**, an agonist of the 5HT$_1$-like receptor, is highly effective in the treatment of migraine (see also Figure 85). **Ondansetron**, granisetron, tropisetron, and batanopride are antagonists of the 5HT$_3$ receptor, and are considered effective in controlling cancer chemotherapy-induced emesis (see also Figure 64). **Clozapine**, an effective antipsychotic agent with little or no extrapyramidal side effects, blocks the 5HT$_2$ receptor (see Table 23).

FLUNISOLIDE
(Nasalide)

Flunisolide nasal spray is indicated for the topical treatment of the symptoms of seasonal rhinitis. Flunisolide, a potent glucocorticoid but weak mineralocorticoid, possesses local antiinflammatory properties. It stimulates the synthesis of enzymes needed to decrease the inflammatory response. The antiinflammatory and vasoconstrictor potency of topically applied flunisolide is several hundred times greater than that of hydrocortisone and about equal to that of an equal weight of triamcinolone. Flunisolide is contraindicated in patients with acute status asthmaticus; in patients with tuberculosis or viral, fungal, or bacterial respiratory infections; and in patients who are hypersensitive to any component of the preparation. It should be used cautiously in patients receiving systemic corticosteroids because of increased risk of hypothalamic-pituitary-adrenal axis suppression; when substituting inhalant for oral systemic administration (because withdrawal symptoms may occur); and in patients with healing nasal septal ulcers, oral or nasal surgery, or trauma (see also Tables 10 and 14).

FLUNISOLIDE
(Nasal Inhalant Nasalide)

Flunisolide, a glucocorticoid with antiinflammatory and antiasthmatic properties (two inhalants b.i.d.) is used in steroid-dependent asthma (see also Table 10).

FLUOCINOLONE ACETONIDE
(Derma-Smoothe/FS, Fluonid, Flurosyn, Neo-Synalar, FS Shampoo Synalar, Synalar-HP, Synemol)

Fluocinolone, a topical adrenocorticoid with antiinflammatory properties (0.01% solution; 0.1% shampoo; 0.025% ointment, 0.01 to 0.2% cream), is used in inflammation of corticoid-responsive dermatoses (see also Table 10).

FLUOCINONIDE
(FAPG, Lidex, Lidex-E)

Fluocinonide, a topical adrenocorticoid with antiinflammatory properties (0.05% cream, gel, ointment, solution), is used in inflammation of corticosteroid-responsive dermatoses (see also Table 10).

FLUORESCEIN SODIUM
(Fluorescite, Fluor-I-Strip, Fluor-I-Strip A.T., Ful-Glo, Funduscein)

Fluorescein, a dye, is used as a diagnostic aid in corneal abrasions and foreign bodies; fitting hard contact lenses; lacrimal patency; fundus photography; and applanation tonometry.

FLUORMETHOLONE

(Fluor-Op, Ophthalmic FML Liquifilm, Opthalamic, FML Ointment)

Fluorometholone, a corticosteroid with ophthalmic antiinflammatory properties (instill 2 drops in conjunctival sac), is used in inflammatory and allergic conditions of cornea, conjunctiva, sclera, and anterior uvea.

FLUORODEOXYURIDINE

(Floxuridine)

Fluorodeoxyuridine, a pyrimidine analog, is an antineoplastic agent. **Fluorouracil** and **fluorodeoxyuridine** inhibit pyrimidine nucleotide biosynthesis and interfere with the synthesis and actions of nucleic acids. To exert its effect, fluorouracil (5-FU) must first be converted to nucleotide derivatives such as **5-fluorodeoxyuridylate** (5-FdUMP). Similarly, floxuridine (FUdR) is also converted to FdUMP.

FdUMP inhibits **thymidylate synthetase**, and this in turn inhibits the essential formation of dTTP, one of the four precursors of DNA. In addition, 5-fluorouracil is sequentially converted to 5-FUTP, which becomes incorporated into RNA, thus inhibiting its processing and functioning. Fluorouracil is used for the following types of cancer:

Breast carcinoma. Cyclophosphamide, methotrexate, fluorouracil, and prednisone (CMP+P). The alternate drugs are doxorubicin and cyclophosphamide.
Colon carcinoma. Fluorouracil.
Gastric adenocarcinoma. Fluorouracil, doxorubicin (Adriamycin), and mitomycin (FAM), or fluorouracil and semustine.
Hepatocellular carcinoma. Fluorouracil alone or in combination with lomustine.
Pancreatic adenocarcinoma. Fluorouracil.

Resistance to 5-fluorouracil occurs as the result of one or a combination of the following factors:

Deletion of uridine kinase.
Deletion of nucleoside phosphorylase.
Deletion of orotic acid phosphoribosyltransferase.
Increased thymidylate kinase.

Because 5-fluorouracil is metabolized rapidly in the liver, it is administered intravenously and not orally. 5-Fluorouracil causes myelosuppression and mucositis.

FLUOROQUINOLONES

The **fluoroquinolones** are bactericidal and considerably more potent against *Escherichia coli* and various species of *Salmonella, Shigella, Enterobacter, Campylobacter,* and *Neisseria.* **Ciprofloxacin** also has good activity against staphylococci, including methicillin-resistant strains.

5-FLUOROURACIL

(5-FU)

5-Fluorouracil (initially 7 to 12 mg/kg IV for 4 days), a cell cycle-phase specific antineoplastic agent, is indicated in colon, rectal, breast, ovarian, cervical, gastric, esophageal, bladder, liver, and pancreatic cancer. Fluorouracil exerts its cytotoxic activity by acting as an antimetabolite, competing for the enzyme that is important in the synthesis of thymidine, an essential substrate

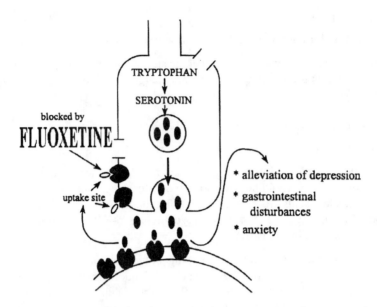

FIGURE 41 Fluoxetine, a specific serotonin uptake site inhibitor, is a second-generation antidepressant, which does not cause sedation or orthostatic hypotension and possesses no anticholinergic properties.

for DNA synthesis. Therefore, DNA synthesis is inhibited. The drug also inhibits RNA synthesis to a lesser extent (see also Figure 2).

5-Fluorouracil is absorbed poorly after an oral administration, and hence is given intravenously. It crosses the blood-brain barrier and is distributed widely in the body. 5-Fluorouracil is metabolized in the urine and the metabolites are primarily excreted through the lung as carbon dioxide. The toxicity of fluorouracil is enhanced by **leucovorin calcium**. 5-Fluorouracil causes stomatitis and esophagopharyngitis leading to ulceration, diarrhea, anorexia, nausea and emesis, leukopenia, and a reversible alopecia.

FLUOXETINE

(Prozac)

Fluoxetine, a selective serotonin uptake inhibitor (SSUI), (20 mg p.o./day) is indicated in the treatment of depression and depressive compulsive disorder (see Figures 41 and 78).

It inhibits the neuronal uptake of serotonin but not that of norepinephrine (Figure 78 and Tables 3 through 5).

Fluoxetine is absorbed well from the GI tract, is bound to plasma proteins to the extent of 95%, is metabolized in the liver to norfluoxetine, and is excreted in the urine. Tryptophan is used as an antidepressant. However, the combined use of tryptophan, which increases the level of serotonin, and fluoxetine, which inhibits the neuronal uptake of serotonin, enhances the side effects of fluoxetine such as gastrointestinal disturbances, anxiety, and insomnia (see Figure 41).

FLUOXYMESTERONE

(Halotestin)

Fluoxymesterone, is a steroid with an androgenic property, which is used in primary hypogonadism and testicular failure due to cryptorchidism, vanishing testes syndrome, or orchidectomy; and in hypogonadotrophic hypogonadism and luteinizing hormone releasing hormone (LHRH) deficiency or pituitary hypothalamic injury from tumors, trauma, or radiation. It mimics the actions of testosterone, which is responsible for normal growth and development of the male sex organs and for the maintenance of secondary sex characteristics. In female postmenopausal patients, fluoxymesterone may be indicated in the palliation of recurrent mammary cancer (see also Table 6 and Figure 87).

Fluoxymesterone is contraindicated in male subjects with known or suspected carcinoma of the prostate gland. Prolonged use of high dosage 17 alpha alkyl androgens is known to have caused hypercalcemia, hepatic adenoma, hepatocellular carcinoma, and hepatitis. Fluoxymesterone, which accelerates bone maturation without producing linear growth, should be used cautiously in males with delayed puberty. Edema and congestive heart failure may occur in patients with pre-existing cardiovascular problems. Androgens cause virilization in female subjects.

FLUPHENAZINE HYDROCHLORIDE
(Prolixin)

Fluphenazine (0.5 to 10 mg p.o. daily in divided doses q. 6 to 8 hours) is indicated in the management of manifestations of psychotic disorders. As depicted in Table 23, its potency equals that of haloperidol. In addition, similar to haloperidol it produces movement disorders such as akathisia, dystonia, parkinsonism, neuroleptic malignant syndrome, and tardive dyskinesia. The drug is available as fluphenazine decanoate and fluphenazine enanthate which are intended for depot injection, with an onset of action of 24 to 72 hours, and a duration of action of two weeks. Neuroleptics are not of any value if patients do not take them at the dosage that has been prescribed, or if their bodies do not absorb the orally administered drug effectively. It has been estimated that 10 to 25% of schizophrenic inpatients somehow fail to ingest the prescribed dosage, and that 25 to 50% of schizophrenic outpatients deviate from or default on their medication regimens. This has obvious consequences in terms of the relapse rate and revolving door syndrome.

The development of long-acting formulations, both injectable and oral, carries the potential to remedy these two treatment liabilities. These new formulations have already made an impact on the treatment of the unreliable drug taker, the poor oral absorbers, and those patients being treated in outpatient settings who are too ill to assume responsibility for their own drug taking. These long-acting psychotropics are remarkably free of side effects when given for extended periods. Full blood counts, urinalysis, and renal function tests are essentially normal, even after years of continuous treatment with these drugs. The only significant hazard that is associated with the continuous, prolonged use of these medications is tardive dyskinesia. There are indications, however, that the injectable psychotropic drugs produce less, or less persistent, tardive dyskinesia than do the orally administered neuroleptics. This is probably due to the fact that the injectable forms can be given in lower dosages. See also **Phenothiazine derivatives**.

FLURANDRENOLIDE
(Cordran, Cordran SP)

Flurandrenolide, a topical adrenocorticoid with antiinflammatory properties (cream, lotion, ointment 0.025 to 0.05%), is used in inflammation of corticosteroid-responsive dermatoses (see also Table 10).

FLURAZEPAM HYDROCHLORIDE

(Dalmane)

Flurazepam (15 to 30 mg p.o. at bedtime) is a benzodiazepine derivative sedative-hypnotic which is used in the management of insomnia. Flurazepam depresses the CNS at the limbic and subcortical levels of the brain. It produces a sedative effect by potentiating the effect of the neurotransmitter gamma-amino-butyric acid on its receptor in the ascending reticular activating system, which increases inhibition and blocks both cortical and limbic arousal (see also Figure 40).

When given orally, flurazepam is absorbed rapidly, is bound to plasma proteins to the extent of 97%, exerts its hypnotic effects within 20 minutes, is metabolized to desalkylflurazepam which is excreted in the urine. Flurazepam potentiates the CNS depressing effects of alcohol, barbiturates, antihistaminics, antidepressants, and several neuroleptics. Cimetidine inhibits the metabolism of flurazepam and hence its duration of action. On the other hand, heavy smoking accelerates the metabolism of flurazepam. The side effects of flurazepam in higher than therapeutic dosage include confusion, depression, drowsiness, lethargy, daytime sedation, disturbed coordination, hangover effect, ataxia, dizziness, syncope, nightmares, fatigue, slurred speech, tremor, vertigo, and headache. The incidence and severity of these side effects are more pronounced in elderly subjects. Since the metabolism and elimination of flurazepam is retarded in elderly subjects, the dosage should be adjusted downward. Flurazepam is excreted in breast milk causing sedation, feeding difficulties, and weight loss in the infants, and hence should be avoided in breast-feeding women (see also Table 8).

FLURBIPROFEN

(Ansaid)

Flurbiprofen is a nonsteroidal antiinflammatory drug of the 2-arylpropionic acid class. The recommended dosages for flurbiprofen are 50 mg q. 4 to 6 hours for analgesia and 100 to 300 mg/day for the treatment of inflammatory conditions (see also Table 2).

Flurbiprofen is indicated for the acute or long-term treatment of rheumatoid arthritis and osteoarthritis. It is a potent inhibitor of prostaglandin synthetase (see Figure 11). Flurbiprofen is absorbed well orally, is bound to plasma proteins to the extent of 99%, metabolized in the liver to pharmacologically active metabolites, and the metabolites are excreted in the urine. Flurbiprofen increases the actions of oral anticoagulants and decreases the effectiveness of diuretics. Flurbiprofen is contraindicated in patients who are allergic to aspirin (see also Table 2).

FLUTAMIDE

(Eulexin)

Flutamide, a nonsteroidal antiandrogen (250 mg p.o. q. 8 hours), is indicated in the treatment of metastatic prostatic carcinoma in combination with LHRH analogs, such as **leuprolide acetate** (see also Table 13).

FLUTICASONE PROPIONATE

(Culivate)

Fluticasone, a topical corticosteroid with antiinflammatory properties (0.05% cream, 0.005% ointment), is used in the relief of inflammation and pruritis of corticosteroid-responsive dermatoses.

FLUVASTATIN SODIUM
(Lescol)

Fluvastatin, a cholesterol-lowering agent which inhibits hydroxy-methylglutaryl-coenzyme A (MHG-CoA) reductase, is effective in the reduction of low-density lipoprotein and total cholesterol levels in patients with primary hypercholesterolemia (types IIa and IIb) when response to diet and other nonpharmacologic measures have been inadequate (see also Figure 25).

FLUVOXAMINE MALEATE

Fluvoxamine, an antidepressant, is a potent and selective serotonin reuptake inhibitor (see Figure 78) which is devoid of anticholinergic, antihistaminic, or cardiotoxic properties. Fluvoxamine offers depressed patients an equivalent level of therapeutic benefit when compared with imipramine (see Tables 3 through 5).

FOLIC ACID
(Folacin; Pteroylglutamic Acid; Folate)

Both **vitamin B_{12}** and **folic acid** are essential for the synthesis of DNA, and this process is impaired in patients with megaloblastic anemia. In the absence of adequate DNA synthesis, cells cannot divide but continue to grow. **Megaloblastic anemia** may also be associated with neurologic disturbances such as paresthesias, diminution of vibration sensation, loss of memory, confusion, irritability, and psychosis, which are due to vitamin B_{12} rather than folic acid deficiency. **Folic acid deficiency** may result from:

Nutritional deficiency.
Malabsorption syndrome.
Reduced folate-binding protein.
Folic acid antagonists (e.g., **methotrexate**).
Drugs reducing the level of folic acid (**anticonvulsants** and **pyrimethamine).**
Agents blocking purine synthesis (e.g., **mercaptopurine, thioguanine**) or pyrimidine synthesis (**5-fluorouracil**).
Hemolytic diseases (accelerated hematopoiesis).
Proliferative diseases and other conditions.
Folic acid is administered orally and should not be used in the treatment of pernicious anemia.

Exogenous folate is required for nucleoprotein synthesis and maintenance of normal erythropoiesis. Folic acid stimulates production of red and white blood cells and platelets in certain megaloblastic anemias. Folic acid is the precursor of tetrahydrofolic acid, which is involved as a cofactor for transformylation reactions in the biosynthesis of purines and thymidylates of nucleic acids. Impairment of thymidylate synthesis in patients with folic acid deficiency is thought to account for the defective deoxyribonucleic acid (DNA) synthesis that leads to megaloblast formation and megaloblastic and macrocytic anemias.

Folic acid is found in liver, dried beans, peas, lentils, oranges, whole-wheat products, asparagus, beets, broccoli, brussel sprouts, and spinach as reduced folate polyglutamate, which undergoes hydrolysis reduction and methylation in the GI tract before it is absorbed. Folic acid is metabolized in the liver to 7,8-dihydrofolic acid and eventually to 5,6,7,8-tetrahydrofolic acid. Tetrahydrofolic acid derivatives are distributed to all body tissues but are stored primarily in the liver. Pregnant women are more prone to develop folate deficiency as reflected in larger dosage recommendations. Folate-deficient mothers may be more prone to complications of pregnancy and fetal abnormalities, including fetal anomalies, placental abruption, toxemia, abortions, placenta previa, low-birth-weight, and premature delivery.

FOLIC ACID ANTAGONISTS

Methotrexate (Amethopterin) is a folic acid antagonist that binds to dihydrofolate reductase, thus interfering with the synthesis of the active cofactor tetrahydrofolic acid, which is necessary for the synthesis of thymidylate, purine nucleotides, and the amino acids serine and methionine. Methotrexate is used for the following types of cancer:

Acute lymphoid leukemia. During the initial phase, vincristine and prednisone are used. Methotrexate and mercaptopurine are used for maintenance therapy. In addition, methotrexate is given intrathecally, with or without radiotherapy, to prevent meningeal leukemia.

Diffuse histiocyte lymphoma. Cyclophosphamide, vincristine, methotrexate, and cytarabine (COMA).

Mycosis fungoides. Methotrexate.

Squamous cell, large-cell anaplastic, and adenocarcinoma. Doxorubicin and cyclophosphamide, or methotrexate.

Head and neck squamous cell. *Cis*-platinum and bleomycin, or methotrexate.

Choriocarcinoma. Methotrexate.

Tumor cells acquire **resistance to methotrexate** as the result of several factors:

The deletion of a high-affinity, carrier-mediated transport system for reduced folates.
An increase in the concentration of dihydrofolate reductase.
The formation of a biochemically altered reductase with reduced affinity for methotrexate.

To overcome this resistance, higher doses of methotrexate need to be administered.

The effects of methotrexate may be reversed by the administration of **leucovorin**, the reduced folate. This leucovorin "rescue" prevents or reduces the toxicity of methotrexate, which is expressed as mouth lesions (stomatitis), injury to the gastrointestinal epithelium (diarrhea), leukopenia, and thrombocytopenia.

FOLINIC ACID

(Leucovorin Calcium, Citrovorum Factor)

Leucovorin is used to reduce the toxicity ("rescue") of high dose **methotrexate** in osteosarcoma; to counteract the action of folic acid antagonists such as **pyrimethamine** or **trimethoprim**; and in combination with 4-fluorouracil to prolong survival in patients with advanced colorectal cancer. In this case, leucovorin enhances the toxicity of 5-fluorouracil (5-FU), and the doses of 5-FU should be reduced.

The adverse reactions following treatment with combination leucovorin/5-fluorouracil in descending order of occurrence are: stomatitis (75%), nausea, leukopenia (69%), diarrhea, vomiting, alopecia (42%), dermatitis, anorexia, fatigue, thrombocytopenia, infection, and constipation (3%).

FORMOTEROL

Formoterol is a selective beta$_2$ adrenergic receptor agonist. The selective beta$_2$-adrenergic stimulants cause bronchodilation without cardiac acceleration. **Metaproterenol** and **terbutaline** are available in tablet form, and terbutaline is also available for subcutaneous injection.

Metaproterenol and **albuterol** are available in metered-dose inhalers. Inhaled selective beta$_2$-adrenergic receptor agonists (**albuterol, terbutaline, fenoterol,** and **bitolterol**) have a rapid onset of action and are effective for 3 to 6 hours. **Formoterol** and **salmeterol** are longer-acting agents (12 hours) and may prove useful in treating nocturnal symptoms. The **side effects** of beta-adrenergic receptor agonists are tremor, tachycardia, and palpitations (see also Figure 86).

FORSKOLIN

Forskolin, which is isolated from *Coleus forskohlii*, stimulates adenylate cyclase (see Figure 42).

FOSCARNET SODIUM

(Phosphonoformic Acid) (Foscavir)

Foscarnet, a pyrophosphate analog with antiviral activity (60 mg/kg IV, is used in cytomegalovirus (CMV) retinitis in patients with acquired immunodeficiency syndrome (AIDS) (see also Figure 3).

FOSINOPRIL SODIUM

(Monopril)

Fosinopril, an angiotensin-converting enzyme (ACE) inhibitor with antihypertensive properties (10 mg p.o. daily), is used in the treatment of hypertension (see also Figure 21).

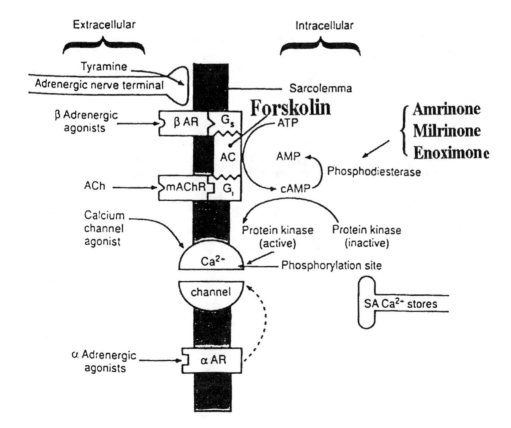

FIGURE 42   **Forskolin**, which is isolated from *Coleus forskohlii*, stimulates adenylate cyclase.

FRUCTOSE

(Levulose)

Fructose, a carbohydrate, is used as a source of carbohydrate calories primarily when fluid replacement is also indicated and as a dextrose substitute for patients with diabetes.

FUROSEMIDE

(Lasix)

The major loop diuretics are furosemide (Lasix) and ethacrynic acid (Edecrin). **Furosemide** is chemically related to the thiazide diuretics, but **ethacrynic acid** is not. These agents inhibit the active resorption of chloride (and sodium) in the thick, ascending medullary portion of the loop of Henle and also in the cortical portion of the loop or the distal tubule. The diuresis they produce, which is similar to that seen with the thiazides, predominantly causes a loss of chloride, sodium, and potassium, but HCO_3 excretion is not increased. Although large volumes of fluid can be excreted with the use of these agents, the ability of the kidney to produce either a dilute or concentrated urine is greatly diminished. These agents are the most efficacious of all the diuretics now on the market, usually producing about a 20% loss in the filtered load of sodium (furosemide, 15 to 30%; ethacrynic acid, 17 to 23%).

Loop diuretics are ordinarily taken orally, but can be given intravenously if a very rapid onset of action is sought, as when used in combination with antihypertensive medications in the management of a **hypertensive crisis**. Furosemide and ethacrynic acid undergo some active renal tubular secretion as well as glomerular filtration. A minor portion is excreted by the liver.

Loop diuretics are used for treating the following conditions:

In the **edema** of cardiac, hepatic, or renal origin, including acute pulmonary edema and hypertensive crisis.
In **acute renal failure**, to maintain urine flow, though an excessive loss of extracellular fluid volume can cause a decrease in the GFR.
In hypercalcemia.

Excessive volume depletion, hyponatremia, and hypotension are major risks associated with the use of loop diuretics, and the side effects of **hypokalemia, hyperuricemia**, and **hyperglycemia** are always present. Loop diuretics should not be used concurrently with **ototoxic aminoglycoside antibiotics** (i.e., streptomycin, gentamicin, kanamycin, tobramycin) (see also Table 25 and Figure 4).

FUNGAL INFECTIONS: TREATMENT OF		
Infections	**Drugs of Choice**	**Alternatives**
Aspergillosis	Amphotericin B	Itraconazole
Blastomycosis	Ketoconazole or Amphotericin B	Itraconazole
Candidiasis oropharyngeal	Clotrimazole troches	Fluconazole Ketoconazole
esophageal systemic	Fluconazole or Ketoconazole Amphotericin B or Flucytosine	Amphotericin B Fluconazole
Chromomycosis	Flucytosine	Itraconazole
Coccidioidomycosis	Ketoconazole or Amphotericin B	Itraconazole Fluconazole

Infections	Drugs of Choice	Alternatives
Cryptococcosis	Amphotericin B ± Flucytosine	Fluconazole
chronic suppression		Itraconazole
	Fluconazole	Amphotericin B
Histoplasmosis	Ketoconazole or Amphotericin B	Itraconazole
chronic suppression	Amphotericin B	Itraconazole
Mucormycosis	Amphotericin B	No dependable alternative
Paracoccidioidomycosis	Ketoconazole or Amphotericin B	Itraconazole, a sulfonamide
Pseudallescheriasis	Ketoconazole or Miconazole	Itraconazole
Sporotrichosis		
cutaneous	Potassium iodide	Local heat
		Itraconazole
systemic	Amphotericin B	Itraconazole

G

GABAPENTIN

(Neurontin)

GABApentin, 1-aminomethylcyclohexoneactic acid possessing anticonvulsant properties (300 mg p.o. initially), is indicated as an adjunctive medication in the treatment of partial seizures with and without secondary generalization (see Figure 43).

GALLAMINE TRIETHIODIDE

(Flaxedil)

Gallamine, a nondepolarizing neuromuscular blocking agent (1 mg/kg IV), is used as an adjunct to anesthesia to induce skeletal muscle relaxation, facilitate intubation and mechanical ventilation, reduce fractures and dislocations, and to weaken muscle contractions in pharmacologically or electrically induced convulsions (see also Figure 92).

GALLIUM NITRATE

(Ganite)

Gallium, a heavy metal with antihypercalcemic effects (200 mg/m^2 IV daily for five consecutive days), is indicated in the treatment of cancer-related hypercalcemia after hydration.

GANCICLOVIR SODIUM

(DHPG, Cytovene)

Ganciclovir is indicated in the treatment of cytomegalovirus (CMV) retinitis in immunocompromised patients and for the prevention of cytomegalovirus disease in transplant patients who may be at risk for developing cytomegalovirus disease. Ganciclovir is a synthetic nucleoside analog of 2'-deoxyguanosine with efficacy against CMV, herpes simplex virus 1 and 2, Epstein-Barr virus, and varicella zoster virus. Ganciclovir, is converted to ganciclovir triphosphate which is preferentially accumulated in CMV inhibiting viral DNA polymerase and by incorporating into viral DNA terminating viral DNA elongation. Ganciclovir, which binds to plasma protein to the extent of 2%, is mostly excreted unchanged in the urine, and hence should be used cautiously in patients with renal impairment. Probenecid reduces the renal clearance of ganciclovir. Ganciclovir has caused granulocytopenia and thrombocytopenia, especially in elderly subjects with reduced glomerular filtration. Cytotoxic drugs that inhibit replication of rapidly dividing cell populations such as bone marrow, spermatogonia, and germinal layers of skin and GI mucosa may have additive toxicity when administered concomitantly with ganciclovir (see also Figure 3).

GASTRIN

Histamine, as a normal constituent of the gastric mucosa, controls both microcirculation and **gastric secretion**. The gastric secretagogues are **acetylcholine, histamine**, and **gastrin**. The action of acetylcholine is blocked by **atropine**, and the action of histamine is blocked by **cimetidine, butrimamide**, and **metiamide**. No specific antagonist is available for gastrin (see Figure 24).

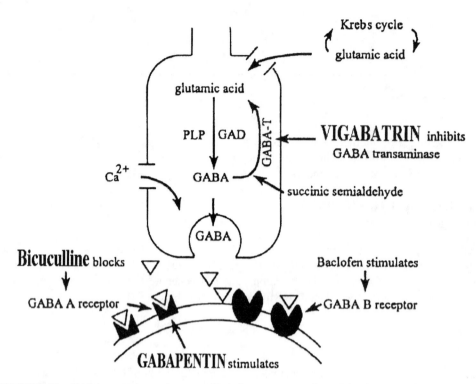

FIGURE 43   GABApentin is used as an adjunctive treatment of partial seizures with and without secondary generalization. (Adapted from Ebadi, M., *Pharmacology, An Illustrated Review with Questions and Answers*, 3rd Edition, Lippincott-Raven Press, Philadelphia, 1996.)

GASTROESOPHAGEAL REFLUX DISEASE (GERD): TREATMENT OF	
Esophagitis results from excessive reflux of gastric juice rather than excessive gastric secretion. The squamous epithelium of the esophagus is intolerant of repetitive exposure to gastric juice for prolonged periods. Low-grade esophagitis is evident only by histopathological examination. High-grade changes are seen endoscopically as erosions and ulcerations. Peptic strictures and Barrett metaplasia result from the response that follows ulceration.	
The goals of drug therapy of reflux esophagitis are to increase the strength and competence of the anti-reflux barrier, to enhance esophageal acid clearance, to improve gastric emptying and pyloric sphincter competence, to prevent reflux of duodenal contents, to coat inflamed and denuded tissue, and, above all, to decrease the volume of pH of gastric contents.	
Prokinetic Agents	
Cisapride is currently considered the drug of choice among the motility modulating agents to treat GERD. It is more potent and has fewer side-effects as compared to the older prokinetics.	
Mucosa Coating Drugs	
Sucralfate is a topically active aluminum hydroxide salt of sucrose octasulfate.	
Histamine₂ Receptor Blocking Agents	
Cimetidine	Ranitidine
Famotidine	Roxatidine
Nizatidine	
Proton Pump Inhibitors	
Omeprazole	

Although usually a mild condition appropriately treated with episodic self-medication and lifestyle modifications, GERD can also result in severe symptoms or in complications. The complications of GERD can be categorized as those involving the esophagus (principally esophagitis, esophageal stricture, or Barrett metaplasia and cancer) or organs other than the esophagus (principally asthma and otolaryngological manifestations).

GAUCHER'S DISEASE: TREATMENT OF

Gaucher's disease is the most prevalent lysosomal storage disorder, caused by an inherited defect in the lysosomal enzyme, glucocerebrosidase, and consequent accumulation of glucocerebrosidase in the cells of the reticuloendothelial system. There is a high incidence of the most common variant, type I, among Ashkenazi Jews. The other two variants, types II and III, are relatively rare and have been described among all ethnic groups.

The earliest sign of Gaucher's disease is generally splenomegaly which may be massive, but even when not palpable, can be demonstrated by ultrasound.

Anemia and thrombocytopenia, resulting in fatigue and bleeding tendencies, respectively, are among the prominent features and are often the initial presenting signs of Gaucher's disease. In type II Gaucher's disease the neurological signs include the classical triad of trismus, strabismus, and retroflexion of the head, as well as spasticity, hyper-reflexia, and seizures during the first year of life. The effective enzyme replacement therapy for Gaucher's disease is the use of a placenta-derived macrophage-targeted glucocerebrosidase.

Of the surgical options available prior to enzyme therapy, splenectomy was most often recommended to combat thrombocytopenia and anemia, mechanical complications, and growth retardation.

It is hoped that in the future, Gaucher's disease, currently a model of enzyme replacement therapy, will prove to be a model of a curative form of gene transfer therapy for inherited metabolic disorders. In this case CD34 cells from the patients' blood, will be genetically corrected *in vitro* and transplanted back into the patient.

GENE THERAPY (e.g., FOR ACQUIRED IMMUNE DEFICIENCY SYNDROME (AIDS)

Gene therapy is defined as the introduction of new genetic material into the cells of an individual that results in a therapeutic benefit. Gene therapy holds considerable potential for the treatment of both hereditary and acquired genetic diseases. Since in its normal life cycle the HIV-1 virus integrates into the host cell's genome, AIDS can be regarded as an acquired genetic disease. Therefore, AIDS may be amenable to treatment by gene therapy approaches.

Gene therapy for HIV-1 infection requires the introduction of genes that will effectively inhibit HIV-1 replication by efficiently inhibiting expression of HIV-1 viral genes or altering the normal function of HIV-1 associated proteins. The ultimate goal of gene therapy is to inhibit HIV-1 viral replication and the resulting AIDS pathogenesis. Anti-HIV-1 gene therapy approaches can be divided into three broad categories: 1) gene therapies based on nucleic acid moieties, including gene vaccines, antisense DNA/RNA, RNA decoys that function by competition for the binding of proteins essential for HIV-1 replication, and catalytic RNA moieties (ribozymes) that inhibit HIV-1 gene expression by cleaving the viral RNA; 2) protein approaches (transdominant negative proteins and single chain antibodies) that are based on the intracellular expression of protein moieties that interfere or inhibit normal viral replication or function; and 3) immunotherapeutic approaches in which HIV-1-specific lymphocytes are generated and used to inhibit HIV replication.

Some other therapeutic gene therapy trials are:
- Gene Therapy for the Treatment of Recurrent Pediatric Malignant Astrocytomas with *in vivo* Tumor Transduction with the Herpes Simplex-Thymidine Kinase Gene.
- Human MDR Gene Transfer in Patients with Advanced Cancer.
- Gene Therapy for Human Brain Tumors Using Episome-Based Antisense cDNA Transcription of Insulin-Like Growth Factor I.
- Immunization of Malignant Melanoma Patients with Interleukin 2-Secreting Melanoma Cells Expressing Defined Allogeneic Histocompatibility Antigens.

- Genetically Engineered Autologous Tumor Vaccines Producing Interleukin-2 for the Treatment of Metastatic Melanoma.
- Intrathecal Gene Therapy for the Treatment of Leptomeningeal Carcinomatosis.
- Retrovirus-Mediated Transfer of the cDNA for Human Glucocerebrosidase into Peripheral Blood Repopulating Cells of Patients with Gaucher's Disease.
- Adoptive Immunotherapy of Melanoma with Activated Lymph Node Cells Primed *in vivo* with Autologous Tumor Cells Transduced with the IL-4 Gene.
- Gene Therapy for Cystic Fibrosis Using Cationic Liposome Mediated Gene Transfer.
- Gene Therapy of Patients with Advanced Cancer Using Tumor Infiltration Lymphocytes Transduced with the Gene Coding for Tumor Necrosis Factor.
- Immunization of Cancer Patients Using Autologous Cancer Cells Modified by Insertion of the Gene for Tumor Necrosis Factor (TNF).
- Immunization of Cancer Patients Using Autologous Cancer Cells Modified by Insertion of the Gene for Interleukin-2 (IL-2).
- Gene Therapy for the Treatment of Recurrent Glioblastoma Multiforme with *in vivo* Tumor Transduction with the Herpes Simplex-Thymidine Kinase Gene/Ganciclovir System.
- Gene Therapy for the Treatment of Brain Tumors Using Intra-Tumoral Transduction with the Thymidine Kinase Gene and Intravenous Ganciclovir.
- Immunization with HLA-A2 Matched Allogeneic Melanoma Cells that Secrete Interleukin-2 in Patients with Metastatic Melanoma.
- Immunization with Interleukin-2 Secreting Allogeneic HLA-A2 Matched Renal Cell Carcinoma Cells in Patients with Advanced Renal Cell Carcinoma.
- Clinical Protocol for Modification of Oncogene and Tumor Suppressor Gene Expression in Non-Small Cell Lung Cancer (NSCLC).
- Cystic Fibrosis Gene Therapy Using an Adenovirus Vector: *In vivo* Safety and Efficacy in Nasal Epithelium.
- Administration of Neomycin Resistance Gene Marked EBV Specific Cytotoxic T Lymphocytes to Recipients of Mismatched-Related or Phenotypically Similar Unrelated Donor Marrow Grafts.
- Retroviral Mediated Gene Transfer of the Fanconi Anemia Complementation Group C Gene to Hematopoietic Progenitors of Group C Patients.
- Clinical Protocol for Modification of Tumor Suppressor Gene Expression and Induction of Apoptosis in Non-Small Cell Lung Cancer (NSCLC) with an Adenovirus Vector Expressing Wildtype p53 and Cisplatin.

GENERAL ANESTHETICS

Anesthesia is the controllable and reversible depression of the central nervous system (CNS) that is characterized by a lack of perception of all sensations, by **analgesia**, and by **amnesia**. An ideal anesthetic is an inexpensive agent that has the following characteristics: It has a fast rate of induction and a rapid rate of emergence; it is nonexplosive and a good muscle relaxant; it has analgesic properties and does not cause respiratory or myocardial depression; it is nontoxic to the liver and kidney; it is inert metabolically and does not interact adversely with other pharmacologic agents used as pre- and postanesthetic medications; and it does not cause any postanesthetic complications. However, the search for this nonexistent ideal anesthetic agent continues.

A patient scheduled for surgery experiences discomfort and much anxiety. This preoperative behavior may be characterized by thoughts of excessive and unrealistic danger of anesthetics or the surgical procedure and by repetitive and redundant inquiries about the preanesthetic and postoperative events. On the other hand, patients may manifest their anxiety by silence, avoidance of eye contact, lack of interest, or lack of communication. A visit by a caring physician or a nurse is extremely useful and supportive for reassuring and allaying a patient's concerns. A reassured patient sleeps easier, requires less anesthetics and analgesics, and shows fewer postanesthetic complications.

The choice of an anesthetic is always made by an anesthesiologist after consultation with the attending physician or surgeon. The anesthetic is selected based on many factors, including the patient's age, complicating and preexisting disease, the nature of the operation, the patient's previous experience with anesthetics, and the nature of nonanesthetic medications to be taken by the patient.

Because general anesthetics alter the **cardiac and respiratory physiology**, those agents causing myocardial irritability, hypotension, circulatory depression, or tachyarrhythmia should be used with extreme caution in patients with preexisting cardiovascular problems. Furthermore, agents causing **respiratory depression** should be used with caution in patients with bronchitis, emphysema, muscular dystrophy, or myasthenia gravis, as well as in those in bronchospastic states. The use of skeletal muscle relaxants should be monitored in conditions of respiratory insufficiency such as kyphoscoliosis. The opioids, which further depress respiration, should also be used with extreme care.

Preexisting **endocrine disorders** such as hypothyroidism, hyperthyroidism, and diabetes mellitus should also dictate the choice of general anesthetics. In patients with hyperthyroidism, agents causing cardiac acceleration (atropine or sympathomimetic amines) should be used carefully.

Because the release of insulin is reduced by sympathomimetic amines and increased by their appropriate blockers, severe **hyperglycemia** or **hypoglycemia** may be caused in susceptible patients who have been given inappropriate anesthetics. Patients who require medications on a permanent basis should be evaluated carefully, and the choice of anesthetics made judiciously.

Antihypertensive medications, diuretics that cause hypokalemia which may predispose to cardiac irritability, and anticoagulants may have to be discontinued or their regimens modified in surgical patients.

The foregoing represents only a brief description of the cautions that should be taken into consideration when choosing an anesthetic.

The preanesthetic medications are given for the following reasons:

To sedate and reduce anxiety (secobarbital, diazepam).
To relieve pain, if present (opiates).
To reduce excess salivation (anticholinergics such as atropine).
To prevent bradycardia during surgery (atropine).
To facilitate intubation (succinylcholine).

The general anesthetics are classified as either inhalational or intravenous. The **inhalational anesthetic** agents include:

Halogenated hydrocarbons
Halothane
Anesthetic ethers
Enflurane
Isoflurane
Methoxyflurane
Anesthetic gases
Nitrous oxide

The **intravenous anesthetic agents** include:

Barbiturates
Thiopental
Methohexital
Nonbarbiturates
Dissociative anesthetics-ketamine (see also Figure 74)
Benzodiazepines — diazepam, midazolam, lorazepam, flumazenil (antagonist)

Neuroleptic anesthetics — droperidol, haloperidol
Imidazole derivatives — etomidate
Phenol derivatives — propofol (see also Figure 74)

Morphine may be used for patients undergoing open-heart surgery. It is given in a dose of 0.5 to 3.0 mg per kilogram administered intravenously over a 15- to 20-minute period, which produces unconsciousness. Morphine is supplemented with nitrous oxide and a muscle relaxant.

Dantrolene is used for patients who are genetically disposed to malignant hyperthermia. **Malignant hyperpyrexia** represents an inherited muscular abnormality that presents clinically as a syndrome of life-threatening complications that arise during general anesthesia. The primary defect in malignant hyperpyrexic susceptible muscle resides in the process that regulates myoplasmic calcium concentrations. Recent investigations have also implicated abnormalities in the phosphoinositide cycle and in the sarcoplasmic-reticular calcium-releasing channels. In the event of anesthetic-induced malignant hyperthermia, the offending anesthetics should be discontinued and dantrolene administered in an initial dose of 1 mg per kilogram (see also Figure 30).

Thiopental is used in patients undergoing **carotid endarterectomy** for whom the maintenance of oxygen and nutrients to the brain during the temporary period of surgical occlusion of the common, internal, and external carotid arteries is essential. Thiopental, given as a bolus of 4 to 5 mg per kilogram or as an intravenous infusion of 10 mg per kilogram over 20 to 30 minutes, protects the brain against ischemia. The general anesthetic may be 0.3 to 0.6% halothane in 50 to 60% nitrous oxide in oxygen.

General anesthetics alter the **excitation of the neuronal membrane** and **modify impulse conduction**. Specifically, the general anesthetics have the following common properties:

They decrease the activity of neurons by increasing their threshold to fire.
By interfering with sodium influx, they prevent the action potential from rising to normal rate.

At the present time, the **depth of anesthesia** is judged by the presence or absence of the eyelash reflex, the respiratory rate, and the response of the heart rate and blood pressure to surgical stimulation.

In the past, the **pupillary signs** have been used to judge the depth of anesthesia; however, premedication with opiate (causing miosis) or with anticholinergics (causing mydriasis) may make these signs unreliable. If both morphine and atropine have been administered, the miotic effect of morphine dominates. In addition, the reaction to light and pupillary signs is less predictable in patients aged 50 and over, and the reaction to light is absent with halothane and enflurane. Nevertheless, the classic signs of general anesthesia following the administration of diethyl ether, as originally described by Guedel, are still valid for educating students of medicine concerning the dose-dependent actions of general anesthetics (see Table 15).

The various stages of anesthesia seem to be sponsored by the dose-dependent alteration of the physiology of different populations of neurons in the CNS. Furthermore, the various anesthetics do indeed show specificity in this respect.

Stage I (analgesia) is brought about by a decrease in the activity of the dorsal horn of the spinal cord, which interferes with the sensory transmission in the spinothalamic tract.
Stage II (excitement or delirium) represents the period of anesthetic-mediated "disinhibition." It is due to the blockade of inhibitory neurons (Golgi type II cells), which then frees up the actions of excitatory neurotransmitters.

Stage III (muscle relaxation and time of surgery) represents the time when a high concentration of anesthetic is reached in the brain, while the reticular activating system and the spinal reflexes are suppressed. The swallowing, retching, and vomiting reflexes are also diminished. This stage, which is divided into four planes, is the time when surgery is performed.

Stage IV (death) occurs when the medullary neurons in the respiratory and vasomotor centers are completely depressed. General anesthetics depress the respiratory center only when given in higher than therapeutic doses; morphine, on the other hand, depresses the respiratory center at a dose that does not cause narcosis.

The states of anesthesia are directly related and dependent on the **concentration of an anesthetic** in the brain; that is, the higher the concentration, the deeper the state of anesthesia. The **administration of general anesthetics** is arbitrarily divided into three phases:

Induction — the time from the onset of administration of an anesthetic to a stage where surgery becomes suitable

Maintenance — the duration of time a patient is kept in a state of surgical anesthesia

Emergence — the time between the discontinuation of an anesthetic agent until the patient regains consciousness

The concentrations of general anesthetics in the brain depend on their solubility, their concentration in the inspired air, the rate of pulmonary ventilation, the rate of pulmonary blood flow, and the concentration gradient of the anesthetic between arterial and mixed venous blood.

The blood-gas partition coefficient is an index of the solubility of an anesthetic or its induction time, as depicted by the following examples.

Anesthetic Agents	Blood-Gas	Induction Time (min)
Nitrous oxide	0.47	2–3
Isoflurane	1.4	5–10
Enflurane	1.9	5–10
Halothane	2.36	10

Similarly, the amount of an anesthetic needed to produce anesthesia depends on the **relative lipid solubility** (oil-gas) of the compound, as denoted by the following examples.

Anesthetic Agents	Oil-Gas	Minimal Anesthetic Concentration (vol%)
Nitrous oxide	1.4	101
Enflurane	98	1.68
Isoflurane	99	1.40
Halothane	224	0.76

Furthermore, the greater the lipid solubility of an anesthetic, the lower the anesthetic tension needed to produce anesthesia. At equilibrium, the concentrations of an anesthetic in the brain and fat cells are high, but are low in the blood. Finally, the **potency** of an anesthetic is inversely related to its **minimum anesthetic concentration**.

GENTAMICIN

(Garamycin)

Gentamicin, an aminoglycoside antibiotic, (3 mg/kg in three equal doses q. 8 hours), is indicated for treatment of serious infections caused by susceptible strains of *Pseudomonas aeruginosa, Proteus sp., Escherichia coli, Klebsiella sp., Enterobacter sp., Serrati sp., Citrobacter sp.,* and *Staphylococcus sp.,* and hence it is used in neonatal sepsis, bacterial septicemia, meningitis, peritonitis, or burns. Gentamicin is bactericidal in nature and binds directly to the 30S ribosomal subunit and hence inhibits bacterial protein synthesis (see Figure 80). Gentamicin is poorly absorbed when given orally, and must be given parenterally. It is distributed widely, but its intraocular penetration and passage across the blood-brain barrier is poor, even in patients with meningitis. Gentamicin is not metabolized and is mostly excreted in the urine, and its half-life of 2 to 3 hours may be lengthened to 24 hours in renal impairment.

Gentamicin, which is ototoxic, should be used cautiously in patients with tinnitus, vertigo, or high-frequency hearing loss. The concomitant administration of methoxyflurane, polymyxin B, vancomycin, capreomycin, cisplatin, cephalosporins, amphotericin B, and other aminoglycosides, may enhance the potential neurotoxicity, nephrotoxicity, and ototoxicity of gentamicin.

GENTIAN VIOLET

Gentian violet, a triphenylmethane (rosaniline) dye, with topical antibacterial and antifungal activities (12% solution), is used in cutaneous or mucocutaneous infections caused by *Candida albicans* and other superficial skin infections.

GEPIRONE HYDROCHLORIDE

Gepirone (30 to 60 mg/day) which interacts with serotonergic systems is an anxioselective agent possessing properties similar to buspirone and ipsapirone. Gepirone is an agonist on presynaptic serotonin (5HT$_1$A) autoreceptors inhibiting the release and firing of **serotonergic neurons**.

Although the benzodiazepines are now viewed as having a direct action at a binding site coupled to the GABA receptor (see Figure 40), this view was predated by the suggestion that serotonergic systems interacted with the benzodiazepines. This view was spawned by the observation that benzodiazepines inhibit the firing of serotonergic neurons in the dorsal raphe nucleus, decrease brain serotonin turnover, and reverse the preconflict effects of direct serotonergic stimulation of the dorsal raphe. As with **buspirone**, lesions of the serotonergic system abolish diazepam's efficacy in a conflict test. A body of data supports the candidacy of serotonin as a mediator of the anxiolytic effects of benzodiazepines downstream from the GABA receptor. There is a convincing body of evidence that several types of serotonin (5-HT) receptors exist in the mammalian brain, two of which are well characterized: 5-HT$_1$ and 5-HT$_2$ sites. The 5-HT$_1$ sites can be further subdivided into at least three distinct subsets, which differ in their regional distribution and functions and are currently termed 5-HT$_{1A}$, 5-HT$_{1B}$, and 5-HT$_{1C}$ sites.

The 5-HT receptors in the hippocampus and other parts of the **limbic system** are primarily of the 5-HT$_{1A}$ type. It is therefore tempting to speculate that drugs that display a high degree of selectivity for these receptor sites can selectively affect anxiety states. A breakthrough in that direction came with the discovery that **buspirone**, a drug with anxiolytic activity in humans, can help elucidate the role of 5-HT in anxiety. **Buspirone, gepirone**, and **ipsapirone** may therefore offer new therapeutic directions in the treatment of anxiety.

Gepirone is absorbed rapidly when given orally and undergoes extensive first-pass metabolism to an active metabolite which is excreted by the kidneys. The most frequently reported adverse effects are dizziness, nausea, headache, drowsiness, and weakness. Gepirone does not impair memory, verbal fluency, or psychomotor performance. Like buspirone, gepirone does not appear to have a potential for causing physical dependence or addiction in humans, and it is expected that gepirone will not interact with alcohol or sedative-hypnotic drugs.

GILLES DE LA TOURETTE'S SYNDROME: TREATMENT OF

Gilles de la Tourette's syndrome is characterized by involuntary movements, echolalia, echopraxia, coprolalia, and strange, uncontrollable sounds. The differential diagnosis includes the various movement disorders that can present in childhood. Other disorders characterized by tics are distinguished by resolution of the tics by early adulthood or by the restricted number of tics.

Wilson's disease can simulate Gilles de la Tourette's syndrome; it must be excluded because it responds well to medical treatment. In addition to a movement disorder, Wilson's disease produces hepatic involvement, Kayser-Fleischer corneal rings, and abnormalities of serum copper and ceruloplasmin, which are absent in Gilles de la Tourette's syndrome.

Sydenham's chorea can be difficult to recognize if there is no recent history of rheumatic fever or polyarthritis and no clinical evidence of cardiac involvement, but this disorder is a self-limiting one, usually clearing in 3 to 6 months.

Bobble-head syndrome which can be difficult to distinguish from Gilles de la Tourette's syndrome, is characterized by rapid, rhythmic bobbing of the head in children with progressive hydrocephalus. Treatment is symptomatic and, if effective, must be continued indefinitely.

Clonidine has been reported to ameliorate motor or vocal tics in roughly 50% of children so treated. It may act by reducing activity in noradrenergic neurons arising in the locus ceruleus.

Haloperidol is often effective. It is started at a low daily dose (0.25 mg), which is gradually increased by 0.25 mg every 4 or 5 days until there is maximum benefit with a minimum of side effects or until side effects limit further increments.

Phenothiazines such as fluphenazine may help, but patients who are unresponsive to haloperidol usually fail with these drugs as well.

Patients occasionally respond favorably to clonazepam or carbamazepine, but diazepam, barbiturates, tricyclic antidepressants, phenytoin, and cholinergic agonists (such as deanol) are usually not helpful.

GLAUCOMA: TREATMENT FOR	
Drugs	**Usual Daily Dosage**
Adrenergic Agonist	
Dipivefrin hydrochloride	1 drop b.i.d.
Beta-blockers	
Betaxolol	1 drop b.i.d.
Levobunolol	1 drop b.i.d.
	1 drop once
Metipranolol	1 drop b.i.d.
Timolol - Timoptic	1 drop b.i.d.
Timoptic-XE	1 drop once
Carbonic Anhydrase Inhibitor	
Dorzolamide	1 drop t.i.d.
Cholinergic Agent	
Pilocarpine hydrochloride	1 drop q.i.d.
Prostaglandin	
Latanoprost	1 drop once

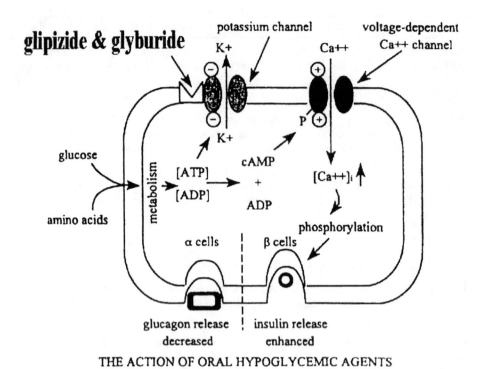

THE ACTION OF ORAL HYPOGLYCEMIC AGENTS

FIGURE 44   Sulfonylureas such as **glyburide** and **glipizide** bind to sulfonylurea receptors located on the surface of beta cells and trigger insulin release. (Adapted from Ebadi, M., *Pharmacology, An Illustrated Review with Questions and Answers*, 3rd Edition, Lippincott-Raven Press, Philadelphia, 1996.)

GLIPIZIDE

(Glucotrol)

Glipizide, a sulfonylurea oral hypoglycemic agent, is used as an adjunct to dieting in order to reduce blood glucose levels in individuals with noninsulin-dependent diabetes mellitus (Type II). Glipizide lowers blood glucose levels by stimulating insulin release from functioning beta cells in the pancreas. After prolonged administration, the drug's hypoglycemic effects appear to reflect extrapancreatic effects, possibly including reduction of basal hepatal glucose production and enhanced peripheral sensitivity to insulin (see Figure 44). The latter may result either from an increase in the number of insulin receptors or from changes in events subsequent to insulin binding. The properties of glipizide are compared with other hypoglycemic agents in Table 1.

Glipizide is absorbed rapidly, is bound to plasma protein to the extent of 92 to 99%, and is metabolized to inactive metabolites which are excreted in the urine.

GLUCAGON

Glucagon (0.5 to 1 mg SC 1 hour after coma) is an antihypoglycemic agent which is indicated in coma of insulin shock therapy. Following ingestion of a meal or the administration of glucose (e.g., in a glucose tolerance test), the glucose level rises, causing the release of insulin and inhibiting the release of hyperglycemic glucagon. Excess glucose is transformed into **glycogen** in the liver and the muscles. The high level of amino acids and fatty free acid fosters the respective formation of **proteins** in the muscles and **triglycerides** in the adipose tissues.

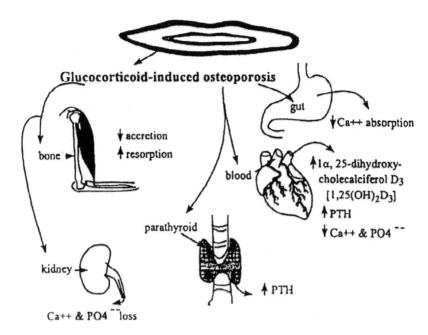

FIGURE 45 The glucocorticoids possess a plethora of physiologic actions, including a role in **differentiation** and **development**. They are vital in the treatment of adrenal insufficiency and are used extensively in large pharmacologic doses as **antiinflammatory** and **immunosuppressive** agents.

In a nondiabetic fasting subject, the ensuing hypoglycemia not only discourages the release of insulin but also activates the homeostatic mechanisms that block the action of insulin and convert the storage forms of fuel into utilizable glucose. Consequently, a number of hormones including **glucagon, epinephrine,** and **glucocorticoid**, are released, and these convert glycogen into glucose, triglyceride into free fatty acid, and proteins into amino acids (gluconeogenesis), respectively. Furthermore, the uptake and utilization of glucose in the peripheral tissue decrease. The muscles and other tissues utilize amino acids and free fatty acid, thus providing the brain with an adequate supply of glucose.

Glucagon increases plasma glucose levels and causes smooth muscle relaxation and an inotropic myocardial effect because of the stimulation of adenylate cyclase to produce cyclic $3',5'$-adenosine monophosphate (AMP). Cyclic AMP initiates a series of reactions that leads to the degradation of glycogen to glucose. Hepatic stores of glycogen are necessary for glucagon to exert an antihypoglycemic effect.

GLUCOCORTICOIDS

The glucocorticoids mainly influence carbohydrate metabolism and, to a certain extent, protein and lipid metabolism (see Figure 45). The main glucocorticoid is **cortisol**, with a daily secretion of 15 mg. Cortisol is synthesized through the 11-beta-hydroxylation of 11-deoxycortisol. Besides cortisol, the adrenal gland also synthesizes and releases a small amount of **corticosterone**, whose synthesis from 11-deoxycorticosterone is catalyzed by 11-beta-hydroxylase. A deficiency of 11-beta-hydroxylase causes:

Diminished secretion of cortisol
Diminished secretion of corticosterone
Enhanced compensatory secretion of ACTH
Enhanced secretion of 11-deoxycortisol and 11-deoxycorticosterone
Enhanced secretion of androgens

TABLE 13
Actions of Glucocorticoids

Steroids	Antiinflammatory Potency (% compared to cortisol)	Sodium Retention (% compared to cortisol)
Betamethasone	20	0
Dexamethasone	20	0
Fludrocortisone	12	100
Paramethasone	6	0
Triamcinolone	5	0
Methylprednisolone	4	0
Prednisolone	3	0.8
Prednisone	2.5	0.8
Cortisol	1	1

The clinical manifestations of 11-beta-hydroxylase deficiency are **virilization,** resulting from the overproduction of androgen, and **hypertension**, stemming from the overproduction of deoxycorticosteroids.

The glucocorticoids work by binding to specific intracellular receptors in target tissues. The receptor hormone complex is then transported into the nucleus where the complex interacts with the DNA, thus augmenting the synthesis of specific RNAs.

Cortisol, corticosterone, aldosterone, and the synthetic steroids used in steroid therapy (e.g., prednisolone, dexamethasone, and triamcinolone) are **glucocorticoid agonists** and therefore elicit glucocorticoid responses. A number of other steroids bind to the glucocorticoid receptor and thus suppress glucocorticoid responses (see Tables 10 and 13).

GLUTETHIMIDE
(Doriden)

Glutethimide (250 to 500 mg at bedtime) is indicated for short-term (few days) relief of insomnia. It exhibits pronounced atropine-like effects including mydriasis and inhibition of secretion and motility of the gastrointestinal tract. Similar to barbiturates, glutethimide depresses the CNS and has addictive effects with alcohol and other CNS drugs. It depresses REM sleep and is associated with REM rebound. Glutethimide induces the activity of hepatic microsomal enzyme and accelerates the metabolism of anticoagulants, and hence reduces their effectiveness, requiring dose adjustment.

Overdosage with glutethimide (10 to 20 g) produces symptoms that are identical to those produced by barbiturates, which include profound CNS depression, hypothermia, altered deep tendon reflexes, absence of corneal and papillary reflexes, absence of response to painful stimulation, hypoventilation, cyanosis, and apnea. Since the absorption of glutethimide from the gastrointestinal tract is erratic, a fluctuating level of alertness may be observed. Glutethimide is a lipid-soluble substance, accumulates in adipose tissues, and is released steadily, which requires careful monitoring of the victim's vital signs even when consciousness has been regained. Glutethimide has been replaced by safer hypnotic-sedative medications (see Table 8).

GLYBURIDE

(Micronase)

Glyburide is a sulfonylurea hypoglycemic agent which is indicated as an adjunct to dieting in order to lower blood glucose levels in patients with noninsulin-dependent diabetes mellitus (Type II).

The release of insulin is enhanced by certain physiologic substances (glucose, leucine, arginine, gastrin, secretin, and pancreozymin) and by certain pharmacologic agents (oral hypoglycemic agents). The release of insulin is also inhibited by some physiologic substances (epinephrine and norepinephrine) as well as by some pharmacologic substances (thiazide diuretics, diazoxide, and chlorpromazine).

Oral hypoglycemic agents have advantages over insulin, because, by releasing insulin and by decreasing the release of glucagon, they mimic physiologic processes and cause fewer allergic reactions. Furthermore, they are effective in an oral form, thus eliminating the need for daily injections. The properties of these agents are described in Table 1 and Figure 44.

Sulfonylureas such as **glyburide** and **glipizide** bind to sulfonylurea receptors located on the surface of beta cells and trigger insulin releases at nanomolar concentrations (Figure 44). Sulfonylureas bind to ATP-sensitive potassium channels and inhibit potassium efflux through these channels. The inhibition of ATP-sensitive potassium channels then leads to depolarization of the beta cell; this opens voltage-dependent calcium channels and allows the entry of extracellular calcium. The rising level of cytosolic free calcium next triggers the release of insulin. An increase in the cyclic adenosine monophosphate levels in the cells can also open the voltage-dependent calcium channels, thus increasing calcium influx into the cells. Glyburide lowers blood glucose levels by stimulating the insulin release from functioning beta cells in the pancreas. After prolonged administration, the drug's hypoglycemic effects appear to be related to extrapancreatic effects, possibly including reduction of basal hepatic glucose production and enhanced peripheral sensitivity to insulin. The latter may result either from an increase in the number of insulin receptors or from changes in events subsequent to insulin binding.

GLYCERIN

(Glycerol)

The osmotic diuretics and related agents consist of **mannitol** (Osmitrol), **urea** (Ureaphil), **glycerin** (Glycerol, Osmoglyn), and **isosorbide** (Hydronol). Mannitol and urea are nonelectrolytes that are freely filterable and undergo very little or no metabolism or renal tubular resorption. When given in sufficient quantities, these drugs increase the osmolarity of plasma and the amount of both the glomerular filtrate and the renal tubular fluid. The presence of such a drug in the lumen prevents the resorption of sodium from the tubular fluid, but some additional sodium is excreted as a normal constituent of the increased volume of urine. Osmotic diuretics are not effective in removing the edematous fluid caused by sodium retention, but can maintain the flow of urine even when the GFR is decreased. Osmotic diuretics are given by intravenous infusion in a hypertonic solution, and they are excreted by glomerular filtration (see Figure 4 and Table 25).

GLYCOPYRROLATE

(Robinul, Robinul Forte)

Glycopyrrolate, an anticholinergic agent with gastrointestinal antispasmodic properties, is used to block the cholinergic effects of anticholinesterase drugs used to reverse neuromuscular blockade. It is used preoperatively to diminish secretions and block cardiac vagal reflexes, as an antiarrhythmic agent, and as adjunctive therapy in peptic ulcers and other GI disorders.

GOLD SALTS

Drugs used in the treatment of arthritis are:

Aurothioglucose (Solganal)
Gold sodium thiomalate (Myochrysine)
Auranofin (Ridaura)

Gold salt therapy is reserved for patients with progressive disease who do not obtain satisfactory relief from therapy with aspirin-like drugs (see Table 2). The principle that underlies this therapy is that gold, which accumulates in lysosomes, decreases the migration and phagocytic activity of macrophages. Aurothioglucose, gold sodium thiomalate, or auranofin may cause toxic effects such as cutaneous reactions (from erythema to exfoliative dermatitis) as well as albuminuria, hematuria, and thrombocytopenia (see Figure 15).

Besides the nonsteroidal antiinflammatory agents and gold, other drugs are also used for the treatment of rheumatoid arthritis. These include immunosuppressive agents, glucocorticoids (see Table 10), penicillamine, and hydroxychloroquine. With the exception of glucocorticoids, these drugs resemble gold salts in that they do not possess antiinflammatory or analgesic properties and their therapeutic effects become evident only after several weeks or months of treatment (see also Table 2).

GOLD SODIUM THIOMALATE

(Myochrysine)

Gold sodium thiomalate (10 mg IM initially) is indicated in the management of rheumatoid arthritis.

GONADORELIN ACETATE

(Lutrepulse)

Gonadorelin, a gonadotropin-releasing hormone (GnRH) with fertility-inducing properties (5 mcg IV q. 90 minutes for 21 days), is used to induce ovulation in women with primary hypothalamic amenorrhea (see Table 14).

GONADORELIN HYDROCHLORIDE

(Factrel)

Gonadorelin, a luteinizing hormone releasing hormone (100 mcg SC), is used in the diagnosis of hypogonadism (see Table 14).

GONADOTROPIN RELEASING HORMONE

The pituitary hormones responsible for regulating gonadal function are **luteinizing hormone** (LH) and **follicle-stimulating hormone** (FSH) (see Figure 46). In **males**, LH stimulates the Leydig's cells to synthesize **testosterone**; FSH stimulates the Sertoli's cells to synthesize **inhibin** and **androgen-binding protein** and, in conjunction with high intratesticular concentrations of testosterone, initiates and maintains **spermatogenesis**. In **females**, LH stimulates **androgen synthesis**, and FSH increases estrogen and inhibin synthesis in the granulosa cells. Both LH and FSH are released from the gonadotroph cells of the anterior pituitary in response to the hypothalamic hormone gonadotropin-releasing hormone (GnRH; also known as **LH-releasing hormone**).

TABLE 14
GnRH Analogs with Agonist Activity

Structures	Generic Names
9-Amino acid analogs	
[D-Trp⁶,Pro⁹Net]GnRH	Deslorelin
[D-Trp⁶,NMeLeu⁷,Pro⁹Net]GnRH	Lutrelin
[D-Leu⁶,Pro⁹Net]GnRH	Leuprolide
[D-His(Bzl)⁶,Pro⁹Net]GnRH	Histerelin
[D-Ser(t-But)⁶,Pro⁹Net]GnRH	Buserelin
10-Amino acid analogs	
Native GnRH	Gonadorelin, Lutrepulse
[D-Naphthyl-Ala(2)⁶]GnRH	Nafarelin
[D-Ser(t-But)⁶,AzaGly¹⁰]GnRH	Goserelin
[D-Trp⁶]GnRH	Tryptorelin

GnRH = gonadotropin-releasing hormone

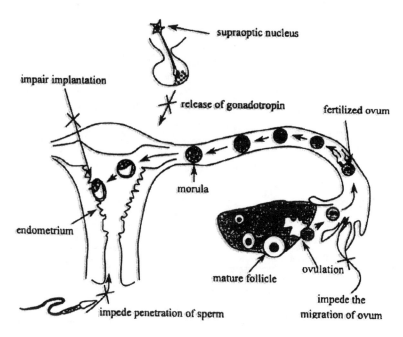

Actions of Oral Contraceptives

FIGURE 46 The antifertility agents suppress ovulation by inhibiting the release of hypophyseal ovulation-regulating gonadotropin, producing thick mucus from the cervical glands and hence impeding the penetration of sperm cells into the uterus, impeding the transfer of the ovum from the oviduct to the uterus, and preventing implantation of the fertilized ovum should fertilization take place.

GnRH is a decapeptide with the following structure: pyro Glu-His-Trp-Ser-Tyr-Gly-Leu-Arg-Pro-Gly-NH₂ (see Table 14).

GnRH is used to induce puberty in males with **idiopathic hypogonadotropic hypogonadism** (IHH). GnRH (15 to 150 ng/kg/hr) is administered by an infusion pump that delivers GnRH as a bolus, but in a pulsatile fashion. This induces the secretion of LH and FSH, the level of testosterone rises, the size of the testes increases, and spermatogenesis commences.

GnRH is used in females to treat **hypothalamic amenorrhea**. A deficit in the synthesis of GnRH has been implicated as the source of menstrual disturbances, hypoprolactinemia, anorexia nervosa, stress- and weight-loss associated amenorrhea, athletes' amenorrhea, some forms of the polycystic ovarian disease syndrome, and infertility associated with hypothalamic tumors (see Table 14).

The GnRH analogs (Table 14) are administered subcutaneously, by nasal spray, or by long-acting depots and may be used to 1) desensitize the gonadotrophs in patients with idiopathic precocious puberty, 2) treat prostate cancer and benign prostatic hypertrophy (androgen-dependent tumor), replacing the old methods of treating patients with castration or with high-dose estrogen therapy, and 3) to ameliorate gynecological diseases such as endometriosis.

The long-term use of GnRH analogs may foster hot flashes, osteoporosis, vaginal dryness, and dyspareunia (difficult coitus). These side effects may result from the prolonged hypoestrogenemia brought about by GnRH use.

GONORRHEA: TREATMENT OF	
Types of Infections	**Regimen of Choice**
Uncomplicated urethral, endocervical, rectal, proctitis, or epididymitis infection	Ceftriaxone 250 mg IM once; or ciprofloxacin 500 mg PO once; or norfloxacin 800 mg PO; or cefuroxime axetil 1 g PO once plus probenecid 1 g; or cefotaxime 1 g IM once or ceftizoxime 500 mg IM once **plus** Doxycycline 100 mg two times daily for 7 days or tetracycline 500 mg four times daily for 7 days
Gonococcal infections in pregnancy	Ceftriaxone 250 mg IM once **plus** Erythromycin base 500 mg PO four times daily for 7 days
Disseminated gonococcal infection	Ceftriaxone 1 g IM or IV every 24 hours **or** ceftizoxime 1 g IV every 8 hours **or** cefotaxime 1 g IV every 8 hours until all symptoms resolve
Gonococcal ophthalmia Adults and children (>20 kg) Neonates	Ceftriaxone 1.0 g IM as a single dose Ceftriaxone 25–50 mg/kg/d IV or IM in a single daily dose for 7 days **or** cefotaxime 25 mg/kg IV or IM two times daily for 7 days
Infants born to mothers with gonococcal infection	Ceftriaxone 50 mg/kg IV or IM, not to exceed 125 mg

GOSSYPOL

Cyproterone inhibits the action of androgens (see Figure 87), and gossypol prevents spermatogenesis without altering the other endocrine functions of the testis (Figure 47).

GOUT: TREATMENT OF
Gout results from the deposition of urate crystals (monosodium urate monohydrate) in joints, leading to an acute inflammatory response, or in soft tissues, such as cartilage, causing no inflammation. Most cases of gout are characterized by the sudden onset of severe acute monarticular arthritis in a peripheral joint in the leg.
Three treatments are available for patients with acute gouty arthritis. **Colchicine** is less favored now than in the past, because its onset of action is slow and it invariably causes diarrhea. **Nonsteroidal antiinflammatory drugs**, which are currently favored, are rapidly effective but may have serious side effects. **Corticosteroids**, administered either intraarticularly or parenterally, are used increasingly in patients with monarticular gout, especially if oral drug therapy is not feasible.

Drugs used in the management of gout are:	
To treat acute gouty arthritis	*To lower serum urate concentrations*
Colchicine	Allopurinol
Corticosteroids	Benzbromarone
NSAIDs	Diflunisal
To prevent acute attacks	Probenecid
Colchicine	Salicylate
NSAIDs	Sulfinpyrazone

GRANISETRON

A new class of antiemetic agents, the serotonin antagonists, has been identified. These agents could be clinically useful in a wide range of areas. Selective antagonists of the serotonin (5-hydroxytryptamine) type 3 (5-HT$_3$) receptor such as **batanopride, granisetron, ondansetron,** or **zancopride** have proved in early clinical trials to be potent antiemetic agents in patients undergoing cytotoxic chemotherapy. Their efficacy has been shown to be comparable or superior to that of conventional phenothiazine antiemetics. The toxic effects observed so far with these agents have been modest, and include headache (14%), asthenia, somnolence and diarrhea (4%) (see Figure 64).

GRANISETRON HYDROCHLORIDE

(Kytril)

Granisetron is indicated for prevention of nausea and vomiting associated with cancer chemotherapy. The recommended dose is 10 mcg/kg infused IV over five minutes beginning within 30 minutes before initiation of chemotherapy and only when chemotherapy is given (see Figure 64).

GRISEOFULVIN

(Fulvicin, Grisactin)

Griseofulvin, a fungistatic agent, is effective against various **dermatophytes**, including *Microsporum, Epidermophyton,* and *Trichophyton*, that produce diseases of the skin, hair,

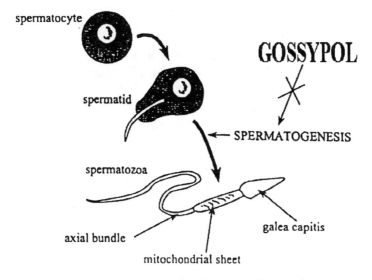

FIGURE 47 **Cyproterone** inhibits the action of androgens, and **gossypol** prevents spermatogenesis without altering the other endocrine functions of the testis.

and nails. It exerts its effect by inhibiting **fungal mitosis**. It is effective in the treatment of ringworm infections of the skin and nails, namely tinea corporis, tinea pedis, tinea cruris, tinea barbae, tinea capitis, and tinea unguium, when caused by one or more of the following genera of fungi: *Trichophyton rubrum, T tonsurans, T. mentagrophytes, T. interdigitalis, T. verrucosum, T. mengini, T. gallinae, T. crateriform, T. sulphureum, T. schoenleini, Microsporum audouini, M. canis, M. gypseum,* and *Epidermophyton floccosum.*

Prior to therapy, the types of fungi responsible for the infection must be identified. The use of this drug is not justified in minor or trivial infections which will respond to topical agents alone.

Griseofulvin is deposited in the keratin precursor cells, which are gradually replaced by healthy tissue. Griseofulvin has caused skin rashes, urticaria, angioneurotic edema, lupus-like syndrome, photosensitivity, and proteinuria. The serum level of griseofulvin is reduced by barbiturates; and griseofulvin reduces the hypoprothrombinemic effects of warfarin and actions of oral contraceptive medications.

GRISEOFULVIN MICROSIZE
(Fulvicin-U/F, Grifulvin V, Grisactin)

GRISEOFULVIN ULTRAMICROSIZE
(Fulvicin P/G, Gris-Peg, Grisactin Ultra)

Griseofulvin, a penicillium antibiotic (330 to 375 mg p.o. daily), is indicated in the treatment of tinea corporis, tinea capitis, or tinea cruris infections.

GROWTH HORMONE-RELEASING HORMONE (GHRH)
Growth hormone is secreted in a pulsatile fashion during sleep by the somatotrophs of the anterior pituitary gland. Two hypothalamic peptides, **growth hormone-releasing hormone** (GHRH) and **somatostatin** (somatotropin release-inhibiting hormone), are the principal stimulatory and inhibitory factors of GHRH, respectively. **Growth hormone deficiency** in children causes short stature, which will respond to GHRH replacement therapy (see also Table 14).

GUANABENZ
Guanabenz (8 to 64 mg given in divided doses) is an orally active central alpha$_2$-adrenergic agonist, which is structurally similar to clonidine (Figure 48) and lowers blood pressure. The major advantages of guanabenz are lack of fluid retention and a beneficial effect on serum lipids.

Guanabenz is rapidly and completely absorbed from the gastrointestinal tract, exerts its effects within two hours, has a duration of action of 10 hours, is metabolized in the liver by hydroxylation followed by glucuronidation, and 2% of it is excreted unchanged by the liver.

Guanabenz has been shown to reduce heart rate and myocardial contractility in animals. However, in hypertensive patients, blood pressure appears to be lowered via a reduction in peripheral resistance with minimal effects on heart rate and contractility. Fluid and electrolyte homeostasis and glomerular filtration rate are not affected by guanabenz. The most noteworthy metabolic action of guanabenz is a reduction in total cholesterol level. In contrast to the other two available alpha-adrenergic agonists, clonidine and methyldopa, glucose intolerance has not been associated with chronic treatment with guanabenz.

Guanabenz is used in the treatment of essential hypertension, and its efficacy compares well with methyldopa, clonidine, propranolol, and hydrochlorothiazide. Similar to other centrally

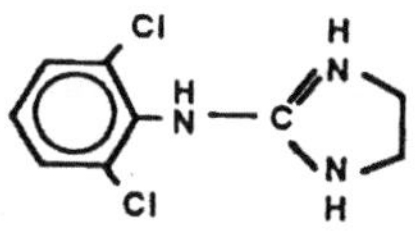

CLONIDINE

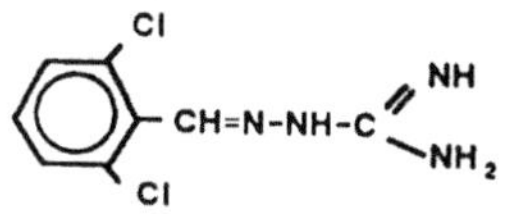

GUANABENZ

FIGURE 48 Guanabenz lowers blood pressure by stimulating the central alpha$_2$-adrenergic receptor, decreasing central sympathetic outflow, and thus decreasing peripheral vascular resistance.

acting alpha$_2$-adrenergic agonists (clonidine, guanfacine, methyldopa), it produces sedation and dry mouth which occur within the first two weeks of therapy and tend to dissipate with long-term administration.

Abrupt cessation of guanabenz therapy may be associated with a discontinuation syndrome similar to that seen with **clonidine**, where the blood pressure may rise 5 to 20 mmHg above pretreatment values. During abrupt withdrawal of guanabenz from patients taking beta-blocking agents, increases in plasma catecholamines may induce marked vasoconstriction because peripheral alpha-receptors are unopposed by peripheral vasodilatory beta-receptors. Consequently, the use of guanabenz in combination with beta-blockers should probably be restricted to patients who are well informed and reliable.

GUANADREL SULFATE

(Hylorel)

Guanethidine, guanadrel, debrisoquin, and bethanidine are all adrenergic neuron blockers with antihypertensive properties. Guanadrel (5 mg twice a day) is transported to presynaptic terminals by the catecholamine uptake mechanism, and then slowly displaces norepinephrine from its storage sites to be metabolized presynaptically. The reduction in neurotransmitter release in response to sympathetic nerve stimulation, leads to reduced arteriolar vasoconstriction, especially the reflex increase in sympathetic tone that occurs with a change in position. Guanadrel is absorbed rapidly from the gastrointestinal tract, has an onset of action of two hours, a duration of action of 10 hours, is metabolized by the liver, and partly excreted unchanged by the kidneys. Morning orthostatic hypotension is less frequent with guanadrel than with guanethidine (see also Figure 27).

GUANETHIDINE MONOSULFATE

(Ismelin)

Guanethidine (initial dose 10 mg daily) is indicated in the management of moderate to severe hypertension. It is transported to presynaptic terminals by the catecholamine uptake mechanism, and then slowly displaces norepinephrine from its storage sites to be metabolized presynaptically.

In contrast to the actions of ganglionic blocking agents, guanethidine suppresses equally the responses mediated by alpha and beta adrenergic receptors but does not produce parasympathetic blockade. It reduces both the systolic and diastolic pressures, and the effect is especially pronounced when the patient is standing.

Guanethidine is absorbed to the extent of 30 to 50%, is metabolized in the liver to a less active compound, and is excreted slowly in the urine. Guanethidine has a half-life of 4 to 8 days, requiring 10 to 14 days to evaluate its antihypertensive effects. Guanethidine causes pronounced orthostatic hypotension. In order to minimize sodium retention, guanethidine is used along with a diuretic. Substances that inhibit the biogenic amine uptake mechanism such as **imipramine** reduce the antihypertensive effects of guanethidine (see also Figures 27 and 31).

GUANFACINE HYDROCHLORIDE

(Tenex)

Guanfacine (1 mg/day at bedtime) is indicated in the management of hypertension. Clonidine, guanfacine, guanabenz, and methyldopa are centrally acting alpha$_2$-adrenergic receptor agonists. Guanfacine reduces sympathetic nerve impulses from the vasomotor center to the heart and blood vessels, resulting in a decrease in peripheral vascular resistance and a reduction in heart rate.

Guanfacine is absorbed orally, is bound to plasma proteins to the extent of 70%, is metabolized in the liver, and 50% of it is excreted unchanged in the urine. The half-life of guanfacine is lengthened in renal impairment. Similar to other centrally acting alpha$_2$-adrenergic receptor agonists, guanfacine causes sedation, especially during the first week, and hence should be given at bedtime.

Similar to clonidine, an abrupt cessation of therapy with guanfacine causes an increase in plasma and urinary catecholamines, nervousness, and rebound hypertension after 2 to 4 days, which is delayed when compared to that of clonidine. The adverse effects of guanfacine are dry mouth, (30%), somnolence, anesthesia, and dizziness (11%).

H

HAEMOPHILUS b VACCINES
(*Haemophilus* b Vaccines)

HAEMOPHILUS b CONJUGATE VACCINE, DIPHTHERIA CRM$_{197}$ PROTEIN CONJUGATE (HbOC)
(HibTITER)

HAEMOPHILUS b CONJUGATE VACCINE, DIPHTHERIA TOXOID CONJUGATE (PRP-D) (ProHIBIT)

HAEMOPHILUS b CONJUGATE VACCINE, MENINGOCOCCAL PROTEIN CONJUGATE (PRP-OMP)
(PedvaxHIB)

Haemophilus vaccine is indicated for routine immunization.

HALAZEPAM
(Paxipam)

Halazepam (20 to 40 mg p.o. t.i.d.) is used as an antianxiety agent. It depresses the CNS by enhancing the effects of gamma-aminobutyric acid (GABA) in the ascending reticular activating system and hence causing inhibition of cortical and limbic arousal (see Figure 40). Halazepam ($t_{1/2}$ of 14 hours) is absorbed orally, distributed widely throughout the body, bound to proteins to the extent of 85 to 90%, metabolized to desmethyldiazepam (an active metabolite with a $t_{1/2}$ of 150 hours), and is excreted as glucuronide conjugate in the urine. Halazepam potentiates the CNS depressant effects of neuroleptics, antidepressants, narcotic analgesics, barbiturates, and ethanol. Disulfiram inhibits the metabolism of halazepam, and heavy smoking accelerates it. Clinical manifestations of overdose include somnolence, confusion, coma, hypoactive reflexes, dyspnea, labored breathing, hypotension, bradycardia, slurred speech, and unsteady gait or impaired coordination. Because of decreased elimination and greater sensitivity to the CNS depressing effects, the dosage of halazepam in elderly subjects should be lower (see also Table 8).

HALCINONIDE
(Halog, Halog-E)

Halcinonide, a topical adrenocorticoid with antiinflammatory properties (cream, ointment, solution 0.025 to 0.1%), is indicated in inflammation of acute and chronic corticosteroid-responsive dermatoses (see also Table 10).

HALOBETASOL PROPIONATE
(Ultravate)

Halobetasol, a topical corticosteroid with antiinflammatory properties (0.05% cream and ointment), is used in the relief of inflammation and pruritus of corticosteroid-responsive dermatoses (see also Table 10).

HALOPERIDOL

(Haldol)

Haloperidol is a butyrophenone derivative with antipsychotic action similar to that of piper-azine phenothiazines such as fluphenazine. Haloperidol (0.5 to 2 mg t.i.d.) is indicated in the management of psychotic disorder; in Tourette's disorder for the control of tics and vocal utterances; in severe behavioral problems of children with combative and explosive nature; in hyperactive impulse disorder in children associated with aggression, low frustration toler-ance, and impulsive behavior, and in elderly subjects with senile dementia (see also Table 23).

Haloperidol blocks dopamine receptors in the brain and hence produces a very high incidence of movement disorders such as parkinsonism (see phenothiazine derivatives). Its mechanism of action in Gilles de la Tourette's syndrome is unknown. In addition to blocking dopamine receptors, haloperidol has many other central and peripheral effects; it has weak peripheral anticholinergic effects and antiemetic effects, produces both alpha and ganglionic blockade, and counteracts histamine- and serotonin-mediated activities.

Haloperidol is absorbed well orally and intramuscularly (haloperidol decanoate), distributed widely in the body while accumulating in adipose tissue, binds to protein heavily (90 to 99%), and is metabolized in the liver. Haloperidol is eliminated unchanged in the feces and urine to the extent of 15% and 40%, respectively.

The highest incidence of adverse effects of haloperidol include the CNS involving extrapyra-midal symptoms such as dystonia, akathisia, parkinsonism, tardive dyskinesia, and neuroleptic malignant syndrome. Overdose with haloperidol causes CNS depression characterized by deep, unarousable sleep and possible coma, hypotension or hypertension, extrapyramidal symptoms, dystonia, abnormal involuntary movements, agitation, seizures, arrhythmias, ECG changes (may show QT prolongation and torsades de pointes), hypothermia or hyperthermia, and autonomic nervous system dysfunction. Overdose with long-acting decanoate requires pro-longed recovery time. Treatment is symptomatic and supportive in nature (see also Table 23).

HALOPROGIN

(Halotex)

Haloprogin is available as a 1% cream or solution, which is applied topically. It is applied twice a day for 2 to 4 weeks. It is used principally in the treatment of tinea pedis, tinea cruris, tinea corporis, tinea manuum, and tinea versicolor. Haloprogin's mechanisms of action in yeast cells are thought to be inhibition of respiration and disruption of yeast cell membranes. Its mechanism of action in dermatophytes is unknown.

HALOTHANE

(Fluothane)

Halothane is 2-bromo-2-chloro-1,1,1-trifluoroethane. Mixtures of halothane with air or oxy-gen are not flammable or explosive.

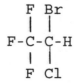

Halothane

TABLE 15
Summary Pharmacology of Nitrous Oxide, Cyclopropane, Halothane, and Ether

Nature and Effects	N₂O	Cyclopropane	Halothane	Ether
Volatile anesthetic	No	No	Yes	Yes
Rate of induction	Fast(2-3 min)	Fast (1-2 min)	Slow (10 min)	Slow (10–20 min)
Potentially explosive anesthetic	No	Yes	No	Yes
Respiration	NC	Depressed	Depressed	Stimulates indirectly, depresses directly
Myocardial depression	NC	Yes	Yes	Yes
Myocardial depression compensated by increased sympathetic activity	—	Yes	No	Yes
Sensitizes heart to catecholamines	No	Yes	Yes	No
Produces excessive salivation and respiratory secretions	No	No	No	Yes
Potentiates neuromuscular blocking agents	No	Yes	Yes	Yes
Nausea and vomiting during emergence	Low	Frequent	Low	Frequent
Liver damage	No	No	Moderate	No
Kidney damage	No	No	No	No
Heat regulatory center	NC	Depressed	Depressed	Depressed
Release of epinephrine from the adrenal gland	No	Increased	Decreased	Increased
Analgesia	Good	Good	Poor	Good
Muscle relaxation	NC	Adequate	Minimal	Good

NC = no change. Nitrous oxide (N₂O) is a nonexplosive and nonflammable gas.

Halothane is a potent anesthetic agent with properties that allow a smooth and rather rapid loss of consciousness that progresses to anesthesia. **Thiopental** is used for induction of anesthesia, and halothane is used for its maintenance (see Table 15).

The signs of depth of anesthesia achieved with halothane that are of the most practical value are blood pressure, which is progressively depressed, and response to surgical stimulation (e.g., pulse rate, blood pressure, movement, or even awakening). Hypotension results from two main effects. First, the myocardium is depressed directly, and cardiac output is decreased; second, the normal baroreceptor-mediated tachycardia in response to hypotension is obtunded.

If the patient anesthetized with halothane is allowed to breathe spontaneously, an increased partial pressure of carbon dioxide in the arterial blood is common and is indicative of ventilatory depression. There also is an increased difference between the partial pressure of oxygen in the alveolar gas and in the arterial blood, indicating less efficient exchange of gas. Halothane thus influences both ventilatory control and the efficiency of oxygen transfer. To compensate for these effects, ventilation frequently is assisted or controlled by manual or mechanical means, and the concentration of inspired oxygen is increased.

Because cerebral blood flow generally increases during halothane anesthesia, cerebrospinal fluid pressure increases. Halothane thus may aggravate conditions in which the intracranial pressure is elevated. The cerebral metabolic consumption of oxygen is reduced. Recovery of mental function after even brief anesthesia with halothane is not complete for several hours, but this phenomenon probably contributes little to the more prolonged impairment of psychological performance that has been reported after major surgery. Shivering during recovery is common and represents both a response to heat loss and an expression of neurological recovery.

Anesthesia with halothane causes some relaxation by central depression; in addition, the duration and magnitude of the muscular relaxation induced by nondepolarizing skeletal muscle relaxants such as tubocurarine or pancuronium are increased (see also Figure 92).

Inhibition of natural or induced uterine contractions by halothane during parturition may prolong the process of delivery, as well as increase blood loss. Thus, other agents or techniques may be preferred for the relief of obstetrical pain.

Halothane causes dose-dependent reductions of renal blood flow and the rate of glomerular filtration.

Halothane-induced hepatitis that occurs in the postoperative period most often is due to transmission of hepatitis virus (e.g., in transfused blood), involvement of the liver by disease processes, or damage by known hepatotoxic drugs. Hepatic necrosis, although rare, does occur with halothane.

Approximately 60 to 80% of absorbed halothane is eliminated unchanged in the exhaled gas in the first 24 hours after its administration, and smaller amounts continue to be exhaled for several days or even weeks. Of the fraction not exhaled, as much as 50% undergoes biotransformation, and the rest is eliminated unchanged by other routes.

In conclusion, the introduction of **enflurane, isoflurane**, and **desflurane**, and the availability of a variety of intravenous agents has dramatically reduced the use of halothane in more recent years (see Table 15).

HEART FAILURE: TREATMENT OF	
ACE Inhibitors	
Captopril	Quinapril
Enalapril	Lisinopril
Enalaprilat	Ramipril
Angiotensin Receptor Antagonist	
Losartan	
Adrenergic Receptor Antagonists	
Bucindolol	Phentolamine
Carvedilol	Prazosin
Labetalol	Quinazoline
Ca^{2+} Channel Blocking Drugs	
Amlodipine	
Nifedipine	
"Direct" Vasodilators	
Hydralazine	
Nicorandil	
Nitrovasodilators	
Isosorbide dinitrate	
Nitroglycerin	
Sodium nitroprusside	
Phosphodiesterase Inhibitors	
Amrinone	
Milrinone	
Vesnarinone	
Sympathomimetics	
Dobutamine	

HEMICHOLINIUM

Acetylcholine receptors are classified as either **muscarinic** or **nicotinic**. The alkaloid muscarine mimics the effects produced by stimulation of the parasympathetic system. These effects are postganglionic and are exerted on exocrine glands, cardiac muscles, and smooth muscle. The alkaloid **nicotine** mimics the actions of acetylcholine, which include stimulation of all autonomic ganglia, stimulation of the adrenal medulla, and contraction of skeletal muscle.

Dimethylphenylpipazinium stimulates the autonomic ganglia; tetraethylammonium and **hexamethonium** block the autonomic ganglia; phenyltrimethylammonium stimulates skeletal muscle end plates; decamethonium produces neuromuscular blockage; and *d*-tubocurarine blocks the autonomic ganglia and the motor fiber end plates.

Among the agents cited, only *d*-tubocurarine is useful as a drug (skeletal muscle relaxant); the rest are useful only as research tools (see Figures 18 and 92).

HEMOSTATIC MECHANISMS AND DRUGS INFLUENCING THEM
Drugs Affecting Platelet Functions
Antiplatelet Agents
Cyclo-oxygenase inhibitors
Aspirin
Sulfinpyrazone
Other nonsteroidal antiinflammatory agents
Phosphodiesterase inhibitors (dipyridamole)
Ticlopidine
Phospholipase inhibitors
Thromboxane synthetase inhibitors
Prostacyclin
Thromboxane receptor blockers
Platelet Promoting Agents
Desmopressin
Estrogens
Drugs Affecting Coagulation
Anticoagulant Agents
Heparin
Vitamin K antagonists
Coumarins (warfarin and dicoumarol)
Indanediones
Ancrod
Procoagulant agents
Vitamin K
Desmopressin
Danazol
Drugs Affecting Fibrinolysis
Antifibrinolytic agents
Lysine analogs
Epsilon amino caproic acid
Tranexamic acid
Profibrinolytic Agents
Urinary plasminogen activator
Urokinase
Streptokinase
Tissue plasminogen activator
Single-chain urinary plasminogen activator
Anistreplase

TABLE 16
Pharmacology of Heparin and Coumarin

Properties Studied	Heparin	Coumarin
Chemistry	High negative charge	
Occurrence	Naturally occurring in most tissues	Synthetic
Mechanism of action	Activates plasma antithrombin, blocks thromboplastin generation, neutralizes tissue thromboplastin	Inhibits the synthesis of factors II, VII, IX, and X by blocking the action of vitamin K
Pharmacokinetics		
Route of administration	Subcutaneously, intravenously	Orally
Onset	Minutes (10–20)	48 hrs
Duration	4 hr (subcutaneously)	2–10 days
Protein binding and metabolism	In liver by heparinase; inactive metabolite is excreted by the kidney	Bound to albumin (99%), side-chain reduction to alcohol (dextrowarfarin), oxidation to 7-hydroxywarfarin (levowarfarin)
Antagonists	Protamine sulfate, a strongly basic protein, forms complex with heparin to an inactive compound; 1 mg protamine for 100 units of heparin	Vitamin K, whole blood, fresh plasma

HEPARIN

Commercial heparin is a sulfated mucopolysaccharide of repeating units of D-glucosamine, D-glucuronic acid, and L-iduronic acid. The comparative pharmacology of heparin and coumarin is shown in Table 16.

The use of heparin and other anticoagulants is contraindicated in the presence of active hemorrhage, potential hemorrhage (acid pepsin disease), and hemorrhagic disorders (hemophilia).

Heparin and other anticoagulants should be used with extreme caution in patients with traumatic injuries to the central nervous system or the eyes because it is very difficult to control hemorrhage in these areas. The possible existence of an aneurysm must be considered in an untreated hypertensive patient.

Anticoagulant therapy during pregnancy is indicated for the treatment and prophylaxis of venous thromboembolic disease and systemic embolism associated with valvular heart disease or prosthetic heart valves. However, there are special problems that need to be considered when deciding on optimal anticoagulant therapy in pregnant women. Heparin does not cross the placenta and is probably safe for the fetus. However, long-term heparin therapy is occasionally associated with maternal hemorrhage and rarely with symptomatic osteoporosis. Coumarin derivatives cross the placenta and are potentially teratogenic, particularly in the first trimester. Neonatal hemorrhage is a risk if warfarin is administered to the pregnant mother near term.

Anticoagulant therapy should be monitored carefully in patients with severe hepatic or renal failure, vitamin K deficiency, or alcoholism, and those with arthritis who are taking acetyl-salicylic acid in large quantities. Furthermore, anticoagulants are extensively metabolized and their metabolites excreted, which can have an important bearing in patients suffering from renal disorders.

HEPARIN CALCIUM

(Calciparine)

HEPARIN SODIUM

(Heparin Lock Flush, Hep-Lock, Heplock U/P, Liquaemin Sodium)

Heparin (5,000 to 7,500 units IV push) is used in the treatment of pulmonary embolism, in prophylaxis of embolism, in open-heart surgery, in disseminated intravascular coagulation, and in an effort to maintain patency of IV indwelling catheters.

HEPATITIS B IMMUNE GLOBULIN, HUMAN (HBIG)

(H-BIG, Hep-B Gammagee, HyperHep)

Hepatitis B immune globulin, a hepatitis B prophylaxis product (0.6 ml/kg IM) is used within seven days of exposure to hepatitis B.

HEPATITIS B VACCINE, RECOMBINANT (INACTIVATED)

(Engerix-B, Recombivax HB, Recombivax HB Dialysis Formulation)

Hepatitis B vaccine (20 mcg IM followed by a second dose of 20 mcg IM 30 days later) is used in immunization against infection from all known subtypes of hepatitis B; primary preexposure prophylaxis against hepatitis B; or postexposure prophylaxis (when given with hepatitis B immune globulin).

HEPOXILINS

Hepoxilins are monohydroxy-epoxide derivatives of arachidonic acid which release intracellular calcium and open potassium channels. Hepoxilins appear to have proinflammatory actions in the skin, but inhibit the actions of inflammatory agents in the human neutrophil. Hepoxilin receptors have recently been identified which are coupled to G-proteins (see Figure 42).

HETASTARCH

(HES, Hydroxyethyl Starch) (Hespan)

Hetastarch, an amylopectin derivative and plasma volume expander (500 to 1000 ml IV), is used in shock and cardiopulmonary bypass surgery.

HICCUP: TREATMENT OF			
Hiccup, or singultus, is a spasmodic, involuntary contraction of the inspiratory muscles, associated with delayed, abrupt glottic closure, causing a peculiar sound, expressed by different words around the world. They are:			
Czkawka	Polish	Hoquet	French
Geehouk	Hebrew	Ikota	Russian
Hakka	Arabic	Lozingas	Greek
Hiccup, hiccough	English	Nac	Vietnamese
Hicka	Swedish	Schluckauf	German
Hiçkirik	Turkish	Sekseke	Parsi
Hik	Dutch	Singhiozzo	Italian
Hikke	Norwegian, Danish	Singultus	Latin
Hipo	Spanish	Sughitz	Romanian
Hirik	Kurd	Tale	Chinese

Hiccup is a forceful, involuntary inspiration commonly experienced by fetuses, children, and adults. Its purpose is unknown and its pathophysiology still poorly understood. Short hiccup bouts are mostly associated with gastric distention or alcohol intake. They resolve spontaneously or with simple folk remedies and do not require medical attention. In contrast, prolonged hiccup is a rare but disabling condition which can induce depression, weight loss, and sleep deprivation. A wide variety of pathological conditions can cause chronic hiccup: myocardial infarction, brain tumor, renal failure, prostate cancer, and abdominal surgery are only a few of these conditions.

Drugs that have been shown to be effective in treating hiccup are:

Amitriptyline	Chlorpromazine	Mephenesin	Orphenadrine
Baclofen	Diphenylhydantoin	Metoclopramide	
Carbamazepine	Haloperidol	Nifedipine	Valproic acid

Baclofen, chlorpromazine, or metoclopramide are most effective.

HIRSUTISM: TREATMENT OF

Hirsutism results from the change of fine, vellus hair to visible, thickened, terminal hair under the influence of dihydrotestosterone, a biologically active form of testosterone. This androgen-dependent hair growth develops in defined patterns. Terminal hair is a normal phenomenon and is often found on the upper lip, the chin, around the nipples and the midline of the lower abdomen.

Drugs causing hirsutism are:

Androgens	**Drugs causing hyperprolactinemia**
Anabolic steroids	High-dose phenothiazines
Some progestogens	Metoclopramide
Danazol	

Patient distress is the prime indication for therapy. Drug treatment should be continued for 12 months before assessing response. Spironolactone is generally the drug tried first. Ovarian hormones, e.g. medroxyprogesterone acetate plus ethinyl estradiol, or cyproterone acetate plus ethinyl estradiol may be added if response is inadequate.

HIRUDIN

The saliva of the medicinal leech contains a battery of substances that interfere with the hemostatic mechanisms of the host. One of these compounds is **hirudin**, a potent anticoagulant that maintains the fluidity of the ingested blood, and the most potent inhibitor of thrombin. Upon binding to thrombin, the cleavage of fibrinogen and subsequent clot formation are prevented. The potency and specificity of hirudin suggest it as a useful antithrombin III-independent alternative to heparin for the control of thrombosis (Table 17).

HISTAMINE

Histamine is synthesized in enterochromaffin-like cells, mucosal mast cells, and nerves, according to the following reaction.

$$\text{Histidine} \xrightarrow{\text{Histidine decarboxylase}} \text{Histamine}$$

Histamine is metabolized by histamine N-methyltransferase to N-methylhistamine, which is then deaminated by monoamine oxidase type B into methylimidazole acetic acid. Histamine

TABLE 17
Comparison of Hirudin and Heparin as Anticoagulants

Heparin	Hirudin
Heteropolysaccharide with various chain lengths (5,000-25,000 Da)	Polypeptide (7,000 Da)
Needs antithrombin III as a cofactor	Direct interaction with thrombin
Heparin/antithrombin III complexes react also with various other factors of the coagulation/fibrinolysis cascades	Selective for thrombin
High affinity for numerous other compounds (e.g., platelets, endothelium)	Pharmacologically inert
May cause thrombocytopenia and bleeding	No side effects observed
Low-molecular-weight heparins (approx. 3,000-5,000 Da) with special properties available	Smaller synthetic hirudin derivatives (approx. 2,000 Da) inhibit thrombin effectively

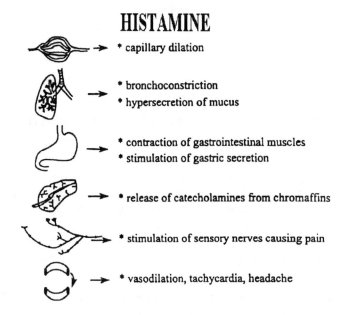

HISTAMINE

* capillary dilation

* bronchoconstriction
* hypersecretion of mucus

* contraction of gastrointestinal muscles
* stimulation of gastric secretion

* release of catecholamines from chromaffins

* stimulation of sensory nerves causing pain

* vasodilation, tachycardia, headache

FIGURE 49   The release of histamine is stimulated by **numerous drugs** including **reserpine, codeine, meperidine, hydralazine, morphine, d-tubocurarine, dextrans,** and **papaverine**. (Adapted from Ebadi, M., *Pharmacology, An Illustrated Review with Questions and Answers*, 3rd Edition, Lippincott-Raven Press, Philadelphia, 1996.)

is also found in platelets, leukocytes, and basophils in the skin, lungs, and gastric mucosa, as well as to a certain extent in blood, plasma, sputum, gastric juice, blister fluid, and pus. Histamine is stored mostly in mast cells.

Histamine may be used **diagnostically** to identify patients with **pheochromocytoma** (it increases the release of catecholamines) and to distinguish **pernicious anemia** (a lack of acid release indicates achlorhydria).

Histamine is involved in the immunoglobulin E-mediated immune responses that initiate and maintain a host of inflammatory and allergic reactions, including lysosomal enzyme release from neutrophils, lymphocyte proliferation in response to mitogens, lymphocyte-mediated cytolysis, and antibody production and secretion (see Figure 49).

Histamine, as a normal constituent of the gastric mucosa, controls both microcirculation and gastric secretion. The gastric secretagogues are acetylcholine, histamine, and gastrin (see Figure 24). The action of acetylcholine is blocked by atropine, and the action of histamine is blocked by **cimetidine, burimamide**, and **metiamide**. No specific antagonist is available for gastrin.

The histamine release in the brain and perhaps other sites involves **exocytosis**, since this potassium-induced release is a calcium-dependent process. Histamine is released by many factors. For example, histamine is released by **numerous drugs** including **reserpine, codeine, meperidine, hydralazine, morphine, d**-tubocurarine, dextrans, papaverine, and **compound 48/80**. However, the different histamine storage sites show certain degrees of **specificity**. For example, the histamine in mast cells is not released following potassium-induced depolarization or by reserpine, factors that release histamine from neurons. Conversely, compound 48/80, which releases histamine from mast cells, is not able to release histamine from neurons.

In the peripheral system, histamine causes capillary dilation and increased permeability, bronchoconstriction and contraction of gastrointestinal muscles, stimulation of chromaffin cells releasing catecholamines, vasodilation, tachycardia, headache, stimulation of exocrine secretion causing hypersecretion of mucus in the lungs, and stimulation of gastric secretion (see Figure 49).

The diversified actions of histamine are brought forth through their interaction with different types of receptors, which are described in the following sections.

Histamine$_1$ (H$_1$) receptors mediate such actions as bronchoconstriction and the contraction of smooth muscles in the gastrointestinal tract. These effects are blocked by classic antihistaminics such as **pyrilamine.**

Stimulation of the H$_2$ receptors elicits a variety of responses, the most widely studied of which is **gastric acid secretion** from the parietal cells of the gastric glands. However, many other effects mediated by H$_2$ receptors are manifested in peripheral tissues. These include the positive chronotropic action in the auricular muscle, the inotropic action in the ventricular muscle, and the lipolytic effect in fat cells. In addition, the extensive use of **cimetidine** has led to the synthesis and marketing of more specific and efficacious analogs with pharmacologic properties (see Table 9).

H$_3$ receptors suppress **gastric acid secretion,** and this is evoked by cholinergic stimuli. H$_3$ receptors exist outside the parietal cells and seem to be located on cholinergic and nonadrenergic neurons of the myenteric plexus, where they inhibit the release of neurotransmitters. The agonist and antagonist for H$_3$ receptors are **alpha-methylhistamine** and **thioperamide**, respectively.

HISTOPLASMIN
(Histolyn-CYL, Histoplasmin Diluted)

Histoplasmin, a histoplasma capsulatum antigen (0.1 ml of 1:100 dilution interdermally 5 to 10 cm apart into the volar surface of the forearm), is used to assess cell-mediated immunity and in suspected histoplasmosis.

HISTRELIN ACETATE
(Supprelin)

Histrelin, a gonadotropin releasing hormone, is used in centrally mediated idiopathic or neurogenic precocious puberty (see also Table 14).

HOMATROPINE HYDROBROMIDE
(Lolab)

Homatropine is a moderately long-acting mydriatic and cycloplegic, which is used for refraction (1 to 2 drops into each eye) in the treatment of inflammatory conditions of uveal tract; for preoperative and postoperative states when mydriasis is required; and in axial lens opacities.

HUMAN IMMUNODEFICIENCY VIRUS (HIV) INFECTION: TREATMENT FOR

HIV is a single-stranded RNA virus which contains a virally encoded DNA polymerase enzyme, reverse transcriptase (RT). The HIV RT is the enzyme responsible for transcribing viral RNA into DNA, a cytoplasmic event. Following reverse transcription, the HIV DNA enters the cell nucleus and, through the action of another viral enzyme (integrase), is incorporated into the host cell genome. It is the event, the incorporation into host DNA, which makes HIV infection a chronic, lifelong disease, since each time the lymphocyte is activated and the DNA transcribed and translated, new HIV virions are created and released.

The classification of antiretroviral agents for HIV infection is primarily based upon the stage of the life cycle which is interrupted by the therapeutic intervention. The primary steps in the life cycle include: 1) viral binding to cell surface receptors; 2) viral entry and uncoating; 3) transcription to DNA via the action of viral reverse transcriptase; 4) integration into the host DNA via the action of viral integrase; 5) transcription of the proviral DNA to mRNA and viral RNA and the translation of other viral proteins; 6) glycosylation of viral proteins; 7) viral assembly; and 8) budding of new viral particles through the host cell membrane (a time during which the action of HIV protease is evident). Each of these stages is currently under investigation in order to examine the potential value at each point of interference with HIV replication.

The medical aspects of HIV infection include:

- AIDS-related complex (weight loss, chronic diarrhea, fever, thrush, herpes zoster, fatigue)
- Opportunistic infections and cancer
- End-stage renal disease
- Blindness (cytomegalovirus)
- HIV encephalopathy and dementia

The psychological aspects of HIV infection include:

- Major depression, regression, and suicidal impulses
- Delirium
- Substance abuse
- Antisocial personality
- Bereavement

Patients with a clinical diagnosis of AIDS should undergo long-term therapy with reverse transcriptase inhibitors such as zidovudine (AZT, 1,200 mg every 4 hours). Protease inhibitors or antiviral agents such as acyclovir may potentiate the beneficial effects of AZT. In addition, patients should be treated prophylactically for *Pneumocystis carinii* pneumonia; such regimens include sulfadoxine and pyrimethamine (Fansidar), dapsone, or aerolized pentamidine. Dextran sulfate is also useful because it blocks the binding of HIV to target cells.

The currently approved reverse transcriptase inhibitors are:
Didanosine
Stavudine
Zalcitabine
Zidovudine

Protease inhibitors are:
Indinavir sulfate (Crixivan)
Ritonavir (Norvir)
Saquinavir mesylate (Invirase)

HUNTINGTON'S DISEASE: THE SEARCH FOR TREATMENT CONTINUES

Huntington's disease (HD) is a progressive degenerative disorder of the central nervous system inherited as an autosomal dominant trait. Clinically, the disorder is characterized by choreoathetosis (with age of onset typically in the late thirties or early forties) and neuropsychiatric disturbance. The striatum is particularly vulnerable to the degenerative disease process, with selective loss of medium spiny neurons and decreased levels of associated neurotransmitters, including substance P, GABA, met-enkephalin and dynorphin. Although the underlying pathophysiology is unknown, recent theories concerning pathogenesis have involved mitochondrial abnormalities and excitotoxin-mediated damage. The gene for HD has recently been discovered and characterized as an unstable CAG trinucleotide repeat sequence on the short arm of chromosome 4 (now known as IT15). The direct test now available for the HD gene has facilitated disease diagnosis, particularly for those with unclear family history or chorea of uncertain origin; presymptomatic testing is also available.

There is no cure for HD, which, as a rule, terminates fatally 10 to 20 years after clinical onset. There is no treatment for the dementia, but the movement disorder may respond to drugs that interfere with dopaminergic inhibition of striatal output neurons. These include dopamine D_2-receptor-blocking drugs such as haloperidol, 0.5 to 4 mg orally four times daily, or chlorpromazine, 25 to 50 mg orally three times daily; and drugs that deplete dopamine from nerve terminals, such as reserpine, 0.5 to 5 mg orally daily, or tetrabenazine (unavailable in the United States), 12.5 to 50 mg orally three times daily. Drugs that potentiate GABAergic or cholinergic neurotransmission are generally ineffective.

HYALURONIDASE

(Wydase)

Hyaluronidase, an enzyme, is used as an adjunct to increase absorption and dispersion of other injected drugs, as an adjunct to increase the absorption rate of fluids given by hypodermoclysis, and as an adjunct in excretion urography.

HYDRALAZINE

(Apresoline)

Hydralazine is the drug most often used in the treatment of **moderate to severe hypertension**. The decrease in total peripheral resistance it brings about causes reflex elevation of the heart rate and enhanced cardiac output. This cardiac acceleration, which may precipitate an **angina attack** in susceptible individuals, can be blocked with beta-adrenergic blocking agents (see Figure 14). **Propranolol** also has a synergistic effect in reducing blood pressure. Hydralazine use can produce headache, palpitations, and gastrointestinal complications. The long-term administration of large doses causes a reversible **lupus erythematosus-like syndrome**. Hydralazine does not alter sympathetic functions.

HYDROCHLOROTHIAZIDE

(Essidrix, Hydro-Diuril)

The thiazide diuretics, also called *sulfonamide* or *benzothiadiazide diuretics*, vary in their actions. For instance, the potency of **hydrochlorothiazide** is ten times greater than that of **chlorothiazide** (Diuril), but the two drugs have equal efficacy. The duration of action of hydrochlorothiazide, which is 6 to 12 hours, is equal to that of chlorothiazide. On the other hand, **chlorthalidone** (Hygroton) has a duration of action lasting 48 hours. Some thiazide derivatives inhibit carbonic anhydrase, which is unrelated to their diuretic activity. Those that are active in this respect may at sufficient dose have the same effect as acetazolamide on bicarbonate excretion. They cause a moderate loss of sodium (5 to 10% of the filtered load), chloride, and water, and the clearance of free water is impaired. They may cause **metabolic alkalosis** (resorption of bicarbonate and loss of hydrogen ions), **hyperuricemia** (enhanced resorption of uric acid), or **hypokalemia**) (see also Figure 4).

Thiazide diuretics are used in the treatment of edema of cardiac and gastrointestinal origin and bring about a state of intravascular volume depletion. Because this depleted intravascular volume is replenished from the interstitial (edematous) sites, the thiazide diuretics should not be administered too frequently. For example, hydrochlorothiazide is given q. other day and chlorthalidone is given once q. 2 to 3 days.

In small doses, thiazide diuretics are extremely effective in controlling essential hypertension. They exert their effects initially by bringing about volume depletion, then reduce the peripheral resistance and sensitivity of vascular receptor sites to catecholamine. Thiazide diuretics are also used in conjunction with antihypertensive medications.

The thiazides decrease the urinary calcium concentration by diminishing glomerular filtration and also enhance the urinary magnesium level.

The thiazide diuretics can reduce free water formation in patients with diabetes insipidus, in whom large amounts of free water are eliminated.

The loss of potassium can produce **hypokalemia**, which is particularly dangerous in patients receiving **digitalis** because it increases the risk of **arrhythmias**. Hypokalemia can be offset either by giving a potassium supplement (potassium chloride), or by the concurrent use of a potassium-sparing diuretic. However, the caregiver should not adopt both measures because **hyperkalemia** will result. **Hyperglycemia** is a potential hazard for patients with **diabetes mellitus. Hyperuricemia** can precipitate an acute attack of **gout**, but usually only in those patients who either have already had gout or have a propensity toward it. Since thiazides can cause a decrease in the GFR, they should not be used in patients whose renal function is less than one-third of normal. The risk of thiazide-induced **hypercalcemia** should be kept in mind in patients with conditions such as **malignancies** or **hyperparathyroidism** that are associated with hypercalcemia (see also Table 25).

HYDROCODONE

(Dicodid; Hycodan)

In this synthetic derivative of codeine, a ketone group replaces the –OH of codeine at position 6, and two H atoms are added at positions 7 and 8. It thus bears the same relation to codeine as dihydromorphinone (Dilaudid) does to morphine. It is marketed as the tartrate under the trade names Dicodid and Hycodan and is used chiefly for the relief of cough.

HYDROCORTISONE

Hydrocortisone is an adrenocorticoid with both glucocorticoid and mineralocorticoid properties. It is a weak antiinflammatory agent but a potent mineralocorticoid, having potency similar to that of cortisone and twice that of prednisone. Hydrocortisone (or cortisone) is usually the drug of choice for replacement therapy in patients with adrenal insufficiency. It is usually not used for immunosuppressant activity because of the extremely large doses necessary and the unwanted mineralocorticoid effects.

Hydrocortisone and hydrocortisone cypionate (**Cortef**) may be administered orally. Hydrocortisone sodium phosphate may be administered by IM, subcutaneous, or IV injection, or by IV infusion, q. 12-hour interval. Hydrocortisone sodium succinate (A-hydroCort, Lifocort, Solu-Cortef) may be administered by IM or IV injection or IV infusion q. 2 to 10 hours, depending on the clinical situation. Hydrocortisone acetate is a suspension that may be administered by intra-articular, intrasynovial, intrabursal, intralesional, or soft tissue injection. It has a slow onset but a long duration of action. The injectable forms are usually used only when the oral dosage forms cannot be used (see also Table 10).

When administered in high doses or for prolonged therapy, hydrocortisone suppresses release of adrenocorticotropic hormone (ACTH) from the pituitary gland, and the adrenal cortex stops secreting endogenous corticosteroids. Since hydrocortisone suppresses immune response, patients should not be given live virus vaccines.

Hydrocortisone should be used with extreme caution in patients with GI ulceration, renal disease, hypertension, osteoporosis, diabetes mellitus, thromboembolic disorders, seizures, myasthenia gravis, congestive heart failure (CHF), tuberculosis, hypoalbuminemia, hypothyroidism, cirrhosis of the liver, emotional instability, psychotic tendencies, hyperlipidemias, glaucoma or cataracts, because the drug may exacerbate these conditions (see Tables 10 and 13).

HYDROCORTISONE (SYSTEMIC)
(Cortef, Cortenema, Hydrocortone)

HYDROCORTISONE ACETATE
(Biosone, Cortifoam)

HYDROCORTISONE CYPIONATE
(Cortef)

HYDROCORTISONE SODIUM PHOSPHATE
(HydroCortone Phosphate)

HYDROCORTISONE SODIUM SUCCINATE
(A-hydroCort, Efcortelan, Lifocort, Solu-Cortef)

Hydrocortisone salts, possessing glucocorticoid-mineralocorticoid properties, are used in severe inflammation or adrenal insufficiency, in shock (other than adrenal crisis), and as an adjunctive treatment of ulcerative colitis and proctitis (see also Table 10).

HYDROCORTISONE (TOPICAL)
(Acticort, CaldeCORT, Cetacort, Cort-Dome, Cortizone, Dermacort, Dermi Cort, Dermolate, Dermtex HC, HC-JEL, HI-COR, H$_2$ Cort, Hydro-Tex, Hytone, Nutracort, Penecort, Racet-SE, Synacort)

HYDROCORTISONE ACETATE
(Cortaid, Cort-Dome, Corticaine, Lanacort, Orabase-HCA, Pharma-Cort, Rhulicort)

Hydrocortisone, a topical glucocorticoid with antiinflammatory properties, is indicated in inflammation of corticosteroid-responsive dermatoses, including those on the face, groin, armpits, and under the breasts; and in seborrheic dermatitis of the scalp.

HYDROFLUMETHIAZIDE
(Diucardin, Saluron)

Hydroflumethiazide, a thiazide diuretic with antihypertensive properties (25 to 200 mg p.o. daily), is used in edema or hypertension (see also Figure 25).

HYDROMORPHONE HYDROCHLORIDE
(Dilaudid, Dilaudid-HP)

Hydromorphone, an opioid analgesic (1 to 6 mg p.o. q. 4 to 6 hours p.r.n.), is used in moderate to severe pain (see also Figure 58).

HYDROXYCHLOROQUINE SULFATE

(Plaquenil Sulfate)

Hydroxychloroquine, a 4-amino-quinoline derivative with antimalarial and antiinflammatory properties (400 mg p.o. weekly), is used in suppressive prophylaxis of malarial attacks.

HYDROXYPROGESTERONE CAPROATE IN OIL

(Delalutin)

Hydroxyprogesterone is a long-acting progestin with a duration of action of 9 to 17 days. It is administered intramuscularly in a dose of 375 mg in primary and secondary amenorrhea, dysfunctional uterine bleeding, and metrorrhagia.

Hydroxyprogesterone suppresses ovulation, causes thickening of cervical mucus, and induces sloughing of the endometrium. It inhibits growth progression of progestin-sensitive uterine cancer tissue by an unknown mechanism.

The concomitant use of hydroxyprogesterone and bromocriptine may cause amenorrhea or galactorrhea, thus interfering with the action of bromocriptine. Concurrent use of these drugs is not recommended.

Hydroxyprogesterone is contraindicated in patients with a history of thromboembolic disorders because of its potential for causing thromboembolic disorders; in patients with severe hepatic disease because impaired hepatic metabolism may cause the drug to accumulate in patients with breast or genital cancer because it may induce tumor growth; in patients with undiagnosed abnormal vaginal bleeding because the origin should be determined; and in pregnant or breast-feeding women.

Hydroxyprogesterone should be used cautiously in patients with existing conditions that might be aggravated by fluid and electrolyte retention, such as cardiac or renal disease, epilepsy, or migraine. Caution is also advised in administering this agent to diabetic patients (because decreased glucose tolerance may occur) or to patients with a history of mental depression.

HYDROXYUREA

(Hydrea)

Hydroxyurea, an antimetabolite with antineoplastic properties (60 to 80 mg/kg p.o. for a minimum of six weeks), is used in the treatment of melanoma; chronic myelocytic leukemia; recurrent, metastatic, or inoperable ovarian cancer; squamous cell carcinoma of the head and neck; polycythemia vera; and essential thrombocytosis (see also Figure 2).

HYDROXYZINE

(Atarax)

Oral hydroxyzine (50 to 100 mg q.i.d.) is indicated for symptomatic relief of anxiety and tension associated with psychoneurosis and as an adjunct in organic disease states in which anxiety is manifest. Hydroxyzine is used for the management of pruritus due to allergic conditions such as chronic urticaria, atopic and contact dermatoses, and in histamine-mediated pruritus. It is also used as a sedative, as a preanesthetic medication, and following general anesthesia.

Intramuscular hydroxyzine (100 mg q. 4 hours) is indicated for the acutely disturbed or hysterical patient; the acute or chronic alcoholic with anxiety withdrawal symptoms or delirium tremens; as pre- and postoperative and pre- and postpartum adjunctive medication to permit reduction in narcotic dosage, allay anxiety and control emesis; and as an adjunctive therapy in asthma.

Hydroxyzine is a piperazine antihistaminic agent that suppresses activity in the subcortical area of the CNS. It has skeletal muscular relaxant properties and exhibits antiemetic, analgesic, and bronchodilating actions.

Hydroxyzine may be teratogenic in experimental animals and should not be used in pregnancy. It causes drowsiness, and caution should be exercised while performing tasks requiring alertness. Hydroxyzine potentiates the CNS depressant effects of narcotics and barbiturates.

HYOSCYAMINE

(Cystospaz)

HYOSCYAMINE SULFATE

(Anaspaz, Bellaspaz, Cystospaz-M, Levsin, Levsin Drops, Levsinex, Timecaps, Neoquess)

Hyoscyamine, a belladonna alkaloid with anticholinergic properties (0.125 to 0.25 mg p.o. t.i.d.), is used in GI tract disorders caused by spasm, and as an adjunctive therapy for peptic ulcers.

HYPERBARIC-OXYGEN THERAPY

Hyperbaric oxygen — 100% oxygen at 2 to 3 times the atmospheric pressure at sea level — can result in arterial oxygen tension in excess of 2000 mmHg and oxygen tension in tissue of almost 400 mmHg. Such doses of oxygen have a number of beneficial biochemical, cellular, and physiologic effects. Hyperbaric oxygen therapy has been used in carbon monoxide poisoning, compromised skin grafts, decompression sickness, anemia, arterial gas embolism, radiation-induced tissue injury, clostridial myonecrosis, necrotizing fascilitis, refractory osteomyelitis, acute traumatic ischemic injury, problem wounds, and thermal burns.

HYPERGLYCEMIA: DRUG-INDUCED	
β_2-Adrenergic receptor agonists	Marijuana
Ca^{2+}-channel blockers	Morphine
Clonidine	Nalidixic acid
Diazoxide	Nicotine
Diuretics	Oral contraceptives
Epinephrine	Pentamidine
Glucocorticosteroids	Phenytoin
H_2-receptor blockers	Sulfinpyrazone
Heparin	

HYPERTENSION: TREATMENT OF	
Drugs	**Adverse Effects**
Angiotensin-Converting Enzyme (ACE) Inhibitors	
Captopril	Cough; hypotension, particularly with a diuretic or volume depletion; loss of taste with anorexia; skin rash; bronchospasm; acute renal failure with bilateral renal artery stenosis or stenosis of the artery to a solitary kidney; cholestatic jaundice; angioedema; hyperkalemia if also on potassium supplements or potassium-retaining diuretics; blood dyscrasias and renal damage are rare except in patients with renal dysfunction, and particularly in patients with collagen-vascular disease; may increase fetal mortality and should not be used during pregnancy
Enalapril	Similar to captopril; pancreatitis

Drugs	Adverse Effects
Lisinopril	Similar to captopril
Ramipril	Similar to captopril
Calcium-Channel Blockers	
Diltiazem	Similar to verapamil, but less likely to cause constipation
Isradipine	Similar to nifedipine
Nicardipine	Similar to nifedipine
Nifedipine	Similar to verapamil, but more likely to cause edema, and less likely to cause constipation or AV block; may cause tachycardia; arthralgias
Verapamil	Heart failure; hypotension; AV block; constipation; dizziness; edema; headache; bradycardia
Diuretics	
Thiazide-Type	
Bendroflumethiazide	
Benzthiazide	
Chlorthalidone	Hyperuricemia; hypokalemia; hypomagnesemia; hyperglycemia; hyponatremia; hypercalcemia; pancreatitis; rashes and other allergic reactions; increased serum low density lipoprotein cholesterol and triglyceride concentrations, may be transient; depression; impotence
Chlorothiazide	
Cyclothiazide	
Hydrochlorothiazide	
Hydroflumethiazide	
Indapamide	
Methyclothiazide	
Metolazone	
Polythiazide	
Quinethazone	
Trichlormethiazide	
Loop Diuretics	
Bumetanide Furosemide	Dehydration; circulatory collapse; thromboembolism; hypokalemia; hypomagnesemia; hypocalcemia; hyperglycemia; metabolic alkalosis; hyperuricemia; blood dyscrasias; rashes; lipid changes as with thiazide-type diuretics
Potassium-Retaining	
Amiloride	Hyperkalemia; GI disturbances; rash; headache
Spironolactone	Hyperkalemia; hyponatremia; gynecomastia; agranulocytosis; menstrual abnormalities; GI disturbances; rash
Triamterene	Hyperkalemia; GI disturbances; increased blood urea nitrogen; metabolic acidosis; nephrolithiasis
Drugs with Peripheral Sympatholytic Action **Beta-Adrenergic Blocking Drugs**	
Acebutolol	Similar to propranolol, but has intrinsic sympathomimetic activity and is relatively cardioselective, with less lipid changes and resting bradycardia and more antinuclear antibodies; occasional drug-induced lupus erythematosus

Drugs	Adverse Effects
Atenolol	Similar to propranolol; relatively cardioselective
Betaxolol	Similar to propranolol; relatively cardioselective
Carteolol	Similar to propranolol, but has intrinsic sympathomimetic activity and less resting bradycardia and lipid changes; asthenia and muscle cramps
Labetalol	Similar to propranolol, but has intrinsic sympathomimetic activity and more orthostatic hypotension; fever; hepatotoxicity
Metoprolol	Similar to propranolol; is relatively cardioselective
Nadolol	Similar to propranolol
Penbutolol	Similar to propranolol, but has intrinsic sympathomimetic activity and fewer bradycardia and lipid changes
Pindolol	Similar to propranolol, but has intrinsic sympathomimetic activity and fewer resting bradycardia and lipid changes
Propranolol	Fatigue; depression; bradycardia; decreased exercise tolerance; congestive heart failure; aggravates peripheral vascular disease; GI disturbances; increased airway resistance; masks symptoms of hypoglycemia; Raynaud's phenomenon; vivid dreams or hallucinations; organic brain syndrome; rare blood dyscrasias and other allergic disorders; increased serum triglycerides, decreased HDL cholesterol; generalized pustular psoriasis; transient hearing loss; sudden withdrawal can lead to exacerbation of angina and myocardial infarction
Timolol	Similar to propranolol

Peripheral Adrenergic Neuron Antagonists

Guanadrel	Similar to guanethidine, but less diarrhea
Guanethidine	Orthostatic hypotension; exercise hypotension; diarrhea; may aggravate bronchial asthma; bradycardia; sodium and water retention; retrograde ejaculation
Reserpine	Psychic depression; nightmares; nasal stuffiness; drowsiness; GI disturbances; bradycardia

Alpha-Adrenergic Blockers

Prazosin	Syncope with first dose; dizziness and vertigo; palpitations; fluid retention; headache; drowsiness; weakness; anticholinergic effects; priapism; urinary incontinence
Terazosin	Similar to prazosin
Doxazosin	Similar to prazosin, but with less hypotension after first dose

Drugs with Central Sympatholytic Action

Clonidine	Severe insomnia and rebound hypertension; headache; cardiac arrhythmias after sudden withdrawal; CNS reactions similar to methyldopa, but more sedation and dry mouth; bradycardia; contact dermatitis from patches
Guanabenz	Similar to clonidine
Guanfacine	Similar to clonidine, but milder
Methyldopa	Sedation and other CNS symptoms; fever; orthostatic hypotension; bradycardia; GI disorders, including colitis; hepatitis; cirrhosis; hepatic necrosis; Coombs' positive hemolytic anemia; lupus-like syndrome; immune thrombocytopenia; red cell aplasia

Direct Vasodilators

Hydralazine	GI disturbances; tachycardia; aggravation of angina; headache and dizziness; fluid retention; nasal congestion; rashes and other allergic reactions; lupus-like syndrome; hepatitis; glomerulonephritis
Minoxidil	Tachycardia; aggravation of angina; marked fluid retention; possible pericardial effusion; hair growth on face and body; coarsening of facial features; thrombocytopenia; leukopenia

HYPERTENSIVE EMERGENCIES: TREATMENT OF

Drugs	Class	Comments
Parenteral		
Nitroprusside	Arteriolar and venous vasodilator	Thiocyanate toxicity with prolonged or too rapid infusion; should not be used in pregnancy
Nitroglycerin	Venous ≫ arteriolar vasodilator	Headache, tachycardia
Diazoxide	Arteriolar vasodilator	Not for patients with angina pectoris, myocardial infarction, dissecting aneurysm or pulmonary edema; can increase blood sugar; will arrest active labor
Trimethaphan	Ganglionic blocker	Preferred by many for emergency treatment of aortic dissection
Labetalol	Alpha- and beta-adrenergic blocker	80-90% response rate; can be followed by same drug taken orally
Hydralazine	Arteriolar vasodilator	May precipitate angina, myocardial infarction; not used for aortic dissection; main use is in pregnancy
Propranolol (Inderal; others)	Beta-adrenergic blocker	Useful as adjunct to potent vasodilators to prevent or treat excessive tachycardia; will not lower blood pressure
Enalaprilat	Angiotensin-converting enzyme inhibitor	Sometimes excessive response; not for use in pregnancy
Oral		
Nifedipine	Calcium entry blocker	Sometimes excessive response
Clonidine	Central sympatholytic	Sedation prominent; rebound hypertension can occur
Captopril	Angiotensin-converting enzyme inhibitor	Excessive response with renal artery stenosis or after diuretics; not for use in pregnancy

HYPNOTICS

Benzodiazepines	Nonbarbiturate, nonbenzodiazepines
Estazolam	Chloral hydrate
Flurazepam	Ethchlorvynol
Quazepam	Methyprylon
Temazepam	
Triazolam	
Barbiturates	**Antihistamines**
Amobarbital	Diphenhydramine
Pentobarbital	Doxylamine
Secobarbital	

HYPOGLYCEMIA: DRUG-INDUCED

Angiotensin-converting enzyme inhibitors	Naproxen
β-Adrenergic receptor antagonists	Pentamidine
Bromocriptine	Pyridoxine
Calcium salts	Salicylates
Clofibrate	Sulbactam/ampicillin
Ethanol	Sulfonamides
Indomethacin	Tetracycline
Lithium salts	Theophylline
Mebendazole	

HYPOTHALAMIC HORMONES	
Agents	**Actions**
Thyrotropin releasing hormone (TRH)	Stimulates both thyrotropin (TSH) and prolactin
Gonadotropin releasing hormone (GnRH) also known as luteinizing hormone releasing hormone (LHRH)	Stimulates both luteinizing hormone (LH) and follicle stimulating hormone (FSH)
Corticotropin releasing hormone (CRH)	Stimulates adrenocorticotropin (ACTH)
Growth hormone releasing hormone (GHRH)	Stimulates growth hormone
Somatostatin	Inhibits growth hormone
Prolactin inhibitory factor (dopamine)	Inhibits prolactin

I

IBOPAMINE

Activation of dopamine$_1$ (DA$_1$) and dopamine$_2$ (DA$_2$) receptors reduces blood pressure. DA is not useful as an antihypertensive agent because of its alpha adrenoreceptor activity. However, extensive studies in patients with hypertension have demonstrated that, after administration of alpha-adrenoreceptor blocking agents, arterial pressure is decreased with maintenance or improvement of renal blood flow.

Ibopamine is the diisobutryic ester of N-methyl dopamine (epinine). Epinine is released from ibopamine by plasma esterases after oral ingestion. Epinine is a DA$_1$-agonist that produces greater alpha-adrenoreceptor actions than DA; in addition, it is a potent beta$_2$-adrenoreceptor agonist. Ibopamine has been studied extensively for the treatment of congestive heart failure. A large number of invasive studies have shown that oral ingestion of 50 to 300 mg of ibopamine increases cardiac index and decreases systemic vascular resistance. Diuretic and natriuretic effects also have been reported in several studies.

Unlike with levodopa, nausea and vomiting do not occur with ibopamine, apparently because ibopamine does not penetrate the chemoreceptor trigger zone in the area postrema. Ibopamine may cause heartburn. Large doses of ibopamine have been shown to produce transient elevations of pulmonary wedge pressure in some patients with severe congestive heart failure, but this effect does not appear to be a serious problem with smaller doses (see Table 12).

IBUPROFEN

(Motrin)

Ibuprofen has analgesic, antipyretic, and antiinflammatory actions. It is indicated in the treatment of primary dysmenorrhea (400 mg q. 4 hours), in the management of fever (5 to 10 mg/kg), and for relief of the signs and symptoms of rheumatoid arthritis and osteoarthritis (300 to 800 mg q.i.d).

Ibuprofen should be administered cautiously to patients with a history of GI disease, hepatic or renal disease, cardiac decompensation, systemic lupus erythematosus, or bleeding abnormalities, because the drug may worsen these conditions.

Patients with known "triad" symptoms (aspirin hypersensitivity, rhinitis/nasal polyps, and asthma) are at high risk of bronchospasm. Concomitant use of ibuprofen with anticoagulants and thrombolytic drugs (coumarin derivatives, heparin, streptokinase, or urokinase) may potentiate anticoagulant effects. Bleeding problems may occur if ibuprofen is used with other drugs that inhibit platelet aggregation, such as azlocillin, parenteral carbenicillin, dextran, dipyridamole, mezlocillin, piperacillin, sulfinpyrazone, ticarcillin, valproic acid, cefamandole, cefoperazone, moxalactam, plicamycin, salicylates, or other antiinflammatory agents. Ibuprofen may displace highly protein-bound drugs from binding sites. Toxicity may occur with coumarin derivatives, phenytoin, verapamil, or nifedipine. Increased nephrotoxicity may occur with gold compounds, other antiinflammatory agents, or acetaminophen. Ibuprofen may decrease the renal clearance of methotrexate and lithium. Antacids may decrease the absorption of ibuprofen. Ibuprofen may decrease effectiveness of diuretics and antihypertensive medications. Concomitant use with diuretics may increase nephrotoxicity. Concomitant use with furosemide and thiazides may decrease their effectiveness. Clinical manifestations of overdose include dizziness, drowsiness, paresthesia, vomiting, nausea, abdominal pain, headache, sweating, nystagmus, apnea, and cyanosis (see also Table 2).

IDARUBICIN
(Idamycin)

Idarubicin, an antibiotic with antineoplastic activity (12 mg/m^2 daily by slow IV injection), is indicated in the treatment of acute myelocytic leukemia in adults, including fragment, antigen-binding, classification M^1 through M^7, in combination with other approved antileukemic agents.

IDOXURIDINE
(IDU; Herplex; Stoxik)

Idoxuridine (1 drop into infected eye/hr during the day and q. 2 hours at night) is indicated for the treatment of herpes simplex keratitis. By altering normal DNA synthesis, idoxuridine inhibits the reproduction of herpes simplex virus. IDU replaces thymidine in the enzymatic step of viral replication, produces faulty DNA, and hence a structure which loses its ability to infect and destroy ocular tissue. Corticosteroids can accelerate the spread of a viral infection and are usually contraindicated in herpes simplex epithelial infections. Idoxuridine occasionally causes irritation, pain, pruritus, inflammation or edema of the eyes or lids; and allergic reactions, photophobia, corneal clouding, stippling, and punctate defects in the corneal epithelium. The punctate defects may be a manifestation of the infection, since healing usually takes place without interruption of therapy.

IFOSFAMIDE
(IFEX)

Ifosfamide, an alkylating agent with antineoplastic properties (1.2 g/m^2/day IV for 5 days), is indicated in the treatment of testicular cancer. In addition, ifosfamide has been used in lung cancer, Hodgkin's and non-Hodgkin's lymphoma, breast cancer, acute and chronic lymphocytic leukemia, ovarian cancer, and sarcomas.

IMIPENEM-CILASTATIN SODIUM
(Primaxin I.M., Primaxin I.V.)

Imipenem, a carbapanem (thienamycin class), beta-lactam antibiotic (750 mg IM q. 12 hours), is indicated in mild to moderate lower respiratory tract, skin and skin-structure, or gynecologic infections; mild to moderate intra-abdominal infections; in serious respiratory and urinary tract infections; intra-abdominal, gynecologic, bone, joint, or skin infections; bacterial septicemia; or endocarditis.

IMIPRAMINE
(Tofranil)

The **dibenzapine derivatives** are called **tricyclic antidepressants** and include **imipramine** (Tofranil), **desipramine** (Norpramin), **amitriptyline** (Elavil), **nortriptyline** (Aventyl), **protriptyline** (Vivactil), and **doxepin** (Adapin).

Imipramine is demethylated to **desipramine**, and **amitriptyline** is demethylated to **nortriptyline.** Both metabolites are active antidepressants. Tricyclic antidepressants bind to plasma proteins to the extent of 90%, and, because of their extensive first-pass metabolism in the liver, they have very low and variable bioavailability. In circumstances when it is desirable to measure the plasma concentrations of these drugs, the concentrations of their active metabolites should also be measured.

They resemble the phenothiazide derivatives such as chlorpromazine in structure and function. Like the phenothiazine derivatives (e.g., chlorpromazine), tricyclic antidepressants (e.g., imipramine) may reduce the seizure threshold and precipitate seizures in epileptic patients, and may cause cholestatic jaundice, movement disorders, and hematologic side effects.

Unlike the phenothiazine derivatives, the tricyclic antidepressants may increase motor activity, are antidepressant, have a very slow onset and long duration of action, and have a relatively narrow margin of safety and a strong anticholinergic effect. In fact, dry mouth is the most common side effect, and other anticholinergic effects, such as tachycardia, loss of accommodation, constipation, urinary retention, and paralytic ileus, have been reported (see Tables 3 and 4).

Tricyclic antidepressants, like some of the phenothiazine derivatives, are **sedative in nature**. Those compounds containing a **tertiary amine** (imipramine, amitriptyline, and doxepin) are the most sedative. Those compounds containing a **secondary amine** (nortriptyline and desipramine) are less so, and protriptyline has no sedative effect (see Tables 4 and 5).

Tricyclic antidepressants, like some of the phenothiazine derivatives (e.g., thoriodazine), have an **anticholinergic property. Amitriptyline** is the strongest in this regard, and **desipramine** is the weakest.

The tricyclic antidepressants also have **cardiovascular actions**. In particular, they cause orthostatic hypotension by obtunding the various reflex mechanisms involved in maintaining blood pressure.

Antidepressants may block the **uptake of norepinephrine** or **serotonin** (see Table 4).

In addition to possessing anticholinergic properties, antidepressants exhibit **affinity** for alpha$_1$ and alpha$_2$-adrenergic receptors, histaminergic (H$_1$) receptors, and dopaminergic (D$_2$) receptors (see Table 5).

The first-generation tricyclic antidepressants, the monoamine oxidase inhibitors, and the newer agents can cause sedation, insomnia, orthostatic hypotension, or nausea. Because of their anticholinergic properties, they may also produce cardiac toxicities. A primary indication for the use of tricyclic antidepressants is **endogenous depression**. Before treating an endogenous depression, however, it should first be differentiated from sadness. Disabling depression and its vegetative symptoms generally respond to tricyclic antidepressants but sadness does not, though it does respond to changes in environmental events. The effective dose of tricyclic antidepressants, which are equivalent drugs, is chosen empirically. The less sedative agents are chosen for apathetic and withdrawn patients. Because the margin of safety for these agents is narrow, they should not be prescribed in large quantities for a depressed patient who may use them to attempt suicide. The anticholinergic effect of **imipramine** has been used successfully in managing **enuresis** (see Figure 50).

The **pain** associated with diabetic peripheral neuropathy, trigeminal neuralgia, or cancer may predispose such patients to depression. Tricyclic antidepressants have been shown to be effective adjuncts in managing these and similar conditions. Some episodic **phobias** are regarded as "masked" depression and thus respond to treatment with tricyclic antidepressants. **Fluoxetine**, in addition to its antidepressant property, has been used as an **appetite suppressant. Imipramine** and **desipramine** have been used as **antibulimic substances. Desipramine** has been used as part of the treatment of **alcoholism**. Because depression has led to relapsed

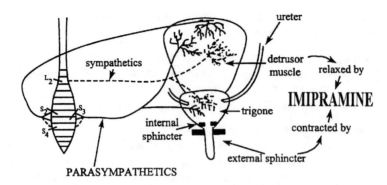

FIGURE 50   The anticholinergic effect of **imipramine** has been used successfully in managing **enuresis**. (Adapted from Ebadi, M., *Pharmacology, An Illustrated Review with Questions and Answers*, 3rd Edition, Lippincott-Raven Press, Philadelphia, 1996.)

drinking in alcoholics striving to maintain sobriety, treatment with antidepressants may reverse or prevent these depressive symptoms. They may also correct the biochemical abnormalities hypothesized to underlie both depression and alcoholism, thus helping to ensure abstinence in recovering alcoholics (see also Figure 31).

Currently, overdoses of tricyclics are one of the most serious types of poisoning encountered in clinical practice because depressed patients who are treated with these drugs are also those who are the most prone to using them for suicidal purposes.

The diagnostic triad of **coma, seizures**, and **cardiac arrhythmias** should raise the suspicion of tricyclic overdose if there is otherwise no verified history of drug intake. Cardiac arrhythmias and conduction abnormalities are the major distinguishing features. A trial dose of intravenously administered **physostigmine** (1 to 4 mg) may suggest the diagnosis, because this will awaken the comatose patient or mitigate the arrhythmias. The effects of physostigmine are transient, and it is not a definitive treatment. Other problems encountered in such poisonings include neuromuscular irritability, delirium, hyperpyrexia, hypotension, and bladder or bowel paralysis. The cardiac arrhythmias are life threatening, so the patient must be closely monitored, with facilities available for possible resuscitation. Drugs such as **quinidine** and **procainamide** are contraindicated, but **lidocaine, propranolol,** or **phenytoin** has been used safely and effectively. The arterial blood gas levels, pH, and electrolyte concentrations should be monitored so that metabolic acidosis or hypokalemia can be identified that would further aggravate the arrhythmias. Electrical pacing may be required if the antiarrhythmic drugs fail. **Hyperpyrexia** is treated by cooling. Seizures may be managed by intravenous doses of **diazepam**.

IMMUNE GLOBULIN
(Gamma Globulin; IG; Immune Serum Globulin; ISG)

IMMUNE GLOBULIN FOR IM USE
(IGIM) (Gamastan, Gammar)

IMMUNE GLOBULIN FOR IV USE
(IGIV) (Gamimune N, Gammagard, Gammar-IV, Iveegam, Sandoglobulin, Venoglobulin-1)

Immune globulin is indicated in patients with agammaglobulinemia or hypogammaglobulinemia.

IMMUNIZATION: AGENTS USED IN	
Passive Immunization	
Antitoxins Botulism Diphtheria Tetanus	
Immunoglobulins Endotoxin (IgM) Hepatitis A or B Pertussis Poliomyelitis Rabies	Rubella Tetanus Vaccinia Varicella
Active Immunization	
Bacterial Cholera Diphtheria Hemophilus Meningococci Pertussis Pneumococci Tetanus Tuberculosis (BCG) Typhoid	***Viral*** Hepatitis B Influenza Measles Mumps Poliomyelitis Rabies Rubella Smallpox Yellow fever

IMMUNOSUPPRESSIVE MEDICATIONS		
Agents	**Actions**	**Side Effects**
Glucocorticoids	Rheumatoid arthritis Systemic lupus erythematosus Autoimmunity Transplantation	Cushing's syndrome Ulcers
Cyclophosphamide	Rheumatoid arthritis Systemic lupus erythematosus	Myelosuppression Alopecia GI symptoms Cystitis Infertility
Azathioprine	Rheumatoid arthritis Systemic lupus erythematosus Polymyositis Collagen diseases Transplantation	Myelosuppression GI symptoms Hepatotoxiciy
Methotrexate	Psoriasis Arthritis Dermatomyositis	Myelosuppression Enteritis Pulmonary fibrosis
Cyclosporine A	Systemic lupus erythematosus Type I diabetes Psoriasis Uveitis Transplantation	Hepatotoxic Renotoxic Neurotoxic Hypertension

INDAPAMIDE
(Lozol)

Indapamide is a sulfonamide diuretic that has been used for treatment of hypertension (2.5 to 5.0 mg/day). It has been proposed as an alternative antihypertensive agent with both diuretic and vasodilatory capability and a more favorable side-effect profile than the thiazides. Indapamide exerts its antihypertensive effect by two mechanisms. It appears to have a modest diuretic effect while also relaxing vascular smooth muscle. As a diuretic, indapamide increases the excretion of sodium, chloride, and water by interfering with the transport of sodium across the renal tubular epithelium. Its principal site of action remains controversial but is probably either at the diluting segment of the loop of Henle or the proximal segment of the distal tubule (see also Table 25 and Figure 4).

In studies with healthy volunteers, the bioavailability of indapamide after a single oral dose is about 90%. Coadministration with food or antacids does not significantly reduce the bioavailability. Peak plasma concentrations occur at 0.5 to 2 hours and remain fairly constant for up to 8 hours. Indapamide is widely distributed throughout the body with an apparent volume of distribution around 25 liters. Indapamide has been shown to cause a significant reduction in total peripheral resistance and mean arterial pressure. Cardiac index and heart rate are essentially unchanged. Compared with the thiazide diuretics, indapamide causes little increase in the percentage of filtered sodium excreted. Indapamide administration causes a significant increase in plasma renin activity. Plasma aldosterone concentrations are increased by around 50%, and urinary aldosterone excretion is more than doubled with chronic indapamide therapy. Unlike the thiazide diuretics, 2.5 mg/day of indapamide has little effect on glomerular filtration rate or effective renal plasma flow in hypertensive patients. Indapamide is indicated as a first-line treatment of the salt and fluid retention associated with congestive heart failure. Studies have shown that it can be as safe and effective in the treatment of pitting edema (both from congestive heart failure and other causes) as hydrochlorothiazide. It has also been shown to decrease urinary calcium excretion in patients with idiopathic hypercalciuria. Indapamide does cause a statistically significant reduction in mean serum potassium value.

INDECAINIDE HYDROCHLORIDE
(Decabid)

Indecainide is a class 1C antiarrhythmic agent structurally similar to aprindine. Similar to **encainide** (Enkaid) and **flecainide** (Tambocor), indecainide suppresses premature ventricular complexes (PVCs) and depresses intramyocardial conduction. Indecainide prolongs the PR and QRS intervals, significantly increasing intraventricular conduction time without significantly affecting atrial or ventricular refractoriness. There appear to be no significant hemodynamic effects. Indecainide is absorbed well orally, is metabolized in the liver to desisopropyl indecainide, and is excreted in the urine. The side effects of indecainide are dizziness, headache, blurry vision, impotence, lightheadedness, confusion, and thought disorders.

INDENOLOL

Indenolol is a new antihypertensive agent with beta$_1$ adrenoceptor antagonist and a beta$_2$ adrenoceptor agonist properties.

INDINAVIR SULFATE (CRIXIVAN)

Indinavir (800 mg/t.i.d.) is an inhibitor of the human immunodeficiency virus (HIV) **protease**, which is an enzyme required for the proteolytic cleavage of the viral polyprotein precursors into the individual functional proteins found in infectious HIV. Indinavir binds to the protease active site and inhibits the activity of the enzyme. This inhibition prevents cleavage of the viral polyproteins resulting in the formation of immature non-infectious viral particles. Cross-resistance between indinavir and HIV reverse transcriptase inhibitors is unlikely because the enzyme targets involved are different. Cross-resistance was noted between indinavir and the protease inhibitor **ritonavir**. Varying degrees of cross-resistance have been noted between indinavir and other HIV protease inhibitors. Indinavir is metabolized in the liver, and seven metabolites have been identified, and 20% of indinavir is excreted unchanged in the urine.

Nephrolithiasis, including flank pain with or without hematuria (including microscopic hematuria), has been reported in approximately 4% of patients receiving **crixivan** in clinical trials. In general, these events were not associated with renal dysfunction and resolved with hydration and temporary interruption of therapy (e.g., 1 to 3 days).

Indinavir should not be administered concurrently with terfenadine, astemizole, cisapride, triazolam, and midazolam because competition for cytochrome P450 3A4 by indinavir could result in inhibition of the metabolism of these drugs and create the potential for serious and/or life-threatening events (i.e., cardiac arrhythmias, prolonged sedation).

INDOMETHACIN
(Indocin)

Indomethacin, which has analgesic, antipyretic, and antiinflammatory actions, is indicated in moderate to severe rheumatoid arthritis (25 mg t.i.d.), in moderate to severe ankylosing spondylitis, in moderate to severe osteoarthritis, in bursitis or tendinitis (75 to 150 mg daily), and in acute gouty arthritis (50 mg t.i.d.) (see Figure 51 and Table 2).

The patency of the ductus arteriosus is maintained in part by prostaglandin. **Indomethacin** induces constriction of the ductus during the neonatal period, whereas infusion of prostaglandin E_1 maintains its patency (Figure 51).

Concomitant use of indomethacin with anticoagulants and thrombolytic drugs (coumarin derivatives, heparin, streptokinase, or urokinase) may potentiate anticoagulant effects. Bleeding problems may occur if indomethacin is used with other drugs that inhibit platelet aggregation, such as azlocillin, parenteral carbenicillin, dextran, dipyridamole, mezlocillin, piperacillin, sulfinpyrazone, ticarcillin, valproic acid, cefamandole, cefoperazone, moxalactam, plicamycin, salicylates, or steroids which may cause increased GI adverse effects, including ulceration and hemorrhage. Aspirin may decrease the bioavailability of indomethacin. Because of the influence of prostaglandins on glucose metabolism, concomitant use with insulin or oral hypoglycemic agents may potentiate hypoglycemic effects. Indomethacin may displace highly protein-bound drugs from binding sites. Toxicity may occur with coumarin derivatives, phenytoin, verapamil, or nifedipine; increased nephrotoxicity may occur with gold compounds, other antiinflammatory agents, or acetaminophen. Indomethacin may decrease the renal clearance of methotrexate and lithium. Concurrent use with antihypertensive medications and diuretics may decrease their effectiveness. Concurrent use with triamterene is not recommended due to potential nephrotoxicity. Other diuretics may also predispose patients to nephrotoxicity. Clinical manifestations of overdose include dizziness, nausea, vomiting, intense headache, mental confusion, drowsiness, tinnitus, sweating, blurred vision, paresthesias, and convulsions. Patients over age 60 may be more susceptible to the toxic effects of indomethacin. The effects of indomethacin on renal prostaglandins may cause fluid retention and edema, a significant drawback for elderly patients and those with congestive heart failure.

INDORAMIN

Indoramin, a vasodilator, is an alpha-adrenergic antagonist and an effective antihypertensive medication. In addition, it has cardiac stabilizing properties. The doses used for the treatment

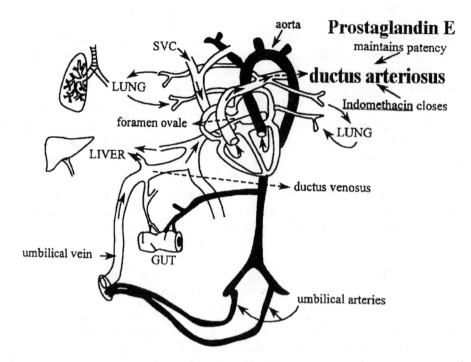

FIGURE 51 The patency of the ductus arteriosus is maintained in part by a prostaglandin. **Indomethacin** induces constriction of the ductus during the neonatal period, whereas infusion of prostaglandin E_1 maintains its patency. (Adapted from Ebadi, M., *Pharmacology, An Illustrated Review with Questions and Answers*, 3rd Edition, Lippincott-Raven Press, Philadelphia, 1996.)

of peripheral vascular disease are lower than those used for the treatment of hypertension. Both these effects are consistent with competitive postsynaptic alpha-adrenoceptor antagonism. Absence of tachycardia can be attributed to a combination of postsynaptic alpha-receptor selectivity and myocardial membrane-stabilizing properties. Cardiac function remains essentially unchanged in humans. The unique mode of action of indoramin suggests that it may be especially beneficial in hypertensive patients with coexisting asthma, migraine, or vasospastic symptoms. Sedation is a side effect that may limit the dose in some patients, but mild sedation can be an advantage in those patients with anxiety, tension headaches, and insomnia among their pretreatment symptomatology. Coprescription with a diuretic reduces the required dose of indoramin and the incidence of sedation. Cerebrovascular accidents due to rebound hypertension after abrupt discontinuation of other antihypertensive agents are not observed with indoramin. No evidence of tolerance has been obtained, and the incidence of postural hypotension appears to be extremely low (see also Figure 27).

INFLUENZA VIRUS VACCINE, TRIVALENT TYPES A&B (PURIFIED SURFACE ANTIGEN)
(Fluvirin)

INFLUENZA VIRUS VACCINE, TRIVALENT TYPES A&B (SPLIT VIRUS)
(Fluogen, Flu-Shield, Fluzone (Split Virus)

INFLUENZA VIRUS VACCINE, TRIVALENT TYPES A&B (WHOLE VIRUS)
(Fluzone) (Whole-Virus)

Influenza viral vaccine is used in annual influenza prophylaxis in high-risk patients.

INHIBIN

The pituitary hormones responsible for regulating gonadal functions are **luteinizing hormone** (LH) and **follicle-stimulating hormone** (FSH). In **males**, LH stimulates the Leydig's cells to synthesize **testosterone;** FSH stimulates the Sertoli's cells to synthesize **inhibin** and **androgen-binding protein**, and, in conjunction with high intratesticular concentrations of testosterone, initiates and maintains **spermatogenesis.** In **females**, LH stimulates **androgen synthesis,** and FSH increases estrogen and inhibin synthesis in the granulosa cells. Both LH and FSH are released from the gonadotroph cells of the anterior pituitary in response to the hypothalamic hormone gonadotropin-releasing hormone (GnRH; also known as LH-releasing hormone). GnRH is a decapeptide with the following structure: pyro Glu-His-Trp-Ser-Tyr-Gly-Leu-Arg-Pro-Gly-NH$_2$ (also see Table 14).

INSOMNIA: TREATMENT WITH BENZODIAZEPINES		
Drugs	**Duration of Action**	**Onset of Action**
Clonazepam	long	intermediate
Diazepam	long	rapid
Estazolam	intermediate	rapid to intermediate
Flurazepam	long	rapid to intermediate
Lorazepam	intermediate	intermediate
Oxazepam	short to intermediate	intermediate to slow
Quazepam	long	rapid
Temazepam	intermediate	intermediate to slow
Triazolam	short	intermediate
Zolpidem	short	rapid

INSULIN

Diabetes mellitus results from disturbances in the metabolism of carbohydrates, lipids, and proteins. Normally, the blood glucose level is maintained within a range of 80 to 130 mg/ml. When the level rises above 180 mg/ml, the glucose spills into the urine, causing **glucosuria**. The utilization of glucose by most tissues, including muscle and adipose tissue, is insulin dependent. The **brain** is an exception in that its utilization of glucose is insulin independent. In the absence of insulin, the organs other than brain are able to make use of amino acids and fatty acids as alternate sources of energy.

The **release of insulin** is closely coupled with the glucose level. **Hypoglycemia** results in a low level of **insulin** and a high level of **glucagon**, and hence favors the processes of **glyco-genolysis** and **gluconeogenesis. Growth hormone** is one of the glucose counterregulatory hormones. It is released in response to hypoglycemia and has intrinsic hyperglycemic actions as well as causing insulin resistance.

Following ingestion of a meal or the administration of glucose (e.g., in a glucose tolerance test), the glucose level rises, causing the release of insulin and inhibiting the release of hyperglycemic glucagon. Excess glucose is transformed into **glycogen** in the liver and the muscles. The high level of amino acids and free fatty acid fosters the respective formation of **proteins** in the muscles and **triglycerides** in the adipose tissues. In a nondiabetic fasting subject, the ensuing hypoglycemia not only discourages the release of insulin but also activates the homeostatic mechanisms that block the action of insulin and convert the storage of forms of fuel into utilizable glucose. Consequently, a number of hormones including **glucagon, epinephrine,** and **glucocorticoid**, are released, and these convert glycogen into glucose, triglyceride into free fatty acids, and proteins into amino acids (gluconeogenesis), respectively.

Furthermore, the uptake and utilization of glucose in the peripheral tissues decrease. The muscles and other tissues utilize amino acids and free fatty acids, thus providing the brain with an adequate supply of glucose. In a diabetic individual who suffers from a deficiency of insulin, all of the aforementioned measures that apply to a fasting individual may also take place. However, the consumption of a meal or the administration of glucose will instead cause pronounced hyperglycemia because the insulin-dependent utilization of glucose by muscles and adipose tissues is lacking. The elevated glucose level thus surpasses the renal threshold, and glucose may appear continuously in the urine. The osmotic diuretic effects of glucose cause **polyuria** and **polydipsia** and the chronic glucosuria may lead to **urinary tract infection**. Because the conversion to triglycerides does not take place, free fatty acids are metabolized to ketone bodies, causing **ketonuria** or **ketoacidosis** (acetone or fruity breath). The continuous destruction of muscular proteins may ultimately lead to muscle wasting and weight loss. There are two types of diabetes mellitus: type I, or **insulin-dependent diabetes mellitus**, and type II, or **non-insulin-dependent diabetes mellitus.** Type I diabetic patients may have islet-cell antibodies and human leukocyte antigens (HLA). They are dependent on insulin to prevent ketosis and have insulinopenia. Affected individuals consist mostly of children and young adults. Type II diabetic patients, who are non-insulin-dependent, are not prone to ketosis. This type of diabetes is not an autoimmune disorder nor associated with HLA. The patients are generally older (>40 years), may or may not be obese, and may or may not have been treated with insulin for the control of their hyperglycemia. The signs and symptoms of diabetes consist of thirst, anorexia, nausea, vomiting, abdominal pain, headache, drowsiness, weakness, coma, severe acidosis, air hunger (Kussmaul's breathing), sweetish odor of the breath, hyperglycemia, decreased blood bicarbonate level, decreased blood pH, and plasma that is strongly positive for ketone bodies. There are a number of complications that arise as the result of poorly treated or unstabilized diabetes. Vascular complications may be manifested by **microangiopathy** (thickening of the capillary basement membrane), **intracapillary glomerulosclerosis** (thickening of the glomerular capillary basement membrane, which leads to a **nephrotic syndrome** characterized by edema, albuminuria, and/or renal failure), and microangiopathy of the blood vessels supplying the **retina** (diabetic retinopathy). In fact, diabetes is still the leading cause of blindness in the world. In addition, there may be **atherosclerosis** of the peripheral arteries. Diabetic neuropathy may be associated with neuropathic ulcer, ptosis, diplopia, stabismus, loss of deep tendon reflexes, ankle drop, wrist drop, paresthesia, hyperalgesia, hyperesthesia, and orthostatic hypotension (because of autonomic dysfunction). When insulin binds to specific membrane receptors on target cells, this initiates a wide spectrum of biologic activities. It enhances the transport of sugar and amino acids, stimulates anabolic pathways, and stimulates growth and development by triggering RNA and DNA synthesis.

The **insulin receptor** is a **disulfide-linked oligomer** consisting of two alpha and two beta chains, with molecular weights of 130,000 and 95,000, respectively. Crosslinking studies using iodine 125-labeled insulin have shown that the **insulin-binding domain** is situated primarily in the alpha subunit. In addition, it has been observed that proteolysis of the beta subunit does not appreciably influence insulin binding. Insulin binding to the alpha subunit was found to induce rapid phosphorylation of the intracellular domain of the beta subunit. The beta subunit contains a putative ATP-binding site and an intrinsic tyrosine-specific kinase as part of the receptor. The enzymatic activity of the receptor is activated by insulin binding, which results in increased tyrosine phosphorylation of the beta subunit as well as the production of a number of other cell proteins (Figure 52). The insulin receptor is internalized, and this action terminates the insulin signal at the surface of the cell. Once internalized, some of the receptors are degraded and others are recycled back to the membrane. In addition, phosphatases are able to dephosphorylate the phosphorylated insulin receptor. This dephosphorylation reduces kinase activity and decreases the responsiveness to insulin. A number of disorders are associated with the development of insulin resistance. Although some cases are due to autoimmune responses,

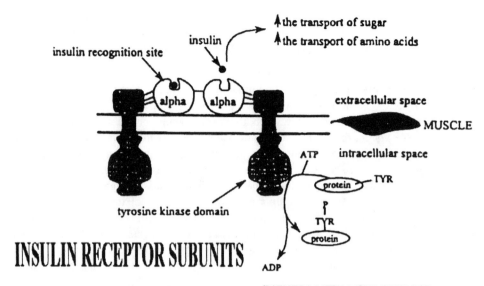

INSULIN-MEDIATED EFFECTS
FOLLOWING TYROSINE PHOSPHORYLATION

FIGURE 52   When insulin binds to specific membrane receptors on target cells, it enhances the transport of sugar and amino acids, stimulates anabolic pathways, and stimulates growth and development by triggering RNA and DNA synthesis. (Adapted from Ebadi, M., *Pharmacology, An Illustrated Review with Questions and Answers*, 3rd Edition, Lippincott-Raven Press, Philadelphia, 1996.)

such as the development of antiinsulin or antiinsulin receptor antibodies, insulin resistance often results from defects at the cellular level in the insulin receptor or in post-receptor function. The drug therapy of diabetes mellitus includes eliminating **obesity** (which causes resistance to both endogenous and exogenous forms of insulin), **exercising** (to promote glucose utilization and reduce insulin requirement), **dieting** (to restrict intake of excess amounts of carbohydrates), and **taking insulin** (primarily in polyuric, polydipsic, and ketonuric patients). **Insulin preparations** are fast-, intermediate-, or long-acting, as summarized in Table 18.

TABLE 18
Properties of Insulin Preparations

Types	Added Protein	Zinc Content (mg/100 U)	Action (hr)* Onset	Action (hr)* Peak	Action (hr)* Duration
Rapid					
Regular (crystalline)	None	0.01–0.04	0.3–0.7	2–4	5–8
Semilente	None	0.2–0.25	0.5–1.0	2–8	12–16
Intermediate					
NPH (Isophane)	Protamine	0.016–0.40	1–2	6–12	18–24
Lente	None	0.2–0.25	1–2	6–12	18–24
Slow					
Ultralente	None	0.2–0.25	4–6	16–18	20–36
Protamine zinc	Protamine	0.2–0.25	4–6	14–20	24–36

*These are approximate figures. There is considerable variation from patient to patient and from time to time in the same patient.

Crystalline (regular) **insulin** may be used as a supplemental injection or for instituting corrective measures in the management of infection and trauma, for postoperative stabilization, and for the rehabilitation of patients recovering from ketoacidosis and coma. In addition, NPH contains regular insulin.

Ultralente or **semilente insulin** is used to eliminate nocturnal and early morning hyperglycemia. **Hypoglycemia** is a primary complication of insulin therapy and may result from either an excess of insulin or a lack of glucose, or both. Severe hypoglycemia may cause headache, confusion, double vision, drowsiness, and convulsions. The treatment of this hypoglycemia may include the administration of glucose or glucagon. **Lipodystrophy** can also result from insulin therapy and is characterized by atrophy of subcutaneous fat. **Insulin edema** is manifested by a generalized retention of fluid. **Insulin resistance** arises when there is an excess insulin requirement that exceeds 200 units per day. The release of insulin is enhanced by certain physiologic substances (glucose, leucine, arginine, gastrin, secretin, and pancreozymin) and by certain pharmacologic agents (oral hypoglycemic agents). The release of insulin is also inhibited by some physiologic substances (epinephrine and norepinephrine) as well as by some pharmacologic substances (thiazide diuretics, diazoxide, and chlorpromazine).

INSULIN PREPARATIONS	
Short-acting insulins	
Standard insulin Regular Iletin I Regular insulin	Semilente Iletin I Semilente insulin
Purified Beef Regular Iletin II Pork Regular Iletin II Regular purified pork insulin	Velosulin Semilente purified pork
Human (purified) Humulin R Humulin BR Velosulin	Novolin R Novolin R PenFill
Intermediate-acting insulins	
NPH (standard) NPH Iletin I NPH insulin	*Lente (purified)* Lente Iletin II Lente purified pork
NPH (purified) Beef NPH Iletin II Pork NPH Iletin II NPH purified pork Insulatard NPH	*Lente (human)* Novolin L Humulin L
NPH (human) Humulin N Insulatard NPH Novolin N Novolin N PenFill	*NPH-regular combination (70%/30%)* *Purified* Mixtard (70% NPH, 30% Regular)
Lente (standard) Lente Iletin I Lente insulin	*Human* Novolin 70/30 Novolin 70/30 PenFill Humulin 70/30 Mixtard 70/30
Long-acting insulins	
Protamine Zinc and Iletin I Ultralente Iletin I Ultralente insulin	*Purified* Protamine Zinc and Iletin II Ultralente purified beef

INSULIN (REGULAR)

(Humulin R, Novolin R, Novolin R PenFill, Pork Regular Iletin II, Regular Insulin, Regular Iletin 1, Regular [Concentrated] Iletin II, Regular Purified Pork Insulin, Velosulin Human)

PROMPT INSULIN ZINC SUSPENSION

(Semilente)

ISOPHANE INSULIN SUSPENSION (NPH)

(Humulin N, NPH Iletin I, NPH-N, Novolin N, Novolin N PenFill, Pork NPH Iletin II)

INSULIN ZINC SUSPENSION (LENTE)

(Humulin l, Lente Iletin I, Lente Lletin II, Lente l, Novolin L

PROTAMINE ZINC INSULIN SUSPENSION (ULTRALENTE)

(Humulin U Ultralente)

ISOPHANE INSULIN SUSPENSION AND INSULIN INJECTION (70% ISOPHANE INSULIN AND 30% INSULIN INJECTION)

(Humulin 70/30, Novolin 70/30, Novolin 70/30 PenFill)

ISOPHANE INSULIN SUSPENSION AND INSULIN INJECTION (50% ISOPHANE INSULIN AND 50% INSULIN INJECTION

(Humulin 50/50)

Insulin, a pancreatic hormone, is used in diabetic ketoacidosis and ketosis-prone and juvenile-onset diabetes mellitus, and in diabetes inadequately controlled by diet and oral hypoglycemics (see Table 18 and Figure 52).

INTERFERON ALFA-n3

(Alteron N)

Interferon, a biological response modifier with antineoplastic properties, is indicated in the treatment of condylomata acuminata (see also Figure 99).

INTERFERON ALFA-2A, RECOMBINANT

(Roferon-A)

INTERFERON ALFA-2B, RECOMBINANT

(Intron A)

Interferon, a biological response modifier with antineoplastic activity, is used in hairy cell leukemia, condylomata acuminata, Kaposi's sarcoma, chronic hepatitis C (non-A, non-B), and chronic hepatitis B (see also Figure 99).

INTERFERON BETA-1B

(Betaseron)

Interferon, a biological response modifier with antiviral and immunoregulating properties, is used to reduce the frequency of exacerbation in patients with relapsing-remitting multiple sclerosis (see also Figure 99).

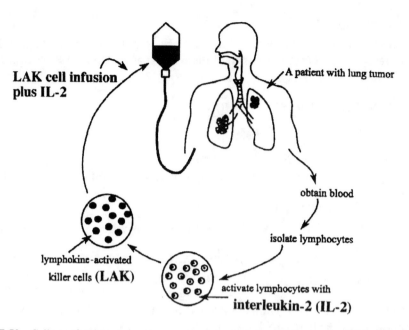

FIGURE 53 Cell transfer therapy is a new approach to strengthening the innate ability of the immune system to fight against cancer. In this therapy, lymphocytes are isolated and cultured with **interleukin 2** for three days to yield **lymphokine-activated killer cells**, which are then administered to patients along with interleukin 2.

INTERFERON GAMMA 1-B

(Actimmune)

Interferon, a biological response modifier with antineoplastic properties, is indicated in the treatment of chronic granulomatous disease (see also Figure 99).

INTERLEUKIN-2

(iL-2)

Interleukin-2 is a lymphokine with immunoregulatory properties which is indicated in metastatic renal cell carcinoma. In addition, interleukin-2 is used in cell transfer therapy in cancer patients. Cell transfer therapy is a new approach to strengthening the innate ability of the immune system to fight against cancer. In this therapy, lymphocytes are isolated and cultured with **interleukin-2** for three days to yield **lymphokine-activated killer cells**, which are then administered to patients along with interleukin-2 (see Figure 53; and **Cytokines**).

INVERT SUGAR

(Travert)

Invert sugar, a carbohydrate (1,000 ml of 5% solution by IV infusion), is indicated for nonelectrolyte fluid replacement and caloric supplementation solution.

IN VITRO FERTILIZATION: DRUGS FOR

In vitro fertilization (IVF) has resulted in thousands of pregnancies for infertile couples. **Clomifene** (clomiphene citrate), human menopausal gonadotrophin (hMG; **menotropins**), and subsequent generations of products are commonly used as stimulation agents. In conjunction with the stimulation agents, gonadotrophin-releasing hormone (GnRH) agonists and human chorionic gonadotrophin (hCG) serve as adjuvants for successful control of all events in the induction process. Midazolam, nuperidine, or fentanyl may be used for oocyte recovery. If full anesthesia is required for gamete intrafallopian tube transfer or zygote intrafallopian tube transfer, balanced anesthesia with nitrous oxide and an opioid appears to be the most appealing option.

TABLE 19
Comparison of Features of Antithyroid Drug and Iodine 131 Therapy for Hyperthyroidism

Features	Drug Therapy	Iodine 131 Therapy
Dosage	Daily	Single dose
Initial response	4–6 wk	8–12 wk
Side effects	Uncommon	Rare
Hypothyroidism	Uncommon	Common
Inadequate therapy	Uncommon	Rare
Need for continuous or repeated therapy	Common	Rare
Long-term outcome	Euthyroidism or hyperthyroidism	Hypothyroidism
Outcome dependent on continued TSab production	Yes	No
Use during pregnancy	Acceptable	Never

TSab = thyroid-stimulating autoantibody.

IODINE

Iodides such as potassium iodide and **Lugol's solution**, which contains 5% iodine and 10% potassium iodide, exert their beneficial effects by inhibiting organification, inhibiting the release of thyroid hormones, and decreasing (inhibiting proteolysis) the size and vascularity of the thyroid gland. This makes them useful for preparing the patient for surgery. Iodine 131 is given orally in **older patients** for the treatment of thyrotoxicosis. It accumulates in the storage follicles and emits beta rays with a half-life of 5 days. Radioactive iodine, which crosses the placental barrier, is contraindicated in pregnant women (see Table 19). The treatment of thyrotoxicosis in **younger patients** may include the administration of an antithyroid drug such as **propylthiouracil** or **methimazole.** These agents are very slow in their onset of action, often taking years for remission to be apparent. The most serious side effect of these drugs is **agranulocytosis.** In the event of **multinodular goiters**, subtotal thyroidectomy may be indicated. Potassium iodide is next administered as a preoperative measure to diminish vascularity of the thyroid. In addition to surgery, radioactive iodine is being used increasingly in younger patients. The major complication following either surgery or treatment with radioactive iodine may be **hypothyroidism**, which then requires replacement therapy with **levothyroxine.**

IODINE-CONTAINING PRODUCTS
Oral Preparations
Amiodarone
Calcium iodide (e.g., calcidrine syrup)
Echothiophate iodide (ophthalmic solution)
Hydriodic acid syrup
Idoxuridine ophthalmic solution
Iodinated glycerol
Iodine-containing vitamins
Iodochlorhydroxyquin
Iodoquinol (diiodohydroxyquin)
Kelp
Lugol's solution
Niacinamide hydroiodide + potassium iodide (e.g., Iodo-Niacin)
Ponaris nasal emollient
Potassium iodide (e.g., Quadrinal)
Saturated solution of potassium iodide

Parenteral Preparations
Sodium iodide, 10% solution
Radiology Contrast Agents
Diatrizoate meglumine sodium
Iohexol
Iopanoic acid
Iothalamate
Ipodate
Metrizamide
Propyliodone
Topical Antiseptics
Iodine tincture
Iodochlorhydroxyquin cream
Iodoform gauze
Iodoquinol (diiodohydroxyquin) cream
Providone iodine

IODIXANOL

Iodixanol, a new isosmotic nonionic contrast agent, similar to **iohexol,** is used in the cardiac catheterization laboratory. Iodixanol and iohexol are safe and effective in patients undergoing cardiac angiography.

IODOQUINOL

(Diiodohydroxyquin) (Amebaquin, Moebiquin, Yodoxin)

Idoquinol, an 8-hydroxyquinoline iodinated compound possessing amebicidic properties (630 to 650 mg p.o. t.i.d. for 20 days), is indicated in the treatment of intestinal amebiasis.

IPECAC SYRUP

(Ipecac fluid extract is 14 times stronger than ipecac syrup.) Ipecac, an emetic, contains **emetine** and **cephaeline.** It is used in a dose of 15 to 30 ml with 200 to 300 ml of water in drug overdosage and certain cases of poisoning. Ipecac may fail to exert its emetic effects on an empty stomach. Ipecac causes vomiting by irritating the stomach and by stimulating the chemotrigger zone for emesis (see also Figure 73). Ipecac exerts its emetic effects in 20 minutes. Activated charcoal will absorb ipecac syrup, and hence they should not be used together. Ipecac syrup is contraindicated in patients with poisoning caused by alkalis or corrosive agents because of hazard of further esophageal or mediastinal injury; in patients with poisoning from petroleum distillates; in patients who are semiconscious, unconscious, comatose, or in shock; and in patients with seizures, severe inebriation, depressed gag reflexes, or strychnine poisoning, because of hazards of aspiration, pneumonitis, bronchospasm, or pulmonary edema. When ipecac syrup does not cause emesis, absorption of the alkaloid emetine may occur and may cause heart conduction disturbances, atrial fibrillation, or fatal myocarditis. Ipecac syrup may be abused by bulimic and anorexic patients. It has been implicated as the causative factor of severe cardiomyopathies, and even death, in several persons with eating disorders who used it regularly to induce vomiting.

IPRATROPIUM BROMIDE

(Atrovent)

Ipratropium (2 inhalations, 36 mcg/q.i.d.) is a bronchodilator which is used in the treatment of bronchospasm associated with chronic obstructive pulmonary diseases including chronic bronchitis and emphysema. Ipratropium is a muscarinic cholinergic receptor blocking agent which inhibits vagally mediated actions in bronchial smooth muscle. Ipratropium exerts its effect locally, is not absorbed in the lung, and is not found in a significant amount in the systemic circulation. The IV-administered ipratropium does not penetrate the blood-brain barrier. Ipratropium does not alter pulmonary gas exchange, pulse rate, or blood pressure. Ipratropium has been used concomitantly with other drugs, including sympathomimetic bronchodilators, methylxanthines, steroids, and cromolyn sodium, commonly used in the treatment of chronic obstructive pulmonary disease, without causing adverse drug reactions. Ipratropium causes dryness of the oropharynx. If sprayed into the eyes, it may cause blurring of vision, and hence could aggravate narrow-angle glaucoma (see also Figure 86).

IPSAPIRONE

The anxiolytic agents consist of **benzodiazepine** derivatives and **azaspirodecanedione** derivatives, which include **buspirone, gepirone,** and **ipsapirone**. The introduction of novel anxiolytic agents such as **buspirone**, which interacts with the serotonergic system, has suggested that serotoninergic fibers may be the final pathway through which anxiolytic effects are expressed. Buspirone has a chemical structure that is distinct from that of the benzodiazepines. Without this structural homology, it is not surprising that buspirone does not interact with the GABA receptors. Furthermore, the clinical profile of buspirone appears to be **anxioselective**, with a much reduced potential for abuse (see also Table 8). Although the benzodiazepines are now viewed as having a direct action at a binding site coupled to the GABA receptor (see Figure 40), this view was predated by the suggestion that serotoninergic systems interacted with the benzodiazepines. This view was spawned by the observation that benzodiazepines inhibit the firing of serotoninergic neurons in the dorsal raphe nucleus, decrease brain serotonin turnover (levels of 5-hydroxyindole acetic acid), and reverse the proconflict effects of direct serotoninergic stimulation of the dorsal raphe. As with buspirone, lesions of the serotoninergic system abolish diazepam's efficacy in a conflict test. A body of data supports the candidacy of serotonin as a mediator of the anxiolytic effects of benzodiazepines downstream from the GABA receptor. There is a convincing body of evidence that several types of serotonin (5-HT) receptors exist in the mammalian brain, two of which are well characterized: 5-HT_1 and 5-HT_2 sites. The 5-HT_1 sites can be further subdivided into at least three distinct subsets, which differ in their regional distribution and functions and are currently termed 5-HT_{1A}, 5-HT_{1B}, and 5-HT_{1C} sites. The 5-HT receptors in the hippocampus and other parts of the **limbic system** are primarily of the 5-HT_{1A} type. It is therefore tempting to speculate that drugs that display a high degree of selectivity for these receptor sites can selectively affect anxiety states. A breakthrough in that direction came with the discovery that **buspirone**, a drug with anxiolytic activity in humans, can help elucidate the role of 5-HT in anxiety. **Buspirone, gepirone**, and **ipsapirone** may therefore offer new therapeutic directions in the treatment of anxiety.

IRON

The iron-deficiency anemias are caused by excessive loss of or an inadequate intake of iron. In women, **menstruation** and **pregnancy** may increase the iron requirement. Iron deficiency in men, as well as women, may be due to blood loss resulting from hemorrhage associated with gastric ulcer or neoplasm. In children, iron deficiency is due to a nutritionally inadequate diet. In the body, the total content of iron in men and women constitutes 50 and 35 mg per kilogram of body weight, respectively. Of this iron content, approximately 60% is associated with **hemoglobin,** 13% is associated with **myoglobin** and iron-containing enzymes, and the remaining 27% is located in the storage sites. Men and women differ with regard to their storage of iron, which is substantially lower in women due to menstruation. Menstrual losses are greater with the use of intrauterine devices and are decreased when estrogen-containing oral contraceptives are used. Iron is primarily obtained from the diet, with an average daily intake of approximately 12 to 15 mg. Under normal circumstances, only 10% (1 mg) of the ingested iron is absorbed. However, in the event of iron-deficiency anemia, this increases to approximately 40%. Of course, the iron requirement is increased during growth and development, as the result of menstruation, pregnancy, and blood donation, and in an extensive number of pathologic conditions causing anemia. In addition, the long-term ingestion of certain drugs such as aspirin may alter the daily requirement. Iron is absorbed better in **ferrous** (Fe^{2+}) than in the ferric (Fe^{3-}) form. The extent of **absorption of iron** from the duodenum is thought to be regulated by mucosal proteins, and this process is referred to as *mucosal block*. The absorbed iron is either stored in mucosal **ferritin**, or is transported to plasma and bound to **transferrin**. Ordinarily, iron excretion and elimination are regulated to equal the amount of iron absorption. A major portion of iron (>60%) in the body is collected by bone marrow and incorporated into hemoglobin in the erythrocytes. In general, four atoms of iron are incorporated into one molecule of hemoglobin. When the erythrocytes are destroyed by the **reticuloendothelium** after 120 days in the circulation, the released iron is returned to transferrin and ferritin. Extensive numbers of oral preparations are available for the treatment of iron deficiency. In general, the **ferrous salts** (ferrous sulfate, ferrous gluconate, and ferrous fumerate) are better absorbed than the **ferric salts** (ferric sulfate). Ferrous calcium citrate is most used in patients during pregnancy to provide iron as well as calcium. The parenteral iron medications available include **iron-dextran** (ferric hydroxide and high-molecular-weight dextran) for intramuscular use, **dextriferron** (a complex of ferric hydroxide and partially hydrolyzed dextran) for intravenous use, and **saccharated iron oxide** (a complex of ferric hydroxide and sucrose) for intravenous use. These preparations are reserved for those cases in which oral preparations are not tolerated, absorbed, or rapid enough in their onset of action, or are otherwise not suitable for noncompliant patients. A lethal dose of iron consists of 12 g of an iron preparation containing 1 or 2 g of elemental iron. Therefore, iron toxicity rarely occurs in adults but is frequently seen in children. The mortality rate among untreated children is high (45%). The initial signs and symptoms of iron poisoning are gastrointestinal and usually consist of nausea, vomiting, and diarrhea. If untreated, **acidosis, cyanosis,** and **circulatory collapse** may ensue. If the patient survives, there may be gastric scarring and pyloric stenosis resulting from the corrosive action of the iron preparation. Treatment should include induced vomiting and lavage if the poisoning is discovered early, catharsis to hasten evacuation, sodium bicarbonate therapy to combat the acidosis, and the administration of **deferoxamine** (Desferal), a specific iron-chelating agent. One hundred milligrams of deferoxamine is able to bind 8.5 mg of iron. The chelating effects of deferoxamine are maximum at an acidic pH; therefore, when given orally, deferoxamine must be administered before the sodium bicarbonate. In the event of iron poisoning, deferoxamine may also be administered intramuscularly. Besides its usefulness in counteracting the effects of iron poisoning, deferoxamine has been used in disorders that involve **iron overload** such as ocular hemosiderosis or hemochromatosis.

ISCHEMIC STROKE: TREATMENT OF

Vascular disorders of the nervous system may be an abnormality of the vessel wall (atheromatous thrombosis), occlusion by embolus, rupture of a vessel, progressive obliteration of the lumen (with or without diminished cardiac output), altered viscosity, or vascular permeability. Whatever the process, the result is one of the ischemic or hemorrhagic stroke syndromes. Here, stroke refers to any sudden focal neurologic deficit, e.g., hemiparesis, loss of consciousness, hemianopia.

In establishing which pathologic process is responsible for a specific stroke syndrome, recognition of the mode of onset of the neurologic deficit is important. The suddenness of onset, rapidity of evolution, and pattern of deficits determined from examination will usually allow an accurate diagnosis.

Thrombotic stroke may be sudden or may have a stuttering onset over hours or several days, often in a stepwise fashion with sudden accumulating increments.

Embolic stroke is almost always abrupt in onset and complete within minutes.

Hemorrhagic stroke may have a sudden onset with evolution to maximal deficit occurring in a smooth fashion over several hours.

Therapy for stroke is undergoing major changes. Many of the changes parallel the advances made in the therapy for myocardial infarction. Acute intervention with cytoprotective and thrombolytic agents is undergoing active investigation. Cytoprotective therapy includes drugs that act to prevent cell death during ischemia and reperfusion. These agents include calpain inhibitors, voltage-sensitive calcium- and sodium-channel antagonists, receptor-mediated calcium-channel antagonists [including N-methyl-D-aspartate (NMDA) and α-amino-3-hydroxy-5-methyl-4-isoxazole propionic acid (AMPA) antagonists], glutamate-synthesis inhibitors, glutamate-release antagonists, γ-aminobenzoic acid (GABA) antagonists, 5-HT (serotonin) receptor agonists, gangliosides, antioxidants, growth factors, antiapoptotic agents, and antiadhesion molecules. Thrombolysis is effective in myocardial infarction. Thrombolysis is undergoing evaluation in stroke with streptokinase, anisoylated plasminogen streptokinase activator complex (APSAC), tissue plasminogen activator (t-PA: including recombinant t-PA), urokinase, and single-chain urokinase (scu-PA). Both systemic and selective administration are being evaluated. Preventive therapy with both antiplatelet and anticoagulant drugs sheds new light on how best to stratify patients in terms of a risk-benefit ratio.

ISOCARBOXAZID
(Marplan)

Isocarboxazid (30 mg/kg) is a monoamine oxidase inhibitor (MAO) indicated for the treatment of depressed patients who have become refractory to tricyclic antidepressants or electroconvulsive therapy and depressed patients in whom tricyclic antidepressants are contraindicated. Isocarboxazid is absorbed rapidly and completely from the GI tract and is excreted primarily in the urine within 24 hours. Isocarboxazid is contraindicated in patients with uncontrolled hypertension and seizure disorders because the drug may precipitate hypertensive reactions and lower the seizure threshold. Isocarboxazid should be used cautiously in patients with a history of severe headaches, angina pectoris or other cardiovascular diseases, Type I and Type II diabetes, Parkinson's disease and other motor disorders, hyperthyroidism, pheochromocytoma, renal or hepatic insufficiency, and bipolar disease (reduce dosage during manic phase). Foods containing high concentrations of tyramine or other pressor amines may precipitate hypertensive crisis. Isocarboxazid enhances the pressor effects of amphetamines, ephedrine, phenylephrine, phenylpropanolamine, and related drugs and may result in serious cardiovascular toxicity. Concomitant use of isocarboxazid with **disulfiram** may cause tachycardia, flushing, or palpitations. Concomitant use with general anesthetics, which are normally metabolized by MAO, may cause severe hypotension and excessive CNS depression; isocarboxazid should be discontinued for at least one week before using these agents. Isocarboxazid decreases the effectiveness of local anesthetics (for example, **procaine** and **lidocaine**), resulting in poor nerve block. Use cautiously and in reduced dosage with alcohol, barbiturates, and other sedatives, narcotics, dextromethorphan, and tricyclic antidepressants. Cocaine and vasoconstrictors in local anesthetics may precipitate a hypertensive response (see also Figure 27).

ISOETHARINE HYDROCHLORIDE
(Arm-a-Med, Beta-2, Bisorine, Bronkosol, Dey-Dose, Dey-Lute, Dispos-a-Med)

ISOETHARINE MESYLATE
(Bronkometer)

Isoetharine, a sympathomimetic agent with bronchodilating properties (aerosol inhaler 340 mcg/metered spray), is indicated in the treatment of bronchial asthma and reversible bronchospasm that may occur with bronchitis and emphysema (see also Figure 86).

ISOFLURANE
(Forane)

Isoflurane is 1-chloro-2,2,2-trifluoroethyl difluoromethyl ether. The chemical and physical properties of isoflurane are similar to those of its isomer enflurane. It is not flammable in air or oxygen. Isoflurane allows a smooth and rapid induction (10 minutes) of, and emergence from, general anesthesia. The clinical signs by which depth of anesthesia is judged include progressive decreases in blood pressure and in respiratory volume and rate, as well as an increase in heart rate. Systemic arterial blood pressure decreases progressively with increasing depth during anesthesia with isoflurane, as it does with halothane and enflurane. However, in contrast to the latter agents, cardiac output is well maintained with isoflurane. Depression of renal blood flow, the rate of glomerular filtration, and urinary flow accompanies anesthesia with isoflurane, as with all the volatile anesthetic agents. However, all changes in renal function observed during anesthesia are rapidly reversed during recovery. Only 0.02% of the isoflurane that enters the body is metabolized; this fraction is markedly less than the extent of metabolism of halothane or enflurane. The small quantities of fluoride and trifluoracetic acid that are generated as degradation products of isoflurane are insufficient to cause cell damage, which accounts for the lack of renal or hepatic toxicity. Isoflurane does not appear to be a mutagen, teratogen, or carcinogen (see also Table 15).

ISONIAZID
(INH)

Isoniazid (300 mg/day in a single dose), which acts against actively growing tubercle bacilli, is indicated for the treatment and chemoprophylaxis of tuberculosis. Isoniazid is bactericidal in nature and interferes with lipid and nucleic acid biosynthesis in the growing organism. It is absorbed completely from the GI tract and diffuses readily into cell body fluids, including cerebrospinal fluid. It is metabolized in the liver by acetylation and is excreted (50%) unchanged in the urine. Isoniazid may cause severe and fatal hepatitis, and the incidence is much higher in elderly subjects. The regular consumption of ethanol enhances the incidence of isoniazid-induced hepatitis. Isoniazid may cause **pyridoxine** deficiency and peripheral neuropathy, which necessitates a daily dose (10 to 50 mg) of pyridoxine. Isoniazid causes **optic neuritis**, and periodic ophthalmologic examinations during isoniazid therapy are recommended even when visual symptoms do not occur. Isoniazid does interact with other medications. Isoniazid inhibits the activity of monoamine oxidase, and adverse interactions may occur with tyramine-containing foods such as aged cheeses. It also inhibits diamine oxidase causing exaggerated responses (e.g., headache, palpitations, sweating, hypotension, flushing, diarrhea, itching) to foods containing histamine (e.g., tuna, sauerkraut juice, yeast extract). Overdosage with isoniazid causes nausea, vomiting, dizziness, slurring of speech, blurring of vision, and visual hallucinations (including bright colors and strange designs). With marked overdosage, respiratory distress and CNS depression, progressing rapidly from stupor to profound coma, are to be expected along with severe, intractable seizures. Ingestion of 80 to 150 mg/kg usually results in severe seizures and a high likelihood of fatality. Severe metabolic acidosis, acetonuria, and hyperglycemia are typical laboratory findings.

ISOPROPAMIDE IODIDE
(Darbid)

Isopropamide (5 mg q. 12 hours) is indicated as an adjunctive therapy in the treatment of peptic ulcer. It is a muscarinic cholinergic receptor antagonist which decreases the motility of the gastrointestinal tract and inhibits gastric acid secretion. Isopropamide is poorly absorbed from the GI tract, does not cross the blood-brain barrier, is excreted in the urine as metabolites, and in the feces as unchanged drug (see also Table 9 and Figure 24).

Isopropamide is contraindicated in patients with narrow-angle glaucoma because drug-induced cycloplegia and mydriasis may increase intraocular pressure; in patients with obstructive uropathy, obstructive GI tract disease, severe ulcerative colitis, myasthenia gravis, paralytic ileus, intestinal atony, or toxic megacolon, because the drug may exacerbate these conditions.

Isopropamide should be administered cautiously to patients with autonomic neuropathy, hyperthyroidism, coronary artery disease, cardiac arrhythmias, congestive heart failure, or ulcerative colitis, because the drug may exacerbate the symptoms of these disorders; to patients with hepatic or renal disease, because toxic accumulation may occur; to patients over age 40, because the drug increases the glaucoma risk; to patients with hiatal hernia associated with reflux esophagitis, because the drug may decrease lower esophageal sphincter tone; and in hot or humid environments, because the drug may predispose the patient to heatstroke. Clinical effects of overdose include curare-like symptoms and such peripheral effects as headache, dilated, nonreactive pupils, blurred vision, flushed, hot, dry skin, dryness of mucous membranes, dysphagia, decreased or absent bowel sounds, urinary retention, hyperthermia, tachycardia, hypertension, and increased respiration.

ISOPROTERENOL
(Aerolone, Isuprel, Vapo-Iso)

ISOPROTERENOL HYDROCHLORIDE
(Isuprel, Isuprel Mistometer, Norisodrine)

ISOPROTERENOL SULFATE
(Medihaler-Iso)

Isoproterenol, a sympathomimetic amine with bronchodilating and cardiac stimulant properties, is indicated in the treatment of complete heart block after closure of ventricular septal defect, to prevent heart block, as maintenance therapy in AV block, as treatment of bronchospasm during mild acute asthma attacks, bronchospasm in chronic obstructive pulmonary disease, bronchospasm during mild acute asthma attacks or in chronic obstructive pulmonary disease, acute asthma attacks unresponsive to inhalation therapy or control of bronchospasm during anesthesia, for bronchodilation, emergency treatment of cardiac arrhythmias, immediate temporary control of atropine-resistant hemodynamically significant bradycardia, and as adjunct therapy in the treatment of shock.

Isoproterenol (aerosol: delivers 131 mcg/dose in fine mist) is indicated in the treatment of bronchospasm associated with acute and bronchial asthma, pulmonary emphysema, bronchitis, and bronchiectasis. Parenteral isoproterenol is indicated as an adjunct to fluid and electrolyte replacement therapy in the treatment of hypovolemic and septic shock, low cardiac output states, congestive heart failure, and cardiogenic shock. Sublingual or rectal isoproterenol is indicated in Adams-Stokes syndrome and atrioventricular heart block. Isoproterenol relaxes bronchial smooth muscle by direct action on beta$_2$-adrenergic receptors, relieving bronchospasm, increasing vital capacity, decreasing residual volume in the lungs, and facilitating passage of pulmonary secretions. It also produces relaxation of GI and uterine smooth muscle via stimulation of beta$_2$ receptors. Peripheral vasodilation, cardiac stimulation, and relaxation of bronchial smooth muscle are the main therapeutic effects. Isoproterenol acts on beta$_1$-adrenergic receptors in the heart, producing a positive chronotropic and inotropic effect. It usually increases cardiac output. In patients with AV block, isoproterenol shortens conduction time and increases the rate and strength of ventricular contraction. Isoproterenol is contraindicated in patients with pre-existing cardiac arrhythmias, especially tachycardia (including tachycardia caused by **digitalis** toxicity) because of the drug's cardiac stimulant effects. Clinical manifestations of overdose include exaggeration of common adverse reactions, particularly cardiac arrhythmias, extreme tremors, nausea and vomiting, and profound hypotension.

ISOSORBIDE

(Ismotic)

Isosorbide, an osmotic diuretic (1 to 5 mg/kg p.o.), is used for short-term reduction of intraocular pressure from glaucoma.

ISOSORBIDE

(Isordil)

Isosorbide dinitrate (sublingual, chewable, and oral medications) is indicated for the treatment and prevention of angina pectoris. Isosorbide dinitrate reduces myocardial oxygen demand through peripheral vasodilation, resulting in decreased venous filling pressure and, to a lesser extent, decreased arterial impedance. These combined effects result in decreased cardiac work and, consequently, reduced myocardial oxygen demands. The drug also redistributes coronary blood flow from epicardial to subendocardial regions. Isosorbide dilates peripheral vessels, helping to manage pulmonary edema and congestive heart failure caused by decreased venous return to the heart. Arterial vasodilatory effects also decrease arterial impedance and thus left ventricular workload, benefiting the failing heart. These combined effects may help some patients with acute myocardial infarction. Clinical effects of overdose result primarily from vasodilation and methemoglobinemia and include hypotension, persistent throbbing headache, palpitations, visual disturbance, flushing of the skin and sweating (with skin later becoming cold and cyanotic), nausea and vomiting, colic and bloody diarrhea, orthostasis, initial hyperpnea, dyspnea, slow respiratory rate, bradycardia, heart block, increased intracranial pressure with confusion, fever, paralysis, and tissue hypoxia from methemoglobinemia, which can lead to cyanosis, metabolic acidosis, coma, clonic convulsions, and circulatory collapse. Death may result from circulatory collapse or asphyxia (see also Figures 59 through 61).

ISOSORBIDE DINITRATE

(Dilatrate-SR, Iso-Bid, Isochron, Isonate, Isonate TR, Isordil, Isotrate, Onset-5, Sorate, Sorbide TD, Sorbitrate, Sorbitrate SA)

Isosorbide, an antianginal nitrate with vasodilating properties (2.5 to 10 mg sublingually), is indicated in the treatment or prophylaxis of acute anginal attacks and treatment of chronic ischemic heart disease (see also Figures 59 through 61).

ISOSORBIDE MONONITRATE

(Imdur, Ismo, Monoket)

Isosorbide, an antianginal nitrate (20 mg p.o. b.i.d.), is indicated in prevention of angina pectoris due to coronary artery disease (see also Figures 59 through 61).

ISOTRETINOIN

(Accutane)

Isotretinoin, a retinoic acid derivative with antiacne properties, is indicated in the treatment of severe cystic acne unresponsive to conventional therapy. In addition, it has been used in keratinization disorders resistant to conventional therapy.

ISRADIPINE

(Dynacirc)

Isradipine, a calcium channel blocking agent with antihypertensive properties (2.5 mg p.o. b.i.d.), is used in the management of hypertension (see also Table 20).

ITRACONAZOLE

(Sporanox)

Itraconazole, a synthetic triazole with antifungal properties, is indicated in the treatment of blastomycosis (pulmonary and extra-pulmonary), histoplasmosis (including chronic cavitary pulmonary disease and disseminated nonmeningeal histoplasmosis) and aspergillosis (pulmonary and extra-pulmonary) in patients who are intolerant of or refractory to amphotericin B therapy. In addition, itraconazole has been used in the treatment of superficial mycoses (dermatophytoses, pityriasis versicolor, sebopsoriasis, candidiasis [vaginal, oral or chronic mucocutaneous], and onychomycosis), systemic mycoses (candidiasis, cryptococcal infections [meningitis, disseminated], dimorphic infections [paracoccidioidomycosis, coccidioidomycosis]), subcutaneous mycoses (sporotrichosis, chromomycosis), cutaneous leishmaniasis, fungal keratitis, alteranariosis, and zygomycosis. Itraconazole is an orally active, broad-spectrum, triazole antifungal agent which has a higher affinity for fungal cytochrome P450 than ketoconazole but a low affinity for mammalian cytochrome P450. Itraconazole has a broader spectrum of activity than other azole antifungals and shows interesting pharmacokinetic features in terms of its tissue distribution. These properties have resulted in reduced treatment times for a number of diseases such as vaginal candidiasis, as well as effective oral treatment of several deep mycoses, including aspergillosis and candidiasis (see also Figure 54).

IVERMECTIN

Ivermectin is a potent macrocyclic lactone causing paralysis in many nematodes and arthropods through an influx of chloride ions across the cell membrane. It is currently the drug of choice for human onchocerciasis and shows potent microfilaricidal activity against the other major filarial parasites of humans (*Wuchereria bancrofti, Brugia malayi, Loa loa,* and *Mansonella ozzardi*) but not against *M. perstans*. Ivermectin also has excellent efficacy in both human strongyloidiasis and cutaneous larva migrans for which good alternative treatments have not been available; and it is as effective as currently available drugs against the intestinal nematodes *Ascaris lumbriocoides, Trichuris trichiura,* and *Enterobius vermicularis*; against the human hookworms, it shows only partial efficacy. Preliminary studies indicate that ivermectin has the potential to become the drug of choice for ectoparasitic infections (mites, lice) of humans as well.

J

JAPANESE ENCEPHALITIS VIRUS VACCINE, INACTIVATED
(Je-Vax)

Japanese encephalitis virus vaccine is indicated for primary immunization (1 ml/SC on days 0, 7, and 30) and booster immunization (1 ml/SC after 2 years) against Japanese encephalitis.

JIMSON WEED

The atropine series contains a number of very closely allied alkaloids of which the chief are atropine, hyoscyamine, and hyoscine or scopolamine. They are found in the roots and leaves of many plants of the **Solanaceae** order, notably belladonna (*Atropa belladonna*), henbane (*Hyoscyamus niger*), the thorn apple or jimson weed (*Datura stramonium*), and some members of the **Duboisia** and **Scopolia** species. These plants were used during the middle ages to form the "sorcerer's drugs" and have been smoked, chewed, or imbibed in the form of decoctions by primitive people for the hallucinations and frenzy which they produce.

Atropine and its allied drugs (hyoscyamine, scopolamine, homatropine, etc.) are autonomic blocking agents which inhibit the action of the postganglionic cholinergic nerves and were, therefore, formerly designated as depressants of the parasympathetic system or as antiparasympathomimetic agents. These drugs differ from nicotine and curare, which are also depressants of the parasympathetic system but which act as blocking agents on preganglionic cholinergic nerves. Atropine in therapeutic doses has no effect on the nicotinic actions of acetylcholine but specifically blocks all muscarinic responses of injected acetylcholine, whether excitatory as in the intestine or inhibitory as in the heart. It fails, however, to block all cholinergic nerve stimulations and also exerts effects which are not explicable on the basis of its antagonism to acetylcholine. In addition to their action in blocking the muscarinic effects of acetylcholine, atropine and its allies exert important effects on the central nervous system (see also Figures 14 and 18).

K

KALLIDIN

As autocoids, bradykinin and kallidin increase vascular permeability, produce vasodilation, increase the synthesis of prostaglandins, and cause edema and pain. Extensive evidence exists that bradykinin and other kallidin substances contribute to the pathogenesis of the inflammatory response that occurs in acute and chronic diseases, including allergic reactions, arthritis, asthma, sepsis, viral rhinitis, and inflammatory bowel diseases. Bradykinin (Arg-Pro-Pro-Gly-Phe-Ser-Pro-Phe-Arg), a nonapeptide, and kallidin, a decapeptide, are derived from **kininogens**. Both tissue and plasma **kallikreins** are involved in the synthesis of bradykinin and kallidin (Figure 19), and both have a short plasma half-life of only 15 seconds. The kinins are catabolized by **kininase II**, which is also known as angiotensin-converting enzyme (see Figure 21). Kinin receptors are classified as either **kinin B$_1$** or **kinin B$_2$**. Kinin B$_1$ receptors, which are located in the aorta and mesenteric veins, respond to kinin agonists in the following order of potency:

$$\text{des Arg}^{10}\text{-kallidin} > \text{des Arg}^{10}\text{-bradykinin} > \text{kallidin} > [\text{try}(\text{Mc}^8)] \text{ bradykinin}$$

Kinin B$_2$ receptors, which are located in the jugular vein and carotid artery, respond to kinin agonists in the following order of potency:

$$\text{kallidin} > [\text{try}(\text{Mc}^8)]\text{bradykinin} > \text{bradykinin} > \text{des Arg}^{10}\text{-kallidin} > \text{des Arg}^{9}\text{-bradykinin}$$

Analogs of des Arg^9-bradykinin or des Arg^{10}-kallidin are selective antagonists for kinin B$_1$ receptors. Analogs of [Dphen^7] bradykinin are antagonists for kinin B$_2$ receptors. Activation of the B$_2$ kinin receptors, in virtually all the tissues so far described, leads to stimulation of phosphatidylinositol (PI)-specific phospholipase C, resulting in the formation of inositol phosphates and diacylglycerol and subsequent elevations in the intracellular calcium concentration. In addition, bradykinin-induced increases in the intracellular calcium concentrations of human airway smooth muscle appear to be mediated both by activation of PLC-PI turnover and by calcium influx via receptor-operated calcium channels.

KANAMYCIN SULFATE

(Kantrex)

The antibacterial activity of gentamicin, tobramycin, kanamycin, netilmicin, and amikacin is primarily directed against aerobic, Gram-negative bacilli. Kanamycin, like streptomycin, has a more limited spectrum compared with other aminoglycosides, and in particular it should not be used to treat infections caused by *Serratia* or *P. aeruginosa*. Kanamycin may be used as an initial therapy for one or more of the following organisms: *Escherichia coli, Proteus sp.* (both indole-positive and indole-negative), *Enterobacter aerogenes, Klebsiella pneumoniae, Serratia marcescens,* and *Acinetobacter sp.* It may be used as initial therapy with a penicillin or cephalosporin before obtaining results of susceptibility testing (see also Figure 80). Aminoglycosides are bactericidal and **inhibit protein synthesis** in susceptible microorganisms. They exert this effect by (1) interfering with the initiation complex of peptide formation, (2) by misreading of the code on the messenger RNA template, which causes the incorporation of inappropriate amino acid into peptide, and (3) rupturing the polysomes into monosomes, which become nonfunctional. Resistance to aminoglycosides may be due to one or a combination of the following mechanisms: interference with the transport of aminoglycoside into bacterial cells, deletion of receptors on the 30S ribosomal subunit, thus preventing the functioning of aminoglycosides, and the bacterial biotransformation of aminoglycosides to inactive forms.

In addition, because the initial transport of aminoglycosides into bacterial cells is an **oxygen-dependent process**, microorganisms that are able to grow under **anaerobic conditions** show or develop resistance. The aminoglycosides are poorly absorbed from the gastrointestinal tract, and, for this reason, they are administered intramuscularly. Furthermore, since they do not penetrate into the central nervous system, they may have to be given intrathecally or intraventricularly in the treatment of meningitis. Aminoglycosides are excreted by glomerular filtration, which is greatly reduced in the presence of renal impairment, thus leading to toxic blood levels. The most serious toxic reactions following aminoglycoside therapy are **cochlear damage** and vestibular impairment, which lead to vertigo and disturb the ability to maintain postural equilibrium. Aminoglycosides given during pregnancy cause **deafness** in the newborn. **Nephrotoxicity** and reversible **neuromuscular blockade** causing respiratory paralysis have also been seen following the use of high doses (see also Table 22).

KAOLIN AND PECTIN MIXTURES
(Kaopectate)

Kaopectate (190 mg kaolin/ml and 4.34 mg pectin/ml) is an antidiarrheal agent. By being absorbent, it recovers excess fluid in bowel dysfunction. It is contraindicated in obstructive bowel dysfunction. When used concomitantly, kaolin/pectin may impair absorption of the following drugs: antidyskinetics, antimuscarinics (especially atropine), chloroquine, dicyclomine, digoxin or digitalis glycosides, lincomycin, phenothiazines, tetracycline antibiotics, and xanthines (especially caffeine, theophylline, aminophylline, dyphylline, and oxtriphylline).

KETAMINE HYDROCHLORIDE
(Ketalar)

Ketamine is used as a sole anesthetic agent for diagnostic and surgical procedures that do not require skeletal muscle relaxation. It is best suited for short procedures, but it can be used with additional doses for longer procedures. Ketamine is also used for the induction of anesthesia prior to the administration of other general anesthetics and to supplement low-potency agents, such as nitrous oxide.

Ketamine is a rapid-acting general anesthetic producing an anesthetic state characterized by profound analgesia, normal pharyngeal-laryngeal reflexes, normal or slightly enhanced skeletal muscle tone, cardiovascular and respiratory stimulation, and occasionally, a transient and minimal respiratory depression.

Emergence from ketamine's anesthesia may be associated with psychological manifestations such as pleasant dream-like states, vivid imagery, hallucinations and emergence delirium sometimes accompanied by confusion, excitement, and irrational behavior. The duration is ordinarily a few hours, however, recurrences have been seen up to 24 hours postoperatively. No residual psychological effects are known. Ketamine should be used cautiously in patients with hypertension and cardiac decompensation. Halothane blocks the cardiovascular stimulatory effects of ketamine. Barbiturates and narcotics prolong the recovery time following ketamine. Ketamine may prolong the action of tubocurarine and cause prolonged respiratory depression (see also Figures 74 and 92).

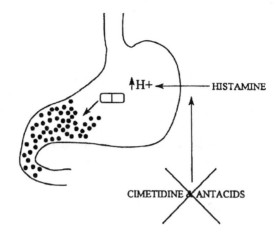

KETOCONAZOLE dissolves in acid media

FIGURE 54   Ketoconazole has a broad therapeutic potential for a number of superficial and systemic fungal infections.

KETANSERINE

Several of the newer antihypertensive medications have multiple sites of action. For example, **labetalol, dilevalol, carvedilol,** and **celiprolol** are beta-adrenergic receptors that also have vasodilating properties. Because serotonin may play a role in the pathogenesis, maintenance, and progression of hypertensive disease, **ketanserine** has been developed as a new antihypertensive medication that exhibits selective antagonism for the serotonin$_2$ receptor and has a somewhat weaker alpha$_1$-adrenergic receptor antagonist activity. **Urapidil** is a vasodilator that elicits central hypotensive activity by stimulating serotonin$_{1A}$ receptors. **Indenolol**, another new antihypertensive agent, is a beta$_1$-receptor antagonist and beta$_2$ vascular adrenergic receptor agonist.

KETOCONAZOLE

(Nizoral)

Ketoconazole (200 mg daily) is indicated in the treatment of the following systemic fungal infections: candidiasis, chronic mucocutaneous candidiasis, oral thrush, candiduria, blastomycosis, coccidiomycosis, histoplasmosis, chromomycosis, and paracoccidioidomycosis. Moreover, it is effective in the treatment of severe recalcitrant cutaneous dermatophyte infections not responding to topical therapy or oral griseofulvin or in patients unable to take griseofulvin. Ketoconazole, a broad-spectrum antifungal agent, impairs the synthesis of ergosterol, the main sterol of fungal cell membranes, allowing increased permeability and leakage of cellular components. Ketoconazole dissolves in an acidic solution. Therefore, antacids, histamine$_2$-receptor blocking agents, or anticholinergic agents reduce its oral absorption and bioavailability (Figure 54). Peak plasma concentration of ketoconazole is achieved within two hours and is bound to albumin to the extent of 95 to 99%. Ketoconazole is metabolized in the liver to inactive metabolites and is excreted mainly (90%) in the bile and feces. Renal failure does not alter the dosing regimen. Since ketoconazole penetrates poorly into CSF, it is not used in fungal meningitis.

Ketoconazole has been associated with hepatic toxicity, hence necessitating the measurement of liver function tests prior, during, and after termination of therapy. Ketoconazole reduces the serum level of testosterone, which returns to normal levels after discontinuation of therapy.

Ketoconazole increases the plasma levels, bioavailability, or actions of oral anticoagulants, astemizole, terfenidine, corticosteroids, and cyclosporine, but decreases that of theophylline.

KETOPROFEN
(Orudis)

Ketoprofen (50 to 75 mg p.o. t.i.d.), an analgesic, antipyretic, and antiinflammatory agent, is indicated in the treatment of rheumatoid arthritis and osteoarthritis. Ketoprofen is absorbed completely from the gastrointestinal tract and is highly protein bound. It is metabolized in the liver, and the metabolites are excreted in the urine. Like other nonsteroidal antiinflammatory agents, ketoprofen should be administered cautiously to patients with a history of peptic ulcer disease, renal dysfunction, or hepatic dysfunction, and to patients predisposed to fluid retention, such as those with congestive heart failure and hypertension, because ketoprofen may increase the risk of fluid retention and edema. Patients with aspirin hypersensitivity, rhinitis/nasal polyps, and asthma are at high risk of bronchospasm. Concomitant use of ketoprofen with anticoagulants and thrombolytic drugs (coumarin derivatives, heparin, streptokinase, or urokinase) may potentiate anticoagulant effects. Bleeding problems may occur if ketoprofen is used with other drugs that inhibit platelet aggregation, such as azlocillin, parenteral carbenicillin, dextran, dipyridamole, mezlocillin, piperacillin, sulfinpyrazone, ticarcillin, valproic acid, cefamandole, cefoperazone, moxalactam, and plicamycin. Because of the influence of prostaglandins on glucose metabolism, concomitant use with insulin or oral hypoglycemic agents may potentiate hypoglycemic effects. Ketoprofen may displace highly protein-bound drugs from binding sites. Toxicity may occur with coumarin derivatives, phenytoin, verapamil, or nifedipine. Increased nephrotoxicity may occur with gold compounds, other antiinflammatory agents, or acetaminophen. Ketoprofen may decrease the renal clearance of methotrexate and lithium. Ketoprofen may decrease the effectiveness of antihypertensive agents and diuretics. Concomitant use with diuretics may increase nephrotoxic potential. Concomitant use with diuretics or antihypertensives may decrease their effectiveness (see also Table 2).

KETOROLAC TROMETHAMINE
(Toradol)

Ketorolac, a nonsteroidal antiinflammatory agent (30 to 60 mg IM), is used in short-term management of pain (see also Table 2).

KETOROLAC TROMETHAMINE (OPHTHALMIC)
(Acular)

Ketorolac, a nonsteroidal antiinflammatory agent (one drop of 0.5% solution instilled in the conjunctival sac), is used as relief of ocular itching caused by seasonal allergic conjunctivitis (see also Table 2).

L

LABETALOL HYDROCHLORIDE
(Normodyne)

Labetalol (100 mg b.i.d.), either by itself or with a thiazide diuretic, may be used in the treatment of hypertension. Labetalol, an alpha$_1$ and beta-adrenergic blocking agent, causes a dose-dependent fall of blood pressure without causing reflex tachycardia or impairing renal function. Labetalol is absorbed completely, reaching peak plasma level in 1 to 2 hours. It undergoes extensive first-pass effects, is conjugated with glucuronic acid, and the metabolite is excreted in the urine and via bile in the feces. Labetalol is contraindicated in bronchial asthma, overt cardiac failure, third-degree heart block, cardiogenic shock, and severe brady-cardia. Labetatol may prevent the premonitory signs and symptoms, such as tachycardia or hypoglycemia, seen in patients with diabetes mellitus. Like other beta-adrenergic blocking agents, labetalol may also reduce the release of insulin in response to hyperglycemia. Therefore, in patients taking labetalol, the dosage of insulin may need to be readjusted. Beta-adrenergic blocking agents may attenuate the effectiveness of adrenergic receptor agonists used in the management of bronchial asthma. Cimetidine increases the bioavailability of labetalol, and halothane augments the myocardial depressant property of labetalol. Labetalol augments the hypertensive effects of nitroglycerine but blocks the nitroglycerine-induced tachycardia.

LACTOFERRIN

Lactoferrin is a 703-amino acid glycoprotein originally isolated from milk. Plasma lactoferrin is predominantly neutrophil derived, but indications are that it may also be produced by other cells. Lactoferrin in body fluids is found in the iron-free form, the monoferric form, and in the diferric form. Three isoforms of lactoferrin have been isolated, i.e., two with RNAse activity (**lactoferrin-beta** and **lactoferrin-gamma**) and one without RNAse activity (**lacto-ferrin-alpha**). Receptors for lactoferrin can be found on intestinal tissue, monocytes/mac-rophages, neutrophils, lymphocytes, platelets, and on certain bacteria. A wide spectrum of functions is ascribed to lactoferrin. These range from a role in the control of iron availability to immune modulation.

LACTOGEN

Early in pregnancy, **glucose homeostasis** is altered by the increasing levels of **estrogen** and **progesterone**, which lead to **beta-cell hyperplasia** and an increased insulin response to a glucose load. During the second half of pregnancy, rising levels of human placental **lactogen** and other **contra-insulin hormones** synthesized by the placenta modify maternal utilization of glucose and amino acids. The actions of lactogen are responsible, in part, for the diabe-togenic state associated with pregnancy.

LACTULOSE

(Cephulac, Cholac, Chronulac, Constilac, Constulose, Duphalac, Enulose, Generiac, Lactulose PSE)

Lactulose, a disaccharide with laxative properties (20 to 30 g p.o. t.i.d.), is used to prevent and treat portal-systemic encephalopathy, including hepatic precoma and coma in patients with severe hepatic disease.

LAMOTRIGINE
(LAMICTAL)

Lamotrigine, a new antiepileptic agent having a long elimination half-life and relative lack of sedation, makes it an attractive drug in patients with refractory epilepsy. The most common dose-related side effects with lamotrigine are headache, nausea, vomiting, diplopia, dizziness, and ataxia.

LANATOSIDE C

The most important and often-used drugs in the treatment of congestive heart failure are the cardiac glycosides, which may exist and occur naturally in the body. Unfortunately, the **margin of safety** for these drugs is very narrow (therapeutic index 3.0). **Toxicity** can develop readily, and careful attention to the pharmacokinetic principles is absolutely crucial. The cardiac glycosides are obtained from numerous natural sources, including *Digitalis lanata* and *Digitalis purpurea* (white and purple foxglove), **squill** (Mediterranean sea onion), **oleander, lily of the valley**, and other plants. Among the useful available cardiac glycosides are the following:

Digitalis purpurea	Digitalis lanata	Strophanthus gratus
Digitoxin	Digoxin	Ouabain
Digoxin	Lanatoside C	
Digitalis leaf	Deslanoside	

Of these, only digoxin and digitoxin and, to a certain extent, ouabain are used extensively. The **molecular structures** of the cardiac glycosides, including digoxin, have three common components: a steroid nucleus (aglycones or genins), a series of sugar residues in the C3 position, and a five- or six-membered lactone ring in the C17 position.

The **sugar residue** in digoxin and digitoxin is –O-digitoxose-digitoxose-digitoxose. Digoxin varies from digitoxin in having a hydroxy group at C12. Glycosides possess both lipophilic residues (a steroid nucleus) and hydrophilic residues (a lactone ring and OH group). These residues and other factors strongly influence the pharmacokinetic profiles of these cardiac glycosides. **Digitoxin** is excreted extensively unchanged by the kidney. Renal insufficiency alters its half-life and safety. An elevated blood urea nitrogen (BUN) level signals the diminished capacity to eliminate digoxin. A direct relationship exists between the clearance of digoxin and that of creatine, which, in addition to BUN, may be used to assess a patient's ability to excrete digoxin (see also Table 11).

LANSOPRAZOLE

Lansoprazole, structurally related to omeprazole, is a benzimidazole derivative with anti-secretory and antiulcer activities. It inhibits the acid pump activity at the final stage of the enzyme process and therefore reduces the acid secretion of parietal cells. Lansoprazole is converted to active metabolites in the acid environment of the cells (see also Figure 63).

LATANOPROST
(Xalatan)

Latanoprost is as effective as other medications in the treatment of glaucoma, which is the second cause of irreversible blindness in the world. Topical beta-adrenergic receptor blocking agents, timolol maleate, betaxolol, levobunolol, and metipranolol, are the most widely used medications. **Apraclonidine**, a new alpha$_2$-adrenergic agonist decreases aqueous humor formation without effect on outflow. Epinephrine and dipivefrin are effective. Systemic carbonic anhydrase inhibitors acetazolamide, dichlorphenamide, and methazolamide are used in chronic glaucoma when topical therapy is insufficient and in acute glaucoma when very high intraocular pressure needs to be controlled quickly. Latanoprost, a phenyl-substituted prostaglandin F_2 alpha, (one drop of 0.006% once or twice daily) has been shown to be effective in the treatment of ocular hypertension, primary open-angle glaucoma, and capsular glaucoma. Latanoprost has been effectively combined with twice daily ophthalmic timolol (0.5%) in patients who are not adequately controlled on timolol alone. Latanoprost reduces intraocular pressure by increasing uveoscleral outflow without effects on aqueous flow. The only apparent side effect is darkening of the pigment of eyes such as hazel which are made up of multiple colors. It will not change the eye color of someone whose eyes are uniformly blue or uniformly brown. Hazel or green eyes may change, and it may cause brown or blue eyes to darken if they have faded with aging.

LAXATIVES AND CATHARTICS

Although often used interchangeably, the terms **laxative** and **cathartic** do have slightly different meanings. A **laxative effect** refers to the excretion of a soft, formed stool; **catharsis** implies a more fluid and complete evacuation.

Irritant agents used in the treatment of constipation include cascara sagrada, castor oil, senna, rhubarb, phenolphthalein, and acetphenolisatin. Phenolphthalein is a constituent of many over-the-counter preparations, including Ex-Lax and Feen-A-Mint. Most of these agents, with the exception of castor oil, are slow in their onset of action (24 hours). **Phenolphthalein** is thought to exert its effect by inhibiting the movement of water and sodium from the colon into the blood and by stimulating mucus secretion. If misused on a prolonged basis, a consequential loss of mucus may lower the plasma protein level. **Castor oil** is hydrolyzed to **ricinoleic acid**, the active cathartic. It has an onset of action of 2 to 6 hours. The **misuse** of any of these agents has been shown to cause hypokalemia, dehydration, and a cathartic colon (resembling ulcerative colitis). Phenolphthalein-containing products may color alkaline urine red.

Bulk saline laxatives fall into two categories: **inorganic salts** (magnesium sulfate, magnesium citrate, milk of magnesia, sodium sulfate, and sodium phosphate), and **organic hydrophilic colloids** (methylcellulose, carboxymethylcellulose [Metamucil], plantago seed, agar, psyllium, bran, and fruits). They exert their effects by absorbing and retaining water, increasing bulk, stimulating colonic peristaltic movements, and lubricating and hydrating the desiccated fecal materials.

These agents are more effective when administered with water. The onset of action of organic salts is relatively fast (2 to 6 hours) and that of colloids is relatively slow (1 to 3 days). These agents, which are very effective and safe, should not be used when the intestinal lumen has been narrowed. The prolonged use of saline cathartics may create problems for certain individuals. For example, magnesium salts have been known to cause hypermagnesemia, coma, and death in patients with renal insufficiency. Sodium salts may also be responsible for causing congestive heart failure. The lubricants consist of mineral oil and dioctyl sodium sulfonsuccinate (Colace). Colace is used in the pharmaceutical industry as an emulsifying and dispersing substance. Both agents are taken orally. These agents, which do not influence peristalsis, soften desiccated stools or delay the desiccation of fecal materials. They are especially useful in patients with painful bowel movements resulting from inspissated stools or inflammation of the anal sphincter such as occurs with hemorrhoids or anal fissures. Colace is also useful for patients in whom the consequences of "straining at stool" may be harmful. When used for a long time, mineral oil may come to interfere with the absorption of fat-soluble vitamins and other essential nutrients. Lipid pneumonitis may evolve if mineral oil is used as a vehicle for drugs that are taken nasally.

Laxatives are used to hasten the elimination and reduce the absorption of a poison that has been taken. Laxatives are used before and after treatment with antihelmintic drugs. Laxatives are used to clean the gastrointestinal tract before radiographic techniques are performed.

LAXATIVES	
Rapid-acting laxatives (2 hrs)	**Intermediate-acting laxatives (6 hrs)**

Osmotive laxatives
Sodium phosphates
Magnesium sulfate
Milk of magnesia
Magnesium citrate
Castor oil
	Stimulant laxatives
	Diphenylmethane derivatives
	  Phenolphthalein
	  Bixacodyl
	Anthraquinone derivatives
	  Senna
	  Cascara sagrada

Slow-acting laxatives (24 hrs)	
Bulk-forming laxatives Bran Psyllium preparations Methylcellulose Calcium polycarbophil	*Surfactant laxatives* Docusates Poloxamers *Lactulose*

LAZAROIDS

The 21-aminosteroids (lazaroids) are inhibitors of lipid membrane peroxidation and appear to function as **oxygen free radical scavengers**. The therapeutic potential of the lazaroid, **tirilazad mesylate**, has been extensively studied in several CNS disorders. Tirilazad and related compounds have been found to be highly beneficial in spinal cord trauma. Clinical studies using tirilazad in subarachnoid hemorrhage have been more promising. It has been shown to be beneficial in terms of reducing vasospasm and cerebral infarction associated with subarachnoid hemorrhage.

LEGIONNAIRES' DISEASE: TREATMENT OF	
Legionnaires' disease is characterized by a nonproductive cough, pulse-temperature dissociation, abnormalities in results of liver function tests, diarrhea, hyponatremia, hypophosphatemia, myalgia, confusion, and multiple rigors.	
The treatment of Legionnaires' disease is summarized below:	
Antimicrobial Agent(s)	*Dosage*
First choice	
Erythromycin (± rifampin)	Intravenous: 500 mg to 1 g every 6 hr
	Oral: 500 mg (base) every 6 hr
Second choices	
Azithromycin	Oral: 500 mg on day 1, then 250 mg daily for another 4 days
or Clarithromycin	Oral: 250 mg every 12 hr
	Intravenous: 400 mg every 12 hr
or Ciprofloxacin	Oral: 500 mg every 12 hr
or Ofloxacin	Oral or intravenous: 400 mg every 12 hr
or Doxycycline (± rifampin)	Intravenous: 200 mg every 12 hr for two doses, then 200 mg every 24 hr
	Oral: 200 mg once, then either 100 mg every 12 hr or 200 mg every 24 hr
Trimethoprim-sulfamethoxazole (TMP-SMZ)	Intravenous or oral: 5 mg of TMP component per kg every 8 hr

LENOGRASTIM

Lenograstim (recombinant glycosylated human granulocyte colony-stimulating factor; rHuG-CSF, is a hematopoietic growth factor (HGF) which acts primarily to stimulate proliferation and differentiation of committed progenitor cells of the granulocyte-neutrophil lineage into functionally mature neutrophils. Lenograstim is a useful adjunct to chemotherapy for the treatment of nonmyelogenous malignancies, including myeloblastive chemotherapy followed by bone marrow transplantation (see also **Cytokines**).

LEUCOVORIN

Tumor cells acquire **resistance to methotrexate** as the result of several factors, which include the deletion of a high-affinity, carrier-mediated transport system for reduced folates, an increase in the concentration of dihydrofolate reductase, and the formation of a biochemically altered reductase with reduced affinity for methotrexate. To overcome this resistance, higher doses of methotrexate need to be administered. The effects of methotrexate may be reversed by the administration of **leucovorin**, the reduced folate. This leucovorin "rescue" prevents or reduces the toxicity of methotrexate, which is expressed as mouth lesions (stomatitis), injury to the gastrointestinal epithelium (diarrhea), leukopenia, and thrombocytopenia.

LEUPROLIDE ACETATE
(Lupron, Lupron Depot)

Leuprolide, a gonadotropic-releasing hormone, with antineoplastic activity, is used (3.75 to 7.5 mg IM once monthly) in the management of advanced prostate cancer and in the treatment of endometriosis.

LEVAMISOLE

In addition to its antiviral actions, interferon has an antiproliferative effect and modifies the functions of macrophages and natural killer cells. **Thymosin**, a protein synthesized by the epitheloid component of the thymus, may be potentially valuable in patients with **DiGeorge's syndrome** or other T-cell deficiency states. **Levamisole** augments T-cell-mediated immunity and may be of value in the immunodeficiency associated with **Hodgkin's disease.**

LEVOBUNOLOL HYDROCHLORIDE
(Betagan)

Levobunolol, a beta-adrenergic receptor blocking agent (instill 1 to 2 drops of 0.25% solution b.i.d. in each eye), is used in the treatment of chronic open-angle glaucoma and ocular hypertension.

LEVOCABASTINE

Levocabastine is a highly specific and potent histamine H_1-receptor antagonist which has been specifically developed for the topical treatment of allergic rhinoconjunctivitis. Levocabastine is some 15,000 times more potent than **chlorpheniramine,** expressing antihistaminic activity at doses below 0.002 mg/kg. In addition, it has a highly specific binding affinity for H_1-receptors with no evidence of anticholinergic, antiserotonergic, or antidopaminergic activity at doses considerably in excess of therapeutically effective concentrations. **Terfenadine, astemizole, loratadine,** and **cetirizine** are **second-generation** antihistaminic agents that are relatively **nonsedating.**

LEVODOPA

In the management of Parkinson's disease, two major precursors of dopamine, namely **L-tyrosine** and **levodopa**, have been investigated. L-Tyrosine has proved ineffective for two reasons: (1) tyrosine hydroxylase is the rate-limiting enzyme, and it must be bypassed in order to raise the concentration of dopamine, and (2) there is some evidence that the action of tyrosine hydroxylase is defective in parkinsonism. Levodopa is an inert chemical, but its metabolite dopamine is pharmacologically active. The amount of levodopa prescribed depends on the severity of the parkinsonism. It is the current practice to give L-dopa in combination with **carbidopa**, a peripheral dopa-decarboxylase inhibitor. In this combination (**Sinemet**), doses of only several hundred milligrams of levodopa daily, instead of several thousand milligrams if given alone, are necessary for achieving the desired control (see also Figure 23).

The first signs of improvement are usually a subjective feeling of well-being accompanied by increased vigor. The symptoms yield in the following sequence: first the akinesia, then the rigidity, and finally the tremor, which disappears slowly and incompletely. If the drug is stopped, the symptoms reappear in the reverse order: tremor, rigidity, and then akinesia. The postural abnormality responds less effectively to medications. Among the adverse reactions encountered during the first months of levodopa therapy is nausea, usually without vomiting. This emetic action of levodopa is often troublesome and seems to be aggravated by the consumption of coffee. Eliminating coffee, or drinking decaffeinated coffee instead, usually overcomes this problem. Enhancing the dose of carbidopa attenuates the emetic actions of levodopa. The use of a phenothiazine antiemetic (such as **clorpromazine**, which blocks the dopamine receptor sites in the brain and therefore counteracts the beneficial effects of levodopa) is discouraged. The development of involuntary movements may limit the usefulness of levodopa. This **peak dose dyskinesia** is usually manifested in the form of choreic movements that involve the hands, arms, legs, and face. Oromandibular dystonia develops in 10% of the patients. In addition, increased oral activity with constant chewing, biting, opening and closing of the mouth, and intermittent protrusions of the tongue are the most frequent side effects. The abnormal involuntary movements usually occur during the period of maximum benefit from levodopa, which is usually 1 to 2 hours after each dose, and may last from several minutes up to 1 to 2 hours. To avoid these involuntary movements, the frequency of drug administration must usually be increased, and the individual dose of levodopa decreased.

The beneficial and side effects of levodopa may be mediated via different receptor sites. For example, the **beneficial effects** of levodopa may be brought about by the **dopamine$_1$ (D$_1$) receptor**, whereas the **dyskinesia** may be brought about by the **dopamine$_2$ (D$_2$) receptor**. D$_2$ receptor-blocking agents such as **oxiperomide** and **tiapride** are able to reduce levodopa-induced dyskinesia without exacerbating the parkinsonian symptomatology. The conventional phenothiazines (such as **chlorpromazine**) and butyrophenones (such as **haloperidol**) block both D$_1$ and D$_2$ receptors. Therefore, these drugs are not suitable for the management of levodopa-induced dyskinesia.

Levodopa should be used with caution in patients with various **cardiovascular disorders**. The peripheral decarboxylation of levodopa markedly increases the concentration of dopamine in the blood. Dopamine is a pharmacologically active catecholamine that influences alpha- and beta-adrenergic receptors.

Therapeutic doses of levodopa produce cardiac stimulation by activating the beta$_1$ receptor site in the heart. In some elderly patients, it may produce cardiac arrhythmias. The cardiac stimulation is blocked by **propranolol**, the beta-adrenergic receptor-blocking agent (see

Figure 75). Propranolol has also been shown to be effective in suppressing tremor. Particular cardiac conditions that warrant careful attention when the use of levodopa is considered are **angina pectoris** and a history of **cardiac arrhythmias. Psychiatric syndromes, peptic ulcer,** and **glaucoma** are also contraindications to its use.

The **on-off phenomenon** is a sudden loss of effectiveness with the abrupt onset of akinesia ("off" effects) that may last for minutes or hours. This is followed by an equally sudden return of effectiveness ("on" effects) which may even be accompanied by hyperkinesia. The effect is so sudden that it has been compared to the action of a light switch being turned on and off. The use of levodopa is associated with a 10 to 20% frequency of the on-off phenomenon, whereas a 50% frequency is seen with levodopa use alone. The mechanism underlying this on-off phenomenon is not known. Most probably it is due to the sudden unavailability of dopamine to its receptor sites. For example, it has been shown that the on-off phenomenon is greatly relieved in patients who are on low protein diets. Dietary amino acids compete with levodopa for absorption from the gut and for transport across the blood-brain barrier. During the "off" period, the plasma level of levodopa is low. Dopamine receptor agonists are able to alleviate the symptoms, indicating that the receptor site is active.

The on-off effect should be differentiated from the **wearing-off** or **end-of-dose response**. Wearing off is clearly related to the dosage and blood level of levodopa. As the disease progresses and the number of nigral striatal neurons decreases, less dopamine can be stored in the striatum. This necessitates the constant replenishment of levodopa from the blood, so that the bioavailability of plasma levodopa becomes an important factor.

The true on-off phenomenon, which is rarely seen before the second year of treatment, probably is related more to the pharmacodynamic properties of the receptors themselves. The receptor mechanisms are turned off as suddenly as they are also turned on.

LEVODOPA-CARBIDOPA
(Sinemet)

Levodopa, a precursor of dopamine (100 mg), and carbidopa, an inhibitor of peripheral dopa decarboxylase (10 mg), in combination are used in the treatment of Parkinson's disease (see also Figure 23).

LEVOMETHADYL ACETATE HYDROCHLORIDE
(Orlaam)

Levomethadyl acetate hydrochloride, a synthetic diphenylheptane derivative and an opioid receptor agonist (20 to 40 mg p.o.), is used in the management of opiate dependence.

LEVONORGESTREL
(Norplant System)

Levonorgestrel, a progestin with contraceptive properties, is used in long-term (up to 5 years), reversible prevention of pregnancy (see also Figure 46).

LEVOPROPOXYPHENE NAPSYLATE
(Novrad)

Unlike dextropropoxyphene (Darvon), levopropoxyphene has no analgesic or respiratory depressant properties.

LEVORPHANOL TARTRATE

(Levo-Dromoran)

Levorphanol (2 to 3 mg p.o.) is a synthetic morphinan derivative which is recommended for moderate to severe pain, often as an adjunct with anesthetics. It exerts its analgesic action in 20 minutes and has a duration of action of 4 hours. Levorphanol is conjugated with glucuronic acid in the liver and is excreted in the urine. Levorphanol should be administered cautiously during labor and delivery, since it crosses the placental barrier and may cause severe respiratory depression in premature infants. Like morphine, levorphanol is contraindicated in severe head injury where the intracranial pressure may be high. Levorphanol should be administered cautiously to patients with renal or hepatic dysfunction, because drug accumulation or prolonged duration of action may occur; to patients with pulmonary disease (asthma, chronic obstructive pulmonary disease), because the drug depresses respiration and suppresses the cough reflex; to patients undergoing biliary tract surgery, because the drug may cause biliary spasm; to patients with convulsive disorders, because the drug may precipitate seizures; to elderly or debilitated patients, who are more sensitive to both therapeutic and adverse drug effects; and to patients prone to physical or psychic addiction, because of the high risk of addiction to this drug (see also Figure 58).

Numerous CNS drugs including narcotics, analgesics, general anesthetics, antihistamines, phenothiazines, barbiturates, benzodiazepines, sedative-hypnotics, tricyclic antidepressants, alcohol, and muscle relaxants, potentiate the respiratory and CNS depression, sedation, and hypotensive effects of levorphanol.

Levorphanol, when combined with anticholinergic medications, may cause paralytic ileus. The most common signs and symptoms of levorphanol overdose are CNS depression, respiratory depression, and miosis. Naloxone will reverse levorphanol-induced respiratory depression. (Because the duration of action of levorphanol is longer than that of naloxone, repeated antagonist dosing is necessary.)

LEVOSULPIRIDE

Levosulpiride is the (–) enantiomer of sulpiride, an antiemetic, antidyspeptic, and antipsychotic drug. However, levosulpiride is a more potent antiemetic compound than sulpiride. Levosulpiride (50 to 300 mg/day) is effective in depressive and somatoform disorders, as well as in the treatment of negative symptoms in schizophrenic patients.

LEVOTHYROXINE SODIUM

(Synthroid)

Levothyroxine is indicated in the treatment of hypothyroidism (0.05 mg initially); of myxedema coma (0.4 mg IV initially); of thyroid stimulating hormone (TSH) suppression in thyroid cancer; of euthyroid and nodules goiter; and of thyroid suppression therapy (2.6 mcg/kg/day for 7 to 10 days). Levothyroxine increases the metabolic rate of tissue. It affects protein and carbohydrate metabolism, promotes gluconeogenesis, increases the utilization and mobilization of glycogen stores, stimulates protein synthesis, and regulates cell growth and differentiation. The orally administered levothyroxine exerts its full effects within one week. It is distributed widely, and the highest levels are found in the liver and the kidneys. Levothyroxine, which is extensively protein bound, becomes metabolized by deiodination. The half-life of levothyroxine is 6 to 7 days. Levothyroxine is contraindicated in patients with thyrotoxicosis, acute myocardial infarction, and uncorrected adrenal insufficiency because the drug increases tissue metabolic demands. Levothyroxine also is contraindicated for treating obesity because it is ineffective and can cause life-threatening adverse reactions.

Levothyroxine should be used cautiously in patients with angina or other cardiovascular disease because of the risk of increased metabolic demands, and in patients with diabetes mellitus because of reduced glucose tolerance. Concomitant use of levothyroxine with tricyclic antidepressants or sympathomimetics may increase the effects of any or all of these drugs and may lead to coronary insufficiency or cardiac arrhythmias. Clinical manifestations of overdose include the signs and symptoms of hyperthyroidism, including weight loss, increased appetite, palpitations, nervousness, diarrhea, abdominal cramps, sweating, tachycardia, increased blood pressure, widened pulse pressure, angina, cardiac arrhythmias, tremor, headache, insomnia, heat intolerance, fever, and menstrual irregularities (see also Figures 56, 90, and 91).

LIDOCAINE HYDROCHLORIDE
(Xylocaine)

Lidocaine is indicated for production of local or regional anesthesia by the infiltration technique, and by central neural techniques such as lumbar and caudal epidural blocks.

Lidocaine produces faster, more intense, longer-lasting, and more extensive anesthesia than does an equal concentration of procaine. Unlike procaine, it is an aminoethylamide and is the prototypical member of this class of local anesthetics. It is a good choice for individuals sensitive to ester-type local anesthetics. Although it is effective when used without any vasoconstrictor, in the presence of epinephrine, the rate of absorption and the toxicity are decreased, and the duration of action usually is prolonged (see also Figure 72).

Lidocaine, given intravenously, is indicated in the acute management of ventricular arrhythmias. Lidocaine blocks both open and inactivated cardiac Na^+ channels. Recovery from block is very rapid, so lidocaine exerts greater effects in depolarized (e.g., ischemic) and/or rapidly driven tissues. Lidocaine is not useful in atrial arrhythmias, probably because atrial action potentials are so short that the Na^+ channel is in the inactivated state only briefly and diastolic (recovery) times are relatively long (see also Figure 76).

Lidocaine decreases automaticity by reducing the slope of phase 4 and altering the threshold for excitability. Action potential duration usually is unaffected or is shortened; such shortening may be due to the block on the few Na^+ channels that inactivate late during the cardiac action potential. Lidocaine usually exerts no significant effect on PR or QRS duration; QT is unaltered or slightly shortened.

Lidocaine is dealkylated in the liver by mixed-function oxidases to monoethylglycine xylidide and glycine xylidide, which can be metabolized further to monoethylglycine and xylidide. Both monoethylglycine and glycine xylidide retain local anesthetic activity. In human beings, about 75% of xylidide is excreted in the urine as the further metabolite, 4-hydroxy-2,6-dimethylaniline. Clinical effects of overdose include signs and symptoms of CNS toxicity, such as convulsions and/or respiratory depression and cardiovascular toxicity.

LINCOMYCIN
(Lincocin)

Lincomycin, which resembles erythromycin, in a dose of 500 mg t.i.d., is indicated in the treatment of serious infections due to susceptible strains of streptococci, pneumococci, and staphylococci resistant to other antibiotics. Lincomycin inhibits protein synthesis by interfering with the formation of initiation complexes and with aminoacyl translocation reactions. The receptor for lincomycins on the 50S subunit of the bacterial ribosome is a 23S rRNA, perhaps identical to the receptor for erythromycins (see also Figure 80). Thus, these two drug classes may block each other's attachment and may interfere with each other. Resistance to lincomycin appears slowly, perhaps as a result of chromosomal mutation. Plasmid-mediated resistance has not been established with certainty. Resistance to lincomycin is not rare among streptococci, pneumococci, and staphylococci. *C. difficile* strains are regularly resistant.

Lincomycin is widely distributed in the body but does not appear in the central nervous system in significant concentrations. It is about 90% protein-bound. Excretion is mainly through the liver, bile, and urine. Lincomycin's common adverse effects are diarrhea, nausea, and skin rashes. Impaired liver function (with or without jaundice) and neutropenia sometimes occur. Severe diarrhea and enterocolitis have followed clindamycin administration and place a serious restraint on its use.

LINDANE
(Gamma Benzene Hexachloride) (G-Well, Kwell, Kwildane, Scabene)

Lindane, a chlorinated hydrocarbon insecticide with scabicidal and pediculicidal properties (1% cream, lotion, shampoo), is used in scabies and pediculosis.

LINOLEIC ACID

All naturally occurring **prostaglandins** are derived through the **cyclization** of 20-carbon unsaturated fatty acids such as **arachidonic acid**, which in turn is synthesized from the essential fatty acid, **linoleic acid.**

Besides serving as a precursor for the synthesis of prostaglandins, arachidonic acid is also a precursor for the synthesis of prostacyclin, thromboxanes, and leukotrienes.

LIOTHYRONINE
(Cytomel; Cytomine)

Liothyronine, a thyroid preparation, has a short half-life and hence is used diagnostically in the T_3 suppression test.

LIOTRIX
(Euthyroid; Thyrolar)

Liotrix, a thyroid preparation, is a combination of T_4 and T_3, and is standardized to yield a T_4 to T_3 ratio of 4 to 1 (see also Figure 56).

LIPID-LOWERING DRUGS	
Drugs	**Actions**
HMG-CoA Reductase Inhibitors	
Fluvastatin Lovastatin Pravastatin Simvastatin	Inhibit HMG-CoA (3-hydroxy-3-methyl-glutaryl-coenzyme A) reductase, the enzyme that catalyzes the rate-limiting step in cholesterol synthesis
Bile Acid-Binding Resins	
Cholestyramine Colestipol	Lower concentration of LDL cholesterol
Fibric Acid Derivatives	
Gemfibrozil Clofibrate Bezafibrate	Lower VLDL and can increase HDL cholesterol concentrations

Nicotinic Acid	
Niacin	Decreases triglyceride

HMG-CoA reductase inhibitors are the drugs of first choice for treatment of most patients with hypercholesterolemia. They are more effective and better tolerated than other lipid-lowering drugs, and have been shown to decrease mortality from coronary artery disease.

LISINOPRIL
(Prinivil, Zestril)

Agents with **positive inotropic actions** that may be used in the management of congestive heart failure include the **cardiac glycosides** (e.g., digoxin and digitoxin), **dopaminergic analogs** (e.g., dobutamine), **phosphodiesterase inhibitors** (e.g., amrinone and milrinone), **angiotensin antagonists** (e.g., captopril, enalapril, and lisinopril), and **vasodilators** (nitrates and hydralazine. Lisinopril, an **angiotensin-converting enzyme** inhibitor, increases the left ventricular ejection fraction in patients with congestive heart failure, and the drug's effectiveness is not diminished in the presence of impaired renal function. Lisinopril (10 mg once a day) may be used in patients with uncomplicated essential hypertension not on diuretic therapy. Lisinopril (5 mg once a day) may be used with diuretics and digitalis in congestive heart failure (see Figure 21).

LITHIUM CARBONATE
(Eskalith)

Lithium is given orally as a salt, and the particular salt does not affect the therapeutic action. Lithium's anionic partner — carbonate, chloride acetate, citrate, or sulfate — serves only as an inert vehicle. Carbonate is by far the most widely used lithium salt. In addition, lithium carbonate contains more lithium, weight for weight, than do the other lithium salts. Because lithium is not bound to any plasma or tissue proteins, it is widely **distributed** throughout the body. Lithium ions are **eliminated** mainly by the kidneys. There is a direct relationship between the amount of **sodium chloride** ingested and the fraction of filtered lithium resorbed, in that the lower the sodium intake, the greater is the lithium retention. The **contraindications** are significant cardiovascular or renal diseases that would compromise its excretion. Lithium is unique among the psychopharmacologic compounds in that it rarely has any undesirable effects on emotional or intellectual functioning. A few unwanted effects are seen in the somatic sphere, and these fall into three overlapping categories.

1. Initially, when the maintenance dose of lithium is being established, the patient may experience **gastrointestinal discomfort** such as nausea, vomiting, diarrhea, stomach pain, muscular weakness, unusual thirst, frequent urination, and a slight feeling of being dazed, tired, and sleepy. These early side effects disappear once the patient is stabilized.
2. From the beginning of treatment, patients exhibit slight and barely noticeable **hand tremors**, which do not respond to antiparkinsonian agents.
3. After several months of continuous therapy with lithium, **diabetes insipidus** and **goiter** may develop. The kidney tubules then become insensitive to the action of **antidiuretic hormone**, and its administration is ineffective. Either a dose reduction or discontinuation of the lithium corrects this side effect without leaving any residual pathology. In the presence of goiter, the patient remains euthyroid. It has been reported that the administration of small amounts of **thyroxine** may counteract this side effect. Lithium is thought to exert its effect by interfering with the

calcium-mediated release of norepinephrine increasing the uptake of norepinephrine, and decreasing the sensitivity of postsynaptic receptor sites to norepinephrine.
In addition, there is increasing evidence that lithium exerts its therapeutic action
by interfering with the polyphosphoinositide metabolism in the brain and by preventing inositol recycling through the uncompetitive inhibition of inositol mono-
phosphatase.

The uses of lithium fall into two categories: established and innovative. Among its **established
uses**, lithium salts are used to treat acute mania and as a prophylactic measure to prevent the
recurrence of bipolar manic-depressive illness. As **innovative** agents, lithium salts have been
used with certain success in the management of the following illnesses or conditions. In
combination with tricyclic antidepressants, lithium is used in treating **recurrent endogenous
depression**. In combination with neuroleptics, it is used in the management of **schizoaffective
disorders**. In combination with neuroleptics, it is used to control **schizophrenia**. Lithium is
also used in the case of patients with **alcoholism** associated with depression and has been
used to correct the **neutropenia** that occurs during cancer chemotherapy. Lithium has been
investigated for use in subduing **aggressive behaviors** in nonpsychotic but possibly brain-
damaged patients. Its use has also been investigated in the management of **inappropriate
secretion of antidiuretic hormone**.

LITOXETINE

Litoxetine is a new selective and potent inhibitor of serotonin receptors which has antiemetic
effects against cisplatin-induced emesis. The clinical use of the majority of serotoninergic
antidepressants such as fluoxetin and fluvoxamine is associated with gastrointestinal discomfort which appears to be due to stimulation of $5-HT_3$ receptors. Litoxetine, by antagonizing
$5-HT_3$ receptors, may limit nausea and vomiting associated with fluoxetin or fluvoxamine
(see also Figure 64).

LOCAL ANESTHETICS	
Ester Compounds	**Amide Compounds**
Chloroprocaine	Bupivacaine
Procaine	Etidocaine
Tetracaine	Lidocaine
	Mepivacaine
	Prilocaine

Epinephrine is used in combination with a local anesthetic to reduce its
uptake, prolong its duration of action, produce a bloodless field of operation,
and protect against systemic effects. Local anesthetic solutions containing
epinephrine should not be used in areas supplied by end-arteries such as in
the digits, ear, nose, and penis, because of the threat of ischemia and
subsequential gangrene. Furthermore, under no circumstances should anesthetic solutions containing epinephrine be used intravenously in patients
with cardiac arrhythmias. In general, solutions designed for multiple doses
should not be used for spinal or epidural anesthesia (see also Figure 72).

LODOXAMIDE TROMETHAMINE

(Alomide)

Lodoxamide, a substance which stabilizes mast cells and has antiallergic properties (1 to
2 drops of 0.1% solution into each affected eye), is used in the treatment of vernal keratoconjunctivitis, vernal conjunctivitis, and vernal keratitis.

LOMEFLOXACIN HYDROCHLORIDE
(Maxaquin)

Lomefloxacin, a fluoroquinolone broad-spectrum antibiotic (400 mg p.o. daily for 10 to 14 days), is used in acute bacterial exacerbations of chronic bronchitis caused by *Haemophilis influenzae* or *Moraxella (Branhamella) catarrhalis*; in uncomplicated urinary tract infections (cystitis) caused by *Escherichia coli, Klebsiella pneumoniae, Proteus mirabilis,* or *Staphylococcus saprophyticus*; in complicated urinary tract infections caused by *E. coli, K. pneumoniae, P. mirabilis,* and *Pseudomonas aeruginosa*; and it is possibly effective against infections caused by *Citrobacter diversus* or *Enterobacter cloacae*; and for the prophylaxis of infections after transurethral surgical procedures (see also Figure 77).

LOMUSTINE
(CCNU)

Carmustine (**BNCU**), lomustine (**CCNU**), and semustine (**methyl-CCNU**) generate alkyl carbonium ions and isocyanate molecules and hence are able to interact with DNA and other macromolecules. These agents, which are lipid soluble, cross the blood-brain barrier and are therefore effective in treating brain tumors. They are bone marrow depressants.

LOOP DIURETICS

The major loop diuretics are furosemide (Lasix) and ethacrynic acid (Edecrin). **Furosemide** is chemically related to the thiazide diuretics, but **ethacrynic acid** is not. These agents inhibit the active resorption of chloride (and sodium) in the thick, ascending medullary portion of the loop of Henle and also in the cortical portion of the loop or the distal tubule. The diuresis they produce, which is similar to that seen with the thiazides, predominantly causes a loss of chloride, sodium, and potassium, but HCO_3 excretion is not increased. Although large volumes of fluid can be excreted with the use of these agents, the ability of the kidney to produce either a dilute or concentrated urine is greatly diminished. These agents are the most efficacious of all the diuretics now on the market, usually producing about a 20% loss in the filtered load of sodium (furosemide, 15 to 30%; ethacrynic acid, 17 to 23%). Loop diuretics are ordinarily taken orally, but can be given intravenously if a very rapid onset of action is sought, as when used in combination with antihypertensive medications in the management of a **hypertensive crisis**. Furosemide and ethacrynic acid undergo some active renal tubular secretion as well as glomerular filtration. A minor portion is excreted by the liver. Loop diuretics are used for treating the following conditions:

In the **edema** of cardiac, hepatic, or renal origin, including acute pulmonary edema and hypertensive crisis

In **acute renal failure**, to maintain urine flow, though an excessive loss of extracellular fluid volume can cause a decrease in the GFR, and

In hypercalemia.

Excessive volume depletion, hyponatremia, and hypotension are major risks associated with the use of loop diuretics, and the side effects of **hypokalemia, hyperuricemia,** and **hyperglycemia** are always present. Loop diuretics should not be used concurrently with **ototoxic aminoglycoside antibiotics** (i.e., streptomycin, gentamicin, kanamycin, tobramycin) (see also Table 25 and Figure 4).

LOPERAMIDE HYDROCHLORIDE
(Imodium)

Loperamide (4 mg initially and not exceeding 16 mg/day) is indicated in the control and symptomatic relief of acute nonspecific diarrhea and chronic diarrhea associated with inflammatory bowel diseases. In addition, it may be used to control traveler's diarrhea or to reduce the volume of discharge from ileostomies. The antidiarrheal agents are codeine, diphenoxylate and atropine (Lomotil), and loperamide. Because it causes less addiction than codeine, **loperamide** is now the most commonly used antidiarrheal agent. These agents achieve their effects by reducing the propulsive activity of the gut, enhancing the contact time between the intestinal mucosal and the luminal contents, and enhancing active chloride absorption, hence opposing the secretory effects of toxin. Loperamide should not be used in acute diarrhea associated with organisms that penetrate the intestinal mucosa (enteroinvasive *Escherichia coli, Salmonella,* and *Shigella*) or in pseudomembranous colitis associated with broad-spectrum antibiotics. Opioid antidiarrheal agents should not be used in cases of severe ulcerative colitis threatened by impending toxic megacolon or in patients with shigellosis, because they prolong duration of the disease.

LORACARBEF
(Lorabid)

Loracarbef, a synthetic beta lactam antibiotic of the carbacephem class (200 to 400 mg p.o. q. 12 hours), is used in the treatment of secondary bacterial infections of acute bronchitis, acute bacterial exacerbations or chronic bronchitis, of pneumonia, pharyngitis, tonsillitis, sinusitis, acute otitis media, uncomplicated skin and skin-structure infections, impetigo, uncomplicated cystitis, and in uncomplicated pyelonephritis.

LORATIDINE
(Claritin)

Terfenadine, astemizole, loratadine, and **cetirizine** are **second-generation** antihistaminic agents that are relatively **nonsedating**. Other H_1-receptor antagonists currently undergoing clinical trials are **azelastine, ebastine,** and **levocabastine.** Loratadine is readily absorbed, with its onset of action beginning within 1 to 3 hours, reaching a maximum at 8 to 12 hours, and lasting in excess of 24 hours. Because peak plasma concentration may be delayed by 1 hour with a meal, the drug should be administered on an empty stomach.

Loratidine is about 98% bound to plasma protein. The drug does not readily cross the blood-brain barrier. Loratidine is extensively metabolized to an active metabolite called descarboethoxyloratadine. Approximately 80% of the total dose administered can be found equally distributed between urine and feces. The mean elimination half-life is 8.4 hours for loratadine. Loratidine overdosage (40 mg) causes somnolence, tachycardia, and headache.

LORAZEPAM
(Ativan)

Lorazepam (2 to 3 mg/day) is indicated for the management of anxiety disorders or for the short-term relief of the symptoms of anxiety or anxiety associated with depressive symptoms. In addition, it may be used as a preanesthetic medication producing sedation, relief of anxiety, and a decreased ability to recall events related to surgery.

The pharmacology of benzodiazepine derivatives differs significantly from that of the neuroleptics, in that the benzodiazepines have no psychoplegic (antipsychotic) activity and cause no extrapyramidal, autonomic, or endocrine side effects. In addition, unlike the neuroleptics, which lower the seizure threshold, these substances are anticonvulsants. In addition, they are anxiolytics, muscle relaxants, and mild sedatives. Although the benzodiazepine derivatives do not produce pronounced autonomic or cardiovascular side effects, they can reduce or block the emotionally induced changes in cardiovascular functions, probably through actions on the limbic system.

Compounds such as **oxazepam** and **lorazepam**, which possess inactive metabolites, are relatively short acting, whereas compounds such as **prazepam**, with several active metabolites, have longer disposition half-lives. Consequently, it may be necessary to reduce the doses of those benzodiazepines with active metabolites.

Lorazepam is absorbed from the gastrointestinal tract at a slightly more rapid rate than oxazepam, with peak plasma concentrations occurring about 2 hours after the administration of a single oral dose. **Steady-state plasma levels** may vary considerably between individuals during repeated dosing, as is the case with other benzodiazepines. Age has no effect on steady-state concentrations, but clearance is slightly reduced in elderly subjects. Unlike diazepam or chlordiazepoxide, the **absorption** of lorazepam from **intramuscular injection sites** is predictable, producing a pattern of absorption similar to that observed with oral doses. Like other benzodiazepines, lorazepam has a relatively large **volume of distribution** of 0.9 L/kg. More than 90% of circulating lorazepam is bound to plasma proteins. As with oxazepam, glucuronidation to an inactive metabolite is the primary **metabolic pathway** of lorazepam, although very small amounts of other metabolites (hydroxylorazepam and quinazolinone derivatives) have been identified in humans. As with oxazepam, **liver disease** does not appreciably alter either the elimination half-life or the plasma clearance of lorazepam. Similarly, in the context of severe renal impairment the elimination half-life of unchanged lorazepam is not altered (see also Table 8).

LOSARTAN

Losartan, a nonpeptide, biphenylimidazole potassium salt, is the first agent in a new class of effective antihypertensive drugs called angiotensin II (Ang II) receptor blockers used for treatment of hypertension. Losartan works by blocking the binding of Ang II selectively at the type 1 Ang II receptor (AT_1), thereby inhibiting all known actions of Ang II that are associated with hypertension (see also Figure 21).

LOVASTATIN

(Mevacor)

Lovastatin (20 mg daily) is indicated for reduction of low-density lipoprotein and total cholesterol levels in patients with primary hypercholesterolemia (types IIa IIb).

Lovastatin, an inactive lactone, is hydrolyzed to the beta-hydroxy acid, which specifically inhibits 3-hydroxy-3-methylglutaryl-coenzyme A reductase (HMG-CoA reductase). This enzyme is an early (and rate-limiting) step in the synthetic pathway of cholesterol. At therapeutic doses, the enzyme is not blocked, and biologically necessary amounts of cholesterol can still be synthesized. These reductase inhibitors are structural analogs of 3-hydroxy-3-methylglutaryl-coenzyme A (HMG-CoA). The first drug in this class was **compactin.** A close congener, **lovastatin**, is widely used. **Simvastatin, pravastatin,** and **fluvastatin** are similar drugs.

Lovastatin is absorbed to the extent of 30% and undergoes an extensive first-pass hepatic extraction. Lovastatin is converted to the active B hydroxy acid form in the liver. Other metabolites include the 6′ hydroxy derivative and two unidentified compounds. About 80% of lovastatin is excreted primarily in feces, about 10% in urine. Concomitant administration with cholestyramine or colestipol may enhance lipid-reducing effects but may decrease bioavailability of lovastatin. Concomitant administration of cyclosporine, erythromycin, gemfibrozil, or niacin may increase risk of severe myopathy or rhabdomyolysis. Lovastatin may increase the anticoagulant effects of warfarin (see also Figure 25).

LOWER RESPIRATORY TRACT INFECTIONS: TREATMENT OF

Lower respiratory tract infections (LRTI) may be grouped according to their clinical picture and differing etiology: bronchitis (acute bronchitis, exacerbation of chronic bronchitis) and pneumonia [primary (community acquired), secondary (nosocomial), atypical]. Additionally, severe cases of LRTIs (mostly pneumonia) should be treated according to the degree of severity.

Acute bronchitis is usually a viral infection which, unless there is a special disposition, does not require antibiotic therapy. For the initial oral chemotherapy of bacterial infections of the lower respiratory tract (chronic bronchitis, pneumonia) the effective and well tolerated cephalosporins, macrolides, and amoxicillin plus β-lactamase-inhibitor are recommended. In complicated cases with severe underlying disease, longer history or frequent exacerbations, quinolones should be given if Gram-negative infections are suspected or if initial therapy with other substances has failed. If *Legionella, Mycoplasma,* or *Chlamydia spp.,* so-called "atypical" pathogens, are involved, macrolide antibiotics are the therapy of first choice. Special attention should be given to the increase in resistance against co-trimoxazole (trimethoprim-sulfamethoxazole) and tetracyclines. In hospitals where primary pneumonias are treated preferentially by intravenous medication, therapy should be switched to oral antibiotics as soon as feasible (follow-up therapy).

For severely ill patients with secondary pneumonia and underlying disease, second-generation cephalosporins with aminoglycosides, or monotherapy with third-generation cephalosporins are recommended. In very severe, high-risk cases, third-generation cephalosporins, combinations with high-dosage quinolones or ureidopenicillins plus β-lactamase-inhibitors are suitable.

LOXAPINE HYDROCHLORIDE
(Loxitane C, Loxitane I.M.)

LOXAPINE SUCCINATE
(Loxitane)

Loxapine, a dibenzoxazepine compound, represents a new subclass of tricyclic antipsychotic agents, chemically distinct from the thioxanthenes, butyrophenones, and phenothiazines. Chemically, it is a 2-Chloro-11-(4-methyl-1-piperazinyl)-dibenz[b,f](1,4)oxazepine. It is present in capsules as the succinate salt, and in the concentrate and parenteral forms primarily as the hydrochloride salt.

Loxapine (10 mg b.i.d.) is indicated for the treatment of psychotic disorders. It exerts its antipsychotic effects in part by blocking postsynaptic dopamine receptors. It causes moderate sedation, possesses anticholinergic properties, and produces extensive movement disorders such as akathisia, dystonia, parkinsonism, tardive dyskinesia, and neuroleptic malignant syndrome.

Loxapine is absorbed rapidly and completely from the GI tract. Sedation occurs in 30 minutes. Loxapine is distributed widely into the body, including breast milk. Peak effect occurs at $1^1/_2$ to 3 hours; steady-state serum level is achieved within 3 to 4 days. The drug is 91 to 99% protein-bound.

The drug is metabolized extensively by the liver, forming a few active metabolites; duration of action is 12 hours. Most of the drug is excreted as metabolites in urine, some is excreted in feces via the biliary tract. About 50% of the drug is excreted in urine and feces within 24 hours. Similar to phenothiazine derivatives such as chlorpromazine, loxapine should be used cautiously in patients with cardiac disease (arrhythmias, congestive heart failure, angina pectoris, valvular disease, or heart block), encephalitis, Reye's syndrome, head injury, respiratory disease, epilepsy and other seizure disorders, glaucoma, prostatic hypertrophy, urinary retention, hepatic or renal dysfunction, Parkinson's disease, or pheochromocytoma. Overdosage with loxapine causes CNS depression characterized by deep, unarousable sleep and possible coma, hypotension or hypertension, extrapyramidal symptoms, abnormal involuntary muscle movements, agitation, seizures, arrhythmias, ECG changes, hypothermia or hyperthermia, and autonomic nervous system dysfunction (see also Table 23).

LUGOL'S SOLUTION

Iodides such as potassium iodide and **Lugol's solution**, which contain 5% iodine and 10% potassium iodide, exert their beneficial effects by inhibiting organification, inhibiting the release of thyroid hormones, and decreasing (inhibiting proteolysis) the size and vascularity of the gland. This makes them useful for preparing the patient for surgery (see also Figure 56).

LUTEINIZING HORMONE

The pituitary hormones responsible for regulating gonadal function are **luteinizing hormone (LH)** and **follicle-stimulating hormone (FSH)**. In males, LH stimulates the Leydig's cells to synthesize **testosterone**; FSH stimulates the Sertoli's cells to synthesize **inhibin** and **androgen-binding protein** and, in conjunction with high intratesticular concentrations of testosterone, initiates and maintains **spermatogenesis.** In females, LH stimulates **androgen synthesis**, and FSH increases estrogen and inhibin synthesis in the granulosa cells. Both LH and FSH are released from the gonadotroph cells of the anterior pituitary in response to the hypothalamic hormone gonadotropin-releasing hormone (GnRH; also known as LH-releasing hormone). GnRH is a decapeptide with the following structure: pyro Glu-His-Trp-Ser-Tyr-Gly-Leu-Arg-Pro-Gly-NH$_2$ (see also Table 14).

LYMPHOCYTE IMMUNE GLOBULIN

(Antithymocyte Globulin [Equine]) (Atgam)

Lymphocyte immune globulin, an immunoglobulin with immunosuppressive properties (15 mg/kg/day IV for 14 days), is used in prevention or treatment of acute renal allograft rejection, in aplastic anemia, skin allotransplantation, and in bone marrow allotransplantation (see also Figure 16).

LYMPHOKINES

Because tumor growth is associated with the progressive impairment of immunologic competence, a therapeutic goal is the enhancement of cell-mediated immunity. Cell-mediated immunity may be augmented by **nonspecific stimulants** such as **levamisole, lymphokines,** and **interferon**, which stimulate the antitumor activity of natural killer cells. Cell-mediated immunity may also be stimulated by **specific stimulants** such as vaccines, which are composed of killed or inactivated tumor cells or tumor cell fragments. The full range of immunotherapy's usefulness remains to be realized (see also Figures 53 and 99).

LYPRESSIN

(Diapid)

Vasopressin (Pitressin) may be administered either subcutaneously or intramuscularly. It has a duration of action of 2 to 8 hours. Vasopressin tannate (pitressin tannate) is a suspension and should be injected intramuscularly only. It has a duration of action of 2 to 3 days. **Desmopressin acetate** (DDAVP) is used topically. **Lypressin** is administered as an intranasal spray. All these agents may be used in the treatment of central diabetes insipidus (vasopressin sensitive) (see also Figure 94).

M

MAFENIDE

(Sulfamylon)

Mafenide, a topical antibacterial agent (8.5% cream) is indicated as an adjunctive treatment of second- and third-degree burns.

MAGALDRATE

(Aluminum-Magnesium Complex) (Lowsium, Riopan, Riopan Plus)

Magaldrate, an antacid (540 mg between meals) by neutralizing gastric acid and inactivating pepsin, is used in the management of acid pepsin disease.

MACROLIDE ANTIBIOTICS
Azithromycin
Clarithromycin
Erythromycin

MAGNESIUM HYDROXIDE

(Milk of Magnesia, Magnesia Magma)

Magnesium hydroxide, an antacid with laxative properties (6 to 20 ml/p.o.), is used as an antacid, as a laxative in constipation and in bowel evacuation before surgery.

MAGNESIUM SALICYLATE

(Analate, Arthrin, Doan's Pills, Efficin, Magan, Mobidin)

Magnesium salicylate (500 mg) is indicated for the relief of the signs and symptoms of rheumatoid arthritis, osteoarthritis, bursitis, and other musculoskeletal disorders. Magnesium salicylate is a nonsteroidal antiinflammatory agent with antipyretic and analgesic properties. Salicylic acid is the active moiety released into the plasma by magnesium salicylate. Salicylic acid is enzymatically biotransformed through two pathways to salicyluric acid and salicylphenolic glucuronide and eliminated in the urine. Oral salicylates are absorbed rapidly, partly from the stomach but mostly from the upper intestine. Salicylic acid is rapidly distributed throughout all body tissues and most transcellular fluids, mainly by pH-dependent passive processes. It can be detected in synovial, spinal and peritoneal fluid, in saliva, and in milk. It readily crosses the placental barrier. From 50 to 90% of salicylic acid is bound to plasma proteins, especially albumin. Magnesium salicylate is contraindicated in patients with advanced chronic renal insufficiency (see also Table 2).

MANIC SYMPTOMS: DRUG-INDUCED	
Alcohol	Disulfiram
Amantadine	Ephedrine
Amphetamines	Hallucinogens
Anabolic steroids	Indomethacin
Anticholinergics	Isoniazid
Anticonvulsants	Levodopa
Antidepressants	Monoamine oxidase inhibitors
Baclofen	Methylphenidate
Benzodiazepines	Metoclopramide
Bromides	Niridazole
Bronchodilators	Phenylpropanolamine
Caffeine	Procainamide
Calcium	Procarbazine
Captopril	Quinacrine
Cimetidine	Sympathomimetics
Cocaine	Theophylline
Corticosteroids (ACTH)	Thyroid supplements
Decongestants	Tolmetin
Diltiazem	Yohimbine

In addition, withdrawal from certain medications, such as baclofen, clonidine, corticosteroids, or tricyclic antidepressants, may cause manic symptoms.

MANNITOL

(Osmitrol)

The osmotic diuretics and related agents consist of **mannitol, urea** (Ureaphil), **glycerin** (Glycerol, Osmoglyn), and **isosorbide** (Hydronol). Mannitol and urea are nonelectrolytes that are freely filterable and undergo very little or no metabolism or renal tubular resorption. When given in sufficient quantities, these drugs increase the osmolarity of plasma and the amount of both the glomerular filtrate and the renal tubular fluid. The presence of such a drug in the lumen prevents the resorption of much of the water, hence the urine volume is increased. They do not prevent the active resorption of sodium from the tubular fluid, but some additional sodium is excreted as a normal constituent of the increased volume of urine. Osmotic diuretics are not effective in removing the edematous fluid caused by sodium retention, but can maintain the flow of urine even when the GFR is decreased. Osmotic diuretics are given by intravenous infusion in a hypertonic solution, and they are excreted by glomerular filtration (see also Figure 4 and Table 25).

MAPROTILINE HYDROCHLORIDE

(Ludiomil)

Maprotiline (75 mg/day), a tricyclic antidepressant, is indicated for the treatment of depressive illness in patients with depressive neurosis (dysthymic disorder) and manic-depressive illness, depressed type (major depressive disorder). Also, it is effective for the relief of anxiety associated with depression. Its properties are compared with that of imipramine and are listed in Tables 3 through 5.

MASOPROCOL
(Actinex)

Masoprocol, a dicatechol compound with antipsoriatic and antineoplastic properties (10% cream), is used in actinic (solar) keratoses.

MAZINDOL
(Mazanor, Sanorex)

Mazindol, an imidazoisoindol, is used as a short-term adjunct regimen in exogenous obesity. In addition, mazindol has been used in the treatment of cocaine misuse and narcolepsy.

MEASLES, MUMPS, AND RUBELLA VIRUS VACCINE, LIVE
(M-M-R-II)

This vaccine is used for measles, mumps, and rubella immunization.

MEASLES AND RUBELLA VIRUS VACCINE, LIVE, ATTENUATED
(M-R-Vax II)

This vaccine is used in measles and rubella immunization.

MEASLES VIRUS VACCINE, LIVE, ATTENUATED
(Attenuvax)

This viral vaccine is used for immunization.

MEBENDAZOLE
(Vermox)

Mebendazole is indicated for the treatment of *Trichuris trichiura* (whipworm), *Enterobius vermicularis* (pinworm), *Ascaris lumbricoides* (roundworm), *Ancylostoma duodenale* (common hookworm), or *Necator americanus* (American hookworm), in single or mixed infections.

Mebendazole inhibits the formation of the worms' microtubules and irreversibly blocks glucose uptake by the susceptible helminths, thereby depleting endogenous glycogen stored within the parasite which is required for survival and reproduction of the helminth. Mebendazole does not affect blood glucose concentrations in the host.

Mebendazole is absorbed poorly after oral administration, and most of it is excreted unchanged in the feces.

Mebendazole exerts its effects slowly (3 days), and effectiveness of treatment depends on the degree of infection or resistance of the parasites to treatment. Phenytoin or carbamazepine reduce the plasma level of mebendazole.

MECAMYLAMINE HYDROCHLORIDE
(Inversine)

Mecamylamine, a ganglionic blocking agent with antihypertensive properties (2 to 5 mg b.i.d.), is used in the treatment of moderately severe to severe essential hypertension and uncomplicated malignant hypertension.

MECHLORETHAMINE HYDROCHLORIDE

(Mustargen)

Mechlorethamine (0.4 mg/kg for each course) is indicated in the palliative treatment of Hodgkin's disease (Stages III and IV), lymphosarcoma, chronic myelocytic or chronic lymphocytic leukemia, polycythemia vera, mycosis fungoides, and bronchogenic carcinoma. Mechlorethamine is an alkylating agent with cytotoxic, mutagenic, and radiomimetic actions which inhibit rapidly proliferating cells. Mechlorethamine is highly toxic and is a potent vesicant. Extravasation of mechlorethamine into subcutaneous tissues results in painful inflammation and induration.

The adverse reactions of mechlorethamine are thrombosis and thrombophlebitis (local toxicity). Bone marrow depression and gastrointestinal problems such as nausea and severe vomiting begin 1 to 3 hours after use and may persist for 24 hours. A maculopapular skin eruption and erythema multiforme have occurred. Alopecia occurs infrequently. Delayed menses, oligomenorrhea, temporary or permanent amenorrhea, and, in male patients, impaired spermatogenesis, azoospermia, and total germinal aplasia have occurred, especially those receiving combination therapy, such as in **MOPP therapy** (mechlorethamine, Oncovin [vincristine], procarbazine, and prednisone). Spermatogenesis may return in patients in remission, but this may occur several years after chemotherapy has been discontinued.

MECLIZINE HYDROCHLORIDE

(Antivert)

Meclizine (25 to 50 mg 1 hour prior to travel) is indicated for prevention and treatment of nausea, vomiting, and dizziness of motion sickness. Meclizine has antiemetic, anticholinergic, and antihistaminic properties. It reduces the sensitivity of the labyrinthine apparatus. The action may be mediated through neuronal pathways to the vomiting center (VC), from the chemoreceptor trigger zone (CTZ), peripheral nerve pathways, or other CNS centers (see also Figure 73).

Meclizine may produce drowsiness and hence should be used cautiously while completing tasks which require alertness. Because of its anticholinergic properties, meclizine should be used cautiously in patients with glaucoma, obstructive disease of the GI or GU tract, and in elderly male subjects with possible prostatic hypertrophy. This drug may have a hypotensive action, which become confusing or dangerous in postoperative patients.

Meclizine may potentiate the CNS depressant effects of alcohol, barbiturates, and anxiolytic agents. The overdosage of meclizine will cause drowsiness, restlessness, excitation, nervousness, insomnia, euphoria, blurred vision, diplopia, vertigo, tinnitus, and auditory and visual hallucinations.

MECLOFENAMATE SODIUM

(Meclomen)

Meclofenamate is indicated in the relief of mild to moderate pain (50 mg/6 hours); in the treatment of primary dysmenorrhea (100 mg t.i.d.); and in acute and chronic rheumatoid arthritis and osteoarthritis (200 to 400 mg/day in 3 to 4 equal doses). Meclofenamate is a nonsteroidal antiinflammatory agent which has analgesic and antipyretic properties. The menstrual cycle is associated with two potentially incapacitating events: **dysmenorrhea** and the **premenstrual syndrome**. Substantial evidence indicates that the excessive production of prostaglandin F_{2a}, is the major source of painful menstruation. The nonsteroidal antiinflammatory drugs such as **aspirin, ibuprofen, meclofenamate, mefenamic acid**, and **naproxen** are used to treat dysmenorrhea.

Meclofenamate is rapidly absorbed, with peak plasma concentration occurring in one hour. It is extensively metabolized to an active metabolite (3-hydroxymethyl metabolite of meclofenamic acid) and at least six other less well-characterized minor metabolites. Only this active metabolite has been shown to inhibit cyclooxygenase activity *in vitro* with approximately one fifth the activity of meclofenamate sodium. The 3-hydroxymethyl metabolite of meclofenamic acid with a mean half-life of approximately 15 hours, does accumulate following multiple dosing. Approximately 70% of the administered dose is excreted by the kidneys, with 8 to 35% excreted as conjugated species of meclofenamic acid and its active metabolite.

Concomitant use of meclofenamate with anticoagulants and thrombolytic drugs (coumarin derivatives, heparin, streptokinase, or urokinase) may potentiate anticoagulant effects. Bleeding problems may occur if used with other drugs that inhibit platelet aggregation, such as azlocillin, parenteral carbenicillin, dextran, dipyridamole, mazlocillin, piperacillin, sulfinpyrazone, ticarcillin, valproic acid, cefamandole, cefoperazone, moxalactam, plicamycin, salicylates, or other antiinflammatory agents. Alcohol, corticotropin, or steroids may increase adverse GI effects caused by meclofenamate which may include ulceration and hemorrhage. Aspirin may decrease the bioavailability of meclofenamate.

Because of the influence of prostaglandins on glucose metabolism, concomitant use with insulin or oral hypoglycemic agents may potentiate hypoglycemic effects. Meclofenamate may displace highly protein-bound drugs from binding sites. Toxicity may occur with coumarin derivatives, phenytoin, verapamil, or nifedipine. Meclofenamate may decrease the renal clearance of methotrexate and lithium. Meclofenamate may decrease the clinical effectiveness of diuretics and antihypertensives. Concomitant use with diuretics may increase nephrotoxicity. Clinical manifestations of meclofenamate overdose include CNS stimulation, irrational behavior, marked agitation, and generalized seizures. Renal toxicity may follow this phase of CNS stimulation.

MEDIUM CHAIN TRIGLYCERIDES

(M.C.T. Oil)

Medium chain triglycerides (15 ml p.o. t.i.d.) are used in conditions of inadequate digestion or absorption of food fats, chylous ascites, or chylous thorax.

MEDROXYPROGESTERONE ACETATE

(Amen, Curretab, Depo-Provera, Provera)

Medroxyprogesterone, a progestin, is used in abnormal uterine bleeding from hormonal imbalance, in secondary amenorrhea, and for female contraception. In addition, it has been used in paraphilia in male subjects.

MEFENAMIC ACID

(Ponstel)

Mefenamic acid (500 mg p.o. initially, then 250 mg every 4 hours), which inhibits prostaglandin synthesis, is indicated in the treatment of moderate pain and in the management of primary dysmenorrhea. The duration of therapy should not exceed one week. It is a nonsteroidal antiinflammatory agent with analgesic and antipyretic properties. Mefenamic acid is absorbed rapidly and completely from the GI tract. It is highly protein-bound and is metabolized in the liver. Mefenamic acid is excreted mainly in urine with some biliary excretion. The plasma half-life is around two hours.

Concomitant use of mefenamic acid with anticoagulants and thrombolytic drugs (coumarin derivatives, heparin, streptokinase, or urokinase) may potentiate anticoagulant effects. Bleeding problems may occur if mefenamic acid is used with other drugs that inhibit platelet aggregation, such as azlocillin, parenteral carbenicillin, dextran, dipyridamole, mezlocillin, piperacillin, sulfinpyrazone, ticarcillin, valproic acid, cefamandole, cefoperazone, moxalactam, plicamycin, aspirin, or other antiinflammatory agents. Alcohol, corticotropin, or steroids may cause increased GI adverse reactions, including ulceration and hemorrhage. Aspirin may decrease the bioavailability of mefenamic acid.

Because of the influence of prostaglandins on glucose metabolism, concomitant use with insulin or oral hypoglycemic agents may potentiate hypoglycemic effects. Mefenamic acid may displace highly protein-bound drugs from binding sites. Toxicity may occur with coumarin derivatives, phenytoin, verapamil, or nifedipine. Increased nephrotoxicity may occur with gold compounds, other antiinflammatory agents, or acetaminophen. Mefenamic acid may decrease the renal clearance of methotrexate and lithium. Mefenamic acid may decrease the clinical effectiveness of diuretics and antihypertensives. Concomitant use with diuretics may increase nephrotoxicity. Clinical manifestations of overdose include CNS stimulation, irrational behavior, marked agitation, and generalized seizures. Renal toxicity may follow this phase of CNS stimulation.

MEGESTROL ACETATE

(Megace)

Megestrol is indicated for the treatment of anorexia, cachexia, or an unexplained significant weight loss in patients with a diagnosis of acquired immunodeficiency syndrome (AIDS). In addition, it has been recommended as a palliative treatment of advanced carcinoma of the breast or endometrium (i.e., recurrent, inoperable, or metastatic disease). Megestrol, a progestin, inhibits growth and causes regression of progestin-sensitive breast and endometrial cancer tissue by an unknown mechanism. An antiluteinizing effect mediated via the pituitary has been postulated. Evidence also suggests a local effect as a result of the marked changes from direct instillation of progestational agents into the endometrial cavity. The precise mechanism by which megestrol produces effects in anorexia and cachexia is unknown.

Megestrol is absorbed from the GI tract, is highly bound to plasma proteins, and is stored in adipose tissue. Megestrol is metabolized in the liver, and the metabolites are eliminated by the kidneys. Megestrol is contraindicated in patients with a history of thromboembolic disorder because the drug may be associated with thromboembolic disease; in patients with severe hepatic disease because drug accumulation may occur; in patients with undiagnosed abnormal vaginal bleeding because the drug may stimulate growth of some tumors; and in pregnant or breast-feeding women because of the potential for adverse effects on the fetus or neonate.

Megestrol should be used cautiously in patients with conditions that might be aggravated by fluid and electrolyte retention such as cardiac or renal disease, epilepsy, or migraine. Caution is also advised in administering this agent to diabetic patients because decreased glucose tolerance may occur, or to patients with a history of mental depression because the drug may exacerbate these effects. Weight gain is a frequent side effect of megestrol acetate. This effect has been associated with increased appetite, not necessarily with fluid retention.

Thromboembolic phenomena, including thrombophlebitis and pulmonary embolism have occurred on rare occasions. Nausea, vomiting, edema, breakthrough bleeding, dyspnea, tumor flare (with or without hypercalcemia), hyperglycemia, alopecia, carpal tunnel syndrome, and rash have been reported.

MELARSOPROL

(Arsobal)

Trypanosomiasis is produced by protozoa of the genus *Trypanosoma* and leads to Gambian or mid-African sleeping sickness (*T. gambiense*), Rhodesian or East African sleeping sickness (*T. rhodesiense*), and Chagas' disease, which is seen in the populations of Central and South America (*T. cruzi*). Agents effective in the treatment of trypanosomiasis are the **aromatic diamidines** (pentamidine, stilbamidine, and propamidine). **Pentamidine** is the preferred drug for the prevention and early treatment of *T. gambiense* infections; however, it cannot penetrate the central nervous system. **Melarsoprol** is the drug recommended for *T. gambiense* infections that do not respond to pentamidine or for managing the late meningoencephalitic stages of infection. It does reach the central nervous system. **Nifurtimox** (Lampit) is the drug of choice for treating the acute form of Chagas' disease. **Suramin** (Naphuride) is effective only in the therapy for African sleeping sickness.

MELATONIN

Melatonin is the major hormone produced in the pineal gland. The concentration of the hormone in blood is increased during the hours of darkness, while a low concentration occurs during daylight. Its secretion is controlled by an endogenous rhythm-generating system that is entrained by light. Melatonin has a role in cuing circadian rhythms (notably the sleep-wake rhythm) and promoting sleep, and it contributes significantly to the circadian rhythm in body temperature.

Administration of melatonin or bright light treatment has established therapeutic actions in circadian rhythm sleep disorders, including disorders associated with jet lag, shift work, delayed phase sleep disorder, periodic sleep disorder in blindness, and sleep and behavioral disorders in children with multiple brain damage. The effects of bright light or melatonin treatment follow a phase-response curve. Evening bright light treatment causes a phase delay in the sleep-wake cycle, and morning light causes a phase advance. Melatonin treatment produces effects that are nearly the mirror image of those caused by bright light.

Few clinical trials have been done in insomnias that are not associated with circadian rhythm disorders. Large doses of melatonin may have a therapeutic effect in chronic insomnia. Insomnia that coincides with diminished melatonin secretion occurs in aging and following treatment with beta-adrenoceptor blockers. Trials of melatonin treatment for these sleep disorders have yet to be published. A decrease in melatonin concentration has been reported in most studies of depressed patients. Treatment with drugs that enhance noradrenergic transmission or with tryptophan or **5-methoxypsoralen** cause both a therapeutic response and an increase in melatonin secretion; however, no treatment trials of melatonin have been reported in depressed patients.

MELPHALAN

(Phenylalanine Mustard) (Alkeran)

Melphalan, an alkylating agent with antineoplastic properties (150 mcg/kg/day p.o. for 7 days), is indicated in the treatment of multiple myeloma, testicular seminoma, non-Hodgkin's lymphoma, osteogenic sarcoma, breast cancer, and nonresectable advanced ovarian cancer.

MEMANTINE

Memantine, an NMDA receptor blocker which neutralizes the effect of glutamate at striatal and subthalamic levels, has shown beneficial effects in the treatment of some parkinsonian patients chronically treated with levodopa, who demonstrated increased motor deterioration.

MENINGITIS VACCINE
(Menomune-A/C/Y/W-135)

Meningitis vaccine, a bacterial vaccine, is used for meningococcal prophylaxis.

MENOTROPINS
(Pergonal)

Menotropins, a gonadotropin with ovulation and spermatogenesis stimulating properties, is used for production of follicular maturation and stimulation of spermatogenesis.

MEPENZOLATE BROMIDE
(Cantil)

Mepenzolate, an anticholinergic agent with gastrointestinal antispasmodic properties (25 to 50 mg p.o. q.i.d.), is used as an adjunctive therapy in peptic ulcer, irritable bowel syndrome, and neurologic bowel disturbances.

MEPERIDINE
(Demerol)

The pharmacology of meperidine resembles that of morphine, with the following exceptions: the antitussive and antidiarrheal effects of meperidine are minimal; meperidine does not produce miosis; and it may even cause mydriasis. Meperidine's **duration of action** is extremely short, and hence it is used as an analgesic during diagnostic procedures such as cystoscopy, gastroscopy, pneumoencephalography, and retrograde pyelography. It is also used as a **preanesthetic medication** and an **obstetric analgesic**. Because meperidine has atropine-like actions, toxic doses produce a mixed picture of morphine and atropine poisoning. In a narcotic addict who has developed tolerance to the depressant effects of morphine, meperidine poisoning resembles that of atropine, and is characterized by mydriasis, tachycardia, dry mouth, excitement, and convulsions. The atropine-like effects of morphine are not reversed by **naloxone**, a narcotic antagonist (see also Figure 58).

MEPHENTERAMINE SULFATE
(Wyamine)

Mephenteramine is indicated in the treatment of hypotension secondary to ganglionic blockage and that occurring following spinal anesthesia. Although not recommended as corrective therapy for shock of hypotension secondary to hemorrhage, mephenteramine may be used as an emergency measure to maintain blood pressure until blood or blood substitutes become available. Mephenteramine sulfate is a mixed-acting sympathomimetic amine that acts both directly and indirectly by releasing norepinephrine. The increase in blood pressure produced by mephenteramine is due to an increase in cardiac output resulting from enhanced cardiac contraction and to a lesser extent due to increased peripheral resistance.

Mephenteramine-induced pressor response occurs almost immediately and persists 15 to 30 minutes after IV injection; after IM injection, onset is within 5 to 15 minutes, persisting 1 to 4 hours. Mephenteramine is metabolized in the liver by N-demethylation and p-hydroxylation. Mephenteramine is excreted in urine within 24 hours as unchanged drug and metabolites.

The antihypertensive effects of guanethidine may be partially or totally reversed by the mixed-acting sympathomimetics. **Halogenated hydrocarbon anesthetics** may sensitize the myocardium to the effects of catecholamines. Use of vasopressors may lead to serious arrhythmias.

Monoamine oxidase (MAO) inhibitors, such as **tranylcypromine**, increase the pressor response to mixed-acting vasopressors. Possible hypertensive crisis and intracranial hemorrhage may occur. This interaction may also occur with **furazolidone**, an antimicrobial with MAO inhibitor activity. In obstetrics, if vasopressor drugs are used either to correct hypotension or are added to the local anesthetic solution, some oxytocics may cause severe persistent hypertension in the presence of mephenteramine. The pressor response of mephenteramine may be attenuated by tricyclic antidepressants, which block the uptake of norepinephrine (see also Figures 27 and 31).

MEPHENYTOIN

(Mesantoin)

Mephenytoin is demethylated to 5-ethyl-5-phenylhydantoin (Nirvanol), which is an active anticonvulsant. Mephenytoin binds to plasma protein to the extent of 40%, with an elimination half-life of 7 hours. Mephenytoin causes sedation, whereas phenytoin does not. The incidence of dose- and time-dependent side effects of mephenytoin is lower than that seen with phenytoin. On the other hand, the incidence of severe and fatal hypersensitivity reactions is far higher than that reported for phenytoin. Therefore, mephenytoin is not the first drug of choice. Mephenytoin is used for the treatment of tonic-clonic, simple partial, and complex partial seizures in patients who have become refractory to phenytoin or other drugs.

MEPHOBARBITAL

(Mebaral)

Mephobarbital is indicated for use as a sedative for the relief of anxiety, tension, and apprehension and as an anticonvulsant for the treatment of grand mal (400 to 600 mg/day) and petit mal epilepsies (6 to 12 mg/kg p.o./day). Mephobarbital, which is more lipid soluble than phenobarbital, becomes metabolized to phenobarbital. The pharmacologic characteristics of mephobarbital are similar to those of phenobarbital, and it is therefore used as an alternate drug. It has been reported that mephobarbital causes less sedation and hypersensitivity reactions than phenobarbital. Similar to phenobarbital, mephobarbital inhibits posttetanic potentiation and especially raises the seizure threshold. The precise mechanism of action of mephobarbital is not known, though two dissimilar mechanisms have been advanced. In the first, phenobarbital and mephobarbital, by inhibiting **aldehyde reductase**, are thought to interfere with the metabolism of aldehyde generated by biogenic amines such as dopamine, norepinephrine, and serotonin. The accumulation of these aldehydes in the CNS has depressing properties, and this reduces the neuronal sensitivity to excitation. In the second theory, phenobarbital and mephobarbital are thought to enhance the presynaptic release of GABA, and at the same time reduce the postsynaptic uptake of GABA. About 50% of an oral dose of mephobarbital is absorbed from the GI tract; action begins within 30 to 60 minutes and lasts 10 to 16 hours. Mephobarbital is distributed widely throughout the body. Mephobarbital is metabolized by the liver to phenobarbital; about 75% of a given dose is converted in 24 hours. Therapeutic blood levels of phenobarbital are 15 to 40 mcg/ml. Mephobarbital is excreted primarily in urine; small amounts are excreted in breast milk. Mephobarbital is contraindicated in pregnancy near term because of the hazard of respiratory depression and neonatal coagulation defects; in patients with severe respiratory disease or status asthmaticus because it may cause respiratory depression; or in patients with a history of porphyria or marked hepatic impairment because it may exacerbate porphyria. The drug should be used with caution in patients taking alcohol, CNS depressants, monoamine oxidase (MAO) inhibitors, narcotic analgesics, or anticoagulants. Symptoms of acute overdose include CNS and respiratory depression, areflexia, oliguria, tachycardia, hypotension, hypothermia, and coma. Shock may occur (see also Figure 40).

MEPIVACAINE HYDROCHLORIDE

(Carbocaine)

Mepivacaine is indicated for production of local or regional analgesia and anesthesia by local infiltration, peripheral nerve block techniques, and central neural techniques including epidural and caudal blocks (see also Figure 20).

Local anesthetics block the generation and the conduction of nerve impulses, presumably by increasing the threshold for electrical excitation in the nerve, by slowing the propagation of the nerve impulse, and by reducing the rate of rise of the action potential. In general, the progression of anesthesia is related to the diameter, myelination, and conduction velocity of affected nerve fibers. Clinically, the order of loss of nerve function is as follows: pain, temperature, touch, proprioception, and skeletal muscle tone. Systemic absorption of local anesthesia produces effects on the cardiovascular and central nervous systems. At blood concentrations achieved with normal therapeutic doses, changes in cardiac conduction, excitability, refractoriness, contractility, and peripheral vascular resistance are minimal. However, toxic concentrations depress cardiac conduction and excitability, which may lead to atrioventricular block and ultimately to cardiac arrest. In addition, myocardial contractility is depressed and peripheral vasodilation occurs, leading to decreased cardiac output and arterial blood pressure. Mepivacaine's potency and speed of action are similar to lidocaine with an onset of action of 5 minutes and a duration of action of 15 to 30 minutes. Local anesthetics rapidly cross the placenta, and when used for epidural, paracervical, caudal, or pudendal block anesthesia, can cause varying degrees of maternal, fetal, and neonatal toxicity.

MEPROBAMATE

(Equanil, Meprospan, Miltown, Neuramate, Neurate, Sedabamate, SK-Bamate, Tranmep)

Meprobamate, a carbamate antianxiety agent (1.2 to 1.6 g p.o. in divided doses), is used in the management of anxiety and tension (see also Table 8).

6-MERCAPTOPURINE

(6-MP)

6-Mercaptopurine (2.5 mg/kg/day) is indicated for remission induction and maintenance therapy of acute lymphatic (lymphocytic, lymphoblastic) leukemia, and for acute myelogenous leukemia. Mercaptopurine competes with hypoxanthine and guanine for the enzyme hypoxanthine-guanine phosphoribosyltransferase and is converted to thioinosinic acid (TIMP). This intracellular nucleotide inhibits several reactions involving inosinic acid (IMP). In addition, 6-methylthioinosinate (MTIMP) is formed by the methylation of TIMP. Both TIMP and MTIMP inhibit *de novo* purine ribonucleotide synthesis. Radiolabeled 6-MP may be recovered from deoxyribonucleic acid (DNA) in the form of deoxythioguanosine. Some mercaptopurine is converted to nucleotide derivatives of 6-thioguanine. The absorption of 6-mercaptopurine is incomplete, averaging 50%, and its entry into cerebrospinal fluid is negligible. Mercaptopurine becomes catabolized by methylation of the sulfhydryl group and oxidation by the enzyme xanthine oxidase. Allopurinol inhibits xanthine oxidase and retards the catabolism of mercaptopurine and its active metabolites. Plasma half-life averages 21 and 47 minutes in children and in adults, respectively. Metabolites of mercaptopurine appear in urine within 2 hours after administration. After 24 hours, >50% of a dose can be recovered in the urine as intact drug and metabolites. There is complete cross-resistance between mercaptopurine and thioguanine. The most consistent dose-related toxicity is bone marrow suppression, which may be manifested by anemia, leukopenia, or thrombocytopenia (see also Figure 2).

The induction of complete remission of acute lymphatic leukemia is frequently associated with marrow hypoplasia. Maintenance of remission generally involves multiple drug regimens whose component agents cause myelosuppression. Anemia, leukopenia, and thrombocytopenia are frequently observed. Dosages and schedules are adjusted to prevent life-threatening cytopenias. Hepatotoxicity occurs with doses of greater than 2.5 mg/kg/day.

MESALAMINE
(Asacol, Pentasa, Rowasa)

Mesalamine, a salicylate antiinflammatory agent (800 mg p.o. t.i.d. for 6 weeks), is used in the treatment of active mild to moderate distal ulcerative colitis, proctosigmoiditis, or proctitis.

MESNA
(Mesnex)

Mesna, a thiol derivative with uroprotectant properties, is used in prevention of ifosfamide-induced hemorrhagic cystitis.

MESORIDAZINE BESYLATE
(Serentil)

Mesoridazine has been used effectively in schizophrenia, behavioral problems in mental deficiency and chronic brain syndrome, alcoholism, and psychoneurotic manifestations associated with neurotic components of personality disorders.

Mesoridazine, a metabolite of thioridazine, is thought to exert its antipsychotic effects by postsynaptic blockade of CNS dopamine receptors, thereby inhibiting dopamine-mediated effects. Mesoridazine has many other central and peripheral affects; it produces both alpha and ganglionic blockade and counteracts histamine- and serotonin-mediated activities. Mesoridazine and thioridazine cause fewer movement disorders (see **Phenotheazine derivatives**). Mesoridazine is metabolized to inactive metabolites which are excreted by the kidneys. Overdosage of mesoridazine causes CNS depression characterized by deep, unarousable sleep, convulsive seizures, and cardiac arrhythmias (see also Table 23).

METAPROTERENOL
(Alupent; Metaprel)

The methylxanthines consist of **aminophylline, dyphylline, enprofylline**, and **pentoxifylline**. Aminophylline (theophylline ethylenediamine) is the most widely used of the soluble theophyllines. Its main therapeutic effect is bronchodilation. In addition, it causes central nervous system stimulation, cardiac acceleration, diuresis, and gastric secretion. Aminophylline is available in an oral, rectal (pediatric), or intravenous solution, which is used in the treatment of status asthmaticus. Although aminophylline is a less effective bronchodilator than beta-adrenergic agonists, it is particularly useful in preventing nocturnal asthma (see also Figure 86).

METARAMINOL
(Aramine)

Metaraminol is indicated for prevention and treatment of the acute hypotensive state occurring with spinal anesthesia, adjunctive treatment of hypotension due to hemorrhage, reactions to medications, surgical complications, and shock associated with brain damage due to trauma or tumor. The pressor effects of metaraminol begin 1 to 2 minutes after IV infusion,

10 minutes after IM injection, and 5 to 20 minutes after SC injection. The effects last from about 20 minutes to 1 hour. Metaraminol is a sympathomimetic amine that increases both systolic and diastolic blood pressure by vasoconstriction, and this effect is accompanied by a marked reflex bradycardia. It has a direct effect on alpha adrenergic receptors, and its prolonged infusions can deplete norepinephrine from sympathetic nerve endings. Metaraminol increases venous tone, causes pulmonary vasoconstriction and elevates pulmonary pressure even when cardiac output is reduced. Pressor effect is decreased, but not reversed, by alpha-adrenergic blocking agents. The antihypertensive effects of guanethidine may be partially or totally reversed by the mixed-acting sympathomimetics. **Halogenated hydrocarbon anesthetics** may sensitize the myocardium to the effects of catecholamines. Use of vasopressors may lead to serious arrhythmias. **Monoamine oxidase (MAO) A inhibitors**, such as **tranylcypromine**, increase the pressor response to mixed-acting vasopressors. Possible hypertensive crisis and intracranial hemorrhage may occur. This interaction may also occur with **furazolidone,** an antimicrobial agent with MAO inhibitory properties. The pressor response of metaraminol is reduced by tricyclic antidepressants such as desipramine (see also Figures 27 and 31).

METAXALONE

(Skelaxin)

Metaxalone (800 mg t.i.d.), a centrally acting muscle relaxant, is indicated as an adjunct to rest, physical therapy, and other measures for the relief of discomfort associated with acute painful musculoskeletal conditions. Metaxalone has no direct action on the contractile mechanism, or myoneural function. It should be administered cautiously to individuals with hepatic impairment. Metaxalone is a CNS depressant and potentiates the CNS depressant effects of ethanol.

METHACYCLINE HYDROCHLORIDE

(Rondomycin)

Methacycline is a broad-spectrum tetracycline antibiotic which is synthetically derived from oxytetracycline. Methacycline (600 mg/day) is indicated in infections caused by Gram-positive bacteria, *Rickettsia*, mycoplasma, amoeba, and *Chlamydia*. Methacycline binds to the 30S subunit of the bacterial ribosome in such a way that the binding of the aminoacyl-transfer RNA to the acceptor site on the messenger RNA ribosome complex is blocked (see also Figure 88). Tetracyclines are effective in the treatment of Rocky Mountain spotted fever, murine typhus, recrudescent epidemic typhus, scrub typhus, Q fever, lymphogranuloma venereum, psittacosis, tularemia, brucellosis, gonorrhea, certain urinary tract infections, granuloma inguinale, chancroid, syphilis, and disease due to *Bacteroides* and *Clostridium.*

Tetracyclines in general cause toxic and hypersensitivity reactions. These consist commonly of gastrointestinal irritations that are disabling and may necessitate discontinuation of the medications. With continuous usage, tetracyclines may alter the normal flora, allowing the growth of *Pseudomonas, Proteus,* staphylococci-resistant coliforms, *Clostridium,* and *Candida* organisms. These superinfections should be recognized and treated appropriately with **vancomycin** and other drugs (see also Figure 93). Tetracyclines have been known to cause hepatic necrosis, especially when given in large intravenous doses or when taken by pregnant women or patients with preexisting liver impairment. Tetracycline preparations whose potency has expired can cause **renal tubular acidosis**. With the exception of doxycycline, tetracyclines accumulate in patients with renal impairment. Tetracyclines also produce **nitrogen retention**, especially when given with diuretics. Tetracyclines bind to calcium and then become deposited in bone, causing damage to developing bone and teeth (see also Figure 80).

METHADONE
(Dolophine)

Pharmacologically, methadone is very similar to morphine, with the following exceptions: methadone is **effective orally**; its onset and duration of action are longer than morphine's; **tolerance** to methadone develops very slowly, and, if abruptly withdrawn, the abstinence syndrome develops more slowly, is less intense, and is more prolonged than the abstinence syndrome of morphine; and the **abuse potential** of methadone is lower than morphine's. Like morphine, methadone is used in the management of pain. It is also used in the **detoxification** and treatment of **narcotic addiction** (see also Figure 58).

METHAMPHETAMINE HYDROCHLORIDE
(Desoxyn)

Methamphetamine (2.5 to 5 mg p.o. daily) has been used in the management of obesity, narcolepsy, and attention deficit hyperactivity impulse disorder. Methamphetamine, which releases norepinephrine and dopamine, stimulates the CNS. It is absorbed from the GI tract after oral administration, is distributed throughout the body, crosses the placenta, and is found in the milk. It is metabolized in the liver and is excreted in the urine. Methamphetamine is contraindicated in patients with hyperthyroidism, glaucoma, angina pectoris, or any degree of hypertension or other severe cardiovascular disease, because it may cause hazardous arrhythmias and changes in blood pressure. The simultaneous use of methamphetamine and a monoamine oxidase inhibitor such as tranylcypromine should be discouraged. Methamphetamine should be used with caution in patients with diabetes mellitus; in patients who are elderly, debilitated, asthenic, or psychopathic; in patients who have a history of suicidal or homicidal tendencies; and in children with Gilles de la Tourette's syndrome. Amphetamine-induced CNS stimulation superimposed on CNS depression can cause seizures. Concomitant use with MAO inhibitors (or drugs with MAO-inhibiting activity, such as **furazolidone**), or within 14 days of such therapy, may cause hypertensive crisis; use with antihypertensives may antagonize their effects. Concomitant use with antacids, sodium bicarbonate, or acetazolamide enhances reabsorption of methamphetamine and prolongs duration of action, whereas use with ascorbic acid enhances methamphetamine excretion and shortens duration of action. Use with phenothiazines or haloperidol decreases methamphetamine effects. Barbiturates antagonize methamphetamine by CNS depression, whereas caffeine or other CNS stimulants produce additive effects. Patients using methamphetamine have an increased risk of arrhythmias during general anesthesia. Methamphetamine may alter insulin requirements. Symptoms of overdose include increasing restlessness, tremor, hyperreflexia, tachypnea, confusion, aggressiveness, hallucinations, and panic; fatigue and depression usually follow the excitement stage. Other symptoms may include arrhythmias, shock, alterations in blood pressure, nausea, vomiting, diarrhea, and abdominal cramps; death is usually preceded by convulsions and coma.

METHANDROSTENOLONE
(Dianabol)

Methandrostenolone is an androgenic steroid with anabolic actions (see also Table 6).

Since androgens have significant effects on muscle mass and on body weight when administered to hypogonadal men, it was assumed, but never proven, that androgens in pharmacological doses could promote growth of muscle above the levels produced by the normal testicular secretion. This assumption was based on the belief that anabolic and androgenic actions are different, and a concerted effort was made to devise pure "anabolic" steroids that have no androgenic effects. In fact, androgenic and anabolic effects do not result from different actions of the same hormone but represent the same action in different tissues; androgen-responsive muscle contains the same receptor that mediates the action of the hormones in other target tissues. *All anabolic hormones tested to date are also androgenic.* In appropriate doses, most anabolic agents can be used for replacement of androgen. For example, meth-androstenolone, which has a greater effect on nitrogen balance per unit weight than does methyltestosterone, is a potent androgen and has been used for replacement therapy in hypogonadal men. Nevertheless, androgens have been tried in a variety of clinical situations other than hypogonadism with the hope that improvement in nitrogen balance and muscle development would outweigh any deleterious side effects.

METHANTHELINE BROMIDE
(Banthine)

Methantheline (50 to 100 mg p.o. q. 6 hours), an anticholinergic agent, is used as an adjunctive therapy in peptic ulcer. It blocks the action of acetylcholine at neuroaffector sites, inhibiting gastric acid secretion and pancreatic secretions. Methantheline is contraindicated in patients with narrow-angle glaucoma, because drug-induced cycloplegia and mydriasis may increase intraocular pressure; in patients with obstructive uropathy, obstructive GI tract disease, severe ulcerative colitis, myasthenia gravis, paralytic ileus, intestinal atony, or toxic megacolon. Meth-antheline should be administered cautiously to patients with autonomic neuropathy, hyperthy-roidism, coronary artery disease, cardiac arrhythmias, congestive heart failure, or ulcerative colitis, because toxic accumulation may occur; in patients over age 40, because the drug increases the glaucoma risk; in patients with hiatal hernia associated with reflux esophagitis, because the drug may decrease lower esophageal sphincter tone; and in hot or humid environments, because the drug may predispose the patient to heatstroke. The concurrent administration of antacids decreases the oral absorption of methantheline, which should be administered at least one hour before antacids. Clinical signs of overdosage with methantheline include curare-like symptoms and such peripheral effects as headache; dilated, nonreactive pupils; blurred vision; flushed, hot, dry skin; dryness of mucous membranes; dysphagia; decreased or absent bowel sounds; urinary retention; hyperthermia; tachycardia; hypertension; and increased respiration.

METHAQUALONE
(Quaalude)

Methaqualone has been used for daytime sedation and in patients with simple insomnia. It is useful for patients who cannot tolerate barbiturates.

METHARBITAL
(Gemonil)

Metharbital, 5,5-diethyl-1-methylbarbituric acid, an N-substituted derivative of barbital, shares the anticonvulsant properties of phenobarbital. It is claimed to be particularly effective in young children for the control of massive spasms resulting from underlying brain damage and in myoclonic seizures. In equivalent doses, it is less depressing than phenobarbital. Metharbital is administered initially in doses of 50 mg (infants and children) and 100 mg (adults) one to three times daily, orally. This dosage may be increased gradually depending on tolerance, 600 to 800 mg if needed to control seizures.

METHAZOLAMIDE
(Neptazane)

Methazolamide (50 to 100 mg p.o. b.i.d. or t.i.d.), a carbonic anhydrase inhibitor, decreases the formation of aqueous humor lowering intraocular pressure, and hence is indicated as an adjunctive treatment for the treatment of open-angle glaucoma. Methazolamide is absorbed orally, and distributes into plasma, erythrocytes, extracellular fluid, bile, aqueous humor, and CSF. It is metabolized partially in the liver and is partially (20 to 30%) excreted in the urine.

Methazolamide is contraindicated in patients with hepatic insufficiency, low potassium or sodium levels, hyperchloremic acidosis, or severe renal impairment, because of the potential for enhanced electrolyte imbalances. Methazolamide should be used cautiously in patients with respiratory acidosis or other severe respiratory problems because the drug may produce acidosis; in patients with diabetes because it may cause hyperglycemia and glycosuria; in patients taking cardiac glycosides because they are more susceptible to digitalis toxicity from methazolamide-induced hypokalemia; and in patients taking other diuretics. Methazolamide alkalizes urine, thus decreasing excretion of amphetamines, procainamide, quinidine, and flecainide. Methazolamide increases excretion of salicylates, phenobarbital, and lithium, lowering plasma levels of these drugs and necessitating dosage adjustments.

METHDILAZINE

METHDILAZINE HYDROCHLORIDE
(Tacacryl)

Methdilazine, a phenothiazine derivative with antihistaminic properties (8 mg p.o. b.i.d.), is used in pruritis.

METHENAMINE HIPPURATE
(Hiprex, Urex)

METHENAMINE MANDELATE
(Mandameth, Mandelamine, Mandelamine Forte Suspension)

Methenamine, a urinary tract antiinfective agent, is used in long-term prophylaxis or suppression of chronic urinary tract infections (methenamine hippurate), and in the treatment of urinary tract infections associated with neurogenic bladder (methenamine mandelate).

METHENAMINE MANDELATE
(Mandelamine)

Methenamine mandelate decomposes in solution to generate **formaldehyde**, which in a concentration of 20 microgram/ml, inhibits all bacteria causing urinary tract infections (see Figure 55). Therefore, methenamine mandelate is indicated for suppression or elimination of bacteriuria associated with pyelonephritis, cystitis, and other chronic urinary tract infections. The nonspecific antibacterial action of formaldehyde is effective against Gram-positive and Gram-negative organisms, and fungi. *Escherichia coli*, enterococci, and staphylococci are usually susceptible. *Enterobacter aerogenes* and *Proteus vulgaris* are generally resistant. Urea-splitting organisms (e.g., *Proteus, Pseudomonas*) may be resistant since they raise the pH of the urine, inhibiting the release of formaldehyde. An effective urine concentration of formaldehyde must persist for a minimum of two hours. Methenamine is effective clinically against most common urinary tract pathogens. It has demonstrable antibacterial activity *in vitro* against *E. coli, Micrococcus pyrogenes, E. aerogenes, P. aeruginosa,* and *P. vulgaris* at pH 5 to 6.8. The minimal inhibitory concentrations are significantly lower in more acidic media; therefore, efficacy can be increased by urine acidification. Methenamine is particularly suited for therapy of chronic infections, since bacteria and fungi do not develop resistance to formaldehyde. **Sodium bicarbonate** and **acetazolamide** can decrease the effectiveness of

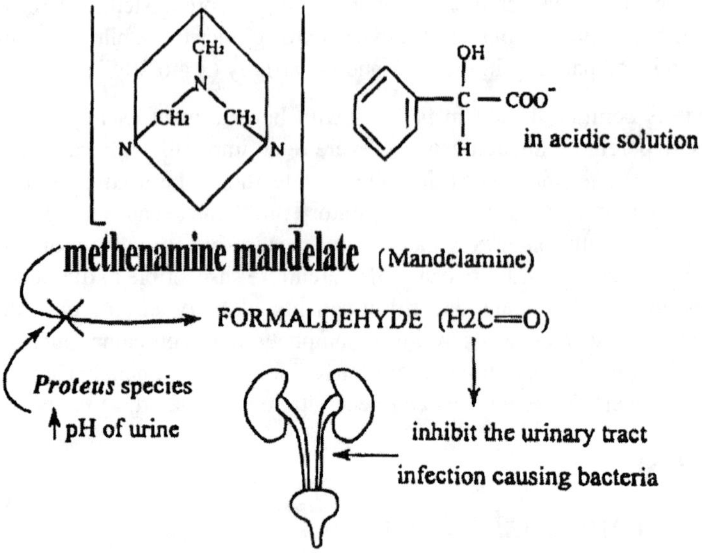

FIGURE 55 **Methenamine mandelate** decomposes in solution to generate **formaldehyde**, which inhibits all bacteria that cause urinary tract infections. Urea-splitting microorganisms raise the pH of the urine and hence inhibit the release of formaldehyde and the action of methenamine.

methenamine by alkalinizing the urine and inhibiting the conversion of methenamine to formaldehyde. Methenamine is absorbed orally. However, because of the ammonia produced, methenamine is contraindicated in patients suffering from hepatic insufficiency (see Figure 55).

METHICILLIN SODIUM

(Staphcillin)

Methicillin, a penicillinase-resistant penicillin (4 to 12 g IM or IV daily), is used in systemic infections caused by susceptible organisms (see also Table 22).

METHIMAZOLE

(Tapazole)

Methimazole (15 to 60 mg p.o. daily until patients are euthyroid), is indicated in the treatment of hyperthyroidism. **Propylthiouracil, carbimazole**, and **methimazole**, thyroid hormone antagonists, exert their effects by inhibiting iodide organification, and by inhibiting the formation of diiodothyronine (DIT) (see Figure 56).

These agents possess a thiocarbamide moiety

$$\begin{array}{c} S \\ \parallel \\ (-N-C-R) \end{array}$$

which is essential for their antithyroid actions. The onset of their beneficial effects is slow and takes 3 to 4 weeks. In preparation for thyroidectomy, methimazole inhibits the synthesis of the thyroid hormone and causes a euthyroid state, reducing surgical problems during

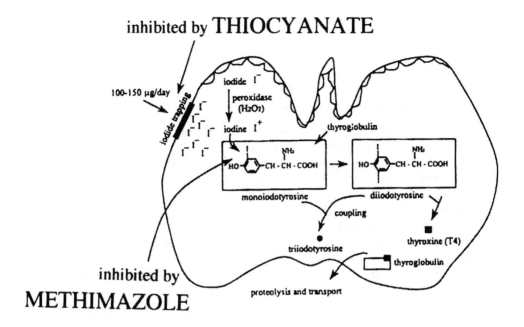

inhibited by THIOCYANATE

100-150 µg/day

iodide trapping

iodide I⁻

peroxidase
(H₂O₂)

iodine I⁺

thyroglobulin

HO—⟨ ⟩—CH·CH·COOH

monoiodotyrosine

diiodotyrosine

coupling

triiodotyrosine

thyroxine (T4)

thyroglobulin

inhibited by
METHIMAZOLE

proteolysis and transport

SYNTHESIS OF THYROXINE

FIGURE 56 Methimazole inhibits the synthesis of thyroid hormone by interfering with the incorporation of iodine into tyrosine, and the formation of iodothyronine.

thyroidectomy; as a result, the mortality for a single-stage thyroidectomy is low. Iodide reduces the vascularity of the gland, making it less friable. For treating thyrotoxic crisis (thyrotoxicosis), propylthiouracil (PTU) theoretically is preferred over methamazole because it inhibits peripheral deiodination of thyroxine to triiodothyronine. Methimazole is absorbed orally, crosses the placental barrier, and is concentrated in the thyroid gland. It is metabolized in the liver and partially (7%) excreted unchanged. Clinical manifestations of overdose include nausea, vomiting, epigastric distress, fever, headache, arthralgia, pruritus, edema, and pancytopenia.

METHOCARBAMOL
(Delaxin, Robamol, Robaxin)

Methocarbamol, a carbamate derivative of **guaifenesin** (1.5 g p.o. q.i.d.), is used as an adjunct in acute, painful musculoskeletal conditions and in supportive therapy in tetanus management.

METHOHEXITAL SODIUM
(Brevital)

Methohexital (1 mg/kg in 1% solution given at a rate of 1 ml/5 seconds) is used for induction of anesthesia lasting 5 to 7 minutes. Maintenance of anesthesia may be accomplished by intermittent injections of 1% solution or by continuous IV drip of a 0.2% solution. Intermittent injections of about 20 to 40 mg (2 to 4 ml of a 1% solution) may be given as required, usually every 4 to 7 minutes. For continuous drip, the average rate of administration is about 3 ml of a 0.2% solution/min (1 drop/sec). Methohexital should not be mixed in the same syringe or administered simultaneously during IV infusion through the same needle with acid solutions, such as atropine sulfate, metocurine iodide, and succinylcholine chloride.

METHOTREXATE

(Amethopterin)

Methotrexate is a folic acid antagonist that binds to dihydrofolate reductase, thus interfering with the synthesis of the active cofactor tetrahydrofolic acid, which is necessary for the synthesis of thymidylate, purine nucleotides, and the amino acids serine and methionine. Methotrexate is used for the following types of cancer:

Acute lymphoid leukemia: During the initial phase, vincristine and prednisone are used. Methotrexate and mercaptopurine are used for maintenance therapy. In addition, methotrexate is given intrathecally, with or without radiotherapy, to prevent meningeal leukemia.

Diffuse histiocytic lymphoma: Cyclophosphamide, vincristine, methotrexate, and cytarbine (COMA).

Mycosis fungoides: Methotrexate.

Squamous cell, large-cell anaplastic, and adenocarcinoma: Doxorubicin and cyclophosphamide, or methotrexate.

Head and neck squamous cell: Cis-platinum and bleomycin, or methotrexate.

Choriocarcinoma: Methotrexate.

Tumor cells acquire **resistance to methotrexate** as a result of several factors which include deletion of a high-affinity, carrier-mediated transport system for reduced folates, an increase in the concentration of dihydrofolate reductase, and the formation of a biochemically altered reductase with reduced affinity for methotrexate. To overcome this resistance, higher doses of methotrexate need to be administered. The effects of methotrexate may be reversed by the administration of **leucovorin**, the reduced folate. This leucovorin "rescue" prevents or reduces the toxicity of methotrexate, which is expressed as mouth lesions (stomatitis), injury to the gastrointestinal epithelium (diarrhea), leukopenia, and thrombocytopenia.

METHOTRIMEPRAZINE HYDROCHLORIDE

(Levoprome)

Methotrimeprazine, a propylamino phenothiazine, with sedative, analgesic, and antipyretic properties, is used to induce preanesthetic sedation and analgesia, and postoperative analgesia.

METHOXAMINE HYDROCHLORIDE

(Vasoxyl)

Methoxamine, a sympathomimetic agent with alpha-adrenergic stimulating effects (3 to 5 mg IV injected slowly), is indicated for supporting, restoring, or maintaining blood pressure during anesthesia. It produces potent and prolonged pressor action without causing cardiac acceleration. Methoxamine occasionally causes bradycardia which is abolished by atropine. It should be used cautiously in patients with hyperthyroidism, bradycardia, partial heart block, myocardial diseases, or severe arteriosclerosis. Bretylium may potentiate the action of methoxamine on adrenergic receptors, possibly resulting in arrhythmias; **guanethidine** may increase the pressor response of methoxamine, possibly resulting in severe hypertension; **halogenated hydrocarbon anesthetics** do sensitize the myocardium to the effects of catecholamines. Methoxamine and halothane may lead to serious arrhythmias. Methoxamine is used in obstetrics to correct hypotension or is added to the local anesthetic solution. Some oxytocics may cause severe and persistent hypertension; and tricyclic antidepressants, such as imipramine, potentiate the pressor effects of methoxamine (see Figure 27).

METHOXSALEN
(8-MOP, Oxsoralen, Oxsoralen-Ultra)

Methoxsalen, a psoralen derivative with pigmenting properties (12 to 20 mg p.o.), is used to induce repigmentation in vitiligo.

METHOXYFLURANE
(Penthrane)

Methoxyflurane is the most potent of the inhalational anesthetics. It is metabolized extensively to fluoride and other nephrotoxic products. Because methoxyflurane does not alter uterine contraction during labor, it is valuable for **obstetric anesthesia**. Its toxic effects on the respiration and cardiovascular systems are similar to those produced by halothane. Methoxyflurane reduces renal blood flow and the glomerular filtration rate (see also Table 15).

METHSCOPOLAMINE BROMIDE
(Pamine)

Methscopolamine, an anticholinergic agent with gastrointestinal antispasmodic properties (2.5 to 5 mg p.o. one-half hour before meals), is used as an adjunctive therapy in peptic ulcer and irritable bowel syndrome.

METHSUXIMIDE
(Celantin)

Methsuximide belongs to the succinimide family (ethosuximide and phensuximide), which share a common heterocyclic (succinimide) ring. Methsuximide is a nonpolar chemical compound that is water soluble and slightly lipophilic. Its exact effects on excitable membranes are not known. Antagonistic against absence and partial seizures, methsuximide may have more than one mechanism of action, including effects on transmitter release, calcium uptake into presynaptic endings, and conductance of sodium, potassium, and chloride. Methsuximide is quickly absorbed through the gastrointestinal tract, and peak plasma levels are achieved in 2 to 4 hours. The drug is distributed evenly throughout the body and penetrates brain and fat tissue better than ethosuximide. Because its protein binding and solubility are poor, methsuximide equilibrates with cerebrospinal fluid. Methsuximide is rapidly metabolized to N-desmethylmethsuximide or 2-methyl-2-phenyl succinimide in hours, and has a mean half-life of 1.4 hours. Methsuximide has a wide spectrum of antiepileptic activity and is effective in complex partial seizures, generalized tonic-clonic seizures, and absence seizures. Furthermore, methsuximide is an effective adjunctive agent in the management of refractory complex partial seizures.

Common adverse experiences such as gastrointestinal disturbance, lethargy, somnolence, fatigue, and headache may be seen with methsuximide, but these usually are transient and dose-related. Other adverse experiences include hiccups, irritability, ataxia, blurred vision or diplopia, inattention, dysarthria, and psychic changes. In some patients, headache, photophobia, and hiccups require withdrawal of methsuximide. Transient leukopenia has been reported. Delayed profound coma after methsuximide overdose has been described.

Methsuximide increases the serum concentrations of phenobarbital and phenytoin and reduces that of carbamezepine.

METHYCLOTHIAZIDE

(Aquatensen, Enduron, Ethon)

Methyclothiazide, a thiazide diuretic with antihypertensive properties (0.05 to 0.2 mg/kg p.o. daily), is used in edema or hypertension (see also Figure 4 and Table 25).

METHYL ALCOHOL

Methyl alcohol is used as an **industrial solvent** and as an **adulterant** that is added to ethyl alcohol to prevent its consumption. Methyl alcohol is metabolized to **formaldehyde** and **formic acid**, according to the following reactions.

$$\text{Methanol} \xrightarrow{\text{Alcohol dehydrogenase}} \text{formaldehyde} \xrightarrow{\text{Aldehyde dehydrogenase}} \text{formic acid}$$

Besides producing all of the CNS effects discussed for ethyl alcohol, methyl alcohol consumption leads to **acidosis** and **blindness**. The treatment of methyl alcohol poisoning may include water and electrolyte replacement along with the administration of sodium bicarbonate to combat the acidosis. Ethyl alcohol may also be administered intravenously, because it is a preferred substrate by liver alcohol dehydrogenase, thus allowing methyl alcohol to be excreted unmetabolized in the urine.

METHYLCELLULOSE

(Cellothyl, Citrucel, Cologel)

Methylcellulose, an absorbent and bulk-forming substance with laxative properties (one tablespoon powder in 240 ml water daily), is indicated in the treatment of chronic constipation.

METHYLDOPA

(Aldomet)

Alpha-methyldopa is used for the control of **mild to severe hypertension.** It is converted to **alpha-methylnorepinephrine**, whose main hypotensive effect is due to stimulation of presynaptic alpha$_2$-adrenergic receptors that leads to a reduction in the release of norepinephrine. In addition, it reduces the peripheral vascular resistance without altering the heart rate or cardiac output. Postural hypotension is mild and infrequent. Alpha-methyldopa can cause sedation, and tolerance to it can develop. **Coomb's test** will be positive (25%) in patients who are taking the drug. Alpha-methyldopa has a long onset and a short duration of action. It is especially useful in the management of hypertension complicated by renal dysfunction, since it does not alter either renal blood flow or the glomerular filtration rate. It is contraindicated in patients with liver disease and may produce hepatitis-like symptoms (see also Figure 27).

METHYLENE BLUE

(Urolene Blue)

Methylene blue, a thiazide dye with urinary tract antiseptic properties (55 mg p.o. t.i.d.), is used in cystitis, urethritis, and chronic urolithiasis; in methemoglobinemia and cyanide poisoning; and in chronic methemoglobinemia.

METHYLERGONOVINE

(Methergine)

Methylergonovine (0.2 mg IM after delivery of placenta) increases the strength, duration, and frequency of uterine contractions and decreases uterine bleeding following placental delivery. It induces a rapid and sustained tetanic uterotonic effect which shortens the third stage of labor and reduces blood loss. The onset of action of methylergonovine when given intramuscularly is 2 to 5 minutes, and a maximum concentration is reached in 30 minutes. The excretion of methylergonovine appears to be both renal and hepatic in nature. Methylergonovine should be given intravenously slowly (within 60 seconds) and cautiously since sudden hypertension may ensue. It may be given orally (0.2 mg t.i.d.) for a maximum of one week to control uterine bleeding. The adverse reactions of methylergonovine include nausea, vomiting, hypertension, dizziness, headache, tinnitus, diaphoresis, palpitations, temporary chest pain, and dyspnea.

METHYLPHENIDATE HYDROCHLORIDE

(Ritalin)

Methylphenidate is indicated for the treatment of children with attention deficit disorder with hyperactivity (5 to 10 mg p.o. daily) and for adults with narcolepsy (10 mg p.o. t.i.d.). Methylphenidate, a CNS stimulant and an analeptic, releases norepinephrine and hence stimulates the reticular activating system and the cerebral cortex. Its actions resemble those produced by amphetamine. Similar to other sympathomimetic agents, methylphenidate should be used with caution in patients with symptomatic cardiovascular disease, hyperthyroidism, angina pectoris, moderate to severe hypertension, or advanced arteriosclerosis because it may cause dangerous arrhythmias and blood pressure changes.

Methylphenidate should not be used with monoamine oxidase inhibitors such as **tranylcypromine**. Symptoms of overdose may include euphoria, confusion, delirium, coma, toxic psychosis, agitation, headache, vomiting, dry mouth, mydriasis, self-injury, fever, diaphoresis, tremors, hyper-reflexia, muscle twitching, seizures, flushing, hypertension, tachycardia, palpitations, and arrhythmias.

METHYLPREDNISOLONE

(Medrol)

Methylprednisolone is an intermediate-acting glucocorticoid with no mineralocorticoid properties (see also Tables 10 and 13).

Glucocorticoids are used in:

Endocrine disorders (e.g., primary or secondary adrenal cortical insufficiency)
Rheumatic disorders (e.g., ankylosing spondylitis, acute or subacute bursitis, or tenosynovitis)
Collagen disease (e.g., lupus erythematosus, acute rheumatic carditis)
Dermatologic diseases (e.g., severe erythema multiforme, bullous dermatitis herpetiformis)
Ophthalmic disorders (e.g., allergic conjunctivitis, keratitis)
Respiratory disorders (e.g., bronchial asthma, seasonal allergic rhinitis)
Hematologic disorders (e.g., idiopathic thrombocytopenic purpura, acquired hemolytic anemia)
Neoplastic diseases (e.g., leukemias and lymphomas)
Edematous states (e.g., nephrotic syndrome)
Gastrointestinal diseases (e.g., ulcerative colitis, Crohn's disease)
Diseases of CNS (e.g., multiple sclerosis)

In addition, glucocorticoids are used in spinal conditions. For example, methylprednisolone (32 mg/day) is used to reduce mortality in severe alcoholism and hepatitis; and methylprednisolone (IV within 8 hours of injury) is used to improve neurogenic function in acute spinal cord injury (see also Table 13).

There are two categories of toxic effects from therapeutic use of glucocorticoids: **Acute adrenal insufficiency** due to too rapid withdrawal of corticosteroids after long-term use, resulting in fever, myalgia, arthralgia, malaise, anorexia, nausea, desquamation of skin, orthostatic hypotension, dizziness, fainting, dyspnea, and hypoglycemia. **Cushingoid changes** from continued use of large doses, resulting in moonface, central obesity, striae, hirsutism, acne, ecchymoses, hypertension, osteoporosis, myopathy, sexual dysfunction, diabetes, hyperlipidemia, peptic ulcer, increased susceptibility to infection, and electrolyte and fluid imbalance.

METHYLPREDNISOLONE

(Systemic) (MedroL)

METHYLPREDNISOLONE ACETATE

(dep-Medalone, Depoject, Depo-Medrol, Depopred, Depo-Predate, Duralone, Durameth, Medralone, Medrone, M-Prednisol, Rep-Ped)

METHYLPREDNISOLONE SODIUM SUCCINATE

(A-MethaPred, Solu-Medrol)

Methylprednisolone, a glucocorticoid with antiinflammatory and immunosuppressant properties, is used in the treatment of severe inflammation or immunosuppression. In addition, methylprednisolone has been used in the treatment or minimization of motor/sensory defects caused by acute spinal cord injury (see also Tables 10 and 13).

METHYLSALICYLATE

(Oil of Wintergreen)

Paraamino salicylic acid has bacteriostatic activity against *Mycobacterium tuberculosis*. **Methyl salicylate** (oil of wintergreen) has been used in the past as a counterirritant. **Salicylic acid** (20% solution) has keratolytic properties and is used to remove cornified epidermis (corn). Because salicylic acid itself is too toxic for systemic use, the various salts of salicylate, including acetylsalicylic acid (aspirin), are used instead (see also Table 2).

METHYLTESTOSTERONE

(Medrol)

Methyltestosterone is used in male and female subjects with the following indications. Hypogonadism, male climacteric, and impotence: 10 to 40 mg/day orally; androgen deficiency: 10 to 50 mg/day orally (5 to 25 mg buccal); postpubertal cryptorchidism: 30 mg/day orally; postpartum breast pain and engorgement: 80 mg/day orally for 3 to 5 days; and breast cancer: 50 to 200 mg/day orally (25 to 100 mg buccal). Methyltestosterone may cause edema. Retention of water in association with sodium chloride appears to be a consistent effect of the administration of androgen and accounts for much of the gain in weight, at least in short-term treatment. In the doses used to treat hypogonadism, retention of fluid usually does not lead to detectable edema, but edema may become troublesome when large doses are given in the treatment of neoplastic diseases. Edema also is common in patients with congestive heart failure or renal insufficiency and in patients prone to edema from some other cause, such as cirrhosis of the liver or hypoproteinemia. Salt and water retention from androgens usually responds to the administration of natriuretics (see Table 25).

Methyltestosterone was the first androgen discovered to cause cholestatic hepatitis, but all androgens with 17 alpha-alkyl substitutions can cause this complication. Jaundice is the prominent clinical feature, and the underlying disturbance is stasis and accumulation of bile in the biliary capillaries of the central portion of the hepatic lobules without obstruction in the larger ducts. The hepatic cells usually exhibit only minor histological changes and remain viable. If jaundice occurs, it generally develops after 2 to 5 months of therapy. Alterations in various tests of hepatic function occur more commonly than jaundice and include increases in the concentration of bilirubin and the levels of aspartate aminotransferase and alkaline phosphatase in the plasma. The severity of the response is dependent on the dose of 17 alpha-alkyl-substituted testosterone analogs administered and is particularly prominent when large amounts are given, as for palliation in neoplastic diseases. Disturbance of hepatic function has not been described with the parenteral use of testosterone esters. Consequently, testosterone esters should be administered instead of 17 alpha-substituted steroids in virtually all clinical situations (except hereditary angioneurotic edema). In particular, the use of 17 alpha-substituted esters should be avoided in patients with liver disease. Patients who have received 17 alpha-alkyl-substituted androgens for prolonged periods may develop hepatic adenocarcinoma. Most of the patients described received the derivatives for 1 to 7 years, and the complication may be more common in subjects with **Fanconi's anemia**. Androgens can decrease the concentration of thyroid-binding globulin in plasma and thereby influence thyroid function tests, increase the excretion of 17-ketosteroids, raise plasma LDL-cholesterol and lower plasma HDL-cholesterol concentrations, and increase the hematocrit. 17 alpha-Alkyl-substituted steroids cause an increase in the hepatic synthesis and plasma concentrations of a variety of glycoproteins.

METHYLXANTHINES

Caffeine, theobromine, and theophylline are purine derivatives closely related to the xanthine bodies found in the urine and tissues of animals. Xanthine is 2:6 dioxypurine; caffeine is 1:3:7 trimethylxanthine; theobromine is 3:7 dimethylxanthine; and theophylline is 1:3 dimethylxanthine. They all resemble each other in most points of their pharmacological action, but they differ markedly in the relative intensity of their action on various functions. Thus caffeine is the most potent central nervous system stimulant of the group; theobromine exerts the greatest action on the muscles; and theophylline is the most effective diuretic and coronary dilator. Theobromine has comparatively little effect on the central nervous system, while theophylline has no action on the muscles. Caffeine stimulates the central nervous system, in particular that part associated with psychical functions. Ideas become clearer; thought flows more easily and rapidly; and fatigue and drowsiness disappear.

METHYSERGIDE MALEATE
(Sansert)

Methysergide (4 to 8 mg daily) is indicated for prophylaxis of vascular headache. In addition, it is used for prevention or reduction of intensity and frequency in patients suffering from one or more severe vascular headaches per week or from vascular headaches that are so severe that preventive therapy is indicated, regardless of the frequency of attack. Methysergide is a semisynthetic ergot derivative which inhibits or blocks the effects of serotonin and ameliorates the attack in 1 to 2 days. Plasma serotonin levels are elevated during the pre-headache phase of classical migraine and decreased during an attack. Without serotonin, the extracranial arteries are dilated and distended, resulting in headache. Methysergide may displace serotonin on receptor pressor sites of the walls of cranial arteries during a migraine attack and thereby preserve the vasoconstriction afforded by serotonin. Methysergide is a peripheral antagonist of serotonin, competitively blocking the serotonin receptor in the blood vessel. It also inhibits histamine release from mast cells and stabilizes platelets against spontaneous or induced release of serotonin. Centrally, methysergide may act as a serotonin agonist, especially in the midbrain. It has very weak uterotonic and emetic actions. Retro-peritoneal fibrosis, pleuropulmonary fibrosis, and fibrotic thickening of cardiac valves may occur in patients receiving long-term methysergide therapy.

The use of methysergide is contraindicated in peripheral vascular disease, severe arteriosclerosis, severe hypertension, coronary artery disease, phlebitis or cellulitis of the lower limbs, pulmonary disease, collagen disease or fibrotic processes, impaired liver or renal function, and valvular heart disease (see also Figure 85).

The concurrent use of beta adrenergic receptor blocking agents and methysergide may result in peripheral ischemia manifested by cold extremities with possible peripheral gangrene.

METIAMIDE

Metiamide, which was developed from **burimamide** by replacing a methylene group with an isoteric thio ether, is a histamine$_2$ (H$_2$) receptor antagonist with high specific activity, low toxicity, and good oral bioavailability in the treatment of acid pepsin disease (see also Table 9).

Histamine, as a normal constituent of the gastric mucosa, controls both **microcirculation** and **gastric secretion**. The gastric secretagogs are **acetylcholine, histamine,** and **gastrin**. The action of acetylcholine is blocked by **atropine,** and the action of histamine is blocked by **cimetidine, burimamide,** and **metiamide**. No specific antagonist is available for gastrin. The histamine release in the brain and perhaps other sites involves **exocytosis**, since this potassium-induced release is a calcium-dependent process. Histamine is released by many factors. For example, histamine is released by **numerous drugs** including reserpine, codeine, meperidine, hydralazine, morphine, *d*-tubocurarine, dextrans, and papaverine (see also Figure 24).

METIPRANOLOL HYDROCHLORIDE

(OptiPranolol)

Metipranolol, a beta-adrenergic blocking agent (instill 1 drop in each affected eye b.i.d.), is used in the treatment of ocular conditions in which lowering of intraocular pressure (LOP) would be beneficial (ocular hypertension, chronic open-angle glaucoma).

METOCLOPRAMIDE

(Reglan)

Oral metoclopramide is indicated for the treatment of diabetic gastroparesis (10 mg 30 minutes before each meal and at bedtime for 2 to 8 weeks) and symptomatic gastroesophageal reflux (10 to 15 mg orally up to 4 times daily 30 minutes before each meal and at bedtime for 4 to 12 weeks). Furthermore, parenteral metoclopramide is indicated for prevention of nausea and vomiting associated with emetogenic cancer chemotherapy, for prophylaxis of postoperative nausea and vomiting when nasogastric suction is undesirable, and as a single dose to facilitate small bowel intubation when the tube does not pass the pylorus with conventional maneuvers.

Metoclopramide stimulates motility of the upper GI tract without stimulating gastric, biliary, or pancreatic secretions. It sensitizes the gastrointestinal tissues to the action of acetylcholine.

The antiemetic properties of metoclopramide appear to be a result of its antagonism of central and peripheral dopamine receptors. Dopamine produces nausea and vomiting by stimulation of the medullary chemoreceptor trigger zone (CTZ), and metoclopramide blocks stimulation of the CTZ by agents like levodopa or apomorphine which are known to increase dopamine levels or to possess dopamine-like effects. Metoclopramide also inhibits the central and peripheral effects of apomorphine and abolishes the slowing of gastric emptying caused by apomorphine.

Metoclopramide is contraindicated in the presence of GI hemorrhage, mechanical obstruction, or perforation. Since metoclopramide is a dopamine receptor blocking agent, it causes extrapyramidal reactions such as dystonia and parkinsonism (see also Figure 73).

Metoclopramide increases gastric transit time enhancing the absorption of substances absorbed in the small intestine (e.g., ethanol, cyclosporin) and decreasing the absorption of substances absorbed in the stomach (e.g., cimetidine, digoxin). Anticholinergic drugs and dopamine-functions-enhancing substances such as levodopa reduce the effectiveness of metoclopramide. Since metoclopramide releases catecholamine, it should be used cautiously with monoamine oxidase inhibitors such as **tranylcypromine.** Since metoclopramide inhibits plasma cholinesterase, it increases the effectiveness of succinylcholine, a skeletal muscle relaxant.

Overdosage with metoclopramide causes drowsiness, disorientation, extrapyramidal reactions, muscle hypertonia, irritability, and agitation. **Diphenhydramine,** possessing anticholinergic and antihistaminic properties may be used to treat the extrapyramidal reactions.

METOCURINE IODIDE

(Metubine)

Metocurine, a skeletal muscle relaxant, is indicated as an adjunct to anesthesia, to facilitate endotracheal intubation (0.2 to 0.4 mg/kg), and to reduce the intensity of muscle contraction in pharmacologically or electrically-induced convulsions. Metocurine is a methyl analog of tubocurarine, which produces nondepolarizing (competitive) neuromuscular blockade.

Histamine release with Metubine iodide occurs less frequently than with d-tubocurarine and is related to dosage and rapidity of administration. Effects on the cardiovascular system (e.g., changes in pulse rate, hypotension) are less than those reported with equivalent doses of d-tubocurarine and gallamine.

Because the main excretory pathway for Metubine iodide is through the kidneys, severe renal disease or conditions associated with poor renal perfusion (shock states) may result in prolonged neuromuscular blockade.

Following intravenous injection in the mother, placental transfer of Metubine iodide occurs rapidly, and, after 6 minutes, the fetal plasma concentration is approximately one tenth the maternal level. Metocurine does not inhibit vagal transmission or sympathetic ganglionic blockade, and therefore produces minimal hemodynamic changes in humans. The relatively stable heart rate and blood pressure associated with its use make it a useful agent for patients with coronary artery disease and hypertension.

Parenteral administration of high doses of certain antibiotics may intensify or resemble the neuroblocking action of metocurine. These include **neomycin, streptomycin, bacitracin, kanamycin, gentamicin, dihydrostreptomycin, polymyxin B, colistin, sodium colistimethate**, and **tetracyclines**. If muscle relaxants and antibiotics must be administered simultaneously, the patient should be observed closely for any unexpected prolongation of respiratory depression. Certain general anesthetics have a synergistic action with neuromuscular blocking agents. **Halothane** and **isoflurane** potentiate the neuromuscular blocking action of other nondepolarizing agents and may be presumed to do so with Metubine iodide.

Administration of **quinidine** shortly after recovery may produce recurrent paranalysis. The use of **magnesium sulfate** in preeclamptic patients potentiates the effects of both depolarizing and nondepolarizing muscle relaxants (see also Figure 92).

The most frequently noted adverse reaction is prolongation of the drug's pharmacologic action. Neuromuscular effects may range from skeletal-muscle weakness to a profound relaxation that produces respiration insufficiency or apnea. Possible adverse reactions include allergic or hypersensitivity reactions to the drug or to its iodide content, and histamine release when large doses are administered rapidly. Signs of histamine release include erythema, edema, flushing, tachycardia, arterial hypotension, bronchospasm, and circulatory collapse. An overdose of Metubine iodide may result in prolonged apnea, cardiovascular collapse, and sudden release of histamine. Massive doses of metocurine are not reversible by the antagonists **edrophonium** or **neostigmine** and **atropine.** Overdosage may be avoided by the careful monitoring of response by means of a peripheral nerve stimulator. The primary treatment for residual neuromuscular blockade with respiratory paralysis or inadequate ventilation is maintenance of the patient's airway and manual or mechanical ventilation. Accompanying derangements of blood pressure, electrolyte imbalance, or circulating blood volume should be determined and corrected by appropriate fluid and electrolyte therapy. Residual neuromuscular blockade following surgery may be reversed by the use of anticholinesterase inhibitors such as neostigmine or pyridostigmine bromide and atropine.

METOLAZONE

(Zaroxolyn)

Metolazone is a quinazoline derivative with thiazide-like diuretic properties which is indicated in the treatment of edema associated with heart failure and hypertension (2.5 to 5 mg p.o./day). Metolazone increases urinary excretion of sodium and water by inhibiting sodium reabsorption in the cortical diluting tubule of the nephron, thus relieving edema. Metolazone may be more effective in edema associated with impaired renal function than thiazide or thiazide-like diuretics. Metolazone is thought to be a direct vasodilator and by decreasing the body sodium, reduces the total peripheral resistance. About 70 to 95% of metolazone is excreted unchanged in urine. Its half-life is about 14 hours in healthy subjects; it may be prolonged in patients with decreased creatinine clearance. Metolazone should be used cautiously in patients with severe renal disease because it may decrease glomerular filtration rate and precipitate azotemia; in patients with impaired hepatic function or liver disease because electrolyte changes may precipitate coma; and in patients taking digoxin, because hypokalemia may predispose them to digitalis toxicity. Metolazone potentiates the hypotensive effects of most other antihypertensive drugs; this may be used to therapeutic advantage. Metolazone may potentiate the hyperglycemic, hypotensive, and hyperuricemic effects of **diazoxide**, and its hyperglycemic effect may increase insulin or sulfonylurea requirements in diabetic patients (see also Figure 4).

Metolazone may reduce renal clearance of lithium, elevating serum lithium levels, and may necessitate a 50% reduction in lithium dosage. Metolazone turns urine slightly more alkaline and may decrease urinary excretion of some amines, such as amphetamine and quinidine; alkaline urine may also decrease therapeutic efficacy of methenamine compounds such as methamine mandelate. **Cholestyramine** and **colestipol** may bind metolazone, preventing its absorption; give drugs 1 hour apart. Clinical signs of overdose include GI irritation and hypermotility, diuresis, and lethargy, which may progress to coma.

METOPROLOL TARTRATE

(Lopressor)

In the treatment of hypertension, a major use of the beta-blockers is in combination with **hydralazine**. The direct vasodilators bring about reflex cardiac stimulation, and the beta-blockers prevent these adverse effects (see also Figure 61). Beta-blockers also reduce blood

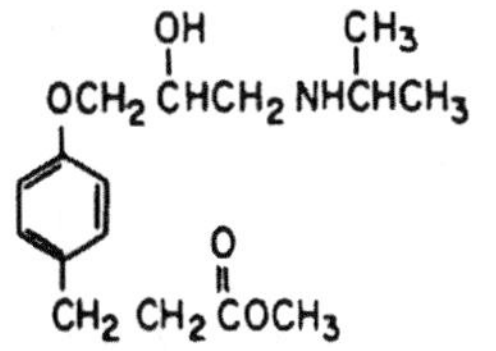

ESMOLOL

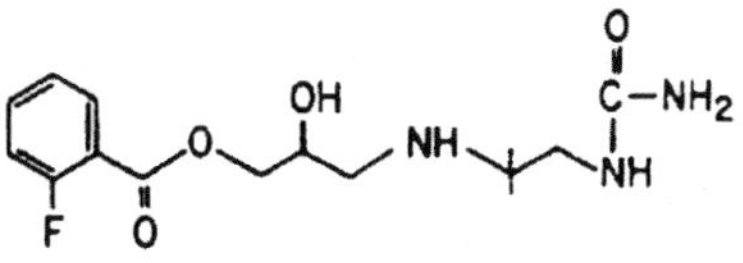

FLESTOLOL

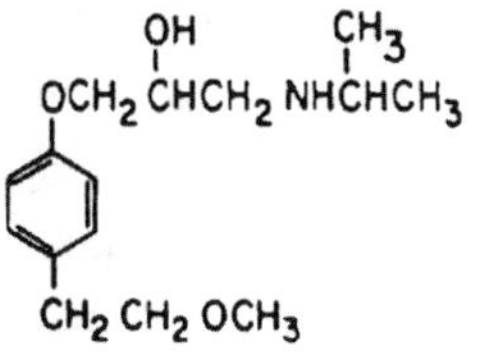

METOPROLOL

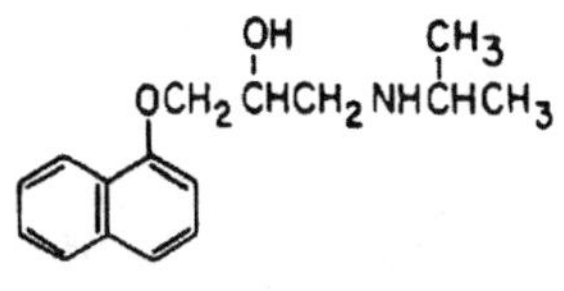

PROPRANOLOL

FIGURE 57 Metoprolol, a cardioselective beta$_1$-adrenergic receptor antagonist, is an antihypertensive agent used in the treatment of acute myocardial infarction.

pressure by exerting a central effect or a peripheral action, or both, that decreases renin activity. **Metoprolol** and **atenolol** are beta$_1$ selective, and they are safer agents in patients with asthma, diabetes mellitus, or low-renin hypertension. Some beta-blocking agents such as **pindolol** have **intrinsic sympathomimetic activity** and may be used in the treatment of pronounced bradycardia (**sick sinus syndrome**). Unlike propranolol, metoprolol is not a very lipid-soluble substance, does not enter the brain, and does not cause central nervous system toxicity (see Figure 57).

In the treatment of hypertension, metoprolol is used in an initial dose of 100 mg/day in single or divided doses, used alone or added to a diuretic. The dosage may be increased at weekly intervals until optimum blood pressure reduction is achieved. In the treatment of angina pectoris, metoprolol is used in an initial dose of 100 mg/day in two divided doses. Dosage may be gradually increased at weekly intervals until optimum clinical response is obtained or a pronounced slowing of heart rate occurs. The effective dosage range is 100 to 400 mg/day. In the treatment of myocardial infarction, treatment with metoprolol should be initiated as soon as possible after the patient's arrival in a coronary care or similar unit immediately after the patient is hemodynamically stable. The patient should receive three intravenous bolus doses of 5 mg each at two-minute intervals. Then 50 mg of metoprolol is given orally every six hours for 48 hours, followed by a maintenance dose of 100 mg b.i.d.

METRIFONATE

(Bilarcil)

Metrifonate is an organophosphorous-inhibiting cholinesterase in *Schistosoma haematobium*. Since the plasma cholinesterase in the host is similarly inhibited, depolarizing neuromuscular blocking agents, other cholinesterase inhibitors, and agents metabolized by plasma cholinesterase should not be administered with metrifonate (see also Figure 71).

METRONIDAZOLE HYDROCHLORIDE

(Protostat)

Metronidazole is indicated for the treatment of symptomatic trichomoniasis in females and males when the presence of the trichomonad has been confirmed by appropriate laboratory procedures; in the treatment of asymptomatic females when the organism is associated with endocervitis, cervicitis, or cervical erosion. Metronidazole is also indicated in the treatment of acute intestinal amebiasis (amebic dysentery and amebic liver abscess). Metronidazole is indicated in the treatment of serious infections caused by susceptible anaerobic bacteria. Indicated surgical procedures should be performed in conjunction with metronidazole therapy. In a mixed aerobic and anaerobic infection, antibiotics appropriate for the treatment of the aerobic infection should be used in addition to metronidazole.

In the treatment of most serious anaerobic infections, metronidazole IV RTU is usually administered initially. This may be followed by oral therapy with metronidazole at the discretion of the physician.

The nitro group of metronidazole is reduced inside the infecting organism; this reduction product disrupts DNA and inhibits nucleic acid synthesis. The drug is active in intestinal and extraintestinal sites. It is active against most anaerobic bacteria and protozoa, including *Bacteroides fragilis, B. metaninogenicus, Fusobacterium, Vellonella, Clostridium, Peptococcus, Peptostreptococcus, Entamoeba histolytica, Trichomonas vaginalis, Giardia lambia,* and *Balantidum coli.* Metronidazole is absorbed orally, and its peak serum concentration occurs in one hour. Metronidazole is distributed into most body tissues and fluids, including cerebrospinal fluid (CSF), bone, bile, saliva, pleural and peritoneal fluids, vaginal secretions, seminal fluids, middle ear fluid, and hepatic and cerebral abscesses. CSF levels approach serum levels in patients with inflamed meninges; they reach about 50% of serum levels in patients with uninflamed meninges. Less than 20% of metronidazole is bound to plasma proteins. It readily crosses the placenta. Metronidazole is metabolized to an active 2-hydroxymethyl metabolite and also to other metabolites. About 60 to 80% of the dose is excreted as the parent compound or its metabolites. About 20% of a metronidazole dose is excreted unchanged in urine; about 6 to 15% is excreted in feces. Metronidazole's half-life is 6 to 8 hours in adults with normal renal function; the half-life may be prolonged in patients with impaired hepatic function.

Concomitant use of metronidazole with oral anticoagulants prolongs prothrombin time. Concomitant use with alcohol inhibits alcohol dehydrogenase activity, causing a disulfiram-like reaction (nausea, vomiting, headache, abdominal cramps, and flushing) in some patients. Concomitant use with disulfiram may precipitate psychosis and confusion and should be avoided. Concomitant use with barbiturates and phenytoin may diminish the antimicrobial effectiveness of metronidazole by increasing its metabolism and may require higher doses of metronidazole. Concomitant use with cimetidine may decrease the clearance of metronidazole, thereby increasing its potential for causing adverse effects. Clinical signs of overdose include nausea, vomiting, ataxia, seizures, and peripheral neuropathy.

METYRAPONE TEST

The level of cortisol is thought to directly control the secretion of ACTH through a negative feedback mechanism that may be directed at both the hypothalamus and the anterior pituitary gland. Conversely, a reduced concentration of cortisol or cortisol-like substances eliminates the negative effect and enhances the release of ACTH (see also Figure 28).

The **metyrapone test** may be used diagnostically to evaluate the proper functioning of the anterior pituitary gland. When administered orally, metyrapone inhibits the activity of 11-beta-hydroxylase, which is necessary for the synthesis of cortisol, corticosterone, and aldosterone, promotes the release of corticotropin, which in turn increases production of the precursors (11-deoxycortisol and 11-deoxycorticosterone), and enhances the appearance of 17-hydroxycorticosteroids and

17-ketogenic steroids. In the event that the pituitary gland is nonfunctional, and therefore cannot stimulate ACTH secretion, the levels of these urinary metabolites will not increase.

MEXILETINE
(Mexitil)

Mexiletine (initially 200 mg/every 8 hours) is indicated for the treatment of documented, life-threatening ventricular arrhythmias, such as sustained ventricular tachycardia. Because of the proarrhythmic effects of mexiletine, its use with lesser arrhythmias is not recommended. The actions of mexiletine resemble those of lidocaine, which inhibits the inward sodium current, thus reducing the rate of rise of the action potential, Phase O. Mexiletine decreases the effective refractory period (ERP) in Purkinje fibers. The decrease in ERP is of lesser magnitude than the decrease in action potential duration (APD), with a resulting increase in ERP/APD ratio. Mexiletine is a local anesthetic and a Class IB antiarrhythmic compound with electrophysiologic properties similar to lidocaine. Mexiletine is contraindicated in cardiogenic shock, and preexisting second- or third-degree AV block. Mexiletine is well absorbed (approximately 90%) from the GI tract. The absorption rate is reduced in situations in which gastric emptying time is increased. Narcotics, atropine, and magnesium-aluminum hydroxide may slow its absorption, whereas, metoclopramide may accelerate its absorption.

Mexiletine is metabolized in the liver. The most active minor metabolite is N-methylmexiletine, which is <20% as potent as mexiletine. The urinary excretion of N-methylmexiletine is <0.5%.

Overdosage with mexiletine causes dizziness, drowsiness, nausea, hypotension, sinus bradycardia, paresthesia, seizures, intermittent left bundle branch block, and temporary asystole. With massive overdoses, coma and respiratory arrest may occur (see also Figure 76).

MEZLOCILLIN SODIUM
(Mezlin)

Carbenicillin cures serious infections caused by *Pseudomonas* species and *Proteus* strains resistant to ampicillin. It is not absorbed from the gastrointestinal tract, and therefore must be administered intraperitoneally. **Carbenicillin indanyl** is acid stable and hence can be given orally. **Ticarcillin** is four times more potent than carbenicillin in treating a *Pseudomonas aeruginosa* infection, and **azlocillin** is ten times more potent than carbenicillin against *Pseudomonas*. **Mezlocillin** and **piperacillin** are more active against *Klebsiella* infection than is carbenicillin.

Mezlocillin is indicated for:

Lower respiratory tract infections, including pneumonia and lung abscess caused by *Haemophilus influenzae, Klebsiella sp.* including *K. pneumoniae, Proteus mirabilis, Pseudomonas sp.* including *P. aeruginosa, E. coli,* and *Bacteroides sp.* including *B. fragilis*

Intra-abdominal infections, including acute cholecystitis, cholangitis, peritonitis, hepatic abscess, and intra-abdominal abscess caused by susceptible *E. coli, P. mirabilis, Klebsiella sp., Pseudomonas sp., Streptococcus faecalis* (enterococcus), *Bacteroides sp., Peptococcus sp.,* and *Peptostreptococcus sp.*

Urinary tract infections caused by susceptible *E. coli, P. mirabilis,* the indole-positive *Proteus sp., Morganella morganii, Klebsiella sp., Enterobacter sp., Serratia sp., Pseudomonas sp., S. faecalis* (enterococcus)

Uncomplicated gonorrhea due to susceptible *Neisseria gonorrhoeae*

Gynecological infections, including endometritis, pelvic cellulitis, and pelvic inflammatory disease associated with susceptible *N. gonorrhoeae, Peptococcus sp., Peptostreptococcus sp., Bacteroides sp., E. coli, P. mirabilis, Klebsiella sp.,* and *Enterobacter sp.*

Skin and skin structure infections caused by susceptible *S. faecalis* (enterococcus), *E. coli, P. mirabilis,* the indole-positive *Proteus sp., P. vulgaris,* and *Providencia rettgeri, Klebsiella sp., Enterobacter sp., Pseudomonas sp., Peptococcus sp.,* and *Bacteroides sp.*

Septicemia, including bacteremia caused by susceptible *E. coli, Klebsiella sp., Enterobacter sp., Pseudomonas sp., Bacteroides sp.,* and *Peptococcus sp.*

Streptococcal infections caused by *Streptococcus sp.* including group A betahemolytic *Streptococcus* and *S. pneumoniae*; however, such infections are ordinarily treated with more narrow-spectrum penicillins.

Mezlocillin's broad spectrum of activity makes it useful for treating mixed infections caused by susceptible strains of both Gram-negative and Gram-positive aerobic and anaerobic bacteria. It is not effective, however, against infections caused by penicillinase-producing *Staphylococcus aureus.*

Mezlocillin is effective in combination with an aminoglycoside for the treatment of life-threatening infections caused by *P. aeruginosa.* For the treatment of febrile episodes in immunosuppressed patients with granulocytopenia, it may be combined with an aminoglycoside or a cephalosporin. The rate of elimination of mezlocillin is dose-dependent and related to the degree of renal function impairment. Dosage adjustments are not required in patients with mild impairment of renal function.

MIANSERIN

Serotonergic antagonists such as methysergide represent the first class of drugs shown to be effective in migraine prophylaxis. Methysergide is an ergot derivative that has complex effects on serotonergic and other neurotransmitter systems. It has been shown to be effective in 60 to 80% of migraine patients and should be given for at least a 6-week trial. This agent is used most frequently for patients who complain of cluster headaches. Common side effects include nausea, vomiting, and diarrhea. A few patients have developed retroperitoneal fibrosis following prolonged use of methysergide. Therefore, it is recommended that this drug be administered for no more than 6 consecutive months. The patient should then discontinue the medication for at least 4 to 8 weeks, after which the drug can be reintroduced safely. **Ergonovine** (Ergotrate) is another ergot alkaloid that has been used prophylactically. Other 5-HT receptor antagonists (i.e., **pizotifen, mianserin**) have also been reported effective in migraine prophylaxis. Mianserin also has shown efficacy as an antidepressant. It does not alter the uptake of norepinephrine, serotonin, or dopamine. Mianserin blocks alpha 1 and 2 adrenergic receptors and H_1 histamine receptors without having any anticholinergic effects. Mianserine is sedative in nature (see also Figure 85).

MICONAZOLE

(Monistat)

Miconazole is indicated in the treatment of the following severe systemic fungal infections: Coccidioidomycosis, candidiasis, cryptococcosis, pseudoallescheriosis (petriellidosis, allescheriosis), paracoccidioidomycosis and for the treatment of chronic mucocutaneous candidiasis.

In the treatment of fungal meningitis or *Candida* urinary bladder infections, IV infusion alone is inadequate. It must be supplemented with intrathecal administration or bladder irrigation.

Miconazole, an imidazole derivative, exerts a fungicidal effect by altering the permeability of the fungal cell membrane. Its mechanism of action may also involve an alteration of RNA and DNA metabolism or an intracellular accumulation of peroxides toxic to the fungal cell.

Miconazole is rapidly metabolized in the liver. About 14 to 22% of the administered dose is excreted in the urine, mainly as inactive metabolites. The terminal elimination half-life is 20 to 25 hours.

Rapid injection of undiluted miconazole may produce transient tachycardia or arrhythmia. **Miconazole** and **amphotericin B** are antagonistic both *in vitro* and *in vivo*. The antifungal activity of the two drugs when used in combination is less than that of either drug used alone. Miconazole enhances the effectiveness of anticoagulants and increases the serum level of phenytoin. Miconazole has caused rash, pruritis, and phlebitis at the site of infusion. A transient decrease in hematocrit has been noted.

MIDAZOLAM

(Versed)

Midazolam (IM) is indicated for causing preoperative sedation and impairment of preoperative events. When given intravenously, it is used for producing conscious sedation prior to short diagnostic or endoscopic procedures, either alone or with a narcotic. It is used for induction of general anesthesia, before administration of other anesthetic agents, and to supplement nitrous oxide and oxygen (balanced anesthesia) for short surgical procedures. Intravenously administered midazolam has been associated with respiratory depression and respiratory arrest, especially when used for conscious sedation. In some cases, where this was not recognized promptly and treated effectively, death or hypoxic encephalopathy resulted. Midazolam, like other members of benzodiazepine derivatives, exerts its CNS depressant effects by enhancing and facilitating GABAergic transmission (see Figure 40). Midazolam decreases cerebrospinal fluid pressure and intraocular pressure. **Barbiturates, alcohol,** or other **CNS depressants** may increase the risk of underventilation or apnea and contribute to prolonged effect when used with midazolam. Narcotic premedication also depresses ventilatory response to carbon dioxide stimulation.

Narcotics (e.g., morphine, meperidine, and fentanyl), **secobarbital**, or **fentanyl** and **droperidol** (Innovar) used as premedications accentuate the hypnotic effect of midazolam (see also Table 8). A moderate (15%) reduction in induction dosage of thiopental is required following IM use of midazolam for premedication. The dosage of inhalational anesthetics may need to be reduced when midazolam is used as an induction agent. The IV administration decreases the minimum alveolar concentration (MAC) of **halothane** required for general anesthesia. Symptoms of overdosage include sedation, somnolence, confusion, impaired coordination and reflexes, coma, and untoward effects on vital signs. **Flumazenil** (Romazicon) may be used to antidote the effects of midazolam (see Figure 40).

MIGRAINE HEADACHES: TREATMENT OF
Drugs and Dosages
Aspirin, 650 mg every 4 hrs
Aspirin, 650 mg with butalbital, 50 mg
Aspirin, 300 mg, with caffeine, 50 mg and butalbital, 50 mg
Acetaminophen, 650 mg every 4 hrs
Acetaminophen, 325 mg, with butalbital, 50 mg
Dihydroergotamine, 1 mg IM or IV at onset and every 1 hr
Ergotamine, 1 mg
Ergotamine, 1 mg plus caffeine, 100 mg
Ergotamine, 2 mg plus caffeine 100 mg (suppository)

Ibuprofen, 400-800 mg three times a day
Indomethacin, 50 mg three times a day
Naproxen sodium, 550 mg then 275 mg every 6 to 8 hrs
Sumatriptan, 6 mg subcutaneously

The medication(s) to be chosen depends on the severity and/or
frequency of attacks and the response of the patients.

MILRINONE LACTATE
(Primacor)

Agents with **positive inotropic actions** that may be used in the management of congestive heart failure include the **cardiac glycosides** (e.g., digoxin and digitoxin), **dopaminergic analogs** (e.g., dobutamine), **phosphodiesterase inhibitors** (e.g., amrinone and milrinone), **angiotensin antagonists** (e.g., captopril, enalapril, and lisinopril), and **vasodilators** (nitrates and hydralazine).

Milrinone is a member of a new class of bipyridine inotropic/vasodilator agents with phosphodiesterase inhibitor activity. It is a positive inotrope and vasodilator, with little chronotropic activity, different in structure and mode of action from either the digitalis glycosides or catecholamines (see also Figures 10 and 42).

At relevant inotropic and vasorelaxant concentrations, milrinone is a selective inhibitor of peak III cAMP phosphodiesterase isozyme in cardiac and vascular muscle. This inhibitory action is consistent with cAMP-mediated increases in intracellular ionized calcium and contractile protein phosphorylation and relaxation in vascular muscle. Additional experimental evidence also indicates that milrinone is not a beta-adrenergic agonist nor does it inhibit sodium-potassium adenosine triphosphatase activity as do the digitalis glycosides.

In patients with congestive heart failure (CHF) milrinone produces dose-related increases in the maximum rate of increase of left ventricular pressure. Milrinone has a direct inotropic effect and a direct arterial vasodilator activity. Both the inotropic and vasodilatory effects occur over the therapeutic range of plasma concentrations of 100 to 300 ng/ml. In addition to increasing myocardial contractility, milrinone improves diastolic function as evidenced by improvements in left ventricular diastolic relaxation.

In patients with depressed myocardial function, milrinone produces a prompt increase in cardiac output and decreases in pulmonary capillary wedge pressure and vascular resistance without a significant increase in heart rate or myocardial oxygen consumption. Overdosage of milrinone, which is a vasodilator, produces hypotension.

MINERALOCORTICOIDS

The mineralocorticoids influence **salt and water metabolism** and in general conserve sodium levels. They promote the resorption of sodium and the secretion of potassium in the cortical collecting tubules and possibly the connecting segment. They also elicit hydrogen secretion in the medullary collecting tubules. The main mineralocorticoid is **aldosterone**, with a daily secretion of 100 micrograms. Aldosterone is synthesized from 18-hydroxycorticocosterone by a dehydrogenase. The consequence of 18-hydroxycorticosterone dehydrogenase deficiency is diminished secretion of aldosterone, and the clinical manifestations consist of sodium depletion, dehydration, hypotension, potassium retention, and enhanced plasma renin levels (see also Figure 21).

MINERAL OIL
(Agoral, Kondremul Plain, Milkinol, Neo-cultol, Nujol, Petrogalar Plain, Zymenol)

Mineral oil, a lubricant, is indicated in constipation or preparation for bowel studies or surgery.

MINOCYCLINE HYDROCHLORIDE
(Minocin)

Minocycline, a tetracycline, is indicated in syphilis or gonorrhea in patients sensitive to penicillin. In addition, it may be used in uncomplicated urethral, endocervical, or rectal infection, and in uncomplicated gonococcal urethritis in men (see also Figure 88). Tetracyclines enter bacterial cells by both passive diffusion and active transport, and then accumulate intracellularly. This does not occur in mammalian cells. The tetracyclines bind to the 30S subunit of the bacterial ribosome in such a way that the binding of the aminoacyl-transfer RNA to the acceptor site on the messenger RNA ribosome complex is blocked (see Figure 80).

Minocycline is active against many Gram-negative and Gram-positive organisms. *Mycoplasma, Rickettsia, Chlamydia,* and spirochetes; it may be more active against staphylococci than other tetracyclines. The potential vestibular toxicity and cost of minocycline limits its usefulness. It may be more active than other tetracyclines against *Nocardia asteroides*; it is also effective against *Mycobacterium marinum* infections. It has been used for meningococcal meningitis prophylaxis because of its activity against *Neisseria meningitidis*. The absorption of tetracyclines from the gastrointestinal tract is **nonuniform**. Up to 30% of chlortetracycline is absorbed. The absorption for tetracycline, oxytetracycline, and demeclocycline ranges between 60 to 80%, whereas as much as 90 to 100% of doxycycline and minocycline is absorbed. The unabsorbed tetracycline may modify the intestinal flora. The absorption of tetracyclines is impaired by **divalent cations** (calcium, magnesium, and ferrous iron), by aluminum, and by extremely alkaline pHs. Tetracyclines are distributed widely throughout the body fluid, cross the placental barrier, and can accumulate in growing bones. The concentrations of chlortetracycline in spinal fluid are only one fourth of those in plasma. Minocycline, a more lipid-soluble tetracycline, reaches a high concentration in tears and saliva and can eradicate the meningococcal carrier state. The tetracyclines are metabolized in the liver and excreted mainly by the bile and urine. The concentrations of tetracyclines in the bile are 10 times higher than those in serum. Tetracyclines in general cause toxic and hypersensitivity reactions. These consist commonly of gastrointestinal irritations that are disabling and may necessitate discontinuation of the medications. With continuous usage, tetracyclines may alter the normal flora, allowing the growth of *Pseudomonas, Proteus*, staphylococci-resistant coliforms, *Clostridium*, and *Candida* organisms. These superinfections should be recognized and treated appropriately with vancomycin and other drugs. Tetracyclines have been known to cause hepatic necrosis, especially when given in large intravenous doses or when taken by pregnant women or patients with preexisting liver impairment. Tetracycline preparations whose potency has expired can cause **renal tubular acidosis** (Fanconi's syndrome). With the exception of doxycycline, tetracyclines accumulate in patients with renal impairment. Tetracyclines also produce **nitrogen retention**, especially when given with diuretics. Tetracyclines bind to calcium and then become deposited in bone, causing damage to developing bone and teeth. The intravenous administration of tetracyclines has been observed to cause venous thrombosis.

MINOXIDIL
(Topical)(Rogaine)

Minoxidil (2% 1 ml of solution b.i.d.) is used in the treatment of male pattern baldness (**alopecia androgenetica**).

MINOXIDIL
(Loniten)

Minoxidil (10 to 40 mg/day) is indicated for severe hypertension that is symptomatic or associated with target organ damage and is not manageable with maximum therapeutic doses of a diuretic plus two other antihypertensives. Topical minoxidil (Rogaine) in 0.3 to 4.5% solution is used to stimulate vertex hair growth in individuals with alopecia androgenetica, expressed in males as baldness of the vertex of the scalp and in females as diffuse hair loss or thinning of the frontoparietal areas. There is no effect in patients with predominantly frontal hair loss. The mechanism is not known, but like minoxidil, some other arterial dilating drugs also stimulate hair growth when given systemically.

Minoxidil is a direct-acting peripheral vasodilator. The exact mechanism of action on the vascular smooth muscle is unknown. It does not interfere with vasomotor reflexes, therefore, it does not produce orthostatic hypotension. The drug does not affect CNS function. It appears to block calcium uptake through the cell membrane. Minoxidil reduces elevated systolic and diastolic blood pressure by decreasing peripheral vascular resistance. The blood pressure response to minoxidil is dose-related and proportional to the extent of hypertension. In humans, forearm and renal vascular resistance decline; forearm blood flow increases, while renal blood flow and glomerular filtration rate (GFR) are preserved.

When used in severely hypertensive patients resistant to other therapy, frequently with an accompanying diuretic and beta-adrenergic blocker, minoxidil decreases the blood pressure and reverses encephalopathy and retinopathy. Minoxidil causes peripheral vasodilation and elicits a reduction of peripheral arteriolar resistance. This action, with the associated fall in blood pressure, triggers sympathetic, vagal inhibitory and renal homeostasis mechanisms, including an increase in renin secretion, that leads to increased cardiac rate and output, and salt and water retention. These adverse effects can usually be minimized by coadministration of a diuretic and a beta-adrenergic blocking agent or other sympathetic nervous system suppressant. Although minoxidil does not cause orthostatic hypotension, its use in patients on **guanethidine** can result in profound orthostatic effects (see also Table 26).

MISOPROSTOL

(Cytotec)

Misoprostol, a prostaglandin E_1 analog with gastric mucosal protectant properties, is used in prevention of gastric ulcer induced by nonsteroidal antiinflammatory agents. In addition, it has been used in the treatment of duodenal or gastric ulcer.

MITHRAMYCIN

(Mithracin)

The mechanism of action of mithramycin is similar to dactinomycin's. It is used in patients with advanced disseminated tumors of the testis and for the treatment of hypercalcemia associated with cancer. Mithramycin may cause gastrointestinal injury, bone marrow depression, hepatic and renal damage, and hemorrhagic tendency.

MITOMYCIN

(Mutamycin)

Mitomycin (20 mg/m^2 IV as a single dose at 6 to 8 week intervals) is indicated in therapy of disseminated adenocarcinoma of stomach or pancreas combined with other chemotherapeutic agents, and as palliative treatment when other modalities fail. Mitomycin has been given by the intravesical route for the management of superficial bladder cancer. Mitomycin as an ophthalmic solution appears beneficial as an adjunct to surgical excision in the treatment of primary or recurrent pterygia. Mitomycin is an antibiotic with antitumor activity isolated from *Streptomyces caespitosus*. It selectively inhibits the synthesis of deoxyribonucleic acid (DNA). The guanine and cytosine content correlates with the degree of mitomycin-induced crosslinking. At high concentrations, cellular ribonucleic acid (RNA) and protein synthesis are also suppressed. *Bone marrow suppression*, notably thrombocytopenia and leukopenia, which may contribute to overwhelming infection in an already compromised patient, is the most serious syndrome of microangiopathic hemolytic anemia. Thrombocytopenia and irreversible renal failure have occurred. Acute shortness of breath and severe bronchospasm have occurred following the use of vinca alkaloids in patients who had previously or simultaneously received mitomycin. Onset of this acute respiratory distress occurs within minutes to hours after the vinca alkaloid injection. Bronchodilators, steroids, or oxygen produce symptomatic relief.

MITOTANE

(Lysodren)

Mitotane, a chlorophenothane (DDT) analog, with antineoplastic properties (1 to 6 g p.o. daily in divided doses) is used in the treatment of inoperable adrenocortical cancer.

MITOXANTRONE HYDROCHLORIDE

(Novantrone)

Mitoxantrone (12 mg/m^2 daily by IV infusion on days 1 to 3) is used as an initial treatment in combination with other approved drugs for acute nonlymphocytic leukemia.

MIVACURIUM CHLORIDE

(Mivacron)

Mivacurium, a nondepolarizing neuromuscular blocking agent (0.15 mg/kg IV push in 5 to 15 sec), is used as an adjunct to general anesthesia to facilitate endotracheal intubation and to provide skeletal muscle relaxation during surgery or mechanical ventilation (see also Figure 92).

MOCLOBEMIDE

Moclobemide is a novel benzamide reversible inhibitor of monoamine oxidase A and has clinical efficacy in a wide spectrum of depressive illness including endogenous and nonendogenous depression in younger adults and in the elderly. Comparisons have shown similar efficacy to all main classes of antidepressants and much greater tolerability and safety in overdose than tricyclic antidepressants. Clinically, it is neither sedative nor alerting. There is no need for dietary restrictions for patients on moclobemide on a normal diet, and drug interactions are few and usually mild. Moclobemide should be used cautiously in patients who may be taking meperidine or serotonin reuptake inhibitors (see Figures 27 and 78).

MOLINDONE HYDROCHLORIDE

(Moban)

Molindone (50 to 75 mg/day) is indicated for the management of the manifestations of psychotic disorders. Molindone is structurally unrelated to the phenothiazines, butyrophenones, or thioxanthenes, but it resembles the piperazine phenothiazines in its clinical action. It causes sedation, possesses anticholinergic properties, and similar to fluphenazine, produces movement disorders. Molindone is metabolized, and the metabolites are excreted in the urine. Molindone lowers the seizure threshold and may cause seizures in patients with epilepsy and other seizure disorders. Concomitant use with sympathomimetics, including epinephrine, phenylephrine, phenylpropanolamine, and ephedrine (often found in nasal sprays), or appetite suppressants may decrease their stimulatory and pressor effects. Because of its alpha-blocking potential, molindone may cause epinephrine reversal — a hypotensive response to epinephrine.

Molindone may inhibit blood pressure response to centrally acting antihypertensive drugs, such as guanethidine, guanabenz, guanadrel, clonidine, methyldopa, and reserpine. Additive effects are likely after concomitant use of molindone with CNS depressants, including alcohol, analgesics, barbiturates, narcotics, tranquilizers, and general, spinal, or epidural anesthetics, or parenteral magnesium sulfate (oversedation, respiratory depression, and hypotension); antiarrhythmic agents, quinidine, disopyramide, or procainamide (increased incidence of cardiac arrhythmias and conduction defects); atropine or other anticholinergic drugs, including antidepressants, monoamine oxidase inhibitors, phenothiazines, antihistamines, meperidine, and antiparkinsonian agents (oversedation, paralytic ileus, visual changes, and severe constipation); nitrates (hypotension); and metrizamide (increased risk of convulsions). Beta-blocking agents may inhibit molindone metabolism, increasing plasma levels and toxicity. Concomitant use with propylthiouracil increases risk of agranulocytosis; concomitant use with lithium may result in severe neurologic toxicity, with an encephalitis-like syndrome and a decreased therapeutic response to molindone. Decreased therapeutic response to molindone may follow concomitant use with calcium-containing drugs such as phenytoin and tetracyclines, aluminum- and magnesium-containing antacids or antidiarrheals (decreased absorption), or caffeine (increased metabolism). Molindone may antagonize the therapeutic effect of bromocriptine on prolactin secretion; it may also decrease the vasoconstricting effects of high-dose dopamine and may decrease effectiveness and increase toxicity of levodopa (by dopamine blockade). Calcium sulfate in molindone tablets may inhibit the absorption of phenytoin or tetracyclines (see Table 23).

MOLSIDOMINE

Molsidomine is a prodrug for the formation of nitric oxide (NO). Its pharmacokinetics are characterized by rapid absorption and hydrolysis, taking a short time to achieve maximal systemic concentration of both the parent compound and its active metabolite. It has been used in the management of angina pectoris (see also Figure 60).

MONOAMINE OXIDASE INHIBITORS

The **monoamine oxidase inhibitors** are used occasionally to treat depression. The **hydrazine** derivatives consist of **isocarboxazid** (Marplan) and **phenelzine sulfate** (Nardil). The **non-hydrazine** derivatives include **tranylcypromine** (Parnate).

Monoamine oxidase can metabolize monoamines by oxidative deamination and convert them to inactive acidic derivatives. Monoamine oxidase inhibitors seem to compete with physiologically active monoamine for the active site of the enzyme. In general, not only do these agents inhibit the oxidase that metabolizes amines, but they also inhibit the oxidase that metabolizes drugs and essential nutrients. Hence, the incidence of drug-drug and drug-food interactions is extremely high with these agents. Monoamine oxidases have various applications. They may be used as a **local anesthetic** (cocaine), an **antihistaminic** (diphenylhydramine), or an **antidepressant** (tranylcypromine). Monoamine oxidase inhibitors have been used in the treatment of hypertension (direct blockade of sympathetic ganglion), angina pectoris (coronary dilation), narcolepsy (stimulating the reticular activating system), and depression (increasing the brain's norepinephrine pool). Needless to say, these agents should be used with extreme caution in conjunction with sympathomimetic amines, ganglionic blocking agents, procaine, and anesthetic agents. They are contraindicated in patients with hyperthyroidism and in combination with tricyclic antidepressants. In the event of poisoning, adrenergic blocking agents such as **phentolamine** may be effective for combating the hypertensive crisis.

The high incidence of drug-food and drug-drug interactions rules out monoamine oxidase inhibitors as antidepressants of first choice. However, there are circumstances in which these agents may be used effectively and successfully. These are: when a patient has not responded to a tricyclic antidepressant for an adequate trial period and with an appropriate dosage; when a patient has developed allergic reactions to tricyclics; and when a patient has had previous depressive episodes that responded well to monoamine oxidase inhibitors (see also Figure 27).

MONOAMINE OXIDASE INHIBITORS: CONTEMPORARY TREATMENT OF DEPRESSION

Monoamine oxidase inhibitor (MAOI) antidepressants have been in use for nearly 40 years. At the present time, they are viewed as second- or third-line antidepressant medications for reasons of both efficacy and safety. The available MAOIs are phenelzine sulfate (Nardil), isocarboxazid (Marplan), and tranylcypromine sulfate (Parnate). Two additional MAOI antidepressants, moclobemide and brofaromine, are approved for use in Europe and/or Canada.

It was initially believed that the antidepressant effectiveness of MAOIs was the direct result of MAO inhibition. This acute effect decreases degradation of monoamines (e.g., norepinephrine, serotonin, or dopamine) stored in presynaptic neurons, thereby resulting in an increased amount of these neurotransmitters available at the synapse. More recent research indicates that this model does not fully explain the mechanism of MAOIs' efficacy. For example, the positive (+) stereoisomer of tranylcypromine is a poor antidepressant despite inhibiting MAO. The main pharmacologic difference between the negative (-) and + isomers of tranylcypromine is that the former has much weaker effects as a norepinephrine reuptake inhibitor in relation to its potency as an MAOI. The other MAOIs may also block the reuptake of selected neurotransmitters. However, like the non-MAOI uptake inhibitors, these acute effects often precede clinical antidepressant effects by weeks. More consistent with the 2- to 4-week lag in therapeutic effect, chronic treatment with a diverse number of MAOIs has been shown to reduce the number of α_2- and β-adrenergic and serotonin (5-HT_2) post-synaptic binding sites in the brain.

The high incidence of drug–food and drug–drug interactions rule out MAOIs as antidepressants of first choice. However, there are circumstances in which these agents may be used effectively and successfully. These are:

> When a patient has not responded to a tricyclic antidepressant for an adequate trial period and with an appropriate dosage.
> When a patient has developed allergic reactions to tricyclics.
> When a patient has had previous depressive episodes that responded well to MAOIs.

MONOCTANOIN
(Moctanin)

Monoctanoin, an esterified glycerol, is used to solubilize cholesterol gallstones that are retained in the biliary tract after cholecystectomy.

MONOIODOTYROSINE
(MIT)

The steps involved in the synthesis of thyroid hormones are depicted in Figure 56. First the ingested iodide (100 to 150 mg/day) is actively transported (**iodide trapping**) and then accumulated in the thyroid gland. Following this, the trapped iodide is oxidized by a peroxidase system to active iodine, which iodinates the tyrosine residue of glycoprotein to yield **monoiodotyrosine** (MIT) and **diiodotyrosine** (DIT). This process is called **iodide organification**. The MIT and DIT combine to form T_4. T_3 and T_4 are released from thyroglobulin through the actions of pinocytosis and the proteolysis of thyroglobulin by lysosomal enzymes. In the circulation, 75% of T_4 is bound to **thyroxine-binding globulin** (TBG), and the remainder is mostly bound to **thyroxine-binding prealbumin** (TBPA). Approximately 0.05% of T_4 remains free. T_3 is similarly bound to TBG, allowing only 0.5% of it to remain in the free form.

MOPP THERAPY

The alkylating agents exert their antineoplastic actions by generating highly reactive carbonium ion intermediates that form a covalent linkage with various nucleophilic components on both proteins and DNA. The 7 position of the purine base **guanine** is particularly susceptible to alkylation, resulting in miscoding, depurination, or ring cleavage. **Bifunctional alkylating agents** are able to crosslink either two nucleic acid molecules or one protein and one nucleic acid molecule. Although these agents are very active from a therapeutic perspective, they are also notorious for their tendency to cause carcinogenesis and mutagenesis. Alkylating agents that have a nonspecific effect on the cell-cycle phase are the most cytotoxic to rapidly proliferating tissues (see also Figure 2).

The activity of nitrogen mustards depends on the presence of a *bis*-(2-chloroethyl) grouping:

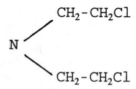

This is present in **mechlorethamine** (Mustargen), which is used in patients with Hodgkin's disease and other lymphomas, usually in combination with other drugs, such as in **MOPP therapy** (mechlorethamine, Oncovin [vincristine], procarbazine, and prednisone). It may cause bone marrow depression.

MORICIZINE HYDROCHLORIDE

(Ethmozine)

Moricizine (600 to 900 mg/day given every 8 hours in three equally divided doses) is indicated in the treatment of documented ventricular arrhythmias, such as sustained ventricular tachycardia, that are life-threatening. Because of the proarrhythmic effects of moricizine, its use should be reserved for patients in whom the benefits of treatment outweigh the risks. Moricizine is a Class 1C antiarrhythmic agent with potent local anesthetic activity and myocardial membrane stabilizing effects. It shares some of the characteristics of the Class 1A (disopyramide, procainamide, or quinidine), of Class 1B (lidocaine, mexiletene, phenytoin, or tocainide), or Class 1C agents (encainide, flecainide, or propafenone) in that it reduces the fast inward current carried by sodium ions. Moricizine shortens Phase 2 and 3 repolarization, resulting in a decreased action potential duration and effective refractory period. A dose-related decrease in the maximum rate of Phase 0 depolarization (V_{max}) occurs without effect on maximum diastolic potential or action potential amplitude. The sinus node and atrial tissue are not affected. Following oral administration, moricizine undergoes significant first-pass metabolism resulting in an absolute bioavailability of ~38%. Moricizine undergoes extensive biotransformation: <1% is excreted unchanged in the urine. There are at least 26 metabolites (see also Figure 76).

Cimetidine increases the plasma level of moricizine, and digoxin and moricizine cause an additive prolongation of the PR interval. Moricizine increases the clearance of theophylline. The most serious adverse reaction of moricizine is its tendency to cause arrhythmias. Palpitation, sustained ventricular tachycardia, cardiac chest pain, congestive heart failure, myocardial infarction, hypotension, hypertension, syncope, supraventricular arrhythmias (including atrial fibrillations/flutter), cardiac arrest, bradycardia, pulmonary embolism, vasodilation, cerebrovascular events, and thrombophlebitis have occurred. CNS problems such as dizziness, headache, fatigue, hypesthesias, asthenia, nervousness, parasthesias, sleep

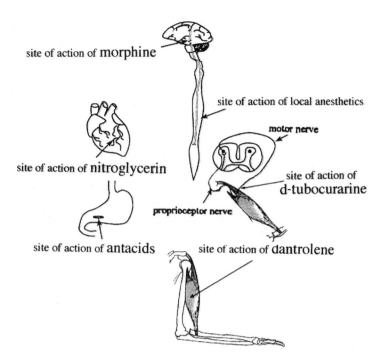

site of action of morphine

site of action of local anesthetics

motor nerve

site of action of nitroglycerin

site of action of
d-tubocurarine

proprioceptor nerve

site of action of antacids   site of action of dantrolene

FIGURE 58   Morphine exerts its analgesic effects by **elevating the pain threshold** and especially by altering the patient's reactions to pain. Morphine induces analgesia by activating the **opioid, adrenergic,** and **serotonergic systems**. (Adapted from Ebadi, M., *Pharmacology, An Illustrated Review with Questions and Answers*, 3rd Edition, Lippincott-Raven Press, Philadelphia, 1996.)

disorders, tremor, anxiety, depression, euphoria, confusion, somnolence, agitation, seizure, coma, abnormal gait, hallucinations, nystagmus, diplopia, speech disorder, akathisia, memory loss, ataxia, abnormal coordination, dyskinesia, vertigo, and tinnitus have been reported. Urinary retention or frequency, dysuria, urinary incontinence, kidney pain, impotence, and decreased libido take place. Abdominal pain, dyspepsia, vomiting, diarrhea, anorexia, bitter taste, dysphagia, flatulence, and ileus are other side effects of moricizine.

MORPHINE SULPHATE

The **opium alkaloids**, which are obtained from *Papaver somniferum*, contain two groups of compounds: those with **phenanthrene derivatives**, consisting of morphine (1 to 10%), codeine (0.7 to 2.5%), and thebaine (0.5 to 1.5%), and those with **isoquinolone derivatives**, consisting of papaverine (1%) and noscapine (5 to 10%). Morphine depresses the cerebral cortex, hypothalamus, and medullary centers. These effects are responsible for suppressing pain perception, including narcosis, depressing the cough center, depressing the vomiting center, and depressing respiration. In horses, morphine stimulates the spinal cord in a predictable fashion. This effect is short-lived in humans and is seldom seen when given in therapeutic doses. Initially, morphine stimulates the vomiting center, and emesis occurs early in cases of intoxication. Depression of the vomiting center then ensues late in intoxication. Morphine stimulates the vagus nerve, causing bradycardia, and stimulates the nucleus of the third cranial nerve (oculomotor), causing miosis.

The relief of pain brought about by morphine is selective, and other sensory modalities such as touch, vibration, vision, hearing, and the like are not obtunded. Morphine does not reduce the responsiveness of nerve endings to noxious stimuli, nor does it impair the conduction of nerve impulses along the peripheral nerves, as seen following the administration of local anesthetics.

Morphine exerts its analgesic effects by elevating the pain threshold and especially by altering the patient's reactions to pain. Morphine induces analgesia by activating the **opioid, adrenergic,** and (see Figure 58) **serotoninergic systems.** Analgesia results from the activation of those systems within the dorsal horn of the spinal cord that depress the transmission of pain sensation to the brain. This is accomplished by decreasing the release of pain transmitters such as substance P or by hyperpolarizing the interneurons within the dorsal horn, or both. Morphine activates these mechanisms by interacting with the mu receptors located on neurons in the dorsal cord. There is considerable evidence suggesting that this action depends on the activation of the adrenergic system within the dorsal horn. This in turn suggests that morphine analgesia could be potentiated by the addition of drugs such as **clonidine** that activate the adrenergic system. In addition, morphine appears to **activate the endogenous supraspinal system** that is normally activated by pain to protect the body from excessive nonessential pain stimulation. It appears that the translocation of calcium is the essential factor and that the basic mechanism of morphine results from alterations in the intracellular calcium concentration. This activity results from the interaction of morphine with mu receptors that, in turn, affect the G protein level, which then activates secondary transmitter systems. Certain antihistaminic substances have analgesic properties.

Morphine also alters a patient's **reaction to pain**. Patients report that the sensation of pain often exists, but, under the influence of morphine, they feel more at ease and comfortable. This **euphoria** is present in 90 to 95% of patients. Morphine may cause **dysphoria** in the remaining 5 to 10%. In a relatively small dose of 5 to 10 mg, morphine relieves the constant but dull pain originating from the viscera, such as that of coronary, pulmonary, and biliary origin. In somewhat larger doses (10 to 20 mg), morphine relieves the sharp, lancinating, and intermittent pain resulting from bone fractures and other physical injuries. Inoperable and terminal causes of neoplastic diseases usually require the administration of morphine or other narcotics in increasing doses that eventually lead to both tolerance and addiction. In the management of **myocardial infarction**, morphine, meperidine, pentazocine, methadone, and heroin have all been used as analgesics. In addition, **streptokinase** (a thrombolytic agent), **atenolol** or **metoprolol** (beta-adrenergic receptor blocking agents), and **nitroglycerin** (a vasodilator) have been advocated.

Chronic idiopathic pain syndrome is a common, disabling, and costly condition. It is believed to be of psychological origin, but may involve both cerebral and peripheral physiologic mechanisms. Because it is often associated with depression, psychotropic drugs, notably the tricyclic **antidepressants**, may be required.

The spinal administration of morphine, with or without a local anesthetic, has been advocated for producing a sustained period of postoperative analgesia. However, adverse side effects from such analgesia include ventilatory depression, itching, and urinary retention. Morphine depresses all phases of respiration (respiratory rate, tidal volume, and minute volume) when given in subhypnotic and subanalgesic doses. In humans, a morphine overdose causes respiratory arrest and death. Therefore, morphine and other narcotic analgesics should be used with extreme caution in patients with asthma, emphysema, or cor pulmonale, and in disorders that may involve hypoxia, such as chest wound, pneumothorax, or bulbar poliomyelitis.

Morphine releases **histamine** and may cause peripheral vasodilation and orthostatic hypotension. The cutaneous blood vessels dilate around the "blush areas" such as the face, neck, and upper thorax. Morphine causes cerebral vasodilation (due to increased carbon dioxide retention secondary to respiratory depression), and hence it increases the cerebrospinal fluid pressure. Therefore, morphine should be used cautiously in patients with either meningitis or recent head injury. When given subcutaneously, morphine is absorbed poorly whenever there is either traumatic or hemorrhagic shock.

Very large doses of morphine can be used to produce anesthesia; however, the consequentially decreased peripheral resistance and blood pressure are troublesome. **Fentanyl** and **sufentanil,** which are potent and selective mu agonists, are less likely to cause hemodynamic instability during surgery, in part because they do not trigger the release of histamine.

Morphine reduces the activity of the entire gastrointestinal tract in that it reduces the secretion of hydrochloric acid, diminishes the motility of the stomach, and increases the tone of the upper part of the duodenum. These actions may delay passage of the stomach contents into the duodenum. Both pancreatic and biliary secretions are diminished, and this may also hinder digestion. In the large intestine, the propulsive peristaltic wave in the colon is reduced, the muscle tone including that of the anal sphincter is increased, and the gastrocolic reflex (defecation reflex) is reduced. These actions, in combination, cause constipation, which seems to be a chronic problem among addicts.

Opiate preparations, usually given as **paregorics**, are effective and fast-acting antidiarrheal agents. These agents are also useful postoperatively to produce solid stool following an ileostomy or colostomy. A meperidine derivative, **diphenoxylate**, is usually dispensed with **atropine** and sold as Lomotil. The atropine is added to discourage the abuse of diphenoxylate by narcotic addicts who are tolerant to massive doses of narcotic but not to the CNS stimulant effects of atropine.

Morphine causes oliguria and this results from (1) pronounced diaphoresis; (2) the relative hypotension and decreased glomerular filtration rate; and (3) the release of antidiuretic hormone from the neurohypophysis. In an elderly patient with prostatic hypertrophy, morphine may cause acute urinary retention. Morphine may reduce the effectiveness of a diuretic when both drugs are used in combination in the treatment of congestive heart failure.

Tolerance develops to the narcotic and analgesic actions of morphine, so that increasingly larger doses are needed to render patients pain free. Tolerance develops to many of morphine's effects such as analgesia, euphoria, narcosis, respiratory depression, hypotension, and antidiuresis. Morphine-induced bradycardia may be experienced. However, no tolerance develops to morphine-induced miosis or constipation. If the administration of morphine is discontinued, the tolerance is lost and the preaddiction analgesic doses of morphine become effective once more.

In subjects who are addicted to morphine, the initial symptoms of the abstinence or withdrawal syndrome usually appear 6 to 12 hours after the last dose and consist of CNS irritability and feeling of fatigue, autonomic hyperactivity such as tachycardia and hypertension, gastrointestinal hyperactivity such as diarrhea, and autonomic supersensitivity such as insomnia and restlessness.

MUZOLIMINE
(Not available in the United States)

Ethacrynic acid, bumetanide, furosemide, and muzolimine are loop diuretics. The most often used and the major loop diuretics are furosemide (Lasix) and ethacrynic acid (Edecrin). **Furosemide** is chemically related to the thiazide diuretics, but **ethacrynic acid** is not. These agents inhibit the active resorption of chloride (and sodium) in the thick, ascending medullary portion of the loop of Henle and also in the cortical portion of the loop or the distal tubule. The diuresis they produce, which is similar to that seen with the thiazides, predominantly causes a loss of chloride, sodium, and potassium, but HCO_3 excretion is not increased. Although large volumes of fluid can be excreted with the use of these agents, the ability of the kidney to produce either a dilute or concentrated urine is greatly diminished. These agents are the most efficacious of all the diuretics now on the market, usually producing about a 20% loss in the filtered load of sodium (furosemide, 15 to 30%; ethacrynic acid, 17 to 23%).

Loop diuretics are ordinarily taken orally but can be given intravenously if a very rapid onset of action is sought, as when used in combination with antihypertensive medications in the management of a **hypertensive crisis**. Furosemide and ethacrynic acid undergo some active renal tubular secretion as well as glomerular filtration. A minor portion is excreted by the liver.

Loop diuretics are used for treating the following conditions:

In the **edema** of cardiac, hepatic, or renal origin, including acute pulmonary edema and hypertensive crisis

In **acute renal failure**, to maintain urine flow, though an excessive loss of extracellular fluid volume can cause a decrease in the GFR

In **hypercalcemia**.

Excessive volume depletion, hyponatremia, and hypotension are major risks associated with the use of loop diuretics, and the side effects of **hypokalemia, hyperuricemia**, and **hyperglycemia** are always present. Loop diuretics should not be used concurrently with **ototoxic aminoglycoside antibiotics** (i.e., streptomycin, gentamicin, kanamycin, tobramycin) (see also Table 25).

MULTIMERIN

Multimerin is a large adhesive protein synthesized by megakaryocytes and stored within platelet alpha-granules. This novel protein was first discovered in platelets, using a monoclonal antibody raised against human platelets. Multimerin is extremely large and is comprised of variably sized, disulfide-linked multimers. The building blocks of the multimers are the p-155 and p-170 subunits. These subunits are derived by proteolysis of a common precursor protein.

Multimerin shares many similarities with von Willebrand factor, but, unlike von Willebrand factor, it is not found in plasma. Within alpha-granules, multimerin is found in an eccentric location, colocalizing with von Willebrand factor. Platelet activation leads to multimerin release with expression of this protein on the activated platelet surface. Increased platelet surface expression of multimerin is a mark of platelet activation, both *in vitro* and *in vivo*. The function of multimerin remains to be discovered.

MULTIPLE SCLEROSIS: TREATMENT OF
Multiple sclerosis (MS) is an inflammatory, demyelinating disease of the white matter of the central nervous system that commonly affects young adults. Two thirds of patients have onset between the ages of 20 and 40 years; the peak period for onset is 25 to 30 years of age.
The disease is characterized by episodes of neurologic symptoms occurring over a period of days to weeks, followed by complete or incomplete remissions of various durations. Early signs and symptoms of MS commonly include fatigue, gait and limb ataxia, spasticity, dizziness, double vision, acute optic neuritis, and numbness and weakness in one or more limbs.
The classical lesions in MS, the plaques, are microscopically characterized by circumscribed demyelination in the presence of intact axons. Macrophages are the main cells involved in myelin destruction; attachment of superficial myelin lamellae to the macrophage surface, immunoglobulin deposition between macrophages and myelin lamellae, and production of complement and proteolytic enzymes all contribute to this process. Furthermore, T lymphocytes, both the CD4 (helper) and CD8 (suppressor) phenotypes, are present in the perivascular lesions.
The initial successes in MS therapy involved the use of **corticosteroid** treatments to induce short-term improvements in neurological function, and symptomatic therapies for some of the complications of MS. More recently, with improved understanding of the immunological events occurring during progression of the disease, therapies that modify the natural history of the disease have become available. **Interferon beta-1b** (Betaseron) is the first new treatment for MS to be licensed by the United States Food and Drug Administration (FDA) in the last 30 years (see Figure 99).

Global immunosuppression with **azathioprine** and **cyclophosphamide** has been utilized with varying benefit for several decades. In addition, there have been recent reports of beneficial effects of immunosuppressive agents such as **methotrexate** and **cladribine** in patients with chronic progressive MS.

Several lines of evidence point to the involvement of immune mechanisms in MS. This suggests that immunotherapy may hold an answer for these patients. The goals of immunotherapy at present are to improve recovery from exacerbations, decrease the number and severity of relapses, and limit progression of the disease. Nonspecific immunosuppressive agents like corticotropin and corticosteroids are beneficial for acute exacerbations, but disease progression still occurs. Attempts to slow progression with azathioprine, cyclophosphamide, intravenous immune globulin, and cyclosporin have been only modestly successful and can cause serious adverse effects. Interferon-β_{1b} can reduce the number and severity of relapses in patients with relapsing-remitting MS; copolymer 1 and cladribine may hold promise as well. Better understanding of the immunologic basis of MS may lead to more specific immunotherapies with more lasting benefits.

MUMPS SKIN TEST ANTIGEN
(MSTA)

Mumps antigen is used to assess cell-mediated immunity.

MUMPS VIRUS VACCINE, LIVE
(Mumpsvax)

Mumps vaccine is used for immunization.

MUPIROCIN
(Pseudomonic Acid A) (Bactroban)

Mupirocin (2% ointment) is used as a topical treatment of impetigo due to *Staphylococcus aureus*, beta-hemolytic *Streptococcus*, and *Streptococcus pyrogenes*.

MUROMONAB-CD3
(Orthoclone OKT3)

Muromonab-CD3, a monoclonal antibody, is used in the treatment of acute allograft rejection in renal transplant patients.

MYASTHENIA GRAVIS: TREATMENT OF

Myasthenia gravis is a neurological disease of autoimmune origin. The basic defect is the reduction of nicotinic acetylcholine receptors (AChR) at the neuromuscular junction, resulting in inadequate transmission through the neuromuscular junction and hence the clinical syndrome of weakness, frequently worsened by exercise or effort.

There are two basic strategies in treating myasthenia gravis. One is to treat symptomatically by increasing the available amount of acetylcholine (ACh) at the neuromuscular junction with a cholinesterase inhibitor compound that inhibits the enzyme acetylcholinesterase, responsible for the breakdown of acetylcholine. This in turn raises the amount of ACh at the neuromuscular junction to stimulate whatever AChR are available. Other strategies include increasing ACh release or its effect.

Immunomodulation is the other important way to treat patients with myasthenia gravis. **Corticosteroid drugs** are the most widely used and some of the most effective agents currently available to treat myasthenic patients. **Azathioprine** is a prodrug that is converted into **mercaptopurine**, a purine analog that in turn is incorporated into nucleotides. These abnormal nucleotides affect synthesis of RNA and DNA, and thus preferentially affect the more actively multiplying cells. Azathioprine can be used in the treatment of generalized myasthenia gravis that is not responding to conventional therapy with cholinesterase inhibitors, thymectomy, and steroid drugs or when the response is limited by side effects of these agents. **Cyclosporin A** and **cyclophosphamide** are used in cases of malignant thymoma with or without myasthenia gravis.

MYCOSES: TREATMENT OF DEEP-SEATED ORGANISMS	
Aspergillosis, invasive	
Immunosuppressed	Amphotericin B
Nonimmunosuppressed	Amphotericin B, itraconazole
Blastomycosis	
Rapidly progressive or CNS	Amphotericin B
Indolent, non-CNS	Itraconazole, ketoconazole
Coccidioidomycosis	
Rapidly progressing	Amphotericin B
Indolent	Itraconazole, ketoconazole, fluconazole
Meningeal	Fluconazole, intrathecal amphotericin B
Cryptococcosis	
Non-AIDS and initial AIDS	Amphotericin B ± flucytosine
Maintenance, AIDS	Fluconazole
Histoplasmosis	
Chronic pulmonary	Itraconazole
Disseminated	
Rapidly progressing or CNS	Amphotericin B
Indolent, non-CNS	Itraconazole
Maintenance, AIDS	Itraconazole
Mucormycosis	Amphotericin B
Pseudallescheriasis	Itraconazole, IV miconazole
Sporotrichosis	
Cutaneous	Iodide, itraconazole
Extracutaneous	Amphotericin B

MYOCLONUS: TREATMENT OF

Myoclonic jerks are sudden, rapid, twitch-like muscle contractions. They can be classified according to their distribution, relationship to precipitating stimuli, or etiology. Generalized myoclonus has a widespread distribution, while focal or segmental myoclonus is restricted to a particular part of the body. Myoclonus can be spontaneous, or it can be brought on by sensory stimulation, arousal, or the initiation of movement (action myoclonus). Myoclonus may occur as a normal phenomenon (physiologic myoclonus) in healthy persons, as an isolated abnormality (essential myoclonus), or as a manifestation of epilepsy (epileptic myoclonus). It can also occur as a feature of a variety of degenerative, infections, and metabolic disorders (symptomatic myoclonus).

Treatments of first choice for cortical myoclonus are **valproic acid** (sodium valproate) and **clonazepam**. **Primidone** and **phenobarbital** may also be useful. **Piracetam** has advantages in these circumstances, as its addition to existing treatments is rarely accompanied by sedation.

In patients with brain stem reticular reflex myoclonus, valproic acid and clonazepam are the most useful agents. In hyperreflexia, treatment is directed against the disabling tonic spasms, rather than jerks. Carbamazepine, phenytoin and clonazepam are useful agents in this respect. Ballistic overflow myoclonus may improve with anticholinergic drugs, such as benztropine or trihexyphenidyl.

Treatment of palatal myoclonus is often unsuccessful, but phenytoin, carbamazepine, clonazepam, trihexyphenidyl, and baclofen have been effective in some patients. Clonazepam is effective in over half of patients with propriospinal myoclonus, but other anticonvulsants are usually not helpful. Segmental spinal myoclonus is often resistant to drug treatment, but diazepam, carbamazepine, tetrabenazine and, particularly, clonazepam are sometimes effective.

N

NABUMETONE
(Relafen)

Nabumetone (1000 mg as a single dose) is indicated for the acute and chronic treatment of osteoarthritis and rheumatoid arthritis. Nabumetone, which has analgesic, antipyretic, and antiinflammatory properties, exerts its effects in part by inhibiting the synthesis of prostaglandin. Nabumetone is absorbed from the GI tract, metabolized to an active metabolite, 6-methoxy 2-naphthylacetic acid, and excreted in the urine. Nabumetone and its metabolite, which are extensively bound to plasma proteins, are able to alter the binding of other drugs such as warfarin possessing the inherent potential to cause toxicity (see also Table 2).

Nabumetone and other antiinflammatory agents impair the synthesis of renal prostaglandin, decreasing reversibly the blood flow, which may become detrimental in individuals with renal impairment. Therefore, individuals with cardiovascular problems taking diuretics and nabumetone should be monitored carefully. The adverse reactions to nabumetone that have been reported, especially in higher than therapeutic doses, include CNS dizziness, headache, fatigue, increased sweating, nervousness, somnolence, pruritis, rash, diarrhea, dyspepsia, abdominal pain, gastric pain, flatulence, and mild gastric bleeding.

NADOLOL
(Corgard)

Nadolol is a nonselective beta-adrenergic receptor blocking agent that possesses no intrinsic sympathomimetic activity. It is indicated in angina pectoris (120 mg/day) and in combination with other antihypertensive medications in the management of hypertension (80 to 600 mg/day) (see also Figure 60).

Nadolol is absorbed modestly (30%) after oral administration, becomes bound to plasma protein to the extent of 20%, and is excreted mostly unchanged (70%) in the urine and feces.

The major hemodynamic effect of nadolol is a decrease in sinus node frequency causing a reduction in the heart rate and cardiac output, and the said effects are more pronounced during exercise. Nadolol decreases sinoatrial impulse formation but does not impair atrial conduction or that of accessory pathways. Similar to propranolol, nadolol causes a mild increase in plasma volume.

Unlike the beta$_1$ selective blockers, nadolol prevents the epinephrine-induced decrease in serum potassium level, an effect that is mediated by beta$_2$-adrenergic stimulation. Like all other beta-adrenergic receptor blockers, nadolol antagonizes the thyroxine-mediated stimulation of beta-adrenergic receptors. Unlike most beta-adrenergic receptor blocking agents, nadolol preserves renal blood flow.

Because of its low lipid solubility, nadolol does not cross the blood-brain barrier, and hence is devoid of any CNS effects seen following administration of propranolol.

Nadolol is contraindicated in severe bradyarrhythmias or bronchospasm. It should be used cautiously in overt congestive heart failure, severe peripheral vascular disorder with claudication, and severe diabetes mellitus. Since nadolol is largely excreted by the kidneys, decreased renal function affects the clearance of the drug. Nadolol concentrates fivefold in human breast milk and that should be taken into consideration in prescribing the drug for a mother nursing an infant.

NAFARELIN ACETATE
(Synarel)

Nafarelin, a synthetic decapeptide and a gonadotropin-releasing hormone (GnRH) analog (200 mcg spray into one nostril in a.m. and in p.m.), is used in the management of endometriosis, pain relief, and reduction of endometriotic lesions (see also Table 14).

NAFCILLIN SODIUM
(Nafcil)

Nafcillin (IV 3 to 6 g/24 hours in severe infections) is indicated for the treatment of infections due to penicillinase-producing staphylococci. It may be used to initiate therapy when a staphylococcal infection is suspected (see also Table 22). Like penicillins, nafcillin, inhibits the formation of cell walls and hence is bactericidal in nature. Penicillin binds to cellular receptors, now identified as **transpeptidation enzymes**, and, by binding to and inhibiting the transpeptidation reactions, the synthesis of cell wall **peptidoglycan** is interrupted. In addition, penicillin removes or inactivates an inhibitor of the lytic enzymes (**autolysin**), resulting in the lysis of microorganisms in an isotonic environment. In general, penicillins are more active against **Gram-positive organisms**.

Nafcillin resists the effects of penicillinases — enzymes that inactivate penicillin — and is thus active against many strains of penicillinase-producing bacteria. This activity is most important against penicillinase-producing staphylococci; some strains may remain resistant. Nafcillin is also active against a few Gram-positive aerobic and anaerobic bacilli but has no significant effect on Gram-negative bacilli (see also Table 22).

Nafcillin is absorbed erratically from the GI tract and distributes poorly into cerebrospinal fluid, but this passage is enhanced by meningeal inflammation. Nafcillin, which is bound to plasma protein to the extent of 90%, crosses the placenta and is found in milk.

Nafcillin and aminoglycosides are chemically inactivated and should not be mixed together. Probenecid blocks renal tubular secretion of penicillins; however, this interaction has only a small effect on the excretion of nafcillin.

Nafcillin should be given with water only, since acid in fruit juices or carbonated water may inactivate it. Furthermore, it should be given on an empty stomach since food decreases its absorption. Clinical signs of overdose include neuromuscular irritability or seizures (see Table 22).

NAFTIFINE HYDROCHLORIDE
(Naftin)

Naftifine (1% cream once a day) is indicated for topical treatment of tinea pedis (athlete's foot), tinea cruris (jock itch), and tinea corporis (ringworm) caused by the organisms *T. rubrum, T. mentagrophytes, T. tonsurans,* and *E. floccosum.*

Naftifine, a broad-spectrum antifungal agent, is a synthetic allylamine derivative that interferes with sterol biosynthesis by inhibiting the enzyme squalene 2,3-epoxidase. This inhibition of enzyme activity results in decreased amounts of sterols, especially ergosterol, and a corresponding accumulation of squalene in the cells.

Naftifine penetrates the stratum corneum to inhibit the growth of dermatophytes. Following a single application of 1% naftifine to the skin, systemic absorption was 5%. Naftifine or its metabolites are excreted via the urine and feces with a half-life of approximately 2 to 3 days.

NALBUPHINE HYDROCHLORIDE

(Nubain)

Nalbuphine, a narcotic agonist-antagonist (10 mg in adult administered SC, IM, or IV every 3 to 6 hours) is indicated for the relief of moderate to severe pain, for preoperative analgesia, as a supplement to balanced analgesia and to surgical anesthesia, and for obstetrical analgesia during labor and delivery.

Nalbuphine is structurally related to both naloxone and oxymorphone. It is an agonist-antagonist opioid possessing a spectrum of effects that resemble those of **pentazocine**; however, nalbuphine is a more potent antagonist at mu receptors and is less likely to produce dysphoria than is pentazocine.

Its analgesic potency is essentially equivalent to that of morphine and about three times that of pentazocine on a milligram basis. Unlike the other agonist-antagonists, nalbuphine does not significantly increase pulmonary artery pressure, systemic vascular resistance, or cardiac work.

Nalbuphine's abuse potential is less than for codeine and propoxyphene. The most common effects of nalbuphine are sleepiness and mild dysphoria. Barbiturate anesthetics increase the respiratory and CNS depressant effects of nalbuphine.

NALIDIXIC ACID

(NegGram)

The quinolones include: **nalidixic acid, cinoxacin** (Cinobac), **norfloxacin** (Noroxin), and **ciprofloxacin** (Cipro). Other members of the quinolone family are **pefloxacin, ofloxacin, enoxacin,** and **fleroxacin** (see also Figure 77).

The bacterial enzyme **DNA gyrase** is responsible for the continuous introduction of negative supercoils into DNA, and the quinolones inhibit this gyrase-mediated DNA supercoiling.

Nalidixic acid and **cinoxacin** are bactericidal against Gram-negative organisms that cause urinary tract infections. The **fluoroquinolones** are bactericidal and considerably more potent against *Escherichia coli* and various species of *Salmonella, Shigella, Enterobacter, Campylobacter,* and *Neisseria*. **Ciprofloxacin** also has good activity against staphylococci, including methicillin-resistant strains.

The quinolones and fluoroquinolones may produce arthropathy, and hence should not be used in prepubertal children or pregnant women.

Nalidixic acid and **cinoxacin** are useful only for treating urinary tract infections. **Ciprofloxacin** is useful for both urinary tract infections and prostatitis.

NALORPHINE

(Nalline)

Nalorphine, a narcotic antagonist, differs from morphine in having an allyl (CH_2–CH=CH_2) group instead of a CH_2 group attached to the N atom. It and levallorphan, which is the corresponding allyl homolog of levorphanol, are effective antagonists against a wide variety of potent analgesics related pharmacologically to morphine. They antagonize many times their molecular equivalent of such narcotics as methadone, isomethadone, heptazone, codeine, dihydromorphinone, metopon, methomorphinan, and meperidine. This antagonism is so complete that administration of nalorphine during addiction leads to an acute abstinence syndrome.

Nalorphine in doses of 5 mg produces side effects that are comparable to those produced by 10 mg of morphine, unaccompanied by any significant analgesic effect. In higher doses, however, particularly in postoperative pain, it exerts analgesic action comparable to that of morphine without the addictive properties of the latter. However, it induces disturbing mental effects and other unpleasant side effects that preclude its use as an analgesic.

NALOXONE HYDROCHLORIDE
(Narcan)

Naloxone a pure narcotic antagonist, (0.4 to 2.0 mg IV) is indicated for the complete or partial reversal of respiratory and CNS depression caused by naturally occurring and synthetic narcotics, including morphine, meperidine, methadone, nalbuphine, butorphanol, and pentazocine.

Naloxone differs from other narcotic analgesics in several respects. Naloxone does not cause respiratory depression, pupillary constriction, sedation, or analgesia. However, it does antagonize the actions of pentazocine. Naloxone neither antagonizes the respiratory-depressant effects of barbiturates and other hypnotics nor aggravates their depressant effects on respiration. Similar to nalorphine and **naltrexone**, naloxone precipitates an abstinence syndrome when administered to patients addicted to opiate-like drugs.

Naloxone is also therefore indicated for the diagnosis of acute opiate overdosage. Since naloxone antagonizes the effects of beta-endorphin, it has been used to improve circulation in refractory shock, allowing prostaglandins and catecholamine to re-establish the control of circulation.

Intravenously administered naloxone is distributed widely, exerts its effects within two minutes, is metabolized in the liver by conjugation with glucuronic acid, and has a short duration of action of 1 to 4 hours depending on the dosage given. Abrupt reversal of narcotic depression may result in nausea, vomiting, sweating, tachycardia, increased blood pressure, and tremulousness.

NALTREXONE HYDROCHLORIDE
(Trexan)

Naltrexone (25 mg initially), a pure narcotic antagonist, is indicated for the treatment of the opioid-free state in formerly opioid dependent individuals who have undergone a methadone detoxification program. Patients taking naltrexone may not benefit from opioid-containing medicines, such as cough and cold preparations, antidiarrheal preparations, and opioid analgesics.

Naltrexone, in a dose of 50 mg, will block the pharmacological effects of 25 mg heroin given intravenously for 24 hours, and the duration of blockade is dose-dependent. Naltrexone undergoes extensive first-pass metabolism, becoming converted to a 6-beta naltrexol, which is an active and pure narcotic receptor antagonist and is excreted by the kidneys. Naltrexone can cause a dose-related hepatic injury.

NANDROLONE DECANOATE

(Deca-Durabolin)

Nandrolone decanoate (women: 50 to 100 mg/week; men: 100 to 200 mg/week), is indicated for the management of anemia of renal insufficiency by increasing hemoglobin and red call mass. Nandrolone stimulates the kidney's production of erythropoietin, leading to increases in red blood cells. Testosterone replacement therapy increases bone mass in hypogonadal men. Androgens also improve bone mass in osteoporotic women, but therapy is limited by virilizing side effects. Nandrolone decanoate (50 mg by injection every three weeks) increases peripheral and axial bone mass without bothersome side effects in osteoporotic women (see also Figure 36).

Nandrolone phenpropionate has antineoplastic action by exerting inhibitory actions on hormone responsive breast tumors and metastases. Nandrolone decanoate is slowly released from the intramuscular depot following injection, and is hydrolyzed to free nandrolone by plasma esterase; peak serum levels of nandrolone are usually observed 8 to 24 hours following intramuscular injection of the decanoate. Nandrolone is subsequently metabolized in the liver; both unchanged nandrolone and its metabolites are excreted in the urine. The elimination half-life of nandrolone is 6 to 8 days after IM administration of nandrolone decanoate.

Androgens such as nandrolone are contraindicated in patients with severe renal or cardiac disease because fluid and electrolyte retention caused by this agent may aggravate these disorders; in patients with hepatic disease because impaired elimination of the drug may cause toxic accumulation; in male patients with prostatic or breast cancer or benign prostatic hypertrophy with obstruction and in patients with undiagnosed abnormal genital bleeding because this drug can stimulate the growth of cancerous breast or prostate tissue in males; and in pregnant or breast-feeding women because animal studies have shown that administration of anabolic steroids during pregnancy causes masculinization of the female fetus. The drug also is contraindicated in females with carcinoma of the breast and with hypercalcemia.

NAPHAZOLINE HYDROCHLORIDE

(Ak-Con, Albalon, Liquifilm, Allerest, Allergy Drops, Clear Eyes, Comfort eye Drops, Degest 2, 1-Naphline, Forte, Muro's Opcon, Naphcon A, Naphcon, Privine Hydrochloride, VasoClear, Vasocon)

Naphazoline, a sympathomimetic agent with decongestant properties, is used in nasal congestion and in ocular congestion, irritation, and itching.

NARCOLEPSY: TREATMENT OF

Narcolepsy is characterized by excessive daytime sleepiness that is typically associated with cataplexy and other rapid eye movement (REM) sleep phenomena such as sleep paralysis and hypnagogic hallucinations. Sleepiness, the main symptom in narcolepsy, leads to repeated daily episodes of naps or lapses into sleep of short duration.

The other main symptom, cataplexy, is characterized by a sudden loss of bilateral muscle tone provoked by strong emotion, typically by laughter. Cataplexy is usually of short duration, ranging from a few seconds to several minutes, and recovery is fast and complete.

The majority of patients need medication for the two main symptoms. Drugs with central nervous system stimulating effects, mostly of the amphetamine-type, are used to alleviate excessive sleepiness and sleep attacks. The resulting increased level of vigilance also decreases or abolishes cataplexy in a number of patients. If this is not achieved, tricyclic antidepressants, in the first instance, and selective serotonin (5-hydroxytryptamine; 5-HT) reuptake inhibitors, in the second instance, can be used to control cataplexy and other rapid eye movement sleep-related symptoms.

Stimulatory drugs used in the treatment of narcolepsy are:	Anticataplectic drugs used in the treatment of narcolepsy are:
Dexamphetamine	Clomipramine
Mazindol	Femoxetine
Methamphetamine	Fluoxetine
Methylphenidate	Imipramine
Modafinil	Protriptyline
Pemoline	
Selegiline	

NAPROXEN SODIUM

(Aleve)

Naproxen (200 mg every 8 to 12 hours with a full glass of liquid) is indicated for the relief of mild to moderate pain, treatment of primary dysmenorrhea, rheumatoid arthritis, osteoarthritis, ankylosing spondylitis, tendinitis, bursitis, and acute gout. Naproxen (Naprosyn) is used in juvenile arthritis. Naproxen, a nonsteroidal antiinflammatory agent, has analgesic and antipyretic actions. It should be used cautiously in patients with a history of angioedema or of GI disease, peptic ulcer, or renal or cardiovascular disease, because the drug may worsen these conditions (see also Table 2).

Concomitant use of naproxen with anticoagulants and thrombolytic drugs (coumarin derivatives, heparin, streptokinase, or urokinase) may potentiate anticoagulant effects. Bleeding problems may occur if used with other drugs that inhibit platelet aggregation such as azlocillin, parenteral carbenicillin, dextran, dipyridamole, mezlocillin, piperacillin, sulfinpyrazone, ticarcillin, valproic acid, cefamandole, cefoperazone, moxalactum, plicamycin, aspirin, or other antiinflammatory agents. Alcohol, corticotropin, or steroids may cause increased GI adverse reactions, including ulceration and hemorrhage. Aspirin may decrease the bioavailability of naproxen.

Because of the influence of prostaglandins on glucose metabolism, concomitant use with insulin or oral hypoglycemic agents may potentiate hypoglycemic effects. Naproxen may displace highly protein-bound drugs from binding sites. Toxicity may occur with coumarin derivatives, phenytoin, verapamil, or nifedipine. Increased nephrotoxicity may occur with gold compounds, other antiinflammatory agents, or acetaminophen. Naproxen may decrease the renal clearance of methotrexate and lithium. Naproxen may decrease the clinical effectiveness of antihypertensive agents and diuretics. Concomitant use may increase risk of nephrotoxicity.

NATAMYCIN

(Natacyn)

Natamycin, a polyene macrolide antibiotic (instill 1 drop of 5% solution in conjunctival sac), is used in conjunctivitis, keratitis, and blepharitis caused by susceptible fungi.

NEDOCROMIL SODIUM

(Tilade)

Nedocromil, a well-tolerated drug (2 inhalations 4 times a day at regular intervals to provide 14 mg/day), is indicated for maintenance therapy in the management of patients with mild to moderate bronchial asthma. Nedocromil has no intrinsic bronchodilating, glucocorticoid, or antihistaminic properties. Therefore, it should not be used in status asthmaticus (see also Figures 29 and 86).

It inhibits the *in vitro* activation of, and mediator release from, a variety of inflammatory cell types associated with asthma, including eosinophils, neutrophils, macrophages, mast cells, monocytes and platelets. *In vitro*, nedocromil inhibits the release of mediators including histamine, leukotriene C_4 and prostaglandin D_2. Similar studies with human bronchoalveolar cells showed inhibition of histamine release from mast cells and beta-glucuronidase release from macrophages.

Nedocromil inhibits the development of early and late bronchoconstriction responses to inhaled antigen. The development of airway hyperresponsiveness to nonspecific bronchoconstrictors was also inhibited in airway microvasculature leakage.

Nedocromil is bound to plasma proteins to the extent of 89%, is not metabolized, and is excreted unchanged.

NEOMYCIN SULFATE
(Mycifradin)

Neomycin is indicated for the suppression of intestinal bacteria of the bowel as a preoperative prophylaxis for elective colorectal surgery. The treatment begins three days prior to surgery with liquid diets with minimum residue, oral capsule of bisacodyl, magnesium sulfate, enema, and repeated oral administration of neomycin and erythromycin (1 gram of each). Neomycin has been used as an adjunctive therapy in hepatic coma by reduction in the ammonia-forming bacteria in the intestinal tract. The subsequent reduction in blood ammonia has resulted in neurologic improvement. Neomycin combined with niacin reduces the cholesterol level.

NEOSTIGMINE
(Prostigmin)

Neostigmine, a cholinesterase inhibitor which is unable to penetrate the blood-brain barrier, does not cause CNS toxicity. However, it may produce a dose-dependent and full range of muscarinic effects, characterized by miosis, blurring of vision, lacrimation, salivation, sweating, increased bronchial secretion, bronchoconstriction, bradycardia, hypotension, and urinary incontinence. Atropine can oppose these muscarinic effects. In addition, neostigmine, which has both a direct action and an indirect action that is mediated by acetylcholine on end-plate nicotinic receptors, may produce muscular fasciculation, muscular cramps, weakness, and even paralysis. These effects are not countered by atropine. Furthermore, neostigmine enhances gastric contraction and secretion. Neostigmine itself is metabolized by plasma acetylcholinesterase.

The therapeutic uses of neostigmine include the treatment of atony of the urinary bladder and postoperative abdominal distention. In addition, it antagonizes the action of d-tubocurarine and curariform drugs. Edrophonium, neostigmine, or pyridostigmine may be used to diagnose myasthenia gravis. Because edrophonium has the shortest duration of action, it is most often used for this purpose.

Neostigmine methylsulfate (2.5 mg) and atropine sulfate (1.2 mg) are given intravenously as an antidote to d-tubocurarine overdosage. The patient should be well ventilated and a patent airway maintained until complete recovery of normal respiration is assured. The optimum time to administer neostigmine methylsulfate is when the patient is being hyperventilated and the carbon dioxide level of the blood is low.

NETILMICIN SULFATE

(Netromycin)

Netilmicin, an aminoglycoside, is similar to gentamicin and tobramycin in its pharmacokinetic properties. It has broad antibacterial activity against aerobic Gram-negative bacilli and causes less ototoxicity and nephrotoxicity (see also Figure 80).

Netilmicin (1.3 to 2 mg/kg IM or IV q. 12 hours in serious systemic infections) is indicated for the short-term treatment of patients with serious or life-threatening bacterial infections caused by susceptible strains of the following organisms:

Complicated urinary tract infections caused by *Escherichia coli, Klebsiella pneumoniae, Pseudomonas aeruginosa, Enterobacter sp., Proteus mirabilis, Proteus sp., Serratia* and *Citrobacter sp.,* and *Staphylococcus aureus*

Septicemia caused by *E. coli, K. pneumoniae, P. aeruginosa, Enterobacter sp., Serratia sp.,* and *P. mirabilis*

Skin and skin structure infections caused by *E. coli, K. pneumoniae, P. aeruginosa, Enterobacter sp., Serratia sp., P. mirabilis, Proteus sp.,* and *S. aureus* (penicillinase- and nonpenicillinase-producing strains)

Intra-abdominal infections including peritonitis and intra-abdominal abscess caused by *E. coli, K. pneumoniae, P. aeruginosa, Enterobacter sp., P. mirabilis, Proteus sp.,* and *S. aureus* (penicillinase- and nonpenicillinase-producing strains)

Lower respiratory tract infections caused by *E. coli, K. pneumoniae, P. aeruginosa, Enterobacter sp., Serratia sp., P. mirabilis, Proteus sp.,* and *S. aureus* (penicillinase- and nonpenicillinase-producing strains)

NEUROLEPTICS

Neuroleptics (see Table 23) are also called **neuroplegics, psychoplegics, psycholeptics, antipsychotics**, and **major tranquilizers**. These agents are classified as follows:

Phenothiazine derivatives (e.g., chlorpromazine)
Thioxanthene derivatives (e.g., thiothixene)
Butyrophenone derivatives (e.g., haloperidol)
Dihydroindolone derivatives (e.g., molindone)
Dibenzoxazepine derivatives (e.g., loxapine)
Atypical neuroleptics (e.g., sulpiride, pimozide, and clozapine)

NEUROTRANSMITTERS AND THEIR RECEPTOR SUBTYPES			
Types	**Subtypes**	**Endogenous Transmitters**	**Ion Channel**
Acetylcholine	Nicotinic Muscarinic: M_1, M_2, M_3, M_4, M_5	Acetylcholine Acetylcholine	Yes
Adrenergic	α_1, α_2 β_1, β_2, β_3	Epinephrine and norepinephrine Epinephrine and norepinephrine	
GABA	A B	GABA GABA	Yes
Acidic amino acids	NMDA, kainate, quisqualate	Glutamate or aspartate	Yes
Opiate	μ, μ_1, κ, δ, ε	Enkephalins	
*Serotonin	$5\text{-}HT_1$, $5\text{-}HT_2$, $5HT_3$ (14 of them)	5-HT	
Dopamine	D_1, D_2, D_3, D_4, D_5	Dopamine	
Adenosine	A_1, A_2	Adenosine	

Types	Subtypes	Endogenous Transmitters	Ion Channel
Glycine	—	Glycine	Yes
Histamine	H_1, H_2, H_3	Histamine	
Insulin	—	Insulin	
Glucagon	—	Glucagon	
ACTH	—	ACTH	
Steroids	—	Several	
* See **Serotonin Receptor Subtypes**.			

NEWBORNS: UNDEVELOPED PHARMACOKINETIC PROFILE

The pharmacokinetic and pharmacodynamic parameters are affected by developmental alterations that require critical evaluation. A few examples are cited to illustrate this concept.

At birth, the gastric pH ranges between 6 and 8, but declines within hours after birth. The most important factor influencing gastric acid secretion is the initiation of enteral feedings. The gastric emptying time in newborns approaches adult values within the first 6 to 8 months of life.

The activities of all pancreatic enzymes are lower at birth, hence decreasing the bioavailability of drugs (e.g., ester formulation of clindamycin or chloramphenicol palmitate) requiring hydrolysis prior to absorption.

The volume of distribution of drugs in newborns is different from that of adults. The percentage of fat that makes up the total body weight is 0.5 percent in the young fetus, increases to 15 percent at birth and 20 percent by the age of 6 months, and then gradually declines until adolescence. The serum albumin and total protein concentrations are lower in infancy and increase to adult values by the age of 10 to 12 months. The concentration of bilirubin in neonates is much higher than the adult level, due to both increased red cell destruction and the limited capacity of the liver to conjugate bilirubin. Therefore, substantial differences exist in the binding of ampicillin, benzylpenicillin, phenobarbital, and phenytoin to plasma proteins of fetal, neonatal, and adult patients.

Postnatally, the hepatic P450 monooxygenase system matures rapidly, with metabolic capacities similar to those in adults achieved by approximately 5 months of age. On the other hand, alcohol dehydrogenase is detectable by 2 months of age (3-4% of adult activity) and approaches adult values after 5 years of age.

The hepatic metabolism of certain drugs has also been found to be different in neonates versus children and adults. The N-methylation of theophylline to caffeine occurs in preterm and full-term infants, whereas in adults theophylline is primarily N-demethylated and C-oxidated to monomethylxanthines and methyluric acid, respectively.

A glomerular filtration rate of 2 to 4 ml per minute in full-term infants increases to 8 to 20 ml per minute by 2 to 3 days of life and approaches adult values by 3 to 5 months of age. Tubular secretory function matures at a much slower rate.

NIACIN

(Vitamin B$_3$, Nicotinic Acid) (NIAC, NICO-400, Nicobid, Nicolar, Nicotinex, Span-Niacin)

Niacin, a B-complex vitamin, is used in the treatment of pellagra, peripheral vascular disease and circulatory disorders, and as an adjunctive treatment of hyperlipidemias, especially those associated with hypercholesterolemia.

NIACINAMIDE

(Nicotinamide)

Niacinamide, a B-complex vitamin (150 to 500 mg p.o. daily), is used in the treatment of pellagra.

NICARDIPINE HYDROCHLORIDE

(Cardene)

Verapamil, nifedipine, diltiazem, and **nicardipine** are used in the treatment of **arrhythmias, ischemic heart disease, hypertrophic cardiomyopathy,** and **hypertension**. The hemodynamic effects of these agents are shown in Table 20.

Nicardipine inhibits the transmembrane flux of calcium ions into cardiac and smooth muscle cells. The drug appears to act specifically on vascular muscle and may cause a smaller decrease in cardiac output than other calcium channel blockers because of its vasodilatory effect (see Figure 95).

Nicardipine is contraindicated in patients with advanced aortic stenosis because the decrease in afterload produced by the drug may worsen myocardial oxygen balance in these patients. Some patients experience worsened severity, frequency, or duration of angina upon initiation of therapy.

Nicardipine should be used cautiously in patients with hepatic dysfunction or with congestive heart failure, because the drug has a negative inotropic effect.

Concomitant administration of cimetidine results in higher plasma levels of nicardipine. Serum levels of dioxin should be carefully monitored because some calcium channel antagonists may increase plasma levels of digitalis preparations.

Concomitant administration of cyclosporine results in increased plasma levels of cyclosporine. Careful monitoring is recommended.

Severe hypotension has been reported in patients taking calcium channel blocking agents who undergo fentanyl anesthesia. Overdosage with nicardipine may produce hypotension, bradycardia, drowsiness, confusion, and slurred speech.

NICLOSAMIDE

(Yomesan)

Niclosamide, which is not absorbed from the gastrointestinal tract, is the safest effective drug in cestode infestations. It inhibits anaerobic metabolism and glucose uptake in *Taenia sodium*, against which it is highly effective. Since lethal doses of niclosamide in adult worms do not destroy the ova, purgation 1 to 2 hours after niclosamide is essential, or the risk of cysticercosis is likely.

NICOTINE POLACRILEX

(Nicorette)

Nicotine transdermal system or nicotine gum is indicated as a temporary aid to the cigarette smoker seeking to give up smoking while participating in a behavior modification program under medical supervision. In general, the smoker with the "physical" type of nicotine dependence is the most likely to benefit from the use of nicotine chewing gum or transdermal system.

Nicotine polacrilex contains nicotine bound to an ion exchange resin in a chewing gum base. The nicotine transdermal system is a multilayered unit containing nicotine as the active agent that provides systemic delivery of nicotine for 24 hours following its application to intact skin.

Nicotine, the chief alkaloid in tobacco products, binds stereoselectively to acetylcholine receptors at the autonomic ganglia, in the adrenal medulla, at neuromuscular junctions, and in the brain. Two types of CNS effects are believed to be the basis of nicotine's positively reinforcing properties. A **stimulating effect**, exerted mainly in the **cortex** via the **locus ceruleus**, produces increased alertness and cognitive performance. A **"reward"** effect via the **"pleasure system"** in the brain is exerted in the **limbic system**. At low doses the stimulant effects predominate, while at high doses the reward effects predominate.

The cardiovascular effects of nicotine include peripheral vasoconstriction, tachycardia, and elevated blood pressure. Nicotine is contraindicated during the immediate postmyocardial infarction period, in life-threatening arrhythmias, and in severe or worsening angina pectoris.

Smoking causes enzyme induction accelerating the metabolism of acetaminophen, caffeine, imipramine, oxazepam, pentazocine, propranolol, and theophylline. Smoking cessation may reverse these actions. Smoking and nicotine can increase circulating cortisol and catecholamines. Therapy with **adrenergic agonists** or with **adrenergic blockers** may need to be adjusted according to changes in nicotine therapy or smoking status.

Smoking may reduce diuretic effects of furosemide and decrease cardiac output. Smoking cessation may reverse these actions.

NICOTINE TRANSDERMAL SYSTEM
(Habitrol, Nicoderm, Nicotrol, Prostep)

Transdermal nicotine is used in the relief of nicotine withdrawal symptoms in patients attempting smoking cessation.

NICOTINIC ACID

Nicotinic acid inhibits the release of free fatty acids, followed by a fall in the VLDL, and then the LDL level. Nicotinic acid may cause intense flushing and itching (vasodilation and histamine release), and tolerance develops to these effects.

NIFEDIPINE
(Procardia)

Nifedipine (10 to 20 mg t.i.d.) is indicated in vasospastic (Prinzmetal's or variant) angina. It may also be used in chronic stable angina (classical effort-associated angina) without vasospasm. Sustained release nifedipine (30 to 60 mg once daily) is used in hypertension.

TABLE 20
Comparison of the Hemodynamic Effects of Calcium Channel Antagonists

Effects	Nifedipine	Nicardipine	Verapamil	Diltiazem
Vasodilation	+++	+++	++	+
Negative inotropic effect	0	0	++	+
Negative chronotropic effect	0	0	+++	+++
Positive chronotropic effect*	+	+	0	0
Negative dromotropic effect (AV conduction)	0	0	+++	+++
Cardiac output increases*	+	+	0	0

*Due to reflex stimulation

AV = atrioventricular; 0 = no effects; + = minor effects; ++ = moderate effects; and +++ = major side effects.

The most common cause of **hypertensive crises** is an abrupt increase in blood pressure in patients with chronic hypertension. Other causes include renovascular hypertension, parenchymal renal disease, scleroderma and other collagen-vascular diseases, the ingestion of drugs such as sympathomimetic agents (cocaine, amphetamines, phencyclidine hydrochloride, lysergic acid diethylmide, and diet pills) and tricyclic antidepressants, withdrawal from antihypertensive drugs (centrally acting agents and beta-antagonists), preeclampsia, eclampsia, pheochromocytoma, acute glomerulonephritis, head injury, the ingestion of tyramine in conjunction with the use of a monoamine oxidase inhibitor, a renin-secreting tumor, vasculitis, and autonomic hyperactivity in patients with Guillain-Barré or other spinal cord syndromes. The parenteral and oral medications used in the treatment of hypertensive emergencies, including nicardipine and nifedipine, are all listed in Table 20.

NIFURTIMOX

(Lampit)

Trypanosomiasis is produced by the protozoa of the genus *Trypanosoma* and leads to Gambian or mid-African sleeping sickness (*T. gambiense*), Rhodesian or East African sleeping sickness (*T. rhodesiense*), and Chagas' disease, which is seen in the populations of Central and South America (*T. cruzi*).

Agents effective in the treatment of trypanosomiasis are the **aromatic diamidines** (pentamidine, stilbamidine, and propamidine). **Pentamidine** is the preferred drug for the prevention and early treatment of *T. gambiense* infections; however, it cannot penetrate the central nervous system. **Melarsoprol** is the drug recommended for *T. gambiense* infections that do not respond to pentamidine or for managing the late meningoencephalitic stages of infection. It does reach the central nervous system. **Nifurtimox** is the drug of choice for treating the acute form of Chagas' disease. **Suramin** (Naphuride) is effective only in the therapy for African sleeping sickness.

NIMODIPINE

(Nimoton)

Nimodipine, a calcium channel blocking agent with cerebrovasodilating properties, is used for improvement of neurological deficits after subarachnoid hemorrhage from ruptured congenital aneurysms. Nimodipine is a calcium channel blocking agent of the 1,4-dihydropyridine family that produces relaxation of smooth muscle. It is marketed as an intravenous infusion for subarachnoid hemorrhage only. Nimodipine exerts its cytoprotective influence by reducing calcium influx into nerve cells. Therefore, it may be useful in stroke, severe head injury, cerebral resuscitation after cardiac arrest, impaired brain functions in old age, and senile dementia.

NIRIDAZOLE

(Ambilhar)

Niridazole possesses both schistosomicidal and amebicidal properties. In addition, it has antiinflammatory properties and is a potent inhibitor of cell-mediated responses. It destroys the vitellogenic gland and egg production in the female and spermatogenesis in the male *Schistosoma haematobium,* against which it is highly effective. Niridazole is extensively metabolized in the liver, and numerous toxicities do occur, especially in patients with impaired liver function. It causes hemolytic anemia in patients with glucose-6-phosphate dehydrogenase deficiency. It should be used cautiously in diseases involving the CNS, such as epilepsy.

NITRATES AND NITRITES

The mechanism underlying the therapeutic actions of nitrates and nitrites may be their ability to relax vascular smooth muscle and consequently **reduce cardiac preload** and **afterload**. The nitrates and nitrites bring about **arterial dilation**, and hence reduce blood pressure and the work of the heart. These agents also produce **venous dilation**, thereby decreasing the venous return and ventricular volume, which in turn diminishes wall tension. The end result of these events is a reduction in the work of the heart. By decreasing blood pressure, the heart rate is increased through the activation of carotid sinus reflexes. However, the extent of the reduction in wall tension is actually of greater benefit than the elevated heart rate (see Figure 59). The nitrate-induced **tachycardia** may be blocked by the administration of propranolol, a beta-adrenergic receptor-blocking agent (see Figure 61).

Collateral vessels are silent blood vessels that become functional during hypoxic emergencies. By dilating, they permit greater blood flow to the ischemic areas, and nitrates accentuate this response. This effect of nitrates, which is greater than that of dipyridamole, seems to be potentiated by propranolol.

Nitrites and nitrates dilate blood vessels in all smooth muscles. When they dilate the cutaneous blood vessels, they cause blushing. When they dilate the cerebral vessels, they cause headache. Thus, the appearance of headache and blushing is an indication of the efficacy of these medications (see Figures 59 and 61).

The nitrates and nitrites are best absorbed through the mucous membrane lining the mouth and nose. Therefore, they are usually administered sublingually or buccally. They may also be inhaled. When administered by these routes, the active ingredient is absorbed into the venous circulation and travels via the vena cava to the heart, aorta, and coronary arteries. If these agents are taken orally, they are metabolized to inactive compounds by nitrate reductase in the liver (see Figure 60).

NITRATES AND NITRITES CAUSE

  Arterial dilation and blood pressure reduction

  Venous dilation and reduced wall tension

  Dilation of coronary vessels

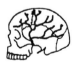 Dilation of cerebral vessels causing headache

FIGURE 59 The mechanism underlying the therapeutic actions of nitrates and nitrites may be their ability to relax vascular smooth muscle and consequently **reduce cardiac preload** and **afterload**.

NITRATE PRODUCTS

Isosorbide dinitrate, sublingual and chewable

Isosorbide dinitrate Isonate 2.5 mg SL Isordil Sorate-2.5 Sorbitrate	Isosorbide dinitrate Isonate 5 mg SL Isordil Sorate-5 Sorbitrate	Isosorbide Isordil Sorbitrate Onset-5 Sorate-5	Sorbitrate Isordil Sorate-10 Sorbitrate

Isosorbide dinitrate, oral

Isosorbide dinitrate Isonage Isordil Titradose Sorbitrate Isosorbide dinitrate Isonate Isordil Titradose	Sorbitrate Isosorbide dinitrate Isonate Isordil Titradose Sorbitrate Isosorbide dinitrate Isordil Titradose	Sorbitrate Isosorbide dinitrate Isordil Titradose Sorbitrate Isosorbide dinitrate Isosorbide dinitrate Isordil Tembids	Sorbitrate SA Isosorbide dinitrate Dilatrate-SR Iso-Bid Isordil Tembids Isotrate Timecelles Sorate-40

Erythritol tetranitrate

Cardilate			

Pentaerythritol tetranitrate (PETN)

PETN Pentylan Peritrate	Naptrate Pentylan Peritrate	Duotrate Plateau Caps Pentritol Tempules Peritrate SA	

Nitroglycerin, intravenous

Tridil Nitrol IV	Nitrostat IV Nitroglycerin	Nitro-Bid IV Nitrol IV Concentrate	Nitrostat IV Tridil

Nitroglycerin, sublingual

Nitroglycerin Nitrostat	Nitroglycerin Nitrostat	Nitroglycerin Nitrostat	Nitroglycerin Nitrostat

Nitroglycerin, translingual

Nitrolingual			

Nitroglycerin, transmucosal

Nitrogard			

Nitroglycerin, sustained release

Nitroglycerin Nitro-Bid Plateau Caps Nitrocap T.D. Nitroglyn Nitrolan Nitrospan Klavikordal	Niong Nitronet Nitrong Nitroglycerin Nitro-Bid Plateau Caps Nitrocap 6.5	Nitroglyn Nitrolan Nitrospan Klavikordal Niong Nitronet	Nitrong Nitroglycerin Nitro-Bid Plateau Caps Nitroglyn Nitrolan Nitrong

Nitroglycerin, transdermal

Nitro-Dur II 2.5 mg/24 h Transderm-Nitro 2.5 Nitrodisc 5 mg/24 h Nitro-Dur 5 mg/24 h Nitro-Dur 5 mg/24 h	NTS 5 mg/24 h Transderm-Nitro 5 Nitrodisc 7.5 mg/24 h Nitro-Dur II 7.5 mg/24 h	Nitrodisc 10 mg/24 h Nitro-Dur 10 mg/24 h Nitro-Dur II 10 mg/24 h Transderm-Nitro 10	Nitro-Dur II 15 mg/24 h NTS 15 mg/24 h NTS 15 mg/24 h Transderm-Nitro 15

Nitroglycerin, topical

Nitroglycerin Nitro-Bid Nitrol	Nitrong Nitrostat		

NITRENDIPINE

Calcium entry blockers include those agents that are **selective for slow calcium channels** in the myocardium (slow channel blockers), and consist of the following categories of substances:

Phenylalkylamines — verapamil, gallopamil, anipamil, desmethoxyverapamil, emopamil, falipamil, and ronipamil

Dihydropyridines — nifedipine, nicardipine, niludipine, nimodipine, nisoldipine, **nitrendipine**, ryosidine, amlodipine, azodipine, dazodipine, felodipine, flordipine, iodipine, isradipine, mesudipine, oxodipine, and riodipine

Nitrendipine is a 1,4-dihydropyridine derivative calcium entry blocker, structurally similar to nifedipine. It is further classified as a Type II calcium antagonist because, at usual doses and concentrations, it is devoid of electrophysiologic effects, but is a potent peripheral vasodilator. Relaxation of peripheral vascular smooth muscle occurs as a result of inhibition of calcium influx across cellular membranes.

Nitrendipine is a potent vasodilator which effectively reduces blood pressure when given 1 to 3 times daily. The drug appears most useful in low-renin hypertensives. Biochemical abnormalities common to other currently used antihypertensives (e.g., hypokalemia, hyperglycemia, increased uric acid and lipids) are not seen with this class of drugs and may represent an advantage over beta-blockers and diuretics. Although most patients will require twice-daily dosing, the only other available dihydropyridine (nifedipine) usually requires dosing 3 to 4 times a day (see Table 20).

NITRIC OXIDE

A number of vasodilators, such as acetylcholine, bradykinin, adenine nucleosides, thrombin, histamine, or serotonin, need an intact vascular endothelium in order to exert their effects. For example, stimulation of endothelial cholinergic receptors causes the release of endothelium-derived relaxing factors (EDRF), which may involve arachidonic acid formation and compartmentalization via the lipoxygenase pathway. EDRF, which is identical to nitric oxide, activates guanylate cyclase and enhances the formation of cyclic guanosine monophosphate (cyclic GMP) in smooth muscle. Tetranoic acid (a vasoconstrictor), thromboxane A_2 (a vasoconstrictor), and prostacyclin (a vasodilator) are formed through the lipoxygenase pathway (Figure 19).

The vasodilating properties of captopril or hydralazine (antihypertensive agents) are mediated by the formation of EDRF or prostaglandin, or both. On the other hand, the vasodilating properties of nitroprusside (an antihypertensive agent) result directly from the formation of cyclic GMP (Figure 62).

NITROFURANTOIN

(Furadantin)

Nitrofurantoin (50 to 100 mg q.i.d.) is indicated in the treatment of urinary tract infections due to susceptible strains of *E. coli, enterococci, S. aureus,* and certain strains of *Klebsiella, Enterobacter,* and *Proteus* species.

Nitrofurantoin is a synthetic nitrofuran that is bacteriostatic in low concentrations (5 to 10 mcg/ml) and bactericidal in higher concentrations. Nitrofurantoin may inhibit acetyl-coenzyme A, interfering with bacterial carbohydrate metabolism. It may also disrupt bacterial cell wall formation.

Nitrofurantoin may cause pulmonary reactions manifested by sudden onset of dyspnea, chest pain, cough, fever, and chills. These reactions may occur rapidly (few hours) or slowly (few weeks). Chest X-rays show alveolar infiltrates or effusions; elevated sedimentation rate and eosinophilia are also present. Resolution of clinical and radiological abnormalities occurs within 24 to 48 hours after discontinuation.

Hemolytic anemia of the primaquine sensitivity type has been induced by nitrofurantoin. The hemolysis appears to be linked to a glucose 6-phosphate dehydrogenase (G-6-PD) deficiency in the red blood cells of affected patients.

Peripheral neuropathy may occur and may become severe or irreversible. Prolonged or repeated therapy with nitrofurantoin may cause superinfection resulting in bacterial or fungal overgrowth of nonsusceptible organisms. Such overgrowth may lead to a secondary infection. *Pseudomonas* is the organism most commonly implicated in superinfections.

Anticholinergic drugs and food increase nitrofurantoin bioavailability by delaying gastric emptying and increasing absorption. Administration of high doses of probenecid with nitrofurantoin decreases renal clearance and increases serum levels of nitrofurantoin. The result could be increased toxic effects. Magnesium trisalicylate may delay or decrease the absorption of nitrofurantoin.

NITROFURANTOIN MACROCRYSTALS
(Macrodantin, Macrobid)

NITROFURANTOIN MICROCRYSTALS
(Furadantin, Furalan, Furan, Furanite, Nitrofan)

Nitrofurantoin, a nitrofuran urinary tract antiinfective agent (50 to 100 mg p.o. q.i.d. with meals), is indicated in initial or recurrent urinary tract infections caused by susceptible organisms, or as a long-term suppression therapy.

NITROGEN MUSTARDS

The activity of nitrogen mustards depends on the presence of a bis-(2-chloroethyl) grouping:

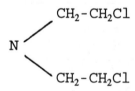

This is present in **mechlorethamine** (Mustargen), which is used in patients with Hodgkin's disease and other lymphomas, usually in combination with other drugs, such as in **MOPP therapy** (mechlorethamine, Oncovin [vincristine], procarbazine, and prednisone). It may cause bone marrow depression.

NITROGLYCERIN
(Transderm-Nitro)

Nitroglycerin is indicated for initial relief of acute angina pectoris and for prophylaxis to prevent or minimize anginal attacks when taken immediately before stressful events. Nitroglycerin has the following molecular structure:

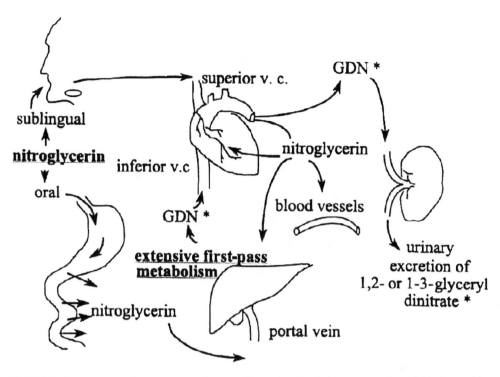

FIGURE 60   Nitroglycerin relaxes vascular smooth muscle of both the venous and arterial beds, resulting in a net decrease in myocardial oxygen consumption. (Adapted from Ebadi, M., *Pharmacology, An Illustrated Review with Questions and Answers,* 3rd Edition, Lippincott-Raven Press, Philadelphia, 1996.)

$$CH_2 - O - NO_2$$
$$|$$
$$CH - O - NO_2$$
$$|$$
$$CH_2 - O - NO_2$$

Nitroglycerin dilates the coronary arteries rapidly (1 to 2 minutes), but the coronary dilatation does not last as long as its antianginal effects (30 minutes). Nitroglycerin also dilates blood vessels in the bronchi, the uterus, and the gastrointestinal tract (see Figure 60). It has a pronounced effect on the meningeal vessels, and blushing and headache are common following administration. Nitroglycerin may also be provided on a continuous 24-hour basis through a transdermal therapeutic system called **Transderm Nitro**. This system releases 5 to 10 mg of nitroglycerin over the course of 24 hours. Using this route of administration, nitroglycerin is absorbed through the skin into the systemic circulation. The beneficial effect is apparent 30 minutes after the pad is applied and ceases 30 minutes after it is removed. Therefore, sublingual nitroglycerin should be used for achieving an immediate effect, followed by Transderm-Nitro as a prophylactic measure.

Nitroglycerin may be applied topically (2% ointment). Its hemodynamic and beneficial effects appear as early as 15 minutes after application and last up to 4 hours. Nitroglycerin ointment may be especially useful for the management of **angina decubitus**, which may develop 3 hours after patients go to sleep.

Due to the first-pass effect, the orally administered nitrates such as isosorbide dinitrite are effective only when given in large doses (30 to 40 mg q.i.d.). Isosorbide is effective in low doses (5 mg) when given sublingually.

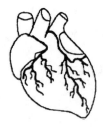

DRUGS	HEART RATE

nitroglycerin ------------------------ increased

propranolol ------------------------ decreased

nitroglycerin + propranolol ------------ no change

THE BENEFICIAL EFFECTS OF β-BLOCKERS IN ANGINA

FIGURE 61   Propranolol is also frequently combined with nitrates to combat nitrate-induced reflex tachycardia.

NITROPRUSSIDE
(Nipride; Nitropress)

Nitroprusside (3 mcg/kg/min) is indicated for immediate reduction of blood pressure in patients in hypertensive crisis. It has also been used to produce controlled hypotension in order to reduce bleeding during surgery (see Table 21).

Nitroprusside, either alone or in combination with dopamine, has been used in patients with severe refractory congestive heart failure. Coadministration of these two agents has also been used in patients with acute myocardial infarction.

The hypotensive effect of nitroprusside is seen within 1 to 2 minutes after the start of an adequate infusion, and it dissipates almost as rapidly after an infusion is discontinued. The effect is augmented by ganglionic blocking agents and inhaled anesthetics. Injudicious use of nitroprusside may cause precipitous decreases in blood pressure leading to irreversible ischemic injuries or death.

Nitroprusside is given by infusion, and its blood pressure-lowering effect is directly related to the rate at which it is administered. When it is discontinued, blood pressure rises rapidly. Lethal **cyanide poisoning** may occur in patients with **rhodanase deficiency**, and thiocyanate may accumulate in patients with renal failure, thus inhibiting **iodine uptake** and causing **hypothyroidism** (see Figure 62).

Nitroprusside is a potent IV antihypertensive agent. The principal pharmacological action of nitroprusside is relaxation of vascular smooth muscle and consequent dilation of peripheral arteries and veins. Other smooth muscle (e.g., uterus, duodenum) is not affected. Nitroprusside is more active on veins than on arteries, but this selectivity is much less marked than that of nitroglycerin. Dilation of the veins promotes peripheral pooling of blood and decreases venous return to the heart, thereby reducing left ventricular end-diastolic pressure and pulmonary capillary wedge pressure (preload). Arteriolar relaxation reduces systemic vascular resistance, systolic arterial pressure, and mean arterial pressure (afterload). Dilation of the coronary arteries also occurs.

TABLE 21
Parenteral Medications Used in the Treatment of Hypertensive Emergencies

Drugs	Administration by IV	Onset	Duration of Action	Dosage	Adverse Effects and Comments
Sodium Nitroprusside	Infusion	Immediate	2-3 min	0.5-10 mcg/kg/min, initial dose; 0.25 mcg/kg/min for eclampsia and renal insufficiency	Hypotension, nausea, vomiting apprehension. Risk of thiocyanate and cyanide toxicity is increased in renal and hepatic insufficiency, respectively. Levels should be monitored. Must shield from light.
Diazoxide	Bolus	1-5 min	6-12 hr	50-100 mg every 5-10 min. up to 600 mg	Hypotension, tachycardia, nausea, vomiting, fluid retention, hyperglycemia. May exacerbate myocardial ischemia, heart failure, or aortic dissection.
	Infusion			10-30 mg/min	May require concomitant use of a beta-antagonist.
Labetalol	Bolus	5-10 min	3-6 hr	20-80 mg every 5-10 min	Hypotension, heart block, heart failure, bronchospasm, nausea, scalp tingling, paradoxical pressor response. May not be
	Infusion			0.5-2 mg/min	effective in patients receiving alpha- or beta-antagonists.
Nitroglycerin	Infusion	1-2 min	3-5 min	5-100 mcg/min	Headache, nausea, vomiting. Tolerance may develop with prolonged use.
Phentolamine	Bolus	1-2 min	3-10 min	5-10 mg every 5-15 min	Hypotension, tachycardia, headache, angina, paradoxical pressor response.
Trimethaphan	Infusion	1-5 min	10 min	0.5-5 mg/min	Hypotension, urinary retention, ileus, respiratory arrest, mydriasis, cycloplegia, dry mouth.
Hydralazine (for treatment of eclampsia)	Bolus	10-20 min	3-6 hr	5-10 mg every 20 min	Hypotension, fetal distress, tachycardia, headache, nausea, vomiting, local thrombophlebitis. Infusion site should be changed after 12 hr.
Nicardipine	Infusion	1-5 min	3-6 hr	5 mg/hr	Hypotension, headache, tachycardia, nausea, vomiting.

IV = intravenous

In association with the decrease in blood pressure, nitroprusside administered IV to hypertensive and normotensive patients produces slight increases in heart rate and a variable effect on cardiac output. In hypertensive patients, moderate doses induce renal vasodilation roughly proportional to the decrease in systemic blood pressure, so there is no appreciable change in renal blood flow or glomerular filtration rate.

In normotensive subjects, acute reduction of mean arterial pressure to 60 to 75 mmHg by infusion of nitroprusside causes a significant increase in renin activity.

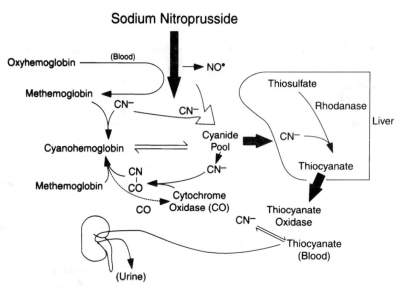

Sodium Nitroprusside

Lethal cyanide poisoning may occur in patients with rhodanase deficiency

FIGURE 62   Nitroprusside is used exclusively in the management of **malignant hypertension** and a **hypertensive crisis**. Nitroprusside is given by infusion, and its blood pressure-lowering effect is directly related to the rate at which it is administered. When it is discontinued, blood pressure rises rapidly. Lethal **cyanide poisoning** may occur in patients with **rhodanase deficiency**, and thiocyanate may accumulate in patients with renal failure, thus inhibiting **iodine uptake** and causing **hypothyroidism**.

Nitroprusside infusions at rates >2 mcg/kg/min generate CN^- faster than the body can normally dispose of it. Since cyanide is metabolized by hepatic enzymes, it may accumulate in patients with severe liver impairment. Nitroprusside infusions can cause sequestration of hemoglobin as methemoglobin. Like other vasodilators, nitroprusside can cause increases in intracranial pressure (see Figure 62).

The adverse reactions of nitroprusside are due to rapid reduction of blood pressure. Abdominal pain, apprehension, diaphoresis, dizziness, headache, muscle twitching, nausea, palpitations, restlessness, retching, and retrosternal discomfort have been noted when the blood pressure was reduced too rapidly. These symptoms quickly disappeared when the infusion was slowed or discontinued, and they did not reappear with a continued (or resumed) slower infusion (see Figure 62).

NITROUREAS
Carmustine (**BCNU**), lomustine (**CCNU**), and semustine (**methyl-CCNU**) generate alkyl carbonium ions and isocyanate molecules and hence are able to interact with DNA and other macromolecules. These agents, which are lipid soluble, cross the blood-brain barrier and are therefore effective in treating brain tumors. They are bone marrow depressants.

NITROUS OXIDE
Nitrous oxide (N_2O) is an inert, colorless, odorless, and tasteless gas. When a mixture of about 40% **nitrous oxide** and air is inhaled for a few seconds, a condition resembling alcoholic intoxication is produced with much hilarity and laughter so that the oxide is known popularly as "laughing gas."

The inhalation of 35 to 70% of nitrous oxide causes, after a few seconds, a rushing, drumming, hammering in the ears, indistinct sight, staggering gait, and swaying of the body from side to side. The patient seems brighter and more lively and often bursts into laughter.

When pure nitrous oxide is inhaled without the admixture of oxygen, the patient loses consciousness completely. The face is cyanotic, the respiration becomes stertorous and dyspneic and ceases after a weak convulsion, while the heart continues to beat for some time afterward. If the mask through which the patient has been inhaling the gas is removed when the cyanosis becomes marked, complete anesthesia lasts for 30 to 60 seconds, and the patient then recovers within a few minutes. The pharmacology of nitrous oxide and that of halothane is compared in Table 15.

NIZATIDINE

(Axid)

Nizatidine, a histamine receptor antagonist (300 mg once daily at bedtime), is indicated in the management of duodenal ulcer, benign gastric ulcer, and gastroesophageal reflux disease (see also Table 9).

Stimulation of H_2 receptors elicits a variety of responses, the most widely studied of which is **gastric acid secretion** from the parietal cells of the gastric glands. However, many other effects mediated by the H_2 receptors are manifested in peripheral tissues. These include the positive chronotropic action in the auricular muscle, the inotropic action in the ventricular muscle, and the lipolytic effect in fat cells. In addition, the extensive use of **cimetidine** has led to the synthesis and marketing of more specific and efficacious analogs with pharmacologic properties that are outlined in Table 9. Examples of the various H_2-receptor blocking agents are:

Imidazole derivatives
  Cimetidine and etintidine
Furan derivatives
  Ranitidine and nizatidine
Guanidinothiazole derivatives
  Famotidine
Piperidinomethylphenoxy derivatives
  Roxatidine acetate and roxatidine

NONDEPOLARIZING NEUROMUSCULAR BLOCKING DRUGS		
Drugs	**Formulations**	**Comments**
Long-acting		
Doxacurium	Solution	Minimal cardiovascular effects; duration of action prolonged in renal failure
Metocurine	Solution	Histamine release may cause hypotension, bronchoconstriction
Pancuronium	Solution	Vagal blocking properties may cause tachycardia
Pipecuronium	Powder	Minimal cardiovascular effects; duration of action prolonged in renal failure
Tubocurarine	Solution	Histamine release may cause hypotension, bronchoconstriction
Intermediate-acting		
Atracurium	Solution	Short duration of action may require repeated doses; no renal excretion; histamine release may cause hypotension, bronchoconstriction
Vecuronium	Powder	Similar to atracurium, but virtually no histamine release; some renal excretion
Halothane, enflurane, and isoflurane potentiate the activity of doxacurium; and phenytoin and carbamazepine shorten the duration of doxacurium block.		

NONSTEROIDAL ANTIINFLAMMATORY AGENTS

Salicylates and allied compounds have **analgesic, antipyretic, uricosuric,** and **antiinflamma-tory** properties. Their mechanisms of action differ from those of the antiinflammatory steroids and the opioid analgesics. They are classified into the following categories (see Table 2).

Salicylate derivatives
   Acetylsalicylic acid (aspirin)
   Diflunisal (Dolobid)
   Salsalate (Arthra-G, Disalcid, Mono-Gesic)
Pyrazolone derivatives
   Phenylbutazone (Butazolidin)
   Oxyphenbutazone (Oxalid, Tandearil)
   Sulfinpyrazone (Anturane)
Paraaminophenol derivatives
   Acetaminophen (Tylenol, Datril)
   Phenacetin (Acetophenetidin)
Propionic acid derivatives
   Ibuprofen (Motrin)
   Naproxen (Naprosyn)
   Fenoprofen (Nalfon)
   Flurbiprofen (Ansaid)
   Ketoprofen (Orudis)
Others
   Indomethacin (Indocin)
   Sulindac (Clinoril)
   Mefenamic acid (Ponstel)
   Tolmetin (Tolectin)
   Piroxicam (Feldene)
   Diclofenac sodium (Voltaren)
   Etodolac
   Nabumetone

In the following pages, the pharmacology of acetylsalicylic acid (aspirin) is discussed in detail as a prototype drug, and all the other drugs are compared to it.

Arachidonic acid, which is stored as a cellular membrane phospholipid, is the precursor for series 2 prostaglandins. Aspirin selectively acetylates the hydroxyl group of a single serine residue at position 530 within the polypeptide chain of prostaglandin G/H synthase, the enzyme that converts arachidonate into prostaglandin cyclic endoperoxide. Aspirin thereby reduces the synthesis of the eicosanoids — **prostaglandins, prostacyclin,** and **thromboxane A.**

Unlike the narcotic analgesics such as morphine, aspirin does not depress respiration, is relatively nontoxic, and lacks addiction liability. Aspirin is a weak or mild analgesic that is effective for ameliorating short, intermittent types of pain such as neuralgia, myalgia, and toothache. It does not have the efficacy of morphine and cannot relieve the severe, prolonged, and lancinating types of pain associated with trauma such as burns or fractures. Like morphine, it produces analgesia by raising the pain threshold in the thalamus, but, unlike morphine, it does not alter the patient's reactions to pain. Because aspirin does not cause hypnosis or euphoria, its site of action has been postulated to be subcortical. In addition to **raising the pain threshold**, the antiinflammatory effects of aspirin may contribute to its analgesic actions.

However, no direct association between the antiinflammatory and analgesic effects of these compounds should be expected. For example, aspirin has both analgesic and antiinflammatory properties, whereas acetaminophen has analgesic but not antiinflammatory properties. Furthermore, potent antiinflammatory agents such as phenylbutazone have only weak analgesic effects.

Aspirin does not alter the normal body temperature, which is maintained by a balance between heat production and dissipation. In a fever associated with infection, increased oxidative processes enhance heat production. Aspirin acts by causing cutaneous vasodilation, which prompts perspiration and enhances heat dissipation. This effect is mediated via the hypothalamic nuclei, as proved by the fact that a lesion in the preoptic area suppresses the mechanism through which aspirin exerts its antipyretic effects. The antipyretic effects of aspirin may be due to its inhibition of hypothalamic prostaglandin synthesis. Although aspirin-induced diaphoresis contributes to its antipyretic effects, it is not an absolutely necessary process, since antipyresis takes place in the presence of atropine.

Numerous agents cause thermoregulatory dysfunction. This dysfunction may occur as the result of decreased sweating (antihistamines and tricyclic depressants), decreased cardiac output (diuretics causing volume depletion and beta-adrenergic receptor-blocking agents causing myocardial depression), decreased vasodilation (sympathomimetic agents and alpha-adrenergic receptor agonists), depression of the hypothalamic centers (neuroleptics such as chlorpromazine or other alpha-adrenergic receptor antagonists), or behavioral dysfunctions (sedatives and opioids).

Small doses (600 mg) of aspirin cause **hyperuricemia**, but large doses (>5 gm) have a uricosuric effect. Aspirin inhibits uric acid resorption by the tubules in the kidneys. However, because of the availability of more effective uricosuric agents, aspirin is no longer used for this purpose.

Aspirin has an **antiinflammatory** action as well as **antirheumatic** and **antiarthritic** effects, and may therefore be used in the treatment of rheumatic fever. However, it cannot alter the cardiac lesion and other visceral effects of the disease. Aspirin is extremely effective in managing rheumatoid arthritis and allied diseases involving the joints, such as ankylosing spondylitis and osteoarthritis. It is thought that aspirin and indomethacin exert their antiinflammatory effects by inhibiting **prostaglandin** synthesis through the inhibition of **cyclooxygenase**. The presynthesized prostaglandins are released during a tissue injury that fosters inflammation and pain. Furthermore, aspirin reduces the formation of prostaglandin in the platelets and leukocytes, which is responsible for the reported hematologic effects associated with aspirin (see also Figure 11).

The current thinking concerning the role of aspirin in the prevention of cardiovascular disease is that it is beneficial in the event of **myocardial infarction** and **stroke**. It is effective because, in platelets, small amounts of aspirin acetylate irreversibly and bind to the active site of thromboxane A_2, a potent promoter of platelet aggregation (see also Figure 12).

The menstrual cycle is associated with two potentially incapacitating events: **dysmenorrhea** and the **premenstrual syndrome**. Substantial evidence indicates that the excessive production of prostaglandin F_{2a} is the major source of painful menstruation. The nonsteroidal antiinflammatory drugs approved for the treatment of dysmenorrhea are **aspirin, ibuprofen, mefenamic acid**, and **naproxen** (see also Table 2).

Aspirin stimulates respiration both directly and indirectly. In analgesic doses, aspirin increases **oxygen consumption** and **carbon dioxide production**. However, increased alveolar ventilation balances the increased carbon dioxide production, thus the partial pressure of CO_2 (PCO_2) in plasma does not change. In the event of salicylate intoxication (e.g., 10 to 12 grams of aspirin given in 6 to 8 hours in adults, and an even smaller dosage in children, whose brains are far more sensitive to salicylate intoxication), salicylate stimulates the medullary centers directly, and this causes **hyperventilation** characterized by an increase in the depth and rate of respiration. The PCO_2 level declines, causing hypocapnia, and the blood pH increases, causing **respiratory alkalosis.** The low PCO_2 then decreases the renal tubular resorption of bicarbonate and compensates for the alkalosis.

If the salicylate level continues to rise, the respiratory centers become depressed, the PCO_2 becomes elevated, and the blood pH becomes more acidic, causing **respiratory acidosis.** Dehydration, reduced bicarbonate levels, and the accumulation of salicylic acid, salicyluric acid resulting from metabolism of aspirin, and lactic and pyruvic acid resulting from deranged carbohydrate metabolism may cause **metabolic acidosis.**

The supportive treatment of aspirin poisoning may include **gastric lavage** (to prevent the further absorption of salicylate), **fluid replenishment** (to offset the dehydration and oliguria), **alcohol and water sponging** (to combat the hyperthermia), the administration of **vitamin K** (to prevent possible hemorrhage), **sodium bicarbonate** administration (to combat acidosis), and, in extreme cases, **peritoneal dialysis** and **exchange transfusion.**

Although innocuous in most subjects, the therapeutic analgesic doses of aspirin may cause epigastric distress, nausea, vomiting, and bleeding. Aspirin can also exacerbate the symptoms of peptic ulcer, characterized by heartburn, dyspepsia, and erosive gastritis. An extensive number of salts have been synthesized from salicylate (e.g., calcium carbaspirin, choline salicylate, alloxiprin, and numerous buffered derivatives) and each has shown some ability to reduce the gastrointestinal toxicity of aspirin. However, other unknown factors may contribute to this undesirable gastrointestinal property of aspirin. In experimental animals, the intravenous administration of sodium salicylate or subcutaneous administration of methyl salicylate has produced petechial hemorrhage of the gastric mucosa. Furthermore, compounds possessing antiinflammatory properties (aspirin, phenylbutazone, and oxyphenbutazone) are associated with a higher incidence of gastrointestinal toxicity than those compounds devoid of antiinflammatory properties (phenacetin and acetaminophen).

Aspirin reduces the **leukocytosis** associated with acute rheumatic fever. When given on a long-term basis, it also reduces the hemoglobin level and the hematocrit. Aspirin use can cause reversible **hypoprothrombinemia** by interfering with the function of **vitamin K** in prothrombin synthesis. Therefore, aspirin should be used with caution in patients with vitamin K deficiency, preexisting hypoprothrombinemia, or hepatic damage; in patients taking anticoagulants; and in patients scheduled for surgery. Aspirin leads to **hemolytic anemia** in individuals with glucose 6-phosphate dehydrogenase deficiency. An **aspirin tolerance test** is used diagnostically in **von Willebrand's disease**, because it will further prolong the bleeding time if the disease exists. Aspirin prevents platelet aggregation and may be helpful in the treatment of thromboembolic disease. In addition to aspirin, indomethacin, phenylbutazone, sulfinpyrazone, and dipyridamole prevent platelet aggregation; whereas epinephrine, serotonin, and prostaglandins promote platelet aggregation and hence are procoagulants. The erythrocyte sedimentation rate is often elevated in infections and inflammations, but aspirin therapy will yield a false negative.

NONSTEROIDAL ANTIINFLAMMATORY DRUGS	
Chemical Classifications	**Generic**
Salicylates	Acetylated Aspirin Aspirin, buffered Enteric coated Sustained release

Chemical Classifications	Generic
	Nonacetylated
	Choline salicylate
	Choline magnesium trisalicylate
	Diflunisal
	Salsalate
	Magnesium salicylate
	Sodium salicylate
Fenamates	Meclofenamic acid
	Mefenamic acid
Acetic acids	Diclofenac
	Etodolac
	Indomethacin
	Oxaprozin
	Sulindac
	Tolmetin
Propionic acids	Fenoprofen
	Flurbiprofen
	Ibuprofen
	Ketoprofen
	Naproxen
Pyrazolones	Phenylbutazone
Oxicam	Piroxicam
Nonacidic	Nabumetone

NOREPINEPHRINE BITARTRATE

(Levophed)

Norepinephrine (8 to 12 mcg/min by IV infusion), an alpha-adrenergic receptor stimulant and vasopressor, is indicated for maintaining blood pressure in acute hypotensive states.

Dopamine, norepinephrine, and epinephrine are classified as **catecholamines**. Tyrosine is converted to dopa by the rate-limiting enzyme, **tyrosine hydroxylase**, which requires tetrahydrobiopterin, and is inhibited by alpha-methyltyrosine. Dopa is decarboxylated to dopamine by **L-aromatic amino acid decarboxylase**, which requires pyridoxal phosphate (vitamin B_6) as a coenzyme. **Carbidopa**, which is used with L-dopa in the treatment of parkinsonism, inhibits this enzyme. Dopamine is converted to norepinephrine by **dopamine beta-hydroxylase**, which requires ascorbic acid (vitamin C), and is inhibited by diethyl-dithiocarbamate. Norepinephrine is converted to epinephrine by **phenylethanolamine N-methyltransferase (PNMT)**, requiring S-adenosylmethionine. The activity of PNMT is stimulated by corticosteroids.

The **catecholamine-synthesizing enzymes** are not only able to synthesize dopamine and norepinephrine from a physiologically occurring substrate such as L-dopa, but also from exogenous substrates such as **alpha-methyldopa**, which is converted to alpha-methyldopamine and in turn to alpha-methylnorepinephrine. Alpha-methyldopamine and alpha-methylnorepinephrine are called **false transmitters** and, in general (except for alpha-methylnorepinephrine), are weaker agonists. Alpha-methyldopa is used in the management of hypertension.

In addition to being synthesized in the peripheral nervous system, dopamine is also synthesized in the corpus striatum and in the mesocortical, mesolimbic, and tuberoinfundibular systems. Norepinephrine is synthesized and stored primarily in sympathetic noradrenergic nerve terminals, as well as in the brain and the adrenal medulla. Epinephrine is synthesized and stored primarily in the adrenal medulla, and, to a certain extent, in the hypothalamic nuclei.

In sympathetic nerve terminals, as well as the brain, the adrenal medulla, and sympathetic postganglionic terminals, there are osmophilic granules (synaptic vesicles) that are capable of storing high concentrations of catecholamine (a complex with adenosine triphosphate [ATP] and protein). The stored amines are not metabolized by the intersynaptosomal mitochondrial enzyme (monoamine oxidase).

Besides releasing norepinephrine (through exocytosis), the stimulation of sympathetic neurons also releases ATP, storage protein, and dopamine beta-hydroxylase. The released norepinephrine interacts with receptor sites located postsynaptically (alpha$_1$) to produce the desired effects

The action of norepinephrine is terminated by reuptake mechanisms, two of which have been identified: **Uptake 1** is located in the presynaptic membrane, requires energy for the transport, is sodium and temperature dependent, and is inhibited by **ouabain** (a cardiac glycoside), **cocaine** (a local anesthetic), and **imipramine** (an antidepressant). **Uptake 2** is located extraneuronally in various smooth muscles and glands, requires energy, and is temperature dependent. Approximately 20% of the amine is either taken up by the Uptake 2 mechanism or is metabolized.

There are two enzymes capable of metabolizing catecholamines. The first is **monoamine oxidase** (MAO), a mitochondrial enzyme that oxidatively deaminates catecholamines, tyramine, serotonin, and histamine. MAO is further subclassified as either **monoamine oxidase A**, which metabolizes norepinephrine and is inhibited by **tranylcypromine**, and **monoamine oxidase B**, which metabolizes dopamine and is inhibited by L-**deprenyl**. **Catechol-O-methyltransferase** (COMT), a soluble enzyme present mainly in the liver and kidney, is also found in postsynaptic neuronal elements. About 15% of norepinephrine is metabolized postsynaptically by COMT.

Epinephrine acts on both alpha and beta receptors. **Norepinephrine** acts on both alpha receptors and primarily on beta receptors. **Isoproterenol** is a pure beta agonist. The functions associated with alpha receptors are vasoconstriction, mydriasis, and intestinal relaxation.

The functions associated with **beta receptors** are vasodilation, cardioacceleration, bronchial relaxation, positive inotropic effect, intestinal relaxation, and glycogenolysis and fatty acid release. The beta$_1$ receptors are responsible for cardiac stimulation and lipolysis. Beta$_2$ receptors are responsible for bronchodilation and vasodepression. Beta$_2$ agonists are especially useful in the treatment of asthma because they produce bronchodilation without causing much cardiac acceleration.

The actions of norepinephrine and epinephrine on the cardiovascular system may be quite different when both drugs are administered in small doses (0.1 to 4.0 microgram/kg/min in a slow intravenous infusion), but are essentially the same when given in large doses.

Following are the effects of **small doses of norepinephrine** in humans:

Systolic pressure — increased
Diastolic pressure — increased
Mean pressure — increased
Heart rate — slightly decreased
Cardiac output — slightly decreased
Peripheral resistance — increased

The effects of **small doses of epinephrine** in humans are:

Systolic pressure — increased
Diastolic pressure — decreased (increased by large dose)

Mean pressure — unchanged
Cardiac output — increased
Peripheral resistance — decreased

Epinephrine increases the heart rate, force of contraction, irritability, and coronary blood flow.

The inherent **chronotropic effect of norepinephrine** is opposed by reflex slowing that is secondary to vasoconstriction and elevated blood pressure.

Epinephrine is a dilator of bronchial smooth muscle (beta$_2$ receptor), whereas norepinephrine is a weak dilator. Isoproterenol is more active than epinephrine.

NORETHINDRONE

(Micronor, Norlutin)

Norethindrone, a progestin with contraceptive properties, is indicated also in amenorrhea, abnormal uterine bleeding, or endometriosis. Norethindrone suppresses ovulation, thickens cervical mucus, and induces sloughing of the endometrium. Norethindrone is contraindicated in patients with a history of thromboembolic disorders, severe hepatic disease, breast cancer, or undiagnosed abnormal vaginal bleeding, and in pregnant and breast-feeding women.

Norethindrone should be used cautiously in patients with existing conditions that might be aggravated by fluid and electrolyte retention, such as cardiac or renal disease; epilepsy or migraine; and in patients with a history of mental depression because norethindrone may worsen this condition. Concomitant use with **bromocriptine** causes amenorrhea or galactorrhea, thus interfering with the action of bromocriptine.

NORETHINDRONE ACETATE

(Aygestin, Norlutate)

NORFLOXACIN

(Noroxin)

Norfloxacin (400 mg once daily for 1 to 20 days depending on the nature of the problem) is indicated for **urinary tract infections:** Uncomplicated (including cystitis), caused by *Enterococcus faecalis, E. coli, K. pneumoniae, P. mirabilis, P. aeruginosa, S. epidermidis, S. saprophyticus, C. freundii, Enterobacter aerogenes, Enterobacter cloacae, P. vulgaris, S. aureus,* or *S. agalactiae;* complicated by *Enterococcus faecalis, E. coli, K. pneumoniae, P. mirabilis, P. aeruginosa,* or *Serratia marcescens.* **Sexually transmitted diseases:** Uncomplicated urethral and cervical gonorrhea caused by *N. gonorrhoeae.*

The quinolones include: **nalidixic acid, cinoxacin** (Cinobac), **norfloxacin** (Noroxin), and **ciprofloxacin** (Cipro). Other members of the quinolone family are **pefloxacin, ofloxacin, enoxacin** and **fleroxacin.** The bacterial enzyme **DNA gyrase** is responsible for the continuous introduction of negative supercoils into DNA, and the quinolones inhibit this gyrase-mediated DNA supercoiling (see also Figure 77).

Nalidixic acid and **cinoxacin** are bactericidal against Gram-negative organisms that cause urinary tract infections. The **fluoroquinolones** are bactericidal and considerably more potent against *Escherichia coli* and various species of *Salmonella, Shigella, Enterobacter, Campylobacter,* and *Neisseria.* **Ciprofloxacin** also has good activity against staphylococci, including methicillin-resistant strains. The quinolones and fluoroquinolones may produce arthropathy, and hence should not be used in prepubertal children or pregnant women. **Nalidixic acid** and

cinoxacin are useful only for treating urinary tract infections. **Ciprofloxacin** is useful for both urinary tract infections and prostatitis.

NORGESTREL

(Ovrette)

Norgestrel (0.075 mg p.o. daily) exerts its contraceptive activity by suppressing ovulation and causing the thickening of cervical mucus (also see Figure 46). Norgestrel is contraindicated in patients with a history of thromboembolic disorders because the drug may induce thromboembolic disorders; in patients with severe hepatic disease because it may worsen liver damage; in patients with breast or genital cancer or undiagnosed abnormal vaginal bleeding because the drug may stimulate growth of hormone-sensitive tumors; and in pregnant and breast-feeding women.

Norgestrel should be used cautiously in patients with existing conditions that might be aggravated by fluid and electrolyte retention, such as in cardiac or renal disease, epilepsy, or migraine. Caution is also advised in administering this agent to diabetic patients (because decreased glucose tolerance may occur) or to patients with a history of mental depression (because norgestrel may worsen this condition). Concomitant use with bromocriptine may cause amenorrhea or galactorrhea, thus interfering with the action of bromocriptine. Concurrent use of these drugs is not recommended.

NORTRIPTYLINE HYDROCHLORIDE

(Aventyl, Pamelor)

Nortriptyline, a tricyclic antidepressant (25 mg p.o. t.i.d. gradually increasing to a dose of 150 mg daily), is indicated for the relief of symptoms of endogenous depression. Nortriptyline blocks the uptake of norepinephrine and to a lesser extent that of serotonin. It blocks cholinergic muscarinic receptors and to a lesser extent, those of alpha$_1$-adrenergic receptor and H$_1$ histamine receptors. Nortriptyline causes mild sedation and possesses anticholinergic properties. Concomitant use of nortriptyline with sympathomimetics, including epinephrine, phenylephrine, phenylpropranolamine, and ephedrine (often found in nasal sprays), may increase blood pressure. Concomitant use with warfarin may increase prothrombin time and cause bleeding. Concomitant use with thyroid medication, pimozide, or antiarrhythmic agents (quinidine, disopyramide, procainamide) may increase incidence of cardiac arrhythmias and conduction defects.

Nortriptyline may decrease hypotensive effects of centrally acting antihypertensive drugs, such as **guanethidine, guanabenz, guanadrel**, **clonidine, methyldopa**, and **reserpine**. Concomitant use with disulfiram or ethchlorvynol may cause delirium and tachycardia.

Additive effects are likely after concomitant use of nortriptyline with CNS depressants, including alcohol, analgesics, barbiturates, narcotics, tranquilizers, and anesthetics (oversedation); atropine and other anticholinergic drugs, including phenothiazines, antihistamines, meperidine, and antiparkinsonian agents (oversedation, paralytic ileus, visual changes, and severe constipation); and metrizamide (increased risk of convulsions).

Barbiturates and heavy smoking induce nortriptyline metabolism and decrease therapeutic efficacy; phenothiazines and haloperidol decrease its metabolism, decreasing therapeutic efficacy, methylphenidate, cimetidine, oral contraceptives, propoxyphene, and beta blockers may inhibit nortriptyline metabolism, increasing plasma levels and toxicity (see Table 3 through 5).

NOSCAPINE

(Nectadon)

Noscapine is a naturally occurring opium alkaloid with a structure and function similar to that of papaverine. It is antitussive and has no analgesic or additive properties. **Diphenhydramine** and **chlorcyclizine** are antihistaminic agents that also have antitussive properties. **Dimethoxanate** (Cothera) and **pipazethate** (Theratuss) are phenothiazine derivatives without analgesic but with weak antitussive and local anesthetic properties.

NURSING INFANTS: PHARMACOLOGY OF

Many drugs are excreted in breast milk, but the actual amount of a drug that appears in the milk depends on many factors. The higher the maternal plasma concentration of a drug, the more drug is likely to appear in the milk. Atropine poisoning has occurred in nursing infants when the mother has taken larger than therapeutic doses of the agent. Un-ionized and nonprotein-bound drugs are excreted more rapidly, and ionized drugs are excreted more slowly. The longer a drug stays in maternal plasma, due to diminished metabolism and excretion, or both, the more it will be excreted in the milk. Because the pH of milk is more acidic (6.7) than that of plasma, a proportionately greater amount of basic drugs than of acidic drugs will accumulate in milk. So in most cases when drugs are used in recommended amounts, the drug concentrations in milk and hence the infant's plasma are lower than those in the maternal plasma, causing no interference with breast-feeding. However, toxicity in the infant has been known to occur, and thus the injudicious use of drugs should be avoided. For example, heavy smokers who intend to breast-feed should expect gastrointestinal, cardiovascular, and central nervous system (CNS) disturbances (anorexia, vomiting, diarrhea, tachycardia, restlessness, and irritability) in their infants. Lactating mothers who are taking medications such as anticonvulsants, neuroleptics, or anxiolytic agents on an ongoing basis should perhaps refrain from breast-feeding their infants. The developing brain is far more susceptible to toxicity than is the developed one. For example, the methyl mercury-contaminated fish ingested by lactating Japanese mothers has been the prime source of neurologic deficits in the infants of these women (Minamata disease).

Mercury has also been implicated in the etiology of acrodynia (pink disease) in children when mercury-containing teething powder was used. The methyl mercury contained in fungicides has been responsible for toxicity in children in Iraq. This toxicity is characterized by phalangeal erythema, muscular weakness, ataxia, hyperirritability, sensory impairment, visual disturbances, involuntary movement, and sometimes unconsciousness.

NYSTATIN

(Mycostatin)

Nystatin (500,000 to 1,000,000 units three times daily) is indicated for the treatment of intestinal candidiasis. Nystatin, a polyene antibiotic with antifungal activity, is poorly absorbed from the gastrointestinal tract. It is both fungistatic and fungicidal but has no effect on bacteria, viruses, or protozoa. It exerts its effect by binding to the sterol moiety and hence damaging the fungal membrane. It is used also as a topical agent to treat candidal infections of the skin and mucous membranes (paronychia, vaginitis, and stomatitis), and so causes no major toxicities.

OBESITY: TREATMENT OF

Obesity is defined as an excess of fat tissue in comparison with normal values for age and sex. In order to compare studies, standard definitions of overweight have been proposed. The most frequently used methods of calculation are ideal body weight and body mass index. The former takes height and sex into account and the individual is said to be obese when the actual weight exceeds 120% of the ideal weight. The latter is calculated with the ratio weight/height^2, and normal values are 23 kg/m^2 for men and 21 kg/m^2 for women.

Individual susceptibility to obesity is recognized to be influenced significantly by genetic inheritance. Recently, candidate obesity genes, such as **the β$_3$-adrenergic receptor leptin**, have been identified that may contribute to the inheritance of body fat mass and the partitioning of fat between central and peripheral fat depots. Nevertheless, overeating and inactive life styles are the direct causes of overweight and obesity.

Drugs that safely control food intake by correcting aberrant hunger and satiety signals, drugs that decrease energy efficiency or increase energy expenditure, and drugs that affect emotional states that have an effect on energy balance are being developed.

Agents Known to Enhance Food Intake

Antidepressant	Glucocorticoids	Neuropeptide Y
Bendorphin	Growth hormone-releasing hormone	Opioid peptides
Dynorphin	Insulin	Testosterone
Galanin	Low serotonin levels	Thyroxine

Agents Known to Suppress Food Intake

Anorectic	High blood glucose	Phenylethylamines
Bombesin	High-fat diet	Satietin
Cholecystokinin	High-protein diets	Serotonin
Corticotropin-releasing hormone	Histidine	Somatostatin
Estrogen	Mazindol	Substance P
Fluoxetine	Neurotensin	Thyrotropin-releasing hormone
Glucagon	Pain	Tryptophane

OCTREOTIDE ACETATE

(Sandostatin)

Octreotide (200 to 300 mcg/day in divided doses) is indicated for the treatment of the following tumors:

Carcinoid Tumors: Symptomatic treatment of patients with metastatic carcinoid tumors where it suppresses or inhibits the associated severe diarrhea and flushing episodes.

Vasoactive Intestinal Peptide Tumors (VIPomas): Treatment of the profuse watery diarrhea associated with VIP-secreting tumors. Significant improvement has been noted in the overall condition of these otherwise therapeutically unresponsive patients. Therapy with octreotide results in improvement in electrolyte abnormalities, (e.g., hypokalemia), often enabling reduction of fluid and electrolyte support.

Somatostatin, a cyclic tetradecapeptide with a disulfide bond between the third and fourteenth amino acid residue, has the following structure:

H-Ala-Gly-Cys-Lys-Asn-Phe-Phe-Trp-Lys-Thr-Phe-Thr-Ser-Cys-OH

The administration of somatostatin inhibits the secretion of a variety of peptides, including:

Hypothalamic hormones
> GHRH (see also Table 14)

Anterior pituitary hormones
> GH
> Thyrotropin (see Figure 90)

Pancreatic hormones
> Insulin (see Table 18)
> Glucagon
> Gastrin
> Cholecystokinin
> Secretin
> Pepsin
> Motilin
> Pancreatic polypeptide
> Gastrointestinal peptide
> Vasoactive intestinal polypeptide

Kidney hormones
> Renin (see Figure 21)

Octreotide, a long-acting somatostatin analog, has been approved for the management of secretory carcinoid tumors and vasoactive intestinal peptide-secreting tumors. Octreotide therapy, like the natural hormone, somatostatin, may be associated with cholelithiasis, presumably by altering fat absorption and possibly by decreasing the motility of the gallbladder.

In patients with severe renal failure requiring dialysis, the half-life of the octreotide may be increased, necessitating adjustment of the maintenance dosage. Octreotide acetate therapy is occasionally associated with mild transient hypo- or hyperglycemia due to alterations in the balance between the counterregulatory hormones: insulin, glucagon, and growth hormone.

OCULOTOXICITY: DRUG-INDUCED			
Antiinflammatory Agents			
Corticosteroids Cyclosporine Gold salts, auranofin	Ibuprofen Indomethacin	Ketoprofen Phenylbutazone	Piroxicam Salicylates
Antimicrobial Agents			
Amiodaquine Clofazimine Chloramphenicol Chloroquine/hydroxychloroquine Diethylcarbamazine	Ethambutol Gentamicin Griseofulvin Isoniazid Minocycline	Nalidixic acid Nitrofurantoin Quinine Rifampin Streptomycin	Sulfonamides Suramin Tetracycline Vaccinations
Antineoplastic Agents			
BCNU/CCNU/MeCCNU Busulfan Carmustine Chlorambucil Cisplatin	Cyclophosphamide Cytosine arabinoside Doxorubicin Fludarabine 5-Fluorouracil	Ifosfamide Methotrexate Mitotane Mitoxanthrone	Nitrogen mustard Procarbazine Tamoxifen Vinca alkaloids
Cardiovascular Agents			
Amiodarone Diazoxide Digitalis glycoside	Ergot alkaloids Flecainide Guanethidine	Metoprolol Minoxidil Nifedipine	Propranolol Quinidine Reserpine

Central Nervous System			
Amantadine	Ethchlorvynol	Phenytoin	
Barbiturates	Lithium	Protriptyline	
Bromocriptine	Narcotic analgesics	Trimethadione	
Carbamazepine	Phenothiazine		
Miscellaneous Agents			
Allopurinol	Dantrolene	Disulfiram	Penicillamine
Amantadine	Deferoxamine	Ganiumnitrate	Thiazide diuretics
Clomiphene	Diphenhydramine	Isotretinoin	

Adverse effects of drugs may involve external ocular functions and structures — oculomotor function, eyelids, lacrimation, conjunctiva, and cornea; or internal structures—trabecular meshwork, ciliary body, iris, lens, retina, and optic nerve. Higher than therapeutic doses and long duration of administration enhance the incidence of drug-induced oculotoxicity.

OFLOXACIN

(Floxin)

Ofloxacin (400 mg p.o.) is indicated for acute bacterial exacerbations of chronic bronchitis and pneumonia caused by susceptible organisms; sexually transmitted diseases, such as acute uncomplicated urethral and cervical gonorrhea, nongonococcal urethritis and cervicitis, and mixed infections of urethra and cervix; mild to moderate skin and skin-structure infections; complicated urinary tract infections; and prostatitis. The quinolones include: **nalidixic acid** (NegGram), **cinoxacin** (Cinobac), **norfloxacin** (Noroxin), and **ciprofloxacin** (Cipro). Other members of the quinolone family are **pefloxacin, ofloxacin, enoxacin**, and **fleroxacin**. The bacterial enzyme **DNA gyrase** is responsible for the continuous introduction of negative supercoils into DNA, and the quinolones inhibit this gyrase-mediated DNA supercoiling (see Figure 77).

Nalidixic acid and **cinoxacin** are bactericidal against Gram-negative organisms that cause urinary tract infections. The fluoroquinolones are bactericidal and considerably more potent against *Escherichia coli* and various species of *Salmonella, Shigella, Enterobacter, Campylobacter*, and *Neisseria*. Ciprofloxacin also has good activity against staphylococci, including methicillin-resistant strains.

The quinolones and fluoroquinolones may produce arthropathy, and hence should not be used in prepubertal children or pregnant women.

Nalidixic acid and **cinoxacin** are useful only for treating urinary tract infections. **Ciprofloxacin** is useful for both urinary tract infections and prostatitis.

OLANZAPINE

Olanzapine, a novel atypical antipsychotic, has properties similar to those exhibited by **clozapine** (see also Table 23).

OLSALAZINE SODIUM

(Dipentum)

Olsalazine (1 g/day in 2 divided doses) is indicated for maintenance of remission of ulcerative colitis in patients intolerant to sulfasalazine (see Figure 82). Olsalazine sodium is a sodium salt of a salicylate compound that is effectively bioconverted to 5-aminosalicylic acid (mesalamine; 5-ASA), which has antiinflammatory activity in ulcerative colitis. Approximately

98 to 99% of an oral dose will reach the colon where each molecule is rapidly converted into two molecules of 5-ASA by colonic bacteria and the low prevailing redox potential found in this environment. More than 0.9 g mesalamine would usually be made available in the colon from 1 g olsalazine. The liberated 5-ASA is absorbed slowly, resulting in very high local concentrations in the colon.

The mechanism of action of mesalamine is unknown, but appears to be topical rather than systemic. It is possible that mesalamine diminishes colonic inflammation by blocking cyclooxygenase and inhibiting colon prostaglandin production in the bowel mucosa.

Symptoms of acute toxicity from olsalazine include diarrhea, vomiting, and decreased motor activity.

OMEGA-CONOTOXIN

Under normal conditions, the extracellular concentration of calcium is in the millimolar range (10^{-3} M), whereas its intracellular concentration is less than 10^{-7} M. The cytoplasmic concentration of calcium is increased through the actions of **receptor-operated channels, voltage-activated channels**, or **ionic pumps**. In addition, calcium can be released from internal stores.

There are two types of voltage-activated channels:

1. **Low-voltage-activated channels** or low-threshold channels, which are also termed T-type channels.
2. **High-voltage-activated channels**, which are further subdivided into L-type, N-type, and P-type channels.

T-Type Channels

T-type calcium channels (with the t standing for "transient") require only a weak depolarization for activation and carry a transient current at negative membrane potentials that inactivates rapidly during a prolonged pulse. In neurons, the T-type channel is responsible for neuronal oscillatory activity and is thought to play a role in the regulation of wakefulness and motor coordination. The pyrazine diuretic, **amiloride**, inhibits the T-type calcium channel.

L-Type Channels

L-type calcium channels (with the l standing for "long lasting") exist in high numbers in the skeletal muscle and require a large depolarization for activation to take place. The channels are phosphorylated prior to opening. Each channel is composed of **five subunits**: $alpha_1$, (molecular weight [MW] = 175 kDa), $alpha_2$ (MW = 143 kDa), beta (MW = 54 kDa), gamma (MW = 30 kDa), and delta (MW = 27 kDa). The $alpha_1$ and beta subunits contain phosphorylation sites for cyclic adenosine monophosphate (AMP)-dependent protein kinase. The $alpha_1$ subunit contains the **dihydropyridine**-binding sites. The L-type calcium channel is involved in the **generation of action potentials** and in **signal transduction** at the cell membrane.

N-Type Channels

The N-type calcium channel (with the n standing for "neither T nor L or neuronal") appears to convey most of the whole-cell calcium current; it is insensitive to dihydropyridine and is blocked by **omega-conotoxin**. The N-type channel is involved in the **release of transmitter** in some, but not all, tissues, with central nervous system (CNS) neurons the exception.

P-Type Channels

The P-type channels were first observed in the Purkinje cells and are inhibited by a toxin derived from a funnel-web spider poison, but not by other calcium channel-blocking agents. P-type channels are widely distributed throughout the CNS and are thought to participate in the generation of **intrinsic activity** as well as serve as modulators of **neuronal integration** and **transmitter release**.

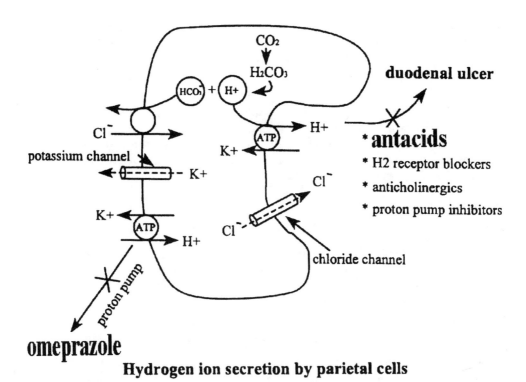

Hydrogen ion secretion by parietal cells

FIGURE 63 Omeprazole inhibits the activity of the acid (proton) pump H+/K+ adenosine triphosphate (ATPase) located at the secretory surface of the gastric parietal cells. (Adapted from Ebadi, M., *Pharmacology, An Illustrated Review with Questions and Answers*, 3rd Edition, Lippincott-Raven Press, Philadelphia, 1996.)

OMEPRAZOLE

(Prilosec)

Omeprazole (20 mg daily for 4 to 8 weeks) is indicated for active duodenal ulcer, gastroe-sophageal reflux disease, and pathological hypersecretory conditions such as Zollinger-Ellison syndrome, multiple endocrine adenomas, and systemic mastocytosis.

Omeprazole belongs to a new class of antisecretory compounds, the substituted benzimida-zoles, that do not exhibit anticholinergic or H_2 histamine antagonistic properties, but that suppress gastric acid secretion by specific inhibition of the H+/K+ ATPase enzyme system at the secretory surface of the gastric parietal cell. Because this enzyme system is the "acid (proton) pump" within the gastric mucosa, omeprazole has been characterized as a gastric acid pump inhibitor; it blocks the final step of acid production. This effect is dose-related and inhibits both basal and stimulated acid secretion irrespective of the stimulus (see Figure 63).

Omeprazole increases the half-life of diazepam by inhibiting its metabolism and reduces the plasma clearance of phenytoin and warfarin.

ONCOGENES

Tumor markers have been used for screening, diagnosing, establishing prognosis, monitoring treatment, and detecting the recurrence of tumors. For example, the measurement of **human chorionic gonadotropin** is used as a marker in patients with high-risk gestational trophoblastic tumors, **alpha-fetoprotein** for hepatocellular carcinoma, **carcinoembryonic antigen** for colon cancer, and **prostatic acid phosphatase** and **prostate-specific antigen** for prostate cancer. In addition, the application of monoclonal antibodies, DNA content analysis, DNA hybridization techniques, and cytogenic analysis has added new dimensions to the diagnosis and classification of hematologic malignancies.

Biotechnologic innovations have fostered the exploitation of **oncogenes** as novel therapeutic targets for the diagnosis, prognosis, and treatment of cancer. The advent of **magnetic resonance imaging** has also advanced the ability to noninvasively visualize smaller pituitary adenomas, and the introduction of computed tomography has led to improvements in the chemotherapy of malignant **mesothelioma**.

ONDANSETRON HYDROCHLORIDE

(Zofran)

Ondansetron, a serotonin (5-HT$_3$) receptor antagonist (0.15 mg/kg IV with the first dose taken infused every 15 minutes before the start of chemotherapy), is used in the prevention of nausea and vomiting associated with initial and repeat courses of emetogenic cancer chemotherapy, including high-dose cisplatin (see Figure 64).

Ondansetron, granisetron, tropisetron, and batanopride are antagonists of the 5-HT$_3$ receptor, and are considered effective in controlling cancer chemotherapy-induced emesis.

Ondansetron is not a dopamine-receptor antagonist. Because serotonin receptors of the 5-HT$_3$ type are present both peripherally on vagal nerve terminals and centrally in the chemoreceptor trigger zone, it is not certain if ondansetron's antiemetic action is mediated centrally, peripherally, or in both sites (see Figure 64).

Ondansetron is metabolized by cytochrome P450; thus, inducers or inhibitors of this enzyme may change the clearance and half-life of ondansetron; however, no dosage adjustment is required. Cisplatin, carmustine, and etoposide do not affect ondansetron's pharmacokinetics.

OPIOID PEPTIDES	
Endogenous Opioid Peptides	
[Leu^5]enkephalin	Tyr-Gly-Gly-Phe-Leu
[Met^5]enkephalin	Tyr-Gly-Gly-Phe-Met
Dynorphin A	Tyr-Gly-Gly-Phe-Leu-Arg-Arg-Ile-Arg-Pro-Lys-Leu-Lys-Trp-Asp-Asn-Gln
Dynorphin B	Tyr-Gly-Gly-Phe-Leu-Arg-Arg-Gln-Phe-Lys-Val-Val-Thr
α-Neoendorphin	Tyr-Gly-Gly-Phe-Leu-Arg-Lys-Tyr-Pro-Lys
β-Neoendorphin	Tyr-Gly-Gly-Phe-Leu-Arg-Lys-Tyr-Pro
β$_h$-Endorphin	Tyr-Gly-Gly-Phe-Met-Thr-Ser-Glu-Lys-Ser-Gln-Thr-Pro-Leu-Val-Thr-Leu-Phe-Lys-Asn-Ala-Ile-Ile-Lys-Asn-Ala-Tyr-Lys-Lys-Gly-Glu
Synthetic Opioid Peptides	
DAMGO	[D-Ala^2,MePhe^4,Gly(ol)^5]enkephalin
DPDPE	[D-Pen^2,D-Pen^5]enkephalin
DSLET	[D-Ser^2,Leu^5]enkephalin-Thr^6
DADL	[D-Ala^2,D-Leu^5]enkephalin
CTOP	D-Phe-Cys-Tyr-D-Trp-Orn-Thr-Pen-Thr-NH$_2$
FK-33824	[D-Ala^2,N-MePhe^4,Met(O)^5-ol]enkephalin
[D-Ala^2]Deltorphin I	Tyr-D-Ala-Phe-Asp-Val-Val-Gly-NH$_2$

[D-Ala²,Glu⁴]Deltorphin (Deltorphin II)	Tyr-D-Ala-Phe-Glu-Val-Val-Gly-NH₂
Morphiceptin	Tyr-Pro-Phe-Pro-NH₂
PL-017	Tyr-Pro-MePhe-D-Pro-NH₂
DALCE	[D-Ala²,Leu⁵,Cys⁶]enkephalin

OPIOIDS: RECEPTOR AGONISTS AND ANTAGONISTS		
Receptor Agonists		
Buprenorphine	Hydromorphine	Nalmefene
Butorphanol	Levallorphan	Nalorphine
Codeine	Levorphanol	Oxycodone
Drocode	Meperidine	Oxymorphone
Fentanyl	Methadone	Pentazocine
Heroin	Morphine	Propoxyphene
Hydrocodone	Nalbuphine	
Receptor Antagonists		
Naloxone		
Naltrexone		

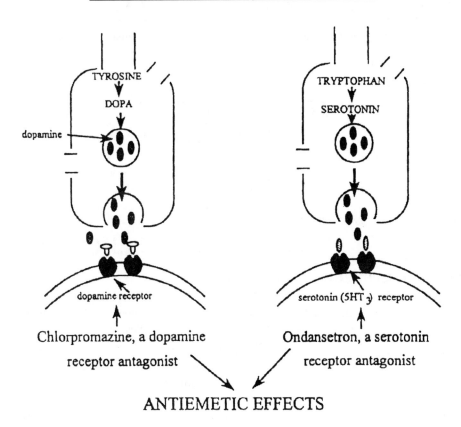

Chlorpromazine, a dopamine receptor antagonist

Ondansetron, a serotonin receptor antagonist

ANTIEMETIC EFFECTS

FIGURE 64 Selective antagonists of the serotonin type 3 (5-HT3) receptor such as **batanopride, granisetron, ondansetron,** or **zacopride** have been shown to be potent antiemetic agents in patients receiving cytotoxic chemotherapy, with efficacy comparable to or superior to that of conventional antiemetics. (Adapted from Ebadi, M., *Pharmacology, An Illustrated Review with Questions and Answers*, 3rd Edition, Lippincott-Raven Press, Philadelphia, 1996.)

OPIATE TINCTURE, CAMPHORATED
(Paregoric)

Opium tincture is used in acute and nonspecific diarrhea.

OPIUM ALKALOIDS

The **opium alkaloids**, which are obtained from *Papaver somniferum*, contain two groups of compounds: compounds with **phenanthrene derivatives**, consisting of morphine (1 to 10%), codeine (0.7 to 2.5%), and thebaine (0.5 to 1.5%), and compounds with **isoquinoline derivatives**, consisting of papaverine (1%) and noscapine (5 to 10%).

Narcotics are divided into naturally occurring, semisynthetic, and synthetic derivatives. The **naturally occurring analgesics** consist of morphine and codeine (methylmorphine). The **semisynthetic analgesics** include hydromorphine (Dilaudid) and hydrocodone (Dicodid). The **synthetic analgesics** consist of meperidine (Demerol), alphaprodine (Nisentil), methadone (Dolophine), propoxyphene (Darvon), and pentazocine (Talwin).

The **narcotic antagonists** are nalorphine (Nalline), naloxone (Narcan), and naltrexone (Trexan). Dextromethorphan (Romilar) is used as an antitussive preparation; apomorphine is used as an **emetic** agent.

Narcotic analgesics may have either a **high potency** (morphine, hydromorphone, oxymorphone, methadone, meperidine, fentanyl, and levorphanol) or **low potency** (codeine, oxycodone, hydrocodone, propoxyphene, and diphenoxylate). These agents may be a pure agonist (morphine), pure antagonist (naloxone), or mixed agonist-antagonist (pentazocine).

OPIUM TINCTURE
(Laudanum)

ORAL HYPOGLYCEMIC AGENTS
First-Generation Agents
Acetohexamide
Chlorpropamide
Tolazamide
Tolbutamide
Second-Generation Agents
Glipizide
Glyburide

ORGANOPHOSPHOROUS COMPOUNDS

The cholinesterase inhibitors are divided into two categories: **organophosphorous compounds**, such as parathion, malathion, and tetraethyl pyrophosphate (TEPP), and the **carbamates**, such as naphthyl-N-methyl carbamate (carbaryl and Sevin).

The clinical manifestations of acute and severe poisoning from the organophosphorous insecticides include **cholinergic crisis**, resulting from the stimulation of muscarine cholinergic receptors (bronchoconstriction, salivation, sweating, lacrimation, bradycardia, hypotension, and urinary and fecal incontinence), from the stimulation of nicotinic cholinergic receptors (muscular fasciculation), and from CNS effects (with initial restlessness, tremors, ataxia, and convulsions, followed by CNS depression and respiratory and circulatory depression). The treatment of a cholinergic crisis caused by organophosphorous compounds includes the administration of a cholinesterase reactivator such as pralidoxine (2-PAM) together with atropine. The poisoning stemming from antidoting with 2-PAM can be avoided in the event of carbaryl toxicity, because this agent is a reversible cholinesterase inhibitor (see Figure 71).

ORPHAN DRUGS: PROPOSED USES OF		
Acetylcysteine	for	Acetaminophen overdose
N-Acetylprocainamide	for	Arrhythmia
Aconiazide	for	Tuberculosis
Adenosine	with	BCNU for treatment of brain tumors
Aldesleukin	for	Metastatic renal cell carcinoma
Alglucerase	for	Gaucher's disease type 1
Allopurinol riboside	for	Chagas' disease
Allopurinol sodium	for	Leukemia and lymphoma
L-Alpha-acetyl-methadol (LAAM)	for	Addiction to narcotics
Alpha-1-antitrypsin (recombinant DNA origin)	for	Alpha-1 antitrypsin deficiency
Alpha-galactosidase A (FABRase)	for	Fabry's disease
Alpha-1-proteinase inhibitor	for	Replacement therapy in the alpha-1-proteinase inhibitor congenital deficiency state
Altretamine	for	Ovarian adenocarcinoma
Amiloride HCl	for	Cystic fibrosis
4-Aminopyridine	for	Multiple sclerosis
Aminosalicylate sodium	for	Crohn's disease
4-Aminosalicylic acid	for	Ulcerative colitis
Aminosidine	for	*Mycobacterium avium* complex
Amiodarone	for	Ventricular tachycardia
Ammonium tetrathiomolybdate	for	Wilson's disease
Amphotericin B lipid complex	for	Cryptococcal meningitis
Amsacrine	for	Leukemia
Anagrelide	for	Polycythemia vera
Ananain, Comosain	for	Enzymatic debridement of severe burns
Anaritide acetate	for	Improving renal functions following transplantation
Ancrod	for	Antithrombotic effects
Antiepilepsirine	for	Epilepsy
Antihemophilic factor	for	Von Willebrand's disease
Antihemophilic factor	for	Hemophilia
Autolymphocyte therapy; ALT	for	Renal cancer
Antimelanoma antibody	for	Imaging melanoma metastasis
Anti-pan T lymphocyte monoclonal antibody (Anti-T)	for	Bone marrow recipients
Antipyrine	for	Diagnostic agent for hepatic function
Anti-Tac	for	Bone marrow transplantation
Anti-TAP-72 immunotoxin	for	Colorectal cancer
Antithrombin III	for	Thromboembolic episodes in genetic AT-III deficiency
Anti-thymocyte serum	for	Transplantation
Antivenin	for	Treatment of snake envenomations
Apomorphine HCl	for	Parkinson's disease

ORPHAN DRUGS: PROPOSED USES OF

Aprotinin	for	Patients undergoing repeat coronary artery bypass graft (CABG) surgery
Arginine butyrate	for	Treatment of beta-hemoglobinopathies
Atovaquone	for	AIDS-associated *Pneumocystis carinii* pneumonia (PCP)
Bacitracin	for	Pseudomembranous enterocolitis
Baclofen, L-Baclofen	for	Spasticity
Benzoate and phenylacetate	for	Prevention of hyperammonemia
Benzylpenicillin	to	Test hypersensitivity to penicillin
Beractant	to	Prevent respiratory distress syndrome in the newborn
Beta-glucocerebrosidase	for	Gaucher's disease
Betaine	for	Homocystinuria
Bethanidine sulfate	for	Prevention of ventricular fibrillation
Biodegradable polymer implant containing carmustine	for	Treatment of malignant glioma
Bispecific antibody 520C9x22	for	Ovarian cancer
Bleomycin sulfate	for	Pleural effusion
Botulinum toxin type A	for	Dystonia
Botulinum toxin type B	for	Cervical dystonia
Botulinum toxin type F	for	Torticollis and blepharospasm
Botulism immune globulin	for	Botulism
Bovine colostrum	for	AIDS-related diarrhea
Bovine whey protein concentrate (Immuno-C)	for	Cryptosporidiosis
Branched chain amino acids	for	Amyotrophic lateral sclerosis
Bromhexine	for	Keratoconjunctivitis sicca in Sjogren's syndrome
Busulfan	for	Malignancies
Butyrylcholinesterase	for	Cocaine toxicity
BW 12C	for	Sickle cell disease
C1-Esterase-inhibitor	for	Hereditary angioedema
Caffeine	for	Apnea
Calcitonin	for	Paget's disease
Calcium acetate	for	Hyperphosphatemia
Calcium carbonate	for	Hyperphosphatemia
Calcium gluconate gel	for	Treatment of hydrogen fluoride (hydrofluoric acid) burns
Carbovir	for	AIDS
CCD 1042	for	Infantile spasms
CD4 human truncated 369 AA polypeptide	for	AIDS
CD4 immunoglobulin G, recombinant human	for	AIDS
CD5-T lymphocyte immunotoxin	for	Bone marrow transplants
CD-45 monoclonal antibodies	for	Organ transplants
Ceramide trihexosidase alpha-galactosidase A	for	Fabry's disease
Chenodiol	for	Gallbladder stones
Chimeric M-T412 IgG monoclonal anti-CD4	for	Multiple sclerosis

Chimeric (murine variable, human constant) Mab to CD20	for	Non-Hodgkin's B-cell lymphoma
Chlorhexidine gluconate mouth rinse	for	Oral mucositis
Choline chloride	for	Choline deficiency
Ciliary neurotrophic factor	for	Amyotrophic lateral sclerosis
Citric acid, glucono-delta-lactone and mag carbonate	for	Renal and bladder calculi
Cladribine	for	Hairy-cell and chronic lymphocytic leukemias; non-Hodgkin's lymphoma; chronic multiple sclerosis
Clindamycin	for	*Pneumocystis carinii* pneumonia associated with AIDS
Clofazimine	for	Lepromatous leprosy
Clonidine HCl	for	Treating pain in cancer
Coagulation factor IX	for	Hemophilia B
Colchicine	for	Multiple sclerosis
Colfosceril palmitate, cetyl alcohol, tyloxapol	for	Hyaline membrane disease
Copolymer 1, (COP 1)	for	Multiple sclerosis
Corticorelin ovine triflutate	to	Diagnose ACTH-dependent Cushing's syndrome
Cromolyn sodium	for	Mastocytosis
Cromolyn sodium 4% ophthalmic solution	for	Vernal keratoconjunctivitis
Cryptosporidium hyperimmune bovine colostrum IgG concentrate	for	Diarrhea in AIDS
Cryptosporidium parvum bovine immunoglobulin concentrate	for	Treatment of *Cryptosporidium parvum* infection of the GI tract in immunocompromised patients
CY-1503	for	Post-ischemic pulmonary reperfusion edema
CY-1899	for	Hepatitis B infection
L-Cycloserine	for	Gaucher's disease
Cyclosporine ophthalmic	for	Keratoconjunctivitis sicca with Sjogren's syndrome
Cyclosporine 2% ophthalmic ointment	following	Keratoplasty
Cyproterone acetate	for	Hirsutism
Cysteamine	for	Nephrophatic cystinosis
L-Cysteine	in	Erythropoietic protoporphyria
Cystic fibrosis gene therapy	in	Cystic fibrosis
Cytarabine	for	Neoplastic meningitis
Cytomegalovirus immune globulin	for	Immunosuppressed recipients of organ transplants
Cytomegalovirus immune globulin (human) IV	with	Ganciclovir sodium for the treatment of CMV pneumonia in bone marrow transplant patients
Dapsone	for	Prophylaxis of *Pneumocystis carinii* pneumonia
Defibrotide	for	Thrombocytopenic purpura
Dehydrex	for	Corneal erosion
Deoxyadenosine, 2-chloro-2′	for	Acute myeloid leukemia
Deoxycytidine, 5-AZA-2′	for	Acute leukemia
Deslorelin	for	Precocious puberty
Desmopressin acetate	for	Hemophilia A and von Willebrand's disease
Dexrazoxane	for	Prevention of doxorubicin-induced cardiomyopathy
Dextran and deferoxamine	for	Iron poisoning

ORPHAN DRUGS: PROPOSED USES OF

Dextran sulfate	for	Cystic fibrosis
Dextran sulfate sodium	for	AIDS
3,4-Diaminopyridine	for	Lambert-Eaton myasthenic syndrome
Dianeal PD-2 peritoneal dialysis soln. with 1.1% amino acid	for	Malnutrition in peritoneal dialysis
Diazepam	for	Status epilepticus
Dibromodulcitol	for	Metastatic squamous cervical carcinoma
Dichloroacetate sodium	for	Lactic acidosis
Diethyldithiocarbamate	for	AIDS
Digoxin immune fab	for	Digitalis intoxication
Dihematoporphyrin ether	for	Therapy of transitional cell carcinoma
24,25 Dihydroxycholecalciferol	for	Uremic osteodystrophy
Dipalmitoylphosphatidylcholine/phosphatidyl-glycerol	for	Neonatal respiratory distress syndrome
Disaccharide tripeptide glycerol dipalmitoyl	for	Pulmonary and hepatic metastases in colorectal adenocarcinoma
Disodium clodronate	for	Hypercalcemia of malignancy
Disodium clodronate tetrahydrate	for	Malignancy-induced bone resorption
Disodium silibinin dihemisuccinate	for	Mushroom poisoning
Dornase (deoxyribonuclease, recombinant human; rhDNase)	for	Cystic fibrosis
Dronabinol	to	Stimulate appetite in AIDS
Dynamine	for	Lambert-Eaton myasthenic syndrome and Charcot-Marie-tooth disease
Eflornithine HCl	for	*Trypanosoma brucei gambiense* (sleeping sickness); *Pneumocystis carinii* pneumonia in AIDS
Enisoprost	with	Cyclosporine in organ transplant recipients
Epidermal growth factor	for	Corneal epithelial regeneration and healing
Epoetin alfa	for	Anemia associated with end-stage renal disease
Epoetin beta	for	Anemia associated with end-stage renal disease
Epoprostenol	for	Primary pulmonary hypertension
Erwinia L-asparaginase	for	Acute lymphocytic leukemia
Erythropoietin	for	Anemia related to HIV infection or anemia associated with end-stage renal disease; anemia of premature infants
Ethanolamine oleate	for	Esophageal varices
Ethinyl estradiol	for	Turner's syndrome
Ethiofos	as	A chemoprotective agent for cisplatin and cyclophosphamide
Etidronate disodium	for	Hypercalcemia of malignancy
Factor VII-a recombinant, DNA origin	for	Hemophilia A and B
Factor XIII	for	Congenital factor XIII deficiency
Felbamate	for	Lennox-Gastaut syndrome
FGN-1	for	Colonic adenomatous polyps
FIAU	for	Treatment of hepatitis B

Fibronectin	for	Corneal ulcers
Filgrastim	for	Myelodysplastic syndrome
Fire ant venom	for	Diagnosing allergy to fire ant
Fludarabine phosphate	for	Non-Hodgkin's lymphoma
Flumecinol	for	Hyperbilirubinemia in newborns unresponsive to phototherapy
Flunarizine	for	Hemiplegia
Fluorouracil	with	Interferon alpha-2a for esophageal colorectal carcinoma
Fluorouracil	with	Leucovorin for metastatic adenocarcinoma of the colon and rectum
Fosphenytoin	for	Status epilepticus
Gallium nitrate injection	for	Hypercalcemia of malignancy
Gangliosides	for	Retinitis pigmentosa
Gelsolin	for	Cystic fibrosis
Gentamicin	for	Osteomyelitis
Glucocerebrosidase	for	Gaucher's disease
L-Glutathione	for	Cachexia
Gonadorelin acetate	to	Induce ovulation
Gossypol	for	Cancer of the adrenal cortex
Granulocyte macrophage colony-stimulating factor	for	AIDS
Growth hormone releasing factor	for	Children who have failed to grow
Guanethidine monosulfate	for	Sympathetic dystrophy and causalgia
Halofantrine	for	Malaria
Heme arginate	for	Acute porphyria; myelodysplastic syndromes
Hemin	for	Porphyria variegata and heredita coproporphyria
Hemin and zinc mesoporphyrin	for	Acute porphyric syndromes
Heparin, 2-0-desulfated	for	Cystic fibrosis
Herpes simplex virus gene	for	Primary and metastatic brain tumors
Histrelin	for	Treatment of acute intermittent porphyria, hereditary coproporphyria, and variegata porphyria
Histrelin acetate	for	Precocious puberty
HIV-neutralizing antibodies	for	AIDS
Human immunodeficiency virus immune globulin	for	AIDS
Hydroxocobalamin/sodium thiosulfate	for	Cyanide poisoning
L-5 Hydroxytryptophan	for	Myoclonus
Hydroxyurea	for	Sickle cell anemia
I-131 radiolabeled B1 monoclonal antibody	for	Non-Hodgkin's B-cell lymphoma
Idarubicin HCl	for	Myelodysplastic syndromes
Ifosfamide	for	Germ-cell testicular cancer; bone sarcomas; soft tissue sarcomas
Iloprost infusion solution	for	Raynaud's phenomenon secondary to systemic sclerosis
Imciromab pentetate	for	Cardiac transplants

ORPHAN DRUGS: PROPOSED USES OF

Immune globulin IV	for	Juvenile rheumatoid arthritis; polymyositis/dermatomyositis; infection prophylaxis in pediatric patients with HIV; acute myocarditis
Indium in 111 altumomab pentetate	for	Tumor detection
Indium in 111 murine monoclonal antibody fab to myosin	for	Diagnosis of myocarditis
Inosine pranobex	for	Subacute sclerosing panencephalitis
Insulin-like growth factor-1	for	Amyotrophic lateral sclerosis
Interferon alfa-2a	for	Chronic myelogenous leukemia
Interferon alfa-2a	with	Fluorouracil for advanced colorectal cancer and esophageal carcinoma
Interferon alfa-2a	with	Teceleukin for metastatic malignant melanoma and renal-cell carcinoma
Interferon alfa-2b	for	AIDS-related Kaposi's sarcoma; acute hepatitis B; chronic myelogenous leukemia
Interferon alfa-NL	for	AIDS-related Kaposi's sarcoma
Interferon beta	for	Multiple sclerosis
Interferon beta	for	Cutaneous T-cell lymphoma; malignant melanoma; metastatic renal-cell carcinoma
Interferon gamma 1-B	for	Chronic granulomatous disease
Interleukin-1 alpha	for	Bone marrow transplantation
Interleukin-1 receptor antagonist	for	Juvenile rheumatoid arthritis
Interleukin-2	for	Cancers of the kidney
Interleukin-3	for	Promotion of erythropoiesis
Iodine I-123 murine monoclonal antibody to alpha-fetoprotein	to	Detect alpha-fetoprotein-producing germ-cell tumors
Iodine I-123 murine monoclonal antibody to hCG	for	Detection of hCG-producing tumors
Iodine I-131 6B-iodomethyl-19-norcholesterol	for	Adrenal cortical imaging
Iodine I-131 metaiodobenzylguanidine sulfate	for	Diagnosis of pheochromocytoma
Iodine I-131 murine monoclonal antibody IgG2a to B cell	for	B-cell lymphoma and B-cell leukemia
Isobutyramide	for	Sickle cell disease; beta-thalassemia; beta-hemoglobinopathies; beta-thalassemia syndromes
Ketoconazole	with	Cyclosporine in organ transplantation
Lactobin	in	AIDS-associated diarrhea
Leucovorin	with	Methotrexate in the treatment of osteosarcoma
Leucovorin	with	5-Fluorouracil for metastatic colorectal cancer
Leukocyte protease inhibitor	for	Congenital alpha-1 antitrypsin deficiency; cystic fibrosis
Leukocyte protease inhibitor	for	Bronchopulmonary dysplasia
Leupeptin	to	Repair peripheral nerve
Leuprolide acetate	for	Precocious puberty
Levocarnitine	for	Carnitine deficiency
Levomethadyl acetate HCl	for	Addiction to narcotics
Liothyronine sodium injection	for	Myxedema coma

Lodoxamide tromethamine	for	Vernal keratoconjunctivitis
Loxoribine	for	Immunodeficiency
Mafenide acetate solution	for	Prevention of graft loss
Matrix metalloproteinase inhibitor	for	Corneal ulcers
Mazindol	for	Duchenne muscular dystrophy
Mefloquine HCl	for	Malaria
Megestrol acetate	for	Anorexia, cachexia or significant weight loss due to AIDS
Melanoma vaccine	for	Melanoma
Melatonin	for	Sleep disorders in blind people
Melphalan	for	Multiple myeloma
Mesna	for	Reducing ifosfamide-induced hemorrhagic cystitis
Methotrexate	for	Juvenile rheumatoid arthritis
Methotrexate sodium	for	Osteogenic sarcoma
Methotrexate with laurocapram	for	Topical treatment of *Mycosis fungoides*
8-Methoxsalen	in	Conjunction with UVAR diffuse systemic sclerosis; prevention of acute rejection of cardiac allografts
6-Methylenandrosta-1,4-diene-3,17-dione	for	Metastatic carcinoma of the breast
4-Methylpyrazole	for	Ethylene glycol poisoning
Metronidazole (topical)	for	Decubitus ulcers; acne rosacea; perioral dermatitis
Microbubble contrast agents	for	Diagnosing intracranial tumors
Midodrine HCl	for	Orthostatic hypotension
Minocycline HCl	for	Malignant pleural effusion
Mitoguazone	for	Non-Hodgkin's lymphoma
Mitoxantrone HCl	for	Acute myelogenous leukemia
Modafinil	for	Narcolepsy
Monoclonal antibodies B-cell lymphoma	for	B-cell lymphoma
Monoclonal antibodies PM-81	for	Acute myelogenous leukemia
Monoclonal antibody 17-1A	for	Pancreatic cancer
Monoclonal antibody to CD4, 5a8	for	Prophylaxis for exposure to HIV
Monoclonal antibody against hepatitis B virus	for	Prophylaxis of hepatitis B reinfection
Monoclonal antibody for lupus nephritis	for	Immunization against lupus nephritis
Monolaurin	for	Congenital primary ichthyosis
Monomercaptoundecahydrocloso-DO decaborate sodium	for	Glioblastoma multiforme
Monoctanoin	for	Dissolution of cholesterol gallstones
Morphine sulfate concentrate	for	Intraspinal administration for intractable chronic pain
Multi-vitamin infusion	for	Parenteral nutrition in low birth weight infants
Myelin	for	Multiple sclerosis
Mytomycin-C	for	Refractory glaucoma
Nafarelin acetate	for	Precocious puberty
Naltrexone HCl	for	Opioid addiction
Nebacumab	for	Opioid-dependent
NG-29	for	Diagnosis of pituitary function
Nifedipine	for	Interstitial cystitis

ORPHAN DRUGS: PROPOSED USES OF

Nitric oxide	for	Pulmonary hypertension
Ofloxacin solution	for	Bacterial corneal ulcers
OM 401	for	Sickle cell disease
OncoRad OV103	for	Ovarian cancer
Oxaliplatin	for	Ovarian cancer
Oxandrolone	for	Turner's syndrome
L-2-Oxothiazolidine-4-carboxylic acid	for	Respiratory distress syndrome
Oxymorphone HCl	for	Relief of severe intractable pain in narcotic-tolerant patients
Papaverine topical gel	for	Sexual dysfunction in spinal cord injury patients
Para-aminosalicylic acid	for	Tuberculosis
Pegademase bovine	for	Severe combined immunodeficiency (SCID)
Pegaspargase	for	Acute lymphocytic leukemia
PEG-Glucocerebrosidase	for	Gaucher's disease
PEG-interleukin-2	for	Immunodeficiencies associated with T-cell defects
PEG-L-asparaginase	for	Acute lymphocytic leukemia
Pentamidine isethionate	for	*Pneumocystis carinii* pneumonia (PCP)
Pentamidine isethionate (inhalation)	for	PCP prevention in high-risk patients
Pentastarch	as	An adjunct in leukapheresis
Pentosan sodium polysulfate	for	Interstitial cystitis
Pentostatin	for	Chronic lymphocytic leukemia
Perfosfamide	in	Bone marrow transplants
Phenylbutyrate sodium	for	Sickling disorders; urea cycle disorders: Carbamylphosphate synthetase deficiency, ornithine transcarbamylase deficiency, and argininosuccinic acid synthetase deficiency
Phosphocysteamine	for	Cystinosis
Physostigmine salicylate	for	Friedreich's ataxias
Pilocarpine HCl	for	Xerostomia and keratoconjunctivitis
Piracetam	for	Myoclonus
Piritrexim isethionate	for	Infection caused by *P. carinii, Toxoplasma gondii,* and *Mycobacterium avium*-intracellulare
Poloxamer 188	for	Sickle cell crisis
Poloxamer 331	for	Toxoplasmosis
Poly I: Poly C12U	for	Renal-cell carcinoma; invasive metastatic melanoma
Polymeric oxygen	for	Sickle cell anemia
Potassium citrate	for	Uric acid nephrolithiasis; calcium renal stones
PPI-002	for	Malignant mesothelioma
PR-122 (Redox-phenytoin)	for	Status epilepticus
PR-225 (Redox-acyclovir)	for	Herpes simplex encephalitis
PR-239 (Redox-penicillin G)	for	Neurosyphilis
PR-320 (Molecusolcarbamazepine)	for	Status epilepticus
Pramiracetam sulfate	for	Cognitive dysfunction
Prednimustine	for	Malignant non-Hodgkin's lymphomas

Primaquine phosphate	with	Clindamycin in the treatment of PCP associated with AIDS
Propamidine isethionate 0.1% ophthalmic soln.	for	Acanthamoeba keratitis
Prostaglandin E1 alpha-cyclodextrin	for	Peripheral arterial occlusive disease
Protein C concentrate	for	Congenital or acquired protein C deficiency
Protirelin	for	Respiratory distress syndrome associated with prematurity
Pseudomonas hyperimmune globulin (mucoid exopolysaccharide) (MEPIG)	for	Pulmonary *Pseudomonas aeruginosa* infections in cystic fibrosis
Pulmonary surfactant replacement	for	Infant respiratory distress syndrome
9-[3-pydidylmethyl]-9-deazaguanine	for	Cutaneous T-cell lymphoma
Respiratory syncytial virus immune globulin	for	Respiratory syncytial virus lower respiratory tract infections
Retinoic acid all-trans	for	Acute promyelocytic leukemia
Retinoic acid, 9-CIS	for	Acute promyelocytic leukemia
Rho(D) immune globulin	for	Immune thrombocytopenic purpura
Ribavirin	for	Hemorrhagic fever with renal syndrome
Ricin conjugated murine MCA (anti-MY9)	for	Acute myelogenous leukemia; myeloid leukemia
Rifabutin	for	Disseminated *Mycobacterium avium* complex disease
Rifampin	for	Tuberculosis
Rifampin, isoniazid, pyrazinamide	for	Tuberculosis
Riluzole	for	Amyotrophic lateral sclerosis
Roquinimex	for	Bone marrow transplantation in leukemic patients
Sargramostim	for	Neutropenia associated with bone marrow transplant
Satumomab pendetide	for	Diagnosis of ovarian carcinoma
SDZ MSL-109	for	Cytomegalovirus disease
Secalciferol	for	Familial hypophosphatemic rickets
Selegiline HCl	for	Neuroprotection in Parkinson's disease
Sermorelin acetate	for	Growth hormone deficiency
Serratia marcescens extract (polyribosomes)	for	Brain malignancies
Short chain fatty acid solution	for	Ulcerative colitis
SK&F 110679	for	Growth hormone deficiency
Sodium benzoate/sodium phenylacetate	for	Urea cycle disorders: Carbamylphosphate synthetase deficiency, ornithine transcarbamylase deficiency and argininosuccinic acid synthetase deficiency
Sodium/Gamma hydroxybutyrate	for	Narcolepsy
Sodium tetradecyl sulfate	for	Bleeding esophageal varices
Somatostatin	for	Non-operative management of secreting cutaneous fistulas of the stomach, duodenum, small intestine, or pancreas
Somatropin	for	Growth hormone deficiency
Sotalol HCl	for	Ventricular tachyarrhythmias
Streptococcus immune globulin group B	for	Disseminated Group B streptococcal infection
ST1-RTA immunotoxin (SR 44163)	for	Lymphocytic leukemia
Succimer	for	Kidney stones
Sucralfate	for	Oral mucositis and stomatitis
Sucrase	for	Sucrase-isomaltase deficiency

ORPHAN DRUGS: PROPOSED USES OF

Sulfadiazine	with	Pyrimethamine for *Toxoplasma gondii*
Superoxide dismutase	for	Protection of donor organ during operative procedures
T4 endonuclease V	for	Cutaneous neoplasma
Teceleukin	with	Interferon alfa-2a for metastatic renal-cell carcinoma and malignant melanoma
Technetium TC-99M antimelanoma murine monoclonal antibody	for	Imaging, metastases of malignant melanoma
Teniposide	for	Acute lymphocytic leukemia
Teriparatide	for	Hypocalcemia due to hypoparathyroidism
Terlipressin	for	Bleeding esophageal varices
Testosterone ointment 2%	for	Vulvar dystrophies
Testosterone sublingual	for	Constitutional delay of growth and puberty in boys
Thalidomide	for	Bone marrow transplantation
L-Threonine	for	Spasticity associated with familial spastic paraparesis; amyotrophic lateral sclerosis
Thymosin alpha-1	for	Active hepatitis B
Thyroid stimulating hormone (TSH)	for	Diagnosis of thyroid cancer
Tiopronin	for	Cystine nephrolithiasis
Tiratricol	with	Levothyroxine to suppress TSH in patients with thyroid cancer
Tizanidine HCl	for	Spasticity associated with multiple sclerosis and spinal cord injury
T-lymphotropic virus type III gp 160 antigens	for	AIDS
Topiramate	for	Lennox-Gastaut syndrome
Toremifene	for	Metastatic breast carcinoma
Tranexamic acid	for	Angioneurotic edema
Transforming growth factor-beta 2	for	Macular holes
Treosulfan	for	Ovarian cancer
Tretinoin	for	Squamous metaplasia of ocular surface epithelia
Tretinoin LF, IV	for	Leukemia
Trientine HCl	for	Wilson's disease
Trifluoroacetyladriamycin-14 valerate	for	Carcinoma of the urinary bladder
Trimetrexate glucuronate	for	Advanced non-small cell carcinoma of the lung
Triptorelin pamoate	for	Ovarian carcinoma
Trisaccharides A and B	for	Hemolytic disease of the newborn
Troleandomycin	for	Asthma
Tumor necrosis factor-binding protein I and II	for	AIDS
Urofollitropin	to	Induce ovulation
Urogastrone	for	Corneal transplant surgery
Ursodeoxycholic acid	for	Cirrhosis
Ursodiol	for	Cirrhosis
Zalcitabine	for	AIDS
Zidovudine	for	AIDS
Zinc acetate	for	Wilson's disease

OSTEOPOROSIS: TREATMENT OF

Osteoporosis is a systemic skeletal disease characterized by a low bone mass and microarchitectural deterioration of bone tissue, with a consequent increase in bone fragility and susceptibility to fracture. It is a major cause of mortality, morbidity, and medical expense worldwide.

In the last few years, the concept of whole-life prevention has emerged. Before menopause, the prevention of osteoporosis may be achieved by increasing the bone mass at maturity. As peak bone mass is influenced by environmental as well as genetic factors, the bone mass at skeletal maturity might be improved during childhood and adolescence and later, in the young adult, by exercise, calcium intake, avoidance of smoking, and/or alcohol, and correction of estrogen-deficiency states.

The treatment of established osteoporosis includes two different approaches in order to prevent the worsening of the bone loss. One uses therapeutic agents which reduce bone resorption, and the other consists in using compounds which can stimulate bone formation. Ideally, these treatments should not only stimulate bone formation and increase bone mass, but also restore a normal bone microarchitecture in order to decrease the occurrence of new fractures. Selective analogs of estrogen, such as **raloxifen** and **droloxifen**, might be alternatives to estrogen in the prevention of late postmenopausal bone loss.

ORPHENADRINE CITRATE

(Norflex)

Orphenadrine citrate, which possesses analgesic and anticholinergic actions (100 mg each morning and evening), is indicated as an adjunct to rest, physical therapy, and other measures for relief of discomfort associated with acute, painful musculoskeletal conditions including leg cramps. Because of its anticholinergic properties, orphenadrine is contraindicated in glaucoma, pyloric or duodenal obstruction, stenosing peptic ulcers, prostatic hypertrophy, obstruction of the bladder neck, cardiospasm (megaesophagus), and myasthenia gravis.

Orphenadrine's anticholinergic property is potentiated by amantadine. Orphenadrine antagonizes the effectiveness of haloperidol or chlorpromazine in managing schizophrenia. The adverse reactions, usually seen with higher than therapeutic doses, are primarily related to orphenadrine's anticholinergic properties and include dry mouth, tachycardia, palpitations, transient syncope, weakness, headache, dizziness, lightheadedness, confusion (in elderly patients), hallucinations, agitation, tremor, drowsiness, vomiting, nausea, constipation, gastric irritation, urinary hesitancy and retention, blurred vision, pupil dilation, and increased ocular tension.

OSMOTIC DIURETICS

The osmotic diuretics and related agents consist of **mannitol** (osmitrol), **urea** (Ureaphil), **glycerin** (glycerol, Osmoglyn), and **isosorbide** (Hydronol). Mannitol and urea are nonelectrolytes that are freely filterable and undergo very little or no metabolism or renal tubular resorption.

When given in sufficient quantities, these drugs increase the osmolarity of plasma and the amount of glomerular filtrate and renal tubular fluid. The presence of such a drug in the lumen prevents the resorption of much of the water, hence the urine volume is increased. They do not prevent the active resorption of sodium from the tubular fluid, but some additional sodium is excreted as a normal constituent of the increased volume of urine. Osmotic diuretics are not effective in removing the edematous fluid caused by sodium retention, but can maintain the flow of urine even when the GFR is decreased. Osmotic diuretics are given by intravenous infusion, in a hypertonic solution, and they are excreted by glomerular filtration.

The osmotic diuretics may be used for any of the following conditions:

In congestive glaucoma, to reduce intraocular pressure.

In neurosurgery, to reduce the pressure and volume of cerebrospinal fluid and hence decrease the intracranial pressure.

In acute renal failure, to maintain urine flow.

In drug poisoning, to prevent nephrotoxicity.

These agents should not be used in edematous states associated with diminished cardiac reserve, because any increase in the extracellular fluid volume constitutes a hazard.

OTITIS MEDIA: TREATMENT OF					
		Haemophilus influenzae		Moraxella catarrhalis	
Antibiotics*	Streptococcus pneumoniae	β-Lactamase		β-Lactamase	
		Negative	Positive	Negative	Positive
Penicillin V	+++++	0	0	0	0
Amoxicillin	++++++	++	0	++++++	0
Ampicillin	++++++	+	0	+++	0
Trimethoprim	+	++	+++	0	0
Sulfamethoxazole	+	++++	++	+	0
Cefaclor	+	+	+	+	+
Erythromycin estolate	+++	0	0	+	+
ethylsuccinate	+	0	0	+	+
* Spectrum of activity					

OTOTOXICITY: DRUG-INDUCED			
Antimicrobials			
Aminoglycosides	Clindamycin	Furazolidone	Rifampin
Antimalarials	Colistin	Metronidazole	Sulfonamides
Ampicillin	Cortimoxazole	Minocycline	Tetracycline
Capreomycin	Doxycycline	Paromomycin	Thiabendazole
Chloramphenicol	Erythromycin	Polymyxin B	Vancomycin
Salicylates and NSAIDs			
Loop diuretics			
Antitumor agents			
Miscellaneous			
Aminophylline	Haloperidol	Morphine	Propylthiouracil
Antihistamines	Levodopa	Penicillamine	Quinidine
Carbamazepine	Lidocaine	Pentazocine	Tocainide
Deferoxamine	Metaproterenol	Propranolol	Tricyclic antidepressants
Diazoxide	Molindone	Propoxyphene	Verapamil

The primary symptoms of drug-induced ototoxicity are the occasional to frequent cochlear signs of tinnitus and in most cases reversible hearing loss; and the vestibular signs of lightheadedness, nystagmus, ataxia, and vertigo.

OUABAIN

The most important and often-used drugs in the treatment of congestive heart failure are the cardiac glycosides, which may exist and occur naturally in the body. Unfortunately, the **margin of safety** for these drugs is very narrow (therapeutic index, 3.0). **Toxicity** can develop readily, and careful attention to the pharmacokinetic principles is absolutely crucial. The cardiac glycosides are obtained from numerous natural sources, including *Digitalis lanata* and *Digitalis purpurea* (white and purple fox-glove), squill (Mediterranean sea onion), oleander, lily of the valley, and other plants. Among the useful available cardiac glycosides are the following:

Digitalis purpurea	Digitalis lanata	Strophanthus gratus
Digitoxin	Digoxin	Ouabain
Digoxin	Lanatoside C	
Digitalis leaf	Deslanoside	

Of these, only digoxin and digitoxin and, to a certain extent, ouabain are used extensively (see Table 11 and Figure 32). Ouabain is a crystalline powder, slowly soluble in water (1:75) and alcohol (1:100) and is available in ampules.

There are only quantitative and no qualitative differences in the actions of any of the above listed digitalis preparations; i.e., they vary only in the rate, intensity, and duration of their action and not in its kind.

OVULATION: DRUGS TO INDUCE	
Categories	**Contents**
Menotropin	FSH and LH
Urofollitropin	FSH
Estrogen agonist/antagonist	Clomiphene citrate
Human chorionic gonadotropin (HCG)	HCG from human placenta
Synthetic GnRH	Gonadorelin acetate Gonadorelin HCl
Synthetic GnRH agonist/analog	Nafarelin acetate Leuprolide acetate Buserelin Goserelin acetate

OXACILLIN SODIUM

(Bactocill)

Oxacillin (500 mg every 4 to 6 hours for a minimum of 5 days) is indicated for the treatment of infections due to penicillinase-producing staphylococci. Furthermore, it may be used to initiate therapy when a staphylococcal infection is suspected (see Table 22).

Oxacillin is bactericidal; it adheres to bacterial penicillin-binding proteins, thus inhibiting bacterial cell wall synthesis. Oxacillin resists the effects of penicillinases — enzymes that inactivate penicillin — and is thus active against many strains of penicillinase-producing bacteria. This activity is most important against penicillinase-producing staphylococci; some strains may remain resistant. Oxacillin is also active against a few Gram-positive aerobic and anaerobic bacilli but has no significant effect on Gram-negative bacilli (see also Figure 65).

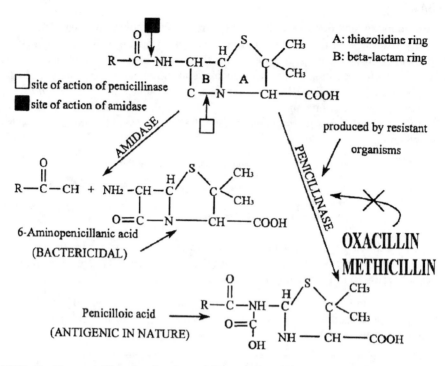

FIGURE 65   The **penicillinase-resistant penicillins** are **oxacillin, cloxacillin, dicloxacillin, methicillin,** and **nafcillin**. These agents are the drugs of choice for treating infections caused by penicillinase-producing *Staphylococci aureus*.

Oxacillin is absorbed rapidly but incompletely from the GI tract; it is stable in an acid environment. Peak serum concentrations occur within $\frac{1}{2}$ to 2 hours after an oral dose and 30 minutes after an IM dose. Food decreases absorption.

Oxacillin is distributed widely. CSF penetration is poor but enhanced by meningeal inflammation. Oxacillin crosses the placenta, and it is 89 to 94% protein-bound. Oxacillin is partially metabolized. Oxacillin and metabolites are excreted primarily in urine by renal tubular secretion and glomerular filtration; it is also excreted in breast milk and in small amounts in bile. Elimination half-life in adults is $\frac{1}{2}$ to 1 hour, extending to 2 hours in severe renal impairment. Dosage adjustments are not required in patients with renal impairment. Concomitant use of oxacillin with aminoglycosides produces synergistic bactericidal effects against *Staphylococcus aureus*. However, the drugs are physically and chemically incompatible and are inactivated when mixed or given together. *In vivo* inactivation has been reported when aminoglycosides and penicillins are used concomitantly. Probenecid blocks renal tubular secretion of penicillins, raising their serum levels. Clinical signs of overdose include neuromuscular sensitivity or seizures.

OXAMNIQUINE

(Vansil)

Oxamniquine, a tetrahydroquinolone with antihelmintic properties, is used in schistosomiasis caused by *Schistosoma mansoni*.

Oxamniquine, which is absorbed following oral administration, is very effective only in *Schistosoma mansoni*. Following treatment, the *S. mansoni* shifts from the mesenteric veins to the liver, where it is destroyed. The male *S. mansoni* is more susceptible to this killing effect than the female, but this will prevent the production of eggs at any rate.

OXANDROLONE
(Oxandrin)

Oxandrolone, an anabolic steroid (2.5 mg 2 to 4 times daily), is indicated as an adjunctive therapy to promote weight gain after weight loss following extensive surgery, chronic infections, or severe trauma, and in some patients who fail to gain or maintain normal weight; to offset the protein catabolism associated with prolonged administration of corticosteroids; for relief of the bone pain frequently accompanying osteoporosis (see also Table 6).

In addition, oxandrolone has been used in short stature associated with Turner's syndrome, constitutional delay of growth and puberty; as adjunctive therapy for AIDS patients with HIV-wasting syndrome; and in moderate/severe acute alcoholic hepatitis and moderate protein calorie malnutrition. The side effects associated with anabolic steroids include cholestatic jaundice; prepubertal phallic enlargement and increased frequency or persistence of erections; postpubertal inhibition of testicular function; testicular atrophy and oligospermia; impotence; chronic priapism; epididymitis and bladder irritability; clitoral enlargement and menstrual irregularities; insomnia, depression, and changes in libido; nausea; vomiting, diarrhea; gynecomastia; potentiation of anticoagulant actions; deepening of voice and hirsutism in female subjects; acne; premature closure of epiphyses in children; disturbed electrolyte balance and edema, and increased serum levels of low-density lipoproteins and decreased level of high-density lipoproteins.

OXAPROZIN
(Daypro)

Oxaprozin, a nonsteroidal antiinflammatory agent with analgesic and antipyretic properties (1200 mg p.o. daily), is used in the management of acute or chronic osteoarthritis or rheumatoid arthritis (see also Table 2).

OXAZEPAM
(Serax)

Oxazepam (10 to 25 mg t.i.d.) is indicated for the management of anxiety disorders, for the symptoms of anxiety associated with depression, for the symptoms of anxiety, tension, agitation, and irritability in older patients, and for the management of alcoholics with acute tremulousness anxiety associated with alcohol withdrawal (see Figure 40 and Table 8).

Oxazepam, which is available only in oral preparations, is metabolized rapidly and hence has a relatively shorter disposition half-life of 5 to 14 hours. Oxazepam is absorbed less rapidly than diazepam after oral administration, limiting its usefulness in the treatment of insomnia. As with diazepam, when alcohol is taken at the same time, the rate of oxazepam absorption is slowed, but food does not affect either the rate or extent of absorption. In healthy subjects, oxazepam is relatively highly protein bound (about 90 to 95%), like other benzodiazepines. Unlike chlordiazepoxide and diazepam, the **biotransformation** of oxazepam involves only simple glucuronidation to an inactive metabolite. In contrast to chlordiazepoxide and diazepam, neither age nor liver disease alters the **elimination half-life** or **plasma clearance** of oxazepam, but the elimination half-life is prolonged to 24 to 91 hours in uremic patients. As might be expected, the elimination of the inactive glucuronide metabolite is greatly prolonged in these patients, its renal clearance being closely related to creatinine clearance. There is evidence that oxazepam may carry a lower abuse liability than diazepam.

OXICONAZOLE NITRATE

(Oxistat)

Oxiconazole, an ergosterol synthesis inhibitor possessing antifungal activity, is used for topical treatment of dermal infections caused by *Trichophyton rubrum* and *T. mentagrophytes* (tinea pedis, tinea cruris, and tinea corporis).

OXTRIPHYLLINE

(Choledyl)

Oxtriphylline, a xanthine derivative with bronchodilating properties (200 mg p.o. q. 6 hours), is used to relieve bronchial asthma and reversible bronchospasm associated with chronic bronchitis and emphysema (see also Figure 86).

OXYBUTYNIN CHLORIDE

(Ditropan)

Oxybutynin possesses anticholinergic and osmolytic properties, which together form the basis for its use as a therapeutic option in patients with overactive detrusor function — either idiopathic detrusor instability (DI) or detrusor hyperreflexia. Of the symptoms of detrusor overactivity, urge incontinence is often the most distressing to the patient. Adverse effects — dry mouth, constipation, blurred vision — related to the anticholinergic activity of oxybutynin occur frequently and can be sufficiently troublesome to necessitate treatment discontinuation in up to 25% of patients depending on the dosage. Increases in residual urine volume suggesting urinary retention (undesirable in patients with idiopathic DI), also can develop in some oxybutynin recipients (see also Figure 50).

OXYCODONE HYDROCHLORIDE

(Roxicodone)

Oxycodone, an opioid analgesic (5 mg p.o. every 3 to 6 hours), is used in the treatment of moderate to severe pain.

OXYMETAZOLLINE HYDROCHLORIDE

(Afrin, Allerest 12-hour Long Lasting Nasal, Coricidin Nasal Mist, Dristan Long Lasting Nasal Mist, Duramist Plus, Duration, 4-Way Long-Acting Nasal Spray, Neo-Synephrine 12-Hour Nasal Spray, Nostrilla Long Acting Nasal Decongestant, NTZ Long Acting Nasal, Sinarest 12-Hour, Sinex Long-Lasting)

Oxymetazolline, a sympathomimetic agent with decongestant properties, is used in nasal congestion.

OXYMETHOLONE

(Anarol-50)

Oxymetholone, an anabolic steroid (1 to 5 mg/kg/day), is indicated for the treatment of anemias caused by deficient red cell production, acquired or congenital aplastic anemia, myelofibrosis, and hypoplastic anemias due to the administration of myelotoxic drugs. Oxymetholone stimulates the kidney production of **erythropoietin**, leading to increases in red blood cell number, mass, and volume (see also Figure 36). Oxymetholone is contraindicated in patients with severe renal or cardiac disease which may be worsened by the fluid and electrolyte retention; and in patients with prostatic hypertrophy with obstruction or prostatic cancer. The side effects associated with anabolic steroids include cholestatic jaundice, prepubertal phallic enlargement, and increased frequency or persistence of erections; postpubertal inhibition of testicular function, testicular atrophy and oligospermia, impotence; chronic priapism, epididymitis, and bladder irritability; clitoral enlargement and menstrual irregularities; insomnia, depression, and changes in libido; nausea, vomiting, diarrhea; gynecomastia; potentiation of anticoagulant actions; deepening of voice and hirsutism in female subjects; acne; premature closure of epiphyses in children; disturbed electrolyte balance and edema; and increased serum levels of low-density lipoproteins and depressed level of high-density lipoproteins (see also Table 6).

OXYMORPHONE HYDROCHLORIDE
(Numorphan)

Oxymorphone, an opioid analgesic (1 to 1.5 mg SC), is used in the management of moderate to severe pain (see also Figure 58).

OXYPHENBUTAZONE
(Oxalid)

Oxyphenbutazone, a nonsteroidal antiinflammatory agent (300 to 600 mg/day in divided doses), is indicated in pain and inflammation of arthritis and ankylosing spondylitis. Oxyphenbutazone, a metabolite of phenylbutazone, has analgesic, antipyretic, antiinflammatory, and uricosuric properties. Oxyphenbutazone is absorbed orally, is bound to plasma proteins to the extent of 98%, has a half-life of 50 to 100 hours, is metabolized in the liver, and is excreted by the kidneys. Oxyphenbutazone is contraindicated in patients with known hypersensitivity to phenylbutazone; in patients in whom aspirin or other nonsteroidal antiinflammatory drugs (NSAIDs) induce symptoms of asthma, urticaria, or rhinitis; in patients under age 14, because safety has not been established; and in patients with senility, GI bleeding, blood dyscrasias, or renal, hepatic, cardiac or thyroid disease, because the drug may mask symptoms associated with these disorders or worsen these conditions. The drug should not be used in patients on long-term anticoagulant therapy because of its potential for adverse hematologic effects. Serious GI toxicity, especially ulceration or hemorrhage, can occur at any time in patients on chronic NSAID therapy. Use with caution in patients with a history of GI disease (especially peptic ulcer disease). Patients with known "triad" symptoms (aspirin hypersensitivity, rhinitis/nasal polyps, and asthma) are at high risk of cross sensitivity to oxyphenbutazone with precipitation of bronchospasm. Because of the potential for serious blood dyscrasias, oxyphenbutazone is not recommended for initial therapy. When used concomitantly, anticoagulants and thrombolytic drugs may be potentiated by the platelet-inhibiting effect of oxyphenbutazone. Concomitant use of oxyphenbutazone with highly protein-bound drugs (phenytoin, sulfonylureas, warfarin) may cause displacement of either drug, and adverse effects. Concomitant use with other GI-irritating drugs (steroids, antibiotics, NSAIDs) may potentiate the adverse GI effects of oxyphenbutazone. Antacids and food delay decrease the absorption of oxyphenbutazone. NSAIDs are known to decrease renal clearance of lithium carbonate, thus increasing lithium serum levels and risks of adverse effects. Oxyphenbutazone is known to induce liver microsomal enzyme activity. Concomitant use with other NSAIDs increases the risk of nephrotoxicity and decreases uricosuric effects.

Clinical manifestations of overdose include nausea, abdominal pain, and drowsiness; vomiting, hematemesis, diarrhea, restlessness, dizziness, agitation, hallucinations, psychosis, coma, convulsions, hyperpyrexia, electrolyte disturbances, hyperventilation, respiratory arrest, and cyanosis (see also Table 2 and Figures 11 and 12).

OXYTETRACYCLINE
(Terramycin)

Oxytetracycline (250 mg/day) is bacteriostatic, has a broad spectrum of activity, and is effective against infections with Gram-positive and Gram-negative bacteria, *Rickettsia*, mycoplasma, amoeba, and *Chlamydia*. Tetracyclines are drugs of choice in brucellosis, glanders, cholera, relapsing fever, meloidosis, leptospirosis, and the early stages of Lyme disease. They are preferred drugs for chlamydial infections, granuloma inguinale, and urethritis due to *Ureaplasma urealyticum* (see also Figures 80 and 88).

Tetracyclines enter bacterial cells by both passive diffusion and active transport, and then accumulate intracellularly. This does not occur in mammalian cells. The tetracyclines bind to the 30S subunit of the bacterial ribosome in such a way that the binding of the aminoacyl-transfer RNA to the acceptor site on the messenger RNA ribosome complex is blocked.

The resistant mutant bacteria do not transport or accumulate tetracycline. This plasmid-controlled resistance is transmitted by transduction or by conjugation.

The absorption of tetracyclines from the gastrointestinal tract is **nonuniform**. Up to 30% of chlortetracycline is absorbed. The absorption for tetracycline, oxytetracycline, and demeclocycline ranges between 60 and 80%, whereas as much as 90 to 100% of doxycycline and minocycline is absorbed. The absorption of tetracyclines is impaired by **divalent cations** (calcium, magnesium, and ferrous iron), by aluminum, and by extremely alkaline pHs. Tetracyclines are distributed widely throughout the body fluid, cross the placental barrier, and can accumulate in growing bones. The concentrations of chlortetracycline in spinal fluid are only one fourth of those in plasma. Minocycline, a more lipid-soluble tetracycline, reaches a high concentration in tears and saliva and can eradicate the meningococcal carrier state. The tetracyclines are metabolized in the liver and excreted mainly by the bile and urine. The concentrations of tetracyclines in the bile are ten times higher than those in serum.

Tetracyclines in general cause toxic and hypersensitivity reactions. These consist commonly of gastrointestinal irritations that are disabling and may necessitate the discontinuation of the medications. With continuous use, tetracyclines may alter the normal flora, allowing the growth of *Pseudomonas, Proteus*, staphylococci-resistant coliforms, *Clostridium*, and *Candida* organisms. These superinfections should be recognized and treated appropriately with vancomycin and other drugs (see also Figure 93).

Tetracyclines have been known to cause hepatic necrosis, especially when given in large intravenous doses or when taken by pregnant women or patients with preexisting liver impairment.

Tetracycline preparations whose potency has expired can cause **renal tubular acidosis**. With the exception of doxycycline, tetracyclines accumulate in patients with renal impairment. Tetracyclines also produce **nitrogen retention**, especially when given with diuretics.

Tetracyclines bind to calcium and then become deposited in bone, causing damage to developing bone and teeth. The intravenous administration of tetracyclines has been observed to cause venous thrombosis.

Oxytetracycline is contraindicated during the second half of pregnancy, and in children under age 8 because of the risk of permanent discoloration of teeth, enamel defects, and retardation of bone growth.

Concomitant use of tetracycline with antacids containing aluminum, calcium, or magnesium decreases absorption of oxytetracycline (because of chelation); concomitant use with food, milk or other dairy products, oral iron products, or sodium bicarbonate also impairs oral absorption.

Tetracyclines may antagonize the bactericidal effects of penicillin, inhibiting cell growth through bacteriostatic action.

Oxytetracycline enhances the risk of nephrotoxicity from methoxyflurane; it also necessitates lowered dosage of oral anticoagulants because of enhanced effects, and lowered dosage of digoxin because of increased bioavailability.

OXYTOCIN

(Pitocin, Syntocinon, and Uteracon)

Oxytocin (0.5 milliunit/min) is indicated to induce term labor, to control postpartum hemorrhage, to prevent postpartum uterine atony, to expel the placenta, and to prevent postpartum breast engorgement.

Oxytocin is a single polypeptide with eight amino acids that are sequenced as follows:

$$
\begin{array}{l}
\text{Gln} - \text{Asn} - \text{Cys} - \text{Pro} - \text{Leu} - \text{Gly} \\
\quad\quad\quad\quad\mid \quad\quad\quad\quad\mid \\
\text{Ile} - - - - - - - \text{Tyr}
\end{array}
$$

Oxytocin is synthesized in the cell bodies of supraoptic and paraventricular neurons and is then transported (complexed with neurophysin) in membrane-bound vesicles to the posterior lobe of the pituitary gland, where it may be released by a reflex mechanism or mechanisms, initiated or amplified by genital stimulation, coitus, parturition, or suckling of the infant. Suckling also releases **prolactin**. The action of oxytocin on the uterus (muscular contraction and parturition) and mammary glands (contraction of myoepithelial cells and milk secretion) is a direct one and is not influenced by the autonomic nervous system.

The uterus contains both **alpha** and **beta$_2$ adrenergic receptor** sites. Stimulation of the alpha receptor site causes contraction; stimulation of the beta$_2$ receptor site causes relaxation. Therefore, beta$_2$ receptor agonists such as **ritodrine hydrochloride** (Yutopar) and **terbutaline sulfate** (Brethine) are used to suppress premature labor.

The promotion of mammary development, lactation, and galactopoiesis requires growth hormone, ovarian estrogen (duct formation), ovarian progesterone (lobule-alveolar development), and adrenal corticoids, as well as prolactin and oxytocin. The secretion of prolactin is modified by substances that stimulate or block dopamine receptor sites. Agents such as **neuroleptics** (chlorpromazine) may cause lactation in a nonpregnant woman. On the other hand, **dopamine receptor agonists** such as bromocriptine (Parlodel) are used to prevent postpartum lactation.

The direct stimulatory effect of oxytocin is prominent in the gravid uterus during the late stage of pregnancy. Its action is augmented by estrogen and inhibited by progesterone. Oxytocin's effect is specific for uterine muscle, as little effect is observed on intestinal muscle or coronary arteries.

P

PACLITAXEL

(Taxol)

Paclitaxel, an antineoplastic agent, is used in the treatment of metastatic ovarian cancer after failure of first-line or subsequent chemotherapy (135 mg/m^2 IV over 24 hours q. three weeks) and breast carcinoma after failure of combination chemotherapy for metastatic disease or relapse within 6 months of adjuvant chemotherapy (175 mg/m^2 IV over 3 hours q. 3 weeks).

PAMIDRONATE DISODIUM

(Aredia)

Pamidronate, a pyrophosphate analog with antihypercalcemic effects, is indicated in the treatment of moderate to severe hypercalcemia associated with malignancy.

PANCREATIC ENZYMES PREPARATIONS			
	Contents (units)		
Agents	Lipase	Protease	Amylase
Cotazym	8000	30,000	30,000
Cotazym-S	5000	20,000	20,000
Creon	8000	13,000	30,000
Entolase	4000	25,000	20,000
Entolase-HP	8000	50,000	40,000
Ilozyme	11,000	30,000	30,000
Pancrease	4000	25,000	20,000
Pancrease MT4	4000	12,000	12,000
Pancrease MT10	10,000	30,000	30,000
Pancrease MT16	16,000	48,000	48,000
Viokase	8000	30,000	30,000
Viokase	16,800	70,000	70,000
Zymase	12,000	24,000	24,000

PANCREATIN

(Creon, Dizymes, Donnazyme, Entozyme, Hi-Vegi-Lip, 4X Pancrezyme, 8X Pancrezyme)

Pancreatin, a pancreatic enzyme, is indicated in exocrine pancreatic secretion insufficiency, as a digestive aid in cystic fibrosis, steatorrhea, and other disorders of fat metabolism secondary to insufficient pancreatic enzymes.

PANCRELIPASE

(Cotazym, Cotazym-S, Ilozyme, Ku-Zyme HP, Pancrease, Pancrease MT4, Pancrease MT10, Pancrease MT16, Pancrelipase, Protilase, Ultrase MT12, Ultrase MT20, Ultrase UT24, Viokase, Zymase)

Pancrelipase, a pancreatic enzyme, is indicated in exocrine pancreatic secretion insufficiency, cystic fibrosis in adults and children, steatorrhea, and other disorders of fat metabolism secondary to insufficient pancreatic enzymes.

PANCURONIUM BROMIDE

(Pavulon)

Pancuronium, a nondepolarizing neuromuscular blocker (initially 0.04 to 0.1 mg/kg IV), is indicated as an adjunct to anesthesia in order to induce skeletal muscle relaxation, to insure the management of patients undergoing mechanical ventilation, and to facilitate tracheal intubation. Agents such as tubocurarine and pancuronium compete with acetylcholine for the cholinergic receptors at the end plate. They combine with the receptors but do not activate them. Competitive or nondepolarizing agents are antagonized by neostigmine (see also Figure 92).

Use of a peripheral nerve stimulator will usually be of value for monitoring the neuromuscular blocking effect, avoiding overdosage and assisting in evaluation of recovery. Patients with severe obesity or neuromuscular disease may pose airway or ventilatory problems requiring special care before, during, and after the use of neuromuscular blocking agents such as pancuronium.

Electrolyte imbalance and diseases which lead to electrolyte imbalance, such as adrenal cortical insufficiency, alter neuromuscular blockade. Depending on the nature of the imbalance, either enhancement or inhibition may be expected. Magnesium sulfate, used in the management of toxemia of pregnancy, enhances the skeletal muscle relaxing effects of pancuronium. Antibiotics such as aminoglycosides, tetracyclines, clindamycin, lincomycin, colistin, and sodium colistimethate, augment the pancuronium-induced neuromuscular blockade. Anesthetics such as halothane, enflurane, and isoflurane enhance the action of pancuronium, whereas azathioprine will cause a reversal of neuromuscular blockade.

PANIC DISORDER: TREATMENT OF
Antihypertensive Medication
Clonidine
Benzodiazepines
Alprazolam
Clonazepam
Diazepam
Monoamine Oxidase Inhibitors
Phenelzine
Tricyclic Antidepressants
Imipramine

PANTOPRAZOLE

Pantoprazole, a substituted benzimidazole sulphoxide, is a proton pump inhibitor recommended for the treatment of acid-related gastrointestinal diseases such as reflux esophagitis and duodenal and gastric ulcers (see also Figure 63).

PAPAVERINE HYDROCHLORIDE

(Cerebid, Cerespan, Delapav, Myobid, Papacon, Pavabid, Pavacap, Pavacen, Pavadur, Pavadyl, Pavagen, Pava-Par, Pava-Rx, Pavased, Pavasule, Pavatine, Paverolan, P-200, Pasal)

Papaverine, a benzylisoquinoline derivative with peripheral vasodilating properties (300 mg p.o. t.i.d.), is indicated in the relief of cerebral and peripheral ischemia associated with arterial spasm and myocardial ischemia; it is used in the treatment of coronary occlusion and certain cerebral angiospastic states.

PARA-AMINOSALICYLATE SODIUM (PAS)

(Parasal Sodium, Pasdium, P.A.S. Sodium, Teebacin)

Para-aminosalicylate, an aminobenzoic acid analog with antituberculant activity (12 to 15 g p.o. daily), is indicated as adjunctive treatment of tuberculosis.

PARALDEHYDE

(Paral)

Paraldehyde (4 to 8 ml in iced fruit juice to mask taste) is used as a sedative and hypnotic, and to calm patients during delirium tremens and other states characterized by excitement. Paraldehyde is a polymer of acetaldehyde (CH_3CHO) in which three molecules of the latter are combined. It is a colorless and transparent liquid with a characteristic pungent odor and a hot burning taste which renders its administration difficult. Paraldehyde is one of the safest of the hypnotics, inducing sleep in moderate doses which is unaccompanied by any marked change in the circulation, respiration, or sensibility. However, its unpleasant odor and hot burning taste militate against its wide use. Paraldehyde is useful in delirium tremens and other forms of **delirium,** and in head injuries with agitation.

PARAMETHADIONE

(Paradione)

Paramethadione, an oxazolidine derivative (300 mg p.o. t.i.d.), is indicated as an alternate drug in the treatment of refractory absence seizures. Paramethadione raises the threshold for cortical seizures but does not modify the seizure pattern. It decreases projection of focal activity and reduces both repetitive spinal cord transmission and spike-and-wave patterns of absence (petit mal) seizures.

Paramethadione is dimethylated to an active anticonvulsant. Paramethadione is contraindicated in patients with severe hepatic or renal disease, severe blood dyscrasias, or diseases of the retina or optic nerve because the drug may exacerbate diseases of the optic nerve.

The concomitant use of mephenytoin and paramethadione, which may cause fatal hypersensitivity reactions, is discouraged.

Symptoms of overdose include nausea, drowsiness, ataxia, and visual disturbances; coma may follow massive overdose.

PARAMETHASONE ACETATE

(Haldrone)

Paramethasone (0.5 to 6 mg p.o. t.i.d.), a glucocorticoid, is used for its antiinflammatory and immunosuppressant properties. It possesses no mineralocorticoid actions.

Paramethasone stimulates the synthesis of enzymes needed to decrease the antiinflammatory response. It suppresses the immune system by reducing activity and volume of the lymphatic system, thus producing lymphocytopenia (primarily of T-lymphocytes), decreasing passage of immune complexes through basement membranes, and possibly by depressing reactivity of tissue to antigen-antibody interactions (see Table 10).

Paramethasone is contraindicated in patients with systemic fungal infections. Patients receiving paramethasone should not be given live-virus vaccines because paramethasone suppresses the immune response.

Paramethasone should be used with extreme caution in patients with GI ulceration, renal disease, hypertension, osteoporosis, diabetes mellitus, thromboembolic disorders, seizures, myasthenia gravis, congestive heart failure (CHF), tuberculosis, hypoalbuminemia, hypothyroidism, cirrhosis of the liver, emotional instability, psychotic tendencies, hyperlipidemias, glaucoma, or cataracts, because the drug may exacerbate these conditions.

Because adrenocorticoids increase the susceptibility to and mask symptoms of infection, paramethasone should not be used (except in life-threatening situations) in patients with viral or bacteria infections not controlled by antiinfective agents.

Glucocorticoids increase the metabolism of isoniazid and salicylates; they cause hyperglycemia, requiring dosage adjustment of insulin or oral hypoglycemic agents in diabetic patients; and they may enhance hypokalemia associated with diuretic or amphotericin B therapy. The hypokalemia may increase the risk of toxicity in patients concurrently receiving digitalis glycosides.

Barbiturates, phenytoin, and rifampin may cause decreased paramethasone effects because of increased hepatic metabolism. Cholestyramine, colestipol, and antacids decrease the corticosteroid effect by absorbing the corticosteroid, decreasing the amount absorbed.

Concomitant use with estrogens may reduce the metabolism of paramethasone by increasing the concentration of transcortin. The half-life of paramethasone is then prolonged because of increased protein binding. Concomitant administration of ulcerogenic drugs, such as nonsteroidal antiinflammatory agents, may increase the risk of GI ulceration (see Table 2).

PARASITIC INFECTIONS: TREATMENT OF		
Infections		**Drugs**
AMEBIASIS (*Entamoeba histolytica*)		
Asymptomatic		
Drugs of choice:		Iodoquinol
	or	Paromomycin
Alternative:		Diloxanide furoate
Mild to moderate intestinal disease		
Drugs of choice:		Metronidazole
	or	Tinidazole
Alternative:		Dehydroemetine
Hepatic abscess		
Drugs of choice:		Metronidazole
	or	Tinidazole
Alternatives:		Dehydroemetine
	followed by	Chloroquine phosphate

Infections	Drugs
AMEBIC MENINGOENCEPHALITIS, PRIMARY	
Naegleria	
Drug of choice:	Amphotericin B
Acanthamoeba	
Drugs of choice:	Pentamidine
or	Ketoconazole
or	Flucytosine
Ancylostoma duodenale, see HOOKWORM	
ANGIOSTRONGYLIASIS	
Angiostrongylus cantonensis	
Drug of choice:	Mebendazole
Angiostrongylus costaricensis	
Drug of choice:	Thiabendazole
ANISAKIASIS (*Anisakis*)	
Treatment of choice:	Surgical or endoscopic removal
ASCARIASIS (*Ascaris lumbricoides*, roundworm)	
Drugs of choice:	Mebendazole
or	Pyrantel pamoate
or	Albendazole
BABESIOSIS (*Babesia Microti*)	
Drugs of choice:	Clindamycin
plus	Quinine
BALANTIDIASIS (*Balantidium coli*)	
Drug of choice:	Tetracycline
Alternatives:	Iodoquinol
	Metronidazole
BAYLISASCARIASIS (*Baylisascaris procyonis*)	
Drugs of choice:	Diethylcarbamazine
or	Levamisole
or	Fenbendazole
BLASTOCYSTIS hominis infection	
Drug of choice:	Metronidazole
CAPILLARIASIS (*Capillaria philippinensis*)	
Drug of choice:	Mebendazole
Alternatives:	Albendazole
	Thiabendazole
Chagas' disease, see Trypanosomiasis	
***Clonorchis sinensis,* see Fluke infection**	
CRYPTOSPORIDIOSIS (*Cryptosporidium*)	
Drug of choice:	Infection is self-limited in immunocompetent patients. Octreotide controls diarrhea
CUTANEOUS LARVA MIGRANS (creeping eruption, dog and cat hookworm)	
Drugs of choice:	Thiabendazole
or	Albendazole

Infections	Drugs
CYCLOSPORA infection	
Drug of choice:	Trimethoprim-sulfamethoxazole
CYSTICERCOSIS, see Tapeworm infection	
DIENTAMOEBA *fragilis* infection	
Drugs of choice:	Iodoquinol
or	Paromomycin
or	Tetracycline
Diphyllobothrium latum, see Tapeworm infection	
DRACUNCULUS *medinensis* (guinea worm) infection	
Drug of choice:	Metronidazole
Alternative:	Thiabendazole
Echinococcus, see Tapeworm infection	
Entamoeba histolytica, see Amebiasis	
ENTAMOEBA *polecki* infection	
Drug of choice:	Metronidazole
ENTEROBIUS *vermicularis* (pinworm) infection	
Drugs of choice:	Pyrantel pamoate
or	Mebendazole
or	Albendazole
Fasciola hepatica, see Fluke infection	
FILARIASIS	
Wuchereria bancrofti, Brugia malayi	
Drug of choice:	Dimethylcarbamazine
Loa loa	
Drug of choice:	Dimethylcarbamazine
Mansonella ozzardi	
Drug of choice:	Ivermectin
Mansonella perstans	
Drug of choice:	Mebendazole
Tropical Pulmonary Eosinophilia (TPE)	
Drug of choice:	Diethylcarbamazine
Onchocerca volvulus	
Drug of choice:	Ivermectin
FLUKE, hermaphroditic, infection	
Clonorchis sinensis (*Chinese liver fluke*)	
Drug of choice:	Praziquantel
Fasciola hepatica **(sheep liver fluke)**	
Drug of choice:	Bithionol
Fasciolopsis buski **(intestinal fluke)**	
Drugs of choice:	Praziquantel
or	Niclosamide
Heterophyes heterophyes **(intestinal fluke)**	
Drug of choice:	Praziquantel

Infections		Drugs
Metagonimus yokogawai (intestinal fluke)		
Drug of choice:		Praziquantel
Nanophyetus salmincola		
Drug of choice:		Praziquantel
Opisthorchis viverrini (liver fluke)		
Drug of choice:		Praziquantel
Paragonimus westermani (lung fluke)		
Drug of choice:		Praziquantel
Alternative:		Bithionol
GIARDIASIS (*Giardia lamblia*)		
Drug of choice:		Metronidazole
Alternatives:		Quinacrine HCl
	or	Tinidazole
	or	Furazolidone
	or	Paromomycin
GNATHOSTOMIASIS (*Gnathostoma spinigerum*)		
Treatment of choice:		Surgical removal
	plus	Albendazole
HOOKWORM infection (*Ancylostoma duodenale, Necator americanus*)		
Drugs of choice:		Mebendazole
	or	Pyrantel pamoate
	or	Albendazole
Hydatid cyst, see Tapeworm infection		
Hymenolepis nana, see Tapeworm infection		
ISOSPORIASIS (*Isospora belli*)		
Drug of choice:		Trimethoprim-sulfamethoxazole
LEISHMANIASIS (*L. mexicana, L. tropica, L major, L. braziliensis, L. donovani* [Kala- azar])		
Drugs of choice:		Sodium stibogluconate
	or	Meglumine antimonate
Alternative:		Pentamidine isethionate
LICE infestation (Pediculus humanus, capitis, Phthirus pubis)		
Drugs of choice:		1% Permethrin (topically)
	or	0.5% Malathion (topically)
Alternatives:		Pyrethrins with piperonyl butoxide
		Lindane (topically)
Loa loa, see Filariasis		
MALARIA, Treatment of (*Plasmodium falciparum, P. ovale, P. vivax,* and *P. malariae*)		
Chloroquine-resistant *P. falciparum*		
ORAL		
Drugs of choice:		Quinine sulfate
	plus	Pyrimethamine-sulfadoxine
	or, plus	Tetracycline
	or, plus	Clindamycin
Alternatives:		Mefloquine
		Halofantrine

Infections	Drugs
PARENTERAL	
Drugs of choice: or	Quinidine gluconate Quinine dihydrochloride
Prevention of relapses: *P. vivax* and *P. ovale* only	
Drug of choice:	Primaquine phosphate
MALARIA, Prevention of	
Chloroquine-sensitive areas	
Drug of choice:	Chloroquine phosphate
Chloroquine-resistant areas	
Drugs of choice: or	Mefloquine Doxycycline
Alternatives: plus or, plus	Chloroquine phosphate Pyrimethamine-sulfadoxine for presumptive treatment Proguanil (in Africa south of the Sahara)
MICROSPORIDIOSIS	
Ocular (*Encephalitozoon hellem, Nosema corneum*)	
Drug of choice:	Fumagillin eyedrops
Intestinal (*Enterocytozoon bieneusi, Septata intestinalis*)	
Drug of choice:	Octreotide
Mites, see Scabies	
MONILIFORMIS *moniliformis* infection	
Drug of choice:	Pyrantel pamoate
***Naegleria* species,** see Amebic Meningoencephalitis, primary	
Necator americanus, see Hookworm infection	
Oesophagostomum bifurcum	
Drugs of choice: or	Albendazole Pyrantel pamoate
Onchocerca volvulus, see Filariasis	
Opisthorchis viverrini, see Fluke infection	
Paragonimus westermani, see Fluke infection	
Pediculus capitis, humanus, Phthirus pubis, see Lice	
Pinworm, see Enterobius	
PNEUMOCYSTIS *carinii* pneumonia	
Drugs of choice: or	Trimethoprim-sulfamethoxazole Pentamidine
Alternatives: plus plus plus	Trimethoprim Dapsone Atovaquone Primaquine Clindamycin Trimetrexate Folinic acid
Primary and secondary prophylaxis	
Drug of choice:	Trimethoprim-sulfamethoxazole
Alternatives: or	Dapsone Aerosol pentamidine
Roundworm, see Ascariasis	

Infections	Drugs
SCABIES (*Sarcoptes scabiei*)	
Drug of choice:	5% Permethrin (topically)
Alternatives: or	Lindane (topically) 10% Crotamiton (topically)
SCHISTOSOMIASIS (*Bilharziasis*)	
S. haematobium	
Drug of choice:	Praziquantel
S. japonicum	
Drug of choice:	Praziquantel
S. mansoni	
Drug of choice:	Praziquantel
Alternative:	Oxamniquine
S. mekongi	
Drug of choice:	Praziquantel
Sleeping sickness, see Trypanosomiasis	
STRONGYLOIDIASIS (*Strongyloids stercoralis*)	
Drugs of choice: or	Thiabendazole Ivermectin
TAPEWORM infection — **Adult (intestinal stage)**	
***Diphyllobothrium latum* (fish), *Taenia saginata* (beef), *Taenia solium* (pork), *Dipylidium caninum* (dog)**	
Drugs of choice: or	Praziquantel Niclosamide
***Hymenolepis nana* (dwarf tapeworm)**	
Drug of choice:	Praziquantel
Alternative: **-Larval (tissue stage)**	Niclosamide
***Echinococcus granulosus* (hydatid cyst)**	
Drug of choice:	Albendazole
Echinococcus multilocularis	
Treatment of choice:	Surgical excision
***Cysticercus cellulosae* (cysticercosis)**	
Drugs of choice: or	Albendazole Praziquantel
Alternative:	Surgery
Toxocariasis, see Visceral Larva Migrans	
TOXOPLASMOSIS (*Toxoplasma gondii*)	
Drug of choice: plus	Pyrimethamine Sulfadiazine
Alternative:	Spiramycin
TRICHINOSIS (*Trichinella spiralis*)	
Drug of choice: plus	Steroids for severe symptoms Mebendazole
TRICHOMONIASIS (*Trichomonas vaginalis*)	
Drugs of choice: or	Metronidazole Tinidazole

Infections	Drugs
TRICHOSTRONGYLUS infection	
Drug of choice:	Pyrantel pamoate
Alternatives:	Mebendazole
or	Albendazole
TRICHURIASIS (*Trichuris trichiura, whipworm*)	
Drugs of choice:	Mebendazole
or	Albendazole
TRYPANOSOMIASIS	
T. cruzi (South American trypanosomiasis, Chagas' disease)	
Drug of choice:	Nifurtimox
Alternative:	Benznidazole
T. brucei gambiense; T.b. rhodesiense (African trypanosomiasis, sleeping sickness)	
Drugs of choice:	Suramin
or	Eflornithine
Alternative:	Pentamidine isethionate
Late disease with CNS involvement	
Drugs of choice:	Melarsoprol
or	Eflornithine
Alternative:	Tryparsamide
plus	Suramin
VISCERAL LARVA MIGRANS	
Drug of choice:	Diethylcarbamazine
Alternatives:	Albendazole
or	Mebendazole
Whipworm, see Trichuriasis	
Wuchereria bancrofti, see Filariasis	

PARATHYROID HORMONE

Four **parathyroid glands** are situated on the lateral lobes of the thyroid. These glands secrete **parathyroid hormone** in response to low serum calcium levels. Parathyroid hormone then increases the serum calcium levels through the functioning of several mechanisms: it stimulates bone resorption; it increases the intestinal absorption of calcium; it increases the resorption of calcium by the renal tubules; and it acts on the kidney to decrease the tubular resorption of phosphate.

A reciprocal relationship exists between the level of calcium and phosphorus, as shown by the following table:

	Serum Calcium	Serum Phosphate
Hyperparathyroidism	Elevated	Low
Hypoparathyroidism	Low	Elevated

Calcitonin is also involved in calcium homeostasis by inhibiting bone resorption and by preventing excess increases in the serum calcium concentration through its monitoring of parathyroid hormone's actions (see Figure 66).

Parathyroid hormone is a single-chain polypeptide composed of 84 amino acids. It has a molecular weight of 9,500 and lacks an intrachain disulfide linkage. Parathyroid hormone is

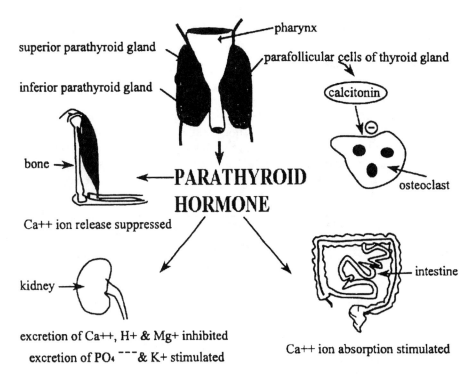

superior parathyroid gland

inferior parathyroid gland

pharynx

parafollicular cells of thyroid gland

calcitonin

⊖

osteoclast

bone →

PARATHYROID HORMONE

Ca++ ion release suppressed

kidney →

intestine

excretion of Ca++, H+ & Mg+ inhibited

excretion of PO₄ ⁻⁻⁻ & K+ stimulated

Ca++ ion absorption stimulated

FIGURE 66 Four **parathyroid glands** are situated on the lateral lobes of the thyroid. These glands secrete **parathyroid hormone** in response to low serum calcium levels. Parathyroid hormone then increases the serum calcium levels by stimulating bone resorption, increasing the intestinal absorption of calcium, increasing the resorption of calcium by the renal tubules, and by acting on the kidney to decrease the tubular resorption of phosphate. (Adapted from Ebadi, M., *Pharmacology, An Illustrated Review with Questions and Answers*, 3rd Edition, Lippincott-Raven Press, Philadelphia, 1996.)

produced by means of two sequential enzymic cleavages from a larger precursor polypeptide, **preparathyroid hormone**.

The organs principally responsible for the peripheral metabolism of parathyroid hormone are the kidneys and liver, and possibly bone. When parathyroid hormones are lacking, the following events take place:

A decreasing serum calcium level (reduced bone resorption)

An increasing serum phosphorus level (increased tubular resorption)

Neuromuscular irritability and tonic-clonic convulsions (low calcium tetany)

Laryngeal stridor, asthma, and other muscular spasms (irritability due to low calcium levels)

Ectopic calcifications in the blood vessels, brain, subcutaneous tissue, muscles, and cartilage (calcium phosphate is an insoluble salt) (see Figure 66).

Other manifestations of hypoparathyroidism include lenticular cataracts, dental defects, dry scaly skin, tendency to monilial infections, impaired mental acuity, and psychiatric disturbances.

Hypocalcemic tetany is treated with the intravenous administration of **calcium gluconate** or **calcium chloride** (5 to 10 ml of 10% solution). The effects of these agents are rapid but transient. Furthermore, a 10-ml solution of calcium chloride and calcium gluconate contains 270 mg and 70 mg of calcium, respectively. Because calcium chloride is a highly irritating substance, it should not be administered intramuscularly. Parathyroid hormone (100 to 300 units) is injected subcutaneously after the initial administration of calcium salt, but its effect is transient and lasts only 3 to 4 weeks. Hypoparathyroidism is also treated with vitamin D (1 to 2 mg = 50,000 to 100,000 units per day) (see also Figure 97).

PAREGORIC

Paregoric (4 to 5 ml 1 tsp.) is a camphorated tincture of opium. Opiate preparations, usually given as **paregorics**, are effective and fast-acting antidiarrheal agents. These agents are also useful postoperatively to produce solid stool following an ileostomy or colostomy. A meperidine derivative, **diphenoxylate**, is usually dispensed with **atropine** and sold as Lomotil. The atropine is added to discourage the abuse of diphenoxylate by narcotic addicts who are tolerant to massive doses of narcotic but not to the CNS stimulant effects of atropine.

PARKINSON'S DISEASE: TREATMENT OF	
Amantadine	100 mg twice a day
Bromocriptine	1.25 mg twice a day
Carbidopa/levodopa	25 to 100 mg three times a day
Carbidopa/levodopa, sustained release	50 to 200 mg twice a day
Pergolide	0.05 mg once a day
Selegiline	5.0 mg twice a day
Trihexyphenidyl HCl	1 mg twice a day

PAROMOMYCIN SULFATE
(Humatin)

Paromomycin, an aminoglycoside with antibacterial and amebicidal properties, is indicated in the treatment of acute and chronic intestinal amebiasis, of tapeworm (fish, beef, pork, and dog) infections in patients who cannot take **praziquantel** or **niclosamide**, and as an adjunctive regimen in the management of hepatic coma.

PAROXETINE HYDROCHLORIDE
(Paxil)

Paroxetin, a selective serotonin uptake inhibitor (20 mg p.o. daily), is indicated in the treatment of depression (see Tables 3 through 5 and Figure 78).

PEFLOXACIN

The quinolones include: **nalidixic acid** (NegGram), **cinoxacin** (Cinobac), **norfloxacin** (Noroxin), and **ciprofloxacin** (Cipro). Other members of the quinolone family are **pefloxacin, ofloxacin, enoxacin,** and **fleroxacin.** The bacterial enzyme **DNA gyrase** is responsible for the continuous introduction of negative supercoils into DNA, and the quinolones inhibit this gyrase-mediated DNA supercoiling (see Figure 77).

Nalidixic acid and **cinoxacin** are bactericidal against Gram-negative organisms that cause urinary tract infections. The **fluoroquinolones** are bactericidal and considerably more potent against *Escherichia coli* and various species of *Salmonella, Shigella, Enterobacter, Campylobacter,* and *Neisseria*. **Ciprofloxacin** also has good activity against staphylococci, including methicillin-resistant strains.

The quinolones and fluoroquinolones may produce arthropathy, and hence should not be used in prepubertal children or pregnant women.

Nalidixic acid and **cinoxacin** are useful only for treating urinary tract infections. **Ciprofloxacin** is useful for both urinary tract infections and prostatitis.

PEGASPARGASE

(Peg-L-Asparaginase) (Oncaspar)

Pegaspargase, an antineoplastic agent with properties similar to those of L-asparaginase (2,500 iu/m^2 IM or IV q. 14 days), is indicated in the management of acute lymphoblastic leukemia (ALL) in patients who require L-asparaginase but have developed hypersensitivity to the native forms of L-asparaginase.

PEMOLINE

(Cylert)

Pemoline, an oxazolidinedione derivative with possible analeptic and CNS stimulating properties (37.5 mg p.o. daily), is indicated in the treatment of attention deficit disorder (ADD).

PENBUTOLOL SULFATE

(Levatol)

Penbutolol (20 mg p.o. daily) is a beta-adrenergic receptor blocking agent which is indicated in the treatment of mild to moderate hypertension. Penbutolol blocks both beta$_1$- and beta$_2$-adrenergic receptors. Its antihypertensive effects may be related to its peripheral antiadrenergic effects that lead to decreased cardiac output, a central effect that leads to decreased sympathetic tone, or decreased renin secretion by the kidneys.

Penbutolol is absorbed well after oral administration, is bound to plasma proteins to the extent of 80 to 90%, and is metabolized in the liver to active and inactive metabolites which are excreted in the urine.

Penbutolol is contraindicated in patients with sinus bradycardia, cardiogenic shock, bronchial asthma, and patients with greater than first-degree heart block. Beta-adrenergic blocking agents should be avoided in patients with pheochromocytoma unless alpha-adrenergic blocking agents are also used. Oral calcium antagonists may enhance the hypotensive effects of beta-adrenergic blocking agents as well as predispose the patient to bradycardia and dysrhythmias. Clonidine may cause paradoxical hypertension when combined with beta-adrenergic blocking agents. Also, beta blockers may enhance rebound hypertension when clonidine is withdrawn. Beta-adrenergic blocking agents may alter the hypoglycemic response to insulin or oral hypoglycemic agents. Beta blockers may enhance the "first dose" orthostatic hypotension seen with **prazocin** and **terazocin**.

Penbutolol has been shown to increase the volume of distribution of lidocaine in normal patients, implying that it may increase the loading dose requirements in some patients. Clinical signs of overdose may include bradycardia, bronchospasm, heart failure, and severe hypotension.

PENICILLAMINE

(Cuprimine, Depen)

Penicillamine (250 mg p.o. q.i.d. 30 to 60 minutes before meals), a metal chelating agent, is indicated in Wilson's disease, in cystinuria, in rheumatoid arthritis, and in heavy metal poisoning. Penicillamine depresses circulating IgM rheumatoid factor (but not total circulating

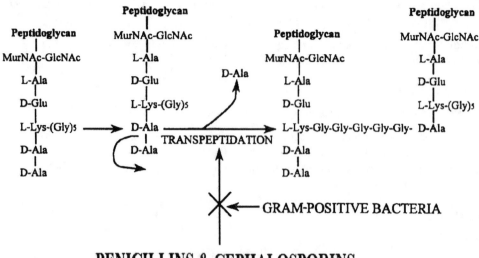

PENICILLINS & CEPHALOSPORINS

FIGURE 67 Penicillins and cephalosporins achieve their effect by inhibiting formation of cell walls, and hence are bactericidal. Penicillin binds to cellular receptors, now identified as **transpeptidation enzymes**, and by binding to and inhibiting the transpeptidation reactions, the synthesis of cell wall **peptidoglycan** is interrupted. (Adapted from Ebadi, M., *Pharmacology, An Illustrated Review with Questions and Answers*, 3rd Edition, Lippincott-Raven Press, Philadelphia, 1996.)

immunoglobulin levels) and depresses T-cell but not B-cell activity. It also depolymerizes some macroglobulins (for example, rheumatoid factors).

Penicillamine forms stable, soluble complexes with copper, iron, mercury, lead, and other heavy metals that are excreted in urine; it is particularly useful in chelating copper in patients with Wilson's disease. Penicillamine also combines with cystine alone, therefore reducing free cystine below the level of urinary stone formation.

Penicillamine is contraindicated in patients with a history of penicillamine-related aplastic anemia or agranulocystosis; in patients with significant renal or hepatic insufficiency; in pregnant women; and in patients receiving gold salts, immunosuppressants, antimalarials, or phenylbutazone because of the increased risk of serious hematologic effects.

PENICILLINS

All penicillins (Figures 65 and 67) are composed of a thiazolidine ring attached to a beta-lactam, which in turn carries a free amide group (O=CNH) on which a substitution and an attachment (R) are made. In the case of benzylpenicillin, the R is a benzyl group. Penicillin may be metabolized by amidase to 6-aminopenicillanic acid, which has antibacterial activity, or by penicillinase (bacterial beta-lactamase) to penicilloic acid, which is devoid of antibacterial activity but is antigenic in nature and acts as a sensitizing structure. The main source of bacterial resistance to penicillin is in fact the production of penicillinase by the microorganisms.

Penicillin is an organic acid, which is commonly supplied as sodium and potassium salts, Penicillin V (Pen-Vee K and V-cillin K) and phenethicillin (Syncillin and Maxipen) are different from penicillin G (benzylpenicillin) in that they are more acid resistant. In addition to the broad-spectrum penicillins such as ampicillin and amoxicillin, there is a newer group of anti-*Pseudomonas* penicillins that are effective against Gram-negative bacilli. These agents include carbenicillin, ticarcillin, azlocillin, and piperacillin. The latter two agents are also useful against *Klebsiella pneumoniae* and *Bacteroides fragilis* (see also Table 22).

The **penicillinase-resistant penicillins** are oxacillin, cloxacillin, dicloxacillin, methicillin, and nafcillin. These agents are the drugs of choice for treating infections caused by penicillinase-producing *Staphylococci aureus*.

One milligram of pure penicillin G sodium is equal to 1,667 units.

Penicillins achieve their effect by inhibiting formation of cell walls, and hence are bactericidal. Penicillin binds to cellular receptors, now identified as **transpeptidation enzymes**, and, by binding to and inhibiting the transpeptidation reactions, the synthesis of cell wall **peptidoglycan** is interrupted. In addition, penicillin removes or inactivates an inhibitor of the lytic enzymes (autolysin), resulting in the lysis of microorganisms in an isotonic environment. In general, penicillins are more active against Gram-positive organisms (see Figure 67).

The penicillin-susceptible organisms are nonpenicillinase-producing strains of most cocci, Gram-positive bacilli, and spirochetes.

Penicillin G may be used either actively or prophylactically in the following clinical settings:

Streptococcal infections
    Streptococcal pharyngitis (including scarlet fever)
    Streptococcal pneumonia, arthritis, meningitis, and endocarditis
    Streptococcal otitis media and sinusitis
    Infectious endocarditis
Pneumococcal infections
Staphylococcal infections (generally resistant to penicillin G)
Meningococcal disease
Gonococcal infections
Syphilis
Actinomycosis, anthrax, and gas gangrene

Thirty percent of an oral dosage of penicillin is absorbed from the gastrointestinal tract. Penicillin G is rapidly destroyed at pH 2 of gastric secretion. Penicillin is widely distributed throughout the body, and, except in the case of meningitis, does not cross the blood-brain barrier. Penicillin is slightly metabolized by the liver but is mainly excreted by the kidney. **Probenecid** blocks the active tubular secretion of penicillin and hence prolongs its action. Penicillin is readily absorbed from intramuscular sites, and long-acting repository forms such as penicillin G procaine and penicillin G benzathine are available.

Penicillins, which are the safest of antibiotics, produce few direct toxic reactions, and most of the serious side effects are hypersensitivity reactions. Penicillins and their by-products, penicilloic acid and penicilloylpolylysine, are antigenic in susceptible individuals who develop immunoglobulin G antibodies to them. Furthermore, all penicillins cross-sensitize and cross-react. Allergic reactions, including **anaphylactoid shock**, occur in sensitized patients following the repeated administration of penicillin. Anaphylactoid reactions, which are more common following the parenteral administration of penicillin, may be reversed by the administration of corticosteroids.

The direct toxicity of penicillin following the administration of large doses may include **phlebitis** if it is given intravenously, **injection site inflammatory reactions** when given intramuscularly, **degeneration of nerve tissue** if injected into a nerve, and **central nervous system excitability** if given intrathecally.

The **broad-spectrum penicillins**, such as **ampicillin** and **amoxicillin**, may cause gastrointestinal irritation. Occasionally, the overgrowth of staphylococci, *Pseudomonas, Proteus*, or yeasts may be responsible for causing **enteritis**. Methicillin and nafcillin may precipitate

TABLE 22
Comparative Pharmacology of Penicillin Derivatives

	Properties		
Drugs	Acid Stability	Penicillinase Resistance	Spectrum of Activity
Penicillin G[a]	No	No	Narrow spectrum
Penicillin V[a]	Yes	No	Narrow spectrum
Oxacillin[a]	Yes	Yes	The isoxazolyl penicillins
Cloxacillin[a]	Yes	Yes	are potent inhibitors of
Dicloxacillin[a]	Yes	Yes	the growth of most penicillinase-producing staphylococci
Nafcillin[b]	No	Yes	Slightly more active than oxacillin against penicillin G-resistant *Staph. aureus*
Ampicillin[c]	Yes	No	Ampicillin and the related
Amoxicillin	Yes	No	aminopenicillins are bactericidal for both Gram-positive and Gram-negative bacteria

[a] Absorbed incompletely from the gastrointestinal tract, attains peak concentration in the plasma in one hour, and is excreted rapidly by the kidneys.

[b] Available for oral and parenteral uses.

[c] Appears in the bile, undergoes enterohepatic circulation, and is excreted in the feces.

granulocytopenia, and methicillin has been known to cause **nephritis**. Carbenicillin may cause **hypokalemic alkalosis**. The properties of the various penicillins are shown in Table 22.

PENICILLIN G BENZATHINE
(Bicillin L-A, Megacillin Suspension, Permapen)

PENICILLIN G POTASSIUM
(Cryspen, Deltapen, Lanacillin, Parcillin, Pensorb, Pentids, Pfizerpen)

PENICILLIN G PROCAINE
(Crysticillin A.S., Duracillin A.S., Fizerpen A.S., Wycillin)

PENICILLIN G SODIUM

Penicillin, a naturally occurring antibiotic, is indicated in the treatment of group A streptococcal upper respiratory infections, prophylaxis of poststreptococcal rheumatic fever, syphilis of less than one year's duration, moderate to severe systemic infections, uncomplicated gonorrhea, pneumococcal pneumonia, and endocarditis prophylaxis for dental surgery (see Table 22).

PENICILLIN V

PENICILLIN V POTASSIUM
(Betapen-VK, Biotic-V Powder, Bopen V-K, Cocillin V-K, Lanacillin VK, Ledercillin VK, LV, Penapar VK, Pen-Vee K, Pfizerpen VK, Robicillin-VK, Uticillin VK, V-Cillin K, Veetids)

Penicillin, a naturally occurring antibiotic, is indicated in the treatment of mild to moderate susceptible infections and endocarditis prophylaxis for dental surgery.

PENICILLINS		
Amoxicillin	Dicloxacillin	Oxacillin
Ampicillin	Floxacillin	Penicillin G
Azlocillin	Methicillin	Penicillin V
Carbenicillin	Mezlocillin	Piperacillin
Cloxacillin	Nafcillin	Ticarcillin

PENTAERYTHRITOL TETRANITRATE
(Peritrate)

Pentaerythritol (10 to 20 mg t.i.d.), a nitric acid ester of a tetrahydric alcohol, is indicated for the relief of angina pectoris and pain associated with coronary artery disease. It is not intended to abort the acute anginal episode but is widely regarded as useful in the prophylactic treatment of angina pectoris (see Figures 59 through 61).

The nitrates and nitrites bring about **arterial dilation**, and hence reduce blood pressure and the work of the heart. These agents also produce **venous dilation**, thereby decreasing the venous return and ventricular volume, which in turn diminishes wall tension. The end result of these events is a reduction in the work of the heart. By decreasing blood pressure, the heart rate is increased through the activation of carotid sinus reflexes. However, the extent of the reduction in wall tension is actually of greater benefit than the elevated heart rate. The nitrate-induced **tachycardia** may be blocked by the administration of propranolol, a beta-adrenergic-receptor blocking agent (see Figure 61).

Collateral vessels are silent blood vessels that become functional during hypoxic emergencies. By dilating, they permit greater blood flow to the ischemic areas, and nitrates accentuate this response. This effect of nitrates, which is greater than that of dipyridamole, seems to be potentiated by propranolol.

Nitrites and nitrates dilate blood vessels in all smooth muscles. When they dilate the cutaneous blood vessels, they cause blushing. When they dilate the cerebral vessels, they cause headache. Thus, the appearance of headache and blushing is an indication of the efficacy of these medications (see Figure 59).

PENTAMIDINE ISETHIONATE
(Pentam-300)

Pentamidine (4 mg/kg once a day for 14 days) is indicated for the treatment of *Pneumocystis carinii* pneumonia (PCP), prevention of PCP in high-risk, HIV-infected patients, and in the treatment of trypanosomiasis and visceral leishmaniasis.

Trypanosomiasis is produced by protozoa of the genus *Trypanosoma* and leads to Gambian or mid-African sleeping sickness (*T. gambiense)*, Rhodesian or East African sleeping sickness (*T. rhodesiense*), and Chagas' disease, which is seen in the populations of Central and South America (*T. cruzi*).

Agents effective in the treatment of trypanosomiasis are the **aromatic diamidines** (pentamidine, stilbamidine, and propamidine). **Pentamidine** is the preferred drug for the prevention and early treatment of *T. gambiense* infections; however, it cannot penetrate the central nervous system. **Melarsoprol** is the drug recommended for *T. gambiense* infections that do not respond to pentamidine or for managing the late meningoencephalitis stages of infection. It does reach the central nervous system. **Nifurtimox** (Lampit) is the drug of choice for treating the acute form of Chagas' disease. **Suramin** (Naphuride) is effective only in the therapy for African sleeping sickness.

PENTAZOCINE

(Talwin)

Pentazocine (50 to 100 mg every 3 to 4 hours) is indicated for relieving moderate to severe pain and for providing preoperative or preanesthetic medications. The analgesia produced by 30 mg of pentazocine, a mixed-narcotic agonist and a weak antagonist, is comparable to that elicited by 10 mg of morphine. Pentazocine will antagonize some of the respiratory depression and analgesia produced by morphine and meperidine. However, the analgesic action and respiratory depression produced by pentazocine can be reversed by a narcotic antagonist. Pentazocine causes tolerance and addiction, but they emerge very slowly compared to those induced by morphine (see Figure 58).

PENTOBARBITAL SODIUM

(Nembutal)

Pentobarbital (200 to 300 mg 1 to 2 hours before surgery) may be used parenterally as a sedative, hypnotic, or preanesthetic medication. Oral pentobarbital may be used as a hypnotic for a short period of time, since it loses its effectiveness after two weeks.

Pentobarbital acts throughout the CNS as a nonselective depressant with a fast onset of action and a short duration of action. Particularly sensitive to this drug is the reticular activating system, which controls CNS arousal. Pentobarbital decreases both presynaptic and postsynaptic membrane excitability by facilitating the action of gamma-aminobutyric acid (GABA) (see also Figure 40).

Pentobarbital is contraindicated in patients with bronchopneumonia, status asthmaticus, or severe respiratory distress, because of the potential for respiratory depression. Pentobarbital should not be used in patients who are depressed or have suicidal ideation because the drug can worsen depression; in patients with uncontrolled acute or chronic pain, because exacerbation of pain and paradoxical excitement can occur, or, in patients with porphyria, because the drug can trigger symptoms of this disease. Pentobarbital should be used cautiously in patients who must perform hazardous tasks requiring mental alertness, because the drug causes drowsiness.

Clinical manifestations of overdose include unsteady gait, slurred speech, sustained nystagmus, somnolence, confusion, respiratory depression, pulmonary edema, and coma.

PENTOSTATIN

(2'-Deoxycoformycin; DCF) (Nipent)

Pentostatin, an antineoplastic agent which inhibits adenosine deaminase (4 mg/m^2 IV every other week), is indicated in the treatment of alpha-interferon-refractory hairy-cell leukemia.

PENTOXIFYLLINE

(Trental)

Pentoxifylline (400 mg t.i.d. p.o. with meals) is indicated in the treatment of intermittent claudication on the basis of chronic occlusive arterial disease of the limbs.

Pentoxifylline, a dimethylxanthine derivative, and its metabolites improve blood flow by decreasing blood viscosity. It produces dose-related hemorrheologic effects, lowering blood viscosity and improving erythrocyte flexibility. In patients with chronic peripheral arterial disease, this increases blood flow to the affected microcirculation and enhances tissue oxygenation.

Pentoxifylline improves deformability of erythrocytes by increasing cellular ATP concentration via a membrane metabolizing action, which in turn reduces the aggregation of erythrocytes and local hyperviscosity. It stimulates prostacyclin formation and release, and inhibits phosphodiesterase degradation of platelet cAMP. The increase of cAMP levels decreases the synthesis of thromboxane A_2, and the net result is reduced platelet aggregation. It increases blood fibrinolytic activity, and decreases fibrinogen concentration.

The overdosage of pentoxifylline has caused flushing, hypotension, nervousness, agitation, tremors, convulsions, somnolence, loss of consciousness, fever, and agitation.

PEPPERMINT OIL

The irritable bowel syndrome is a functional bowel disorder exhibiting the following characteristics: abdominal pain, symptoms of disturbed defecation (urgency, straining, and feeling of incomplete evacuation), altered stool consistency, and altered stool frequency and timing. There are also symptoms of bloatedness (distention).

If **diarrhea** is the chief complaint, it is treated with **loperamide** or **cholestyramine. Pain** is treated with **dicyclomine, amitriptyline,** and **peppermint oil. Bran** and **psyllium** are used to treat the **constipation** that may occur in irritable bowel syndrome. **Flatulence** is treated with **simethicone.**

Many volatile oils on passing into the stomach cause a sensation of warmth in the gullet accompanied by a sense of well-being and comfort, the appetite is often increased, and any feeling of distention after meals is relieved. This is often attended by the eructation of gas. Substances which produce these effects are known as **carminatives.** They are used to relieve intestinal flatulence and distention, to lessen the spasms which cause colic, and as stimulants to the appetite. Those used for this purpose include camphor, cinnamon, fennel, peppermint, spearmint, wintergreen, bitter almond, and anise.

PEPTIC ULCER: TREATMENT OF	
The pathogenesis of peptic ulceration is not yet clear. It could be due to an imbalance between acid secretion and mucosal defensive and/or protective mechanisms, but the association between *Helicobacter pylori* and peptic ulceration has questioned this hypothesis. Therefore, drugs inhibiting acid secretion and/or eradicating *H. pylori* are of major interest.	
Inhibition of Acid Secretion Histamine H_2-receptor antagonists inhibit acid secretion by blocking the stimulation of H_2-receptors in the gastric parietal cell. They are: Cimetidine Nizatidine Ranitidine Roxatidine	**Proton Pump Inhibitors** They are: Lansoprazole Omeprazole Pantoprazole **Cytoprotective Agents** They are: Antacids Bismuth salts Prostaglandin derivatives (misoprostol) Sucralfate
Histamine H_2-receptor antagonists can still be considered as a king of a "gold" standard for the treatment of peptic lesions based on their large therapeutic margins, extensive safety records, and well-documented clinical efficacy.	

PERGOLIDE MESYLATE

(Permax)

Pergolide (0.05 mg initially in divided doses) is indicated as an adjunctive treatment to levodopa/carbidopa in the management of Parkinson's disease. Pergolide mesylate is a potent dopamine receptor agonist at both D_1 and D_2 receptor sites. It is 10 to 1000 times more potent than bromocriptine on a mg per mg basis. In patients with Parkinson's disease, it exerts its therapeutic effect by directly stimulating postsynaptic dopamine receptors in the nigrostriatal system. In addition, pergolide inhibits the secretion of prolactin; it causes a transient rise in serum concentrations of growth hormone and a decrease in serum concentrations of luteinizing hormone.

Pergolide is absorbed orally, is bound to plasma proteins to the extent of 90%, metabolized to N-despropylpergolide, pergolide sulfoxide, and pergolide sulfone, and the metabolites are excreted by the kidneys.

Dopamine receptor antagonists, having antipsychotic properties such as phenothiazine, butyrophenone, and thioxanthene derivatives, and gastrointestinal stimulant drugs, such as metoclopramide, are contraindicated with pergolide. The most common side effects of pergolide, especially in higher than recommended doses, are dyskinesia, hallucinations, somnolence, insomnia, nausea, constipation, diarrhea, dyspepsia, and rhinitis.

PERMETHRIN

(Elimite, Nix)

Permethrin, a synthetic pyrethroid with scabicidal and pediculocidal properties, is indicated in the treatment of pediculosis.

PERPHENAZINE

(Trilafon)

Perphenazine, a phenothiazine (4 to 8 mg t.i.d.), is indicated in the management of psychotic disorders, in the control of nausea and vomiting in adults, and for the relief of intractable hiccoughs.

Perphenazine is thought to exert its antipsychotic effects by postsynaptic blockade of CNS dopamine receptors, thus inhibiting dopamine-mediated effects. The antiemetic effects of perphenazine are attributed to dopamine receptor blockade in the medullary chemoreceptor trigger zone (see Figure 73). Perphenazine has many other central and peripheral effects; it produces both alpha and ganglionic blockade and counteracts histamine- and serotonin-mediated functions. It produces a very high incidence of movement disorders including akathisia, dystonia, parkinsonism, tardive dyskinesia, and neuroleptic malignant syndrome. Perphenazine possesses anticholinergic properties and hence should be used cautiously in patients with arrhythmias, congestive heart failure, angina pectoris, valvular disease, heart block, encephalitis, Reye's syndrome, head injury, respiratory disease, epilepsy and other seizure disorders (the drug may lower the seizure threshold), glaucoma (the drug may raise intraocular pressure), prostatic hypertrophy, Parkinson's disease, urinary retention (the drug may worsen these conditions), and hepatic or renal dysfunction (impaired metabolism and excretion may cause drug accumulation).

Concomitant use of perphenazine with sympathomimetics, including epinephrine, phenylephrine, phenylpropanolamine, and ephedrine (often found in nasal sprays), and with appetite suppressants may decrease their stimulatory and pressor effects. Phenothiazines can cause epinephrine reversal and a hypotensive response when epinephrine is used for its pressor effects.

Perphenazine may inhibit blood pressure response to centrally acting antihypertensive drugs, such as guanethidine, guanabenz, guanadrel, clonidine, methyldopa, and reserpine. Additive effects are likely after concomitant use of perphenazine with CNS depressants, including alcohol, analgesics, barbiturates, narcotics, tranquilizers, and general, spinal, or epidural anesthetics, or parenteral magnesium sulfate (oversedation, respiratory depression, and hypotension); antiarrhythmic agents, quinidine, disopyramide, and procainamide (increased incidence of cardiac dysrhythmias and conduction defects); atropine or other anticholinergic drugs, including antidepressants, monoamine oxidase inhibitors, phenothiazines, antihistamines, meperidine, and antiparkinsonian agents (oversedation, paralytic ileus, visual changes, and severe constipation); nitrates (hypotension) and metrizamide (increased risk of convulsions). Beta-blocking agents may inhibit perphenazine metabolism, increasing plasma levels and toxicity (see also Table 23).

PERTUSSIS TOXIN

The secretory product of *Bordetella pertussis* interferes with the ability of agonists to inhibit adenylate cyclase. It catalyzes the transfer of the ADP-ribose moiety of NAD^+ to a cysteine residue close to the carboxy terminus of G_{ia}.

Forskolin, which is isolated from *Coleus forskohlii*, stimulates adenylate cyclase. **Choleragen**, the secretory product of *Vibrio cholerae*, can persistently activate adenylate cyclase by catalyzing the transfer of the ADP-ribose moiety of nicotinamide adenine dinucleotide (NAD^+) to G_{sa} (see also Figure 42).

PHENACEMIDE
(Phenurone)

Phenacemide, a substituted acetylurea derivative with anticonvulsant properties (500 mg p.o. t.i.d.), is indicated in the treatment of refractory, complex-partial, generalized tonic-clonic, absence, and atypical absence seizures.

PHENACETIN
(Acetaphenetidin)

Phenacetin has analgesic and antipyretic but no antiinflammatory properties. Phenacetin and its deethylated metabolite, acetaminophen, are superior to aspirin in that they do not cause hypoprothrombinemia, gastrointestinal irritation, or disturbances of acid-base balance. The serious, but rare, side effects of phenacetin are **methemoglobinemia, hemolytic anemia, fatal hepatic necrosis,** and **hypoglycemic coma**. Both interstitial nephritis and renal papillary necrosis can be caused by phenacetin and acetaminophen. The less toxic acetaminophen should be used only in patients who cannot tolerate aspirin or in whom aspirin is contraindicated (see also Table 2).

PHENAZOPYRIDINE HYDROCHLORIDE
(Pyridium; Urodine)

Phenazopyridine (200 mg t.i.d.) is indicated for symptomatic relief of pain, burning, urgency, frequency, and other discomforts arising from irritation of the lower urinary tract mucosa caused by infections, trauma, surgery, endoscopic procedures, or passage of sounds or catheters. Its analgesic action may reduce or eliminate the need for systemic analgesics or narcotics.

Overdosage of phenazopyridine is known to have caused headache, rash, pruritis, occasional GI disturbances; anaphylactoid-like reaction, methemoglobinemia, hemolytic anemia, and renal and hepatic toxicity.

PHENDIMETRAZINE HYDROCHLORIDE

(Adipost, Anorex, Bacarate, Bontril, Delcozine, Di-ap-trol, Obalan, Obezine, PDM, Phenzine, Prelu-2, SPRX-1, SPRX-2, SPRX-3, Statobex, Trimtabs, Wehless-105)

Phendimetrazine, an indirect acting sympathomimetic agent with amphetamine-like action (35 mg p.o. b.i.d.), is indicated as a short-term adjunct in the treatment of obesity.

PHENELZINE SULFATE

(Nardil)

Phenelzine, a monoamine oxidase A inhibitor (15 mg t.i.d.), is indicated for the treatment of depressed patients clinically characterized as "atypical," "nonendogenous," or "neurotic." These patients often have mixed anxiety and depression and phobic or hypochondriacal features (see also Tables 3 through 5).

Monoamine oxidase can metabolize monoamines by oxidative deamination and convert them to inactive acidic derivatives. Monoamine oxidase inhibitors seem to compete with physiologically active monoamine for the active site of the enzyme. In general, not only do these agents inhibit the oxidase that metabolizes amines but they also inhibit the oxidase that metabolizes drugs and essential nutrients. Hence, the incidence of drug-drug and drug-food interactions is extremely high with these agents. Monoamine oxidases have various applications. They may be used as a local **anesthetic** (cocaine), an **antihistaminic** (diphenylhydramine), or an **antidepressant** (tranylcypromine, phenelzine). Monoamine oxidase inhibitors have been used in the treatment of hypertension (direct blockade of sympathetic ganglion), angina pectoris (coronary dilation), narcolepsy (stimulating the reticular activating system), and depression (increasing the brain's norepinephrine pool). Needless to say, these agents should be used with extreme caution in conjunction with sympathomimetic amines, ganglionic blocking agents, procaine, and anesthetic agents. They are contraindicated in patients with hyperthyroidism and in combination with tricyclic antidepressants. In the event of poisoning, adrenergic blocking agents such as **phentolamine** may be effective for combating the hypertensive crisis (see also Figure 27).

PHENOBARBITAL

(Luminal)

Phenobarbital is indicated as a hypnotic agent for the short-term treatment of insomnia, as an anticonvulsant for the treatment of partial and generalized tonic-clonic and cortical focal seizures; and for emergency control of certain acute convulsive episodes (e.g., those associated with status epilepticus, eclampsia, tetanus, and toxic reactions to strychnine or local anesthetics).

Phenobarbital is absorbed from the small intestine. As much as 50% binds to albumin, and it is metabolized in the liver to **hydroxyphenobarbital**. Approximately 20 to 25% of phenobarbital is excreted in the urine unchanged. It has a very long elimination half-life of up to 140 hours. Therefore, it is administered orally in a dose of 2 to 3 mg/kg once a day. The renal excretion of phenobarbital is enhanced by the alkalinization of urine, which favors its ionization and excretion. $NaHCO_3$ has been used in the management of phenobarbital toxicity.

Phenobarbital induces hepatic microsomal drug metabolizing enzymes. The sudden withdrawal of phenobarbital may precipitate withdrawal seizures. Therefore, the doses should be tapered gradually whenever discontinuation is contemplated.

Phenobarbital inhibits posttetanic potentiation and especially raises the seizure threshold. The precise mechanism of action of phenobarbital is not known, though two dissimilar mechanisms have been advanced.

In the first, phenobarbital, by inhibiting **aldehyde reductase**, is thought to interfere with the metabolism of aldehyde generated by biogenic amines such as dopamine, norepinephrine, and serotonin. The accumulation of these aldehydes in the CNS has depressing properties, and this reduces the neuronal sensitivity to excitation.

In the second theory, phenobarbital is thought to enhance the presynaptic release of GABA, and at the same time reduce the postsynaptic uptake of GABA (see also Figure 40).

Compared to phenytoin, phenobarbital is a relatively safe compound. Rarely a morbilliform rash occurs. However, in some patients, heavy sedation, reduction in activity, and impairment in cognition may be pronounced.

Phenobarbital has a broad spectrum of antiepileptic activity and efficacy. It is often used by itself or in combination with phenytoin. **Advantages** of phenobarbital are:

It has a long history of usage with few serious systemic and no dysmorphic side effects.
It is inexpensive and widely available.
It can be used both orally and parenterally.
Its long elimination half-life allows simple single daily administration; missed doses have little clinical impact.
It has broad-spectrum antiepileptic properties and is useful for febrile, toxic metabolic, and withdrawal seizures.
The teratogenicity risk is less than that of phenytoin.

Disadvantages of phenobarbital are:

It produces annoying sedative effects in many patients, even within the therapeutic range.
Significant disturbance of cognitive function, mood, or behavior is seen in some patients, especially children and the elderly.
Rapid manipulation to raise or lower serum levels is somewhat difficult due to slow accumulation and elimination.
Accidental or purposeful overdose may be lethal.

PHENOLPHTHALEIN

Although often used interchangeably, the terms **laxative** and **cathartic** do have slightly different meanings. A **laxative effect** refers to the excretion of a soft, formed stool; **catharsis** implies a more fluid and complete evacuation.

Irritant agents used in the treatment of constipation include cascara, sagrada, castor oil, senna, rhubarb, phenolphthalein, and acetphenolisatin. Phenolphthalein is a constituent of many over-the-counter preparations, including Ex-Lax and Feen-A-Mint. Most of these agents, with the exception of castor oil, are slow in their onset of action (24 hours). **Castor oil** is hydrolyzed to ricinoleic acid, the active cathartic. It has an onset of action of 2 to 6 hours.

Phenolphthalein is thought to exert its effect by inhibiting the movement of water and sodium from the colon into the blood and by stimulating mucus secretion. If misused on a prolonged basis, a consequential loss of mucus may lower the plasma protein level.

The **misuse** of any of these agents has been shown to cause hypokalemia, dehydration, and a cathartic colon (resembling ulcerative colitis). Phenolphthalein-containing products may color alkaline urine red.

PHENOTHIAZINE DERIVATIVES

The phenothiazine-derivative antipsychotics are classified according to their **chemical structures**. These are (see Table 23):

TABLE 23
Antipsychotic Agents

Drugs	Injectable Form	Equivalent Dose (mg)	Daily Dosage (mg)[a]	Sedation	Incidence of Movement Disorders	Anticholinergic Effects
Phenothiazines						
Aliphatic						
Chlorpromazine	Yes	50	30–800	+++	++	++
Triflupromazine	Yes	12.5	60–150	+++	++	+++
Piperidine						
Mesoridazine	Yes	25	30–400	+++	+	++
Thioridazine	No	50	150–800	+++	+	+++
Piperazine						
Acetophenazine	No	10	60–120	++	+++	++
Fluphenazine	Yes	1	1–40	+	+++	+
Perphenazine	Yes	4	12–64	+	+++	++
Prochlorperazine	Yes	8	15–150	++	+++	+
Trifluperazine	Yes	2.5	2–40	+	+++	+
Thioxanthenes						
Chlorprothixene	Yes	50	75–600	+++	++	++
Thiothixene	Yes	2	8–30	+	+++	+
Butyrophenone						
Haloperidol	Yes	1	1–15	+	+++	+
Dihydroindolone						
Molindone	No	5	15–225	+	+++	+
Dibenzoxazepine						
Loxapine	Yes	5	20–250	++	+++	+
Diphenylbutylpiperidine						
Pimozide	No	2	1–25	++	+++	++
Dibenzodiazepine						
Clozapine	No	Not Available	100–900	+	–	+

[a] Dosages of oral medications only.

+++ = high; ++ = moderate; + = low; – = not present

Propylamine derivatives, which include chlorpromazine (Thorazine), promazine (Sparine), and triflupromazine (Vesprin).

Propylpiperazine derivatives, which include fluphenazine (Permitil, Prolixin), perphenazine (Trilafon), prochlorperazine (Compazine), trifluoperazine (Stelazine), and acetophenazine (Tindal).

Methylpiperidyl derivatives, which include thioridazine (Mellaril).

These agents differ in their potency but not their efficacy. Long-acting injectable drugs such as **fluphenazine decanoate** or **fluphenazine enanthate**, which need to be given only once every two or three weeks, are increasingly used in outpatients and in those patients who are uncooperative and noncompliant. Phenothiazine derivatives devoid of neuroleptic activity also exist. **Promethazine** (Phenergan) is an **antihistaminic; ethopropazine** (Parsidol) has a **muscle relaxant** effect and, because of its anticholinergic action, may be used in **parkinsonism.** Methotrimeprazine (Levoprome) is claimed to be a nonaddictive analgesic that does not cause respiratory depression (see Table 23).

PHENOXYBENZAMINE HYDROCHLORIDE
(Dibenzyline)

Phenoxybenzamine (5.0 to 60.0 mg/day) is used in order to control episodes of hypertension and sweating. If tachycardia is excessive, it may also be necessary to use a beta-blocker concomitantly. In addition, phenoxybenzamine has been tested for its efficacy in micturition disorders resulting from neurogenic bladder, functional outlet obstruction, and partial prostatic obstruction.

Phenoxybenzamine is a noncompetitive alpha-adrenergic receptor blocker, and its action cannot be nullified by increasing the amount of agonist, or agonists. It causes **epinephrine reversal** in that the administration of epinephrine after pretreatment with phenoxybenzamine elicits vasodilation, and, conversely, phenoxybenzamine reverses epinephrine-mediated vasoconstriction to vasodilation (see also Figure 27).

The adverse effects of phenoxybenzamine include nasal congestion, miosis, postural hypotension, tachycardia, and inhibition of ejaculation.

PHENSUXIMIDE
(Milontin)

Phensuximide (500 to 1000 mg p.o. b.i.d.) suppresses the paroxysmal three cycles per second spike-and-wave activity associated with lapses of consciousness common in absence (petit mal) seizures. The frequency of epileptiform attacks is reduced, apparently by motor cortex depression and elevation of the threshold of the CNS to convulsive stimuli.

Phensuximide may increase the incidence of generalized tonic-clonic seizures if used alone to treat mixed seizures; and abrupt withdrawal may precipitate petit mal seizures.

Concomitant use of phensuximide and other CNS depressants (alcohol, narcotics, anxiolytics, antidepressants, antipsychotics, and other anticonvulsants) may increase sedative effects.

Symptoms of overdose may include dizziness and ataxia, which may progress to stupor and coma.

PHENTERMINE HYDROCHLORIDE
(Adipex-P, Anoxine, Dapex, Fastin, Donamin, Ionamin, Obe-Nix, Obermine, Obiphen, Phentrol, Rolaphent, Unicelles, Wilpower)

Phentermine, an indirect-acting sympathomimetic agent with amphetamine-like actions (8 mg p.o. t.i.d.), is indicated as a short-term adjunct in the treatment of exogenous obesity.

PHENTOLAMINE
(Regitine)

Phentolamine (5 mg IV or IM 1 to 2 hours before surgery) is indicated for prevention or control of hypertensive episodes that may occur in a patient with pheochromocytoma as a result of stress or manipulation during preoperative preparation and surgical excision; for prevention and treatment of dermal necrosis and sloughing following IV administration or extravasation of norepinephrine or dopamine. Phentolamine has been used to treat hypertensive crisis secondary to MAO inhibitors/sympathomimetic amine interactions and rebound hypertension on withdrawal of clonidine, propranolol, or other antihypertensives. It has also been used in combination with papaverine as an intracavernous injection for impotence.

Phentolamine is a competitive alpha-adrenergic blocker, and its action can be nullified by increasing the amount of agonist, or agonists. The vasoconstricting and hypertensive effects of epinephrine and ephedrine are antagonized by phentolamine (see also Figure 27).

The dose-dependent adverse effects of phentolamine include nausea, vomiting, diarrhea, nasal stuffiness, hypotension, tachycardia, dizziness, flushing, and weakness.

Myocardial infarction, cerebrovascular spasm and cerebrovascular occlusion have followed phentolamine administration, usually in association with marked hypotensive episodes with shock-like states which occasionally follow parenteral use.

PHENYLBUTAZONE

(Butazolidin)

Phenylbutazone is indicated for relieving the symptoms of acute gouty arthritis, active rheumatoid arthritis, and active ankylosing spondylitis, acute attacks of degenerative joint disease of the hips and knees, painful shoulder (peritendinitis, capsulitis, bursitis, and acute arthritis of that joint). However, because of the risk of agranulocytosis and aplastic anemia, it should be used only when other nonsteroidal antiinflammatory substances have proven unsatisfactory.

Phenylbutazone and its analog, oxyphenbutazone, are closely related chemically and pharmacologically to the pyrazolines, aminopyrine and antipyrine. These drugs have antiinflammatory, antipyretic, analgesic and mild uricosuric actions resulting in symptomatic relief only; the disease process is unaltered.

The exact mechanism of the antiinflammatory effect is unknown, but these agents inhibit factors believed to be involved in the inflammatory process, including prostaglandin synthesis, leukocyte migration, and release and activity of lysosomal enzymes.

The antiinflammatory effect of phenylbutazone is greater than aspirin's but less than that of the steroid antiinflammatory agents. Phenylbutazone causes sodium and chloride retention, and edema may result. In addition, fatal **aplastic anemia** and **agranulocytosis** have occurred following the use of phenylbutazone. The activation of and perforation of hemorrhagic **ulcer** can also take place, and hypersensitivity reactions are common. Consequently, phenylbutazone should be used only in the treatment of inflammatory conditions (rheumatoid arthritis, ankylosing spondylitis, or osteoarthritis) when the safer antiinflammatory agents are no longer effective.

Antiinflammatory agents, oral anticoagulants, oral antidiabetics, sulfonamides, sodium valproate, and phenytoin are competitively displaced by phenylbutazone from serum-binding sites. The activity, duration of effect, and toxicity of the displaced drugs may be increased.

Barbiturates, promethazine, chlorpheniramine, rifampin, and corticosteroids, inducers of microsomal enzymes, may decrease the half-life of phenylbutazone. Cholestyramine reduces the enteral absorption of phenylbutazone (see also Table 2).

PHENYLEPHRINE HYDROCHLORIDE

(Neo-Synephrine; Allerest; Sinex)

Phenylephrine is indicated in the treatment of vascular failure in shock, shock-like states, drug-induced hypotension, or hypersensitivity; to overcome paroxysmal supraventricular tachycardia; to prolong spinal anesthesia; as a vasoconstrictor in regional analgesia; and to maintain an adequate level of blood pressure during spinal and inhalation anesthesia.

Phenylephrine is a powerful postsynaptic alpha-receptor stimulant with little effect on the beta receptors of the heart (see also Figure 27).

The predominant actions of phenylephrine are on the cardiovascular system. Parenteral administration causes a rise in systolic and diastolic pressures due to peripheral vasoconstriction. Accompanying the pressor response to phenylephrine is a marked reflex bradycardia that can be blocked by atropine; after atropine, large doses of the peripheral resistance is considerably increased. Circulation time is slightly prolonged, and venous pressure is slightly increased; venous constriction is not marked. Most vascular beds are constricted; renal, splanchnic, cutaneous, and limb blood flows are reduced, but coronary blood flow is increased. Pulmonary vessels are constricted, and pulmonary arterial pressure is raised.

The drug is a powerful vasoconstrictor, with properties very similar to those of norepinephrine, but almost completely lacking the chronotropic and inotropic actions on the heart. Cardiac irregularities are seen only very rarely, even with large doses. In contrast to epinephrine and ephedrine, phenylephrine produces longer-lasting vasoconstriction, a reflex bradycardia, and increases the stroke output, producing no disturbance in the rhythm of the pulse.

In therapeutic doses, it produces little if any stimulation of either the spinal cord or cerebrum. An advantage is that repeated injections produce comparable effects.

PHENYTOIN SODIUM

(Dilantin)

Phenytoin (2 to 3 mg/kg p.o. daily divided b.i.d.) is indicated for generalized tonic-clonic seizures, for status epilepticus, and for post head-injury trauma.

Phenytoin, which has a pK_a of 8.3 to 9.2, is insoluble at the pH of gastric juice and therefore is not absorbed to a significant degree from the stomach. On passage into the small intestine, where the pH is basic (7.0 to 7.5), phenytoin exists in a nonionized form that favors its absorption. Absorption is highest from the duodenum and decreases rapidly in the lower parts of the small intestine. Because phenytoin is not absorbed well from the large intestine, the rectal administration of phenytoin is of little therapeutic value and should not be encouraged.

When used on a long-term basis, phenytoin is always given orally. To abort **status epilepticus**, it is given intravenously. Because the injectable form of phenytoin has a pH of 12.0, it should not be injected intramuscularly.

After absorption, as much as 92 to 93% of phenytoin becomes bound to plasma proteins, allowing only 7 to 8% of the drug to remain free. Circumstances or drugs that alter the extent of protein binding will significantly affect phenytoin's therapeutic usefulness and may also precipitate phenytoin toxicity. For example, in **uremic patients**, whose free phenytoin level may reach as high as 30%, the dosage of phenytoin should be reduced. Similarly, in patients with **hypoalbuminemia** resulting from numerous disorders, the doses of phenytoin should be adjusted downward.

Phenytoin becomes metabolized in the liver to **hydroxyphenytoin,** which is an inactive metabolite. Hydroxyphenytoin is then conjugated with glucuronic acid and excreted by the kidneys. Hydroxphenytoin inhibits the metabolism of phenytoin, and the half-life of phenytoin may be altered if doses exceed the therapeutic level, as shown in the following example:

Oral Dose of Phenytoin (mg/kg)	Plasma Level of Phenytoin (microgram/ml)	Half-Life (hr)
4	10–15	24
12	>25	60

Clinical evidence indicates that epileptic patients are either **slow or rapid metabolizers of phenytoin.** In the slow metabolizers, 4 mg/kg of phenytoin may produce toxicity, whereas, in the rapid metabolizers, this may be a subtherapeutic dose. In addition, the results of

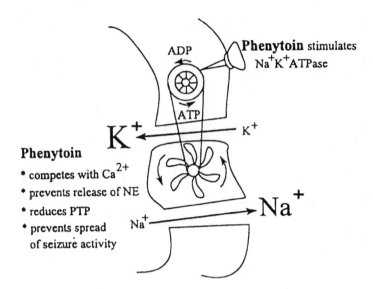

FIGURE 68   The mode of action of phenytoin has been attributed to its **membrane-stabilizing effects**, because it (1) limits the development of maximal seizure activity, and (2) reduces the spread of the seizure process from an epileptic focus. (Adapted from Ebadi, M., *Pharmacology, An Illustrated Review with Questions and Answers*, 3rd Edition, Lippincott-Raven Press, Philadelphia, 1996.)

randomized, double-blind, controlled clinical trials of antiepileptic drugs conducted in adult patients with mostly partial onset or generalized tonic-clonic seizures, or both, have shown that there are considerable individual differences between patients' responses to the same drug. Side effects are common with all of the antiepileptic drugs.

The mode of action of phenytoin has been attributed to its **membrane-stabilizing effects**, because it (1) limits the development of maximal seizure activity, and (2) reduces the spread of the seizure process from an epileptic focus. The precise mechanisms responsible for stabilization of the neuronal membrane are uncertain, though several concepts have been advanced (Figure 68).

One of these concerns phenytoin's interference with calcium action. Phenytoin inhibits the development of and reverses **posttetanic potentiation**, or posttetanic facilitation. It is thought that this is an important mechanism in the development of the high-frequency train of impulses that takes place in cerebral excitatory feedback circuits and in the spread of such activity to neighboring loops, resulting in maximal seizure activity. Phenytoin reduces calcium transport at the outer nerve membrane by blocking its high-affinity binding sites. This prevents the release of norepinephrine, which is necessary for the generation of posttetanic potentiation, and the spread of the impending seizure process is curtailed.

A second concept that attempts to explain the mechanism of phenytoin's activity is its interference with **sodium movement**. In a hyperexcitable state, the intracellular concentration of sodium is elevated. Phenytoin decreases the inward sodium current. Furthermore, when the intracellular concentration of sodium is elevated, phenytoin is thought to stimulate **Na^+K^+-ATPase** to reestablish the ionic gradient. The activity of Na^+, K^+-ATPase is reduced in the brains of epileptic patients (see Figure 68).

The membrane-stabilizing effect of phenytoin is not limited to neurons but is also seen in other excitable tissues, such as skeletal muscle and heart. Furthermore, phenytoin is effective in treating **myotonia** and **cardiac arrhythmias**.

A third concept is that phenytoin enhances **GABAergic transmission**. Chloride ions enhance the binding of phenytoin to a specific but unknown receptor site in the brain. It has been postulated that this binding may enhance GABA-mediated chloride conductance in the postsynaptic membrane (see Figure 40).

Phenytoin may cause **nystagmus, diplopia, staggering**, and **ataxia**. These side effects are generally regarded as dose dependent and usually appear whenever the plasma concentration of phenytoin exceeds 20 microgram/ml. These side effects are reversible with dose reduction.

Phenytoin causes **gingival hyperplasia** which occurs with much greater frequency in children (60%) than in adults (40%), shows no race or sex predilection, and may appear 2 to 3 months after the initiation of therapy. Gingival hyperplasia, which does not occur in the toothless portion of the gum, regresses gradually on discontinuation of the medication. Other medications causing gingival hyperplasia include **cyclosporin, nifedipine, diltiazem, verapamil**, and **nitrendipine** (see also Table 20).

Phenytoin causes **hypertrichosis** in 5% of patients, which occurs several months after the initiation of therapy and is either slowly reversible or irreversible, even after discontinuation of medication. Phenytoin may also cause a **hypersensitivity reaction**, characterized by rashes, Stevens–Johnson syndrome, lymphoid hyperplasia, blood dyscrasias, and serum sickness. If any of these reactions occur, the medications must be discontinued.

Long-term phenytoin therapy carries several drawbacks. It may **impair cognitive functions**, cause bilateral **peripheral neuropathy** that is characterized by decreased reflexes and sensory deficits, and produce **hypokalemia** and **osteomalacia**, resulting in accelerated vitamin D metabolism.

Advantages of phenytoin are:

It is relatively nonsedating.
Serious toxicity is rare.
Parenteral administration is possible.
A loading dose may be given by the oral or intravenous route.
It only needs to be taken once a day by most adults.
It is relatively inexpensive.

Disadvantages of phenytoin are:

It may cause some sedation and/or impairment of higher intellectual function.
There is a relatively high incidence of annoying side effects with long-term administration, including gingival hyperplasia, hypertrichosis, acne, and coarsening of the facial features.

PHOTOSENSITIVITY: MEDICATION-INDUCED			
Anticancer Drugs			
Dacarbazine Fluorouracil Flutamide	Methotrexate Vinblastine		
Antidepressants			
Amitriptyline Amoxapine Clomipramine	Desipramine Doxepin Imipramine	Maprotiline Nortriptyline Phenelzine	Protriptyline Trazodone Trimipramine
Antihistamines			
Cyproheptadine Diphenhydramine			

Antihypertensives

Captopril	Minoxidil		
Diltiazem	Nifedipine		
Methyldopa			

Antimicrobials

Ciprofloxacin	Enoxacin	Nalidixic acid	Pyrazinamide
Clofazimine	Flucytosine	Norfloxacin	Sulfonamides
Dapsone	Griseofulvin	Ofloxacin	Tetracycline
Demeclocycline	Lomefloxacin	Oxytetracycline	Trimethoprim
Doxycycline	Minocycline		

Antiparasitic Drugs

| Chloroquine |
| Quinine |
| Thiabendazole |

Antipsychotic Drugs

Chlorpromazine	Perphenazine	Thioridazine	Trifluoperazine
Fluphenazine	Prochlorperazine	Thiothixene	Triflupromazine
Haloperidol			

Diuretics

Acetazolamide	Chlorothiazide	Hydroflumethiazide	Polythiazide
Amiloride	Furosemide	Methyclothiazide	Triamterene
Bendroflumethiazide	Hydrochlorothiazide	Metolazone	Trichlormethiazide
Benzthiazide			

Hypoglycemics

| Acetohexamide | Glipizide | Tolazamide | |
| Chlorpropamide | Glyburide | Tolbutamide | |

Nonsteroidal Antiinflammatory Drugs

Diflunisal	Ketoprofen	Naproxen	Piroxicam
Ibuprofen	Nabumetone	Phenylbutazone	Sulindac
Indomethacin			

Others

Alprazolam	Chlordiazepoxide	Fluorescein	Promethazine
Amantadine	Clofibrate	Gold salts	Quinidine sulfate and
Amiodarone	Desoximetasone	Hexachlorophene	gluconate
Benzocaine	Disopyramide	Isotretinoin	Tretinoin
Carbamazepine	Etretinate		Trimeprazine

The frequency of photosensitivity reactions is nonuniform and may not be related either to the structure or the functions of the drugs. For example, the highest incidence of photosensitivity reactions have occurred following administration of amiodarone, chlorpromazine, chlorothiazide, demeclocycline, doxycycline, furosemide, hydrochlorothiazide, piroxicam, promethazine, or tolbutamide. Many chemicals are activated to toxic metabolites by enzymatic biotransformation. However, some chemicals can be activated in the skin by ultraviolet and/or visible radiation. In photoallergy, radiation absorbed by the drug, such as sulfonamide, results in its conversion to a product that is a more potent allergen than the parent compound. The clinical manifestations may range from acute urticarial reactions, which develop a few minutes after exposure to sunlight, to eczematous or papular lesions, which appear after 24 hours or more. Phototoxic reactions to drugs, in contrast to photoallergic ones, do not have an immunological component. Drugs, either absorbed locally into the skin or that have reached the skin through the systemic circulation, may be the object of photochemical reactions within the skin. This can lead directly either to chemically induced photosensitivity reactions or to enhancement of the usual effects of sunlight. Tetracyclines, sulfonamides, chlorpromazine, and nalidixic acid are examples of phototoxic chemicals; generally, they are innocuous to skin if not exposed to light.

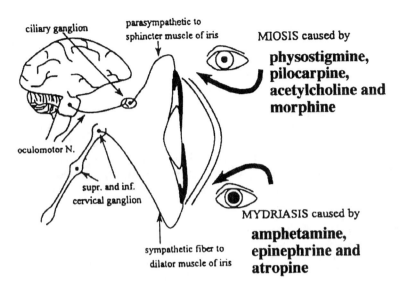

ciliary ganglion

parasympathetic to
sphincter muscle of iris

MIOSIS caused by

**physostigmine,
pilocarpine,
acetylcholine and
morphine**

oculomotor N.

supr. and inf.
cervical ganglion

sympathetic fiber to
dilator muscle of iris

MYDRIASIS caused by

**amphetamine,
epinephrine and
atropine**

FIGURE 69 **Physostigmine** causes miosis and spasm of accommodations; it also lowers intraocular pressure and hence can be used in the treatment of wide-angle glaucoma. (Adapted from Ebadi, M., *Pharmacology, An Illustrated Review with Questions and Answers*, 3rd Edition, Lippincott-Raven Press, Philadelphia, 1996.)

PHYSOSTIGMINE SULFATE

(Eserine)

Physostigmine sulfate and **physostigmine salicylate** (Antilirium) are cholinesterase inhibitors which are indicated as antidotes to poisoning from substances possessing anticholinergic properties such as imipramine, a tricyclic antidepressant. In addition, it has been used in open-angle glaucoma (see Figure 69).

Physostigmine competitively blocks acetylcholine hydrolysis by cholinesterase, resulting in acetylcholine accumulation at cholinergic synapses that antagonizes the muscarinic effects of overdose with antidepressants and anticholinergics. With ophthalmic use, miosis and ciliary muscle contraction increases aqueous humor outflow and decreases intraocular pressure.

The **reversible inhibitors**, which have a short to moderate duration of action, fall into two categories. **Type one**, exemplified by **edrophonium**, forms an ionic bond at the anionic site and a weak hydrogen bond at the esteratic site of acetylcholinesterase. **Type two**, exemplified by **neostigmine**, forms an ionic bond at the anionic site and a hydrolyzable covalent bond at the esteratic site.

The **irreversible inhibitors**, exemplified by organophosphorous compounds (diisopropyl fluorophosphate [DFP], parathion, malathion, diazinon), have long durations of action and form a covalent bond with acetylcholinesterase, which is hydrolyzed very slowly and negligibly, but the inhibition may be overcome by cholinesterase activators such as **pralidoxime** (see also Figure 71).

Cholinesterase inhibitors may also be classified according to agents that possess **tertiary nitrogens** (e.g., physostigmine and most organophosphorous compounds) and those that contain **quaternary nitrogens** (e.g., neostigmine, pyridostigmine, and some organophosphorous compounds such as echothiphate). The following summarizes the comparative properties of these agents.

	Physostigmine	Neostigmine
Oral absorption	Good	Poor
Crosses the blood-brain barrier	Well	No
Stimulates nicotinic receptors (skeletal muscle)	Yes	Yes
Used to combat the CNS toxicity of numerous anticholinergic drugs	Yes	No

Physostigmine causes miosis and spasm of accommodation; it also lowers intraocular pressure and hence can be used in the treatment of wide-angle glaucoma. Being lipid-soluble, it penetrates into the brain rapidly, raises the acetylcholine concentration, and, in toxic amounts, may cause cholinergic CNS toxicity, which is characterized by restlessness, insomnia, tremors, confusion, ataxia, convulsions, respiratory depression, and circulatory collapse. These effects are reversed by atropine.

Neostigmine, which is unable to penetrate the blood-brain barrier, does not cause CNS toxicity. However, it may produce dose-dependent and full-range muscarinic effects, characterized by miosis, blurring of vision, lacrimation, salivation, sweating, increased bronchial secretion, bronchoconstriction, bradycardia, hypotension, and urinary incontinence. Atropine is able to oppose these muscarinic effects. In addition, neostigmine, which has both a direct action as well as an indirect action that is mediated by acetylcholine on end-plate nicotinic receptors, may produce muscular fasciculation, muscular cramps, weakness, and even paralysis. These effects are not countered by atropine. Furthermore, neostigmine enhances gastric contraction and secretion. Neostigmine itself is metabolized by plasma acetylcholinesterase.

The therapeutic uses of neostigmine include the treatment of atony of the urinary bladder and postoperative abdominal distention. In addition, it antagonizes the action of *d*-tubocurarine and curariform drugs. Edrophonium, neostigmine, or pyridostigmine may be used to diagnose myasthenia gravis. Because edrophonium has the shortest duration of action, it is most often used for this purpose.

PILOCARPINE NITRATE
(Pilagan)

Pilocarpine (1 to 2 drops of 2% solution 2 to 4 times daily) is used to control intraocular pressure in glaucoma. In addition, it is used for emergency relief of mydriasis in an acutely glaucomatous situation or to reverse mydriasis caused by cycloplegic agents. It may be applied topically in the form of a drug reservoir (Ocusert) (see Figure 70).

Pilocarpine is a naturally occurring (active ingredient of poisonous mushrooms, *Amanita muscaria)* cholinomimetic agent possessing both muscarinic and nicotinic properties (stimulates autonomic ganglia).

PIMOZIDE
(ORAP)

Pimozide (diphenyl-butylpiperidine, an antipsychotic, 1 to 2 mg daily in divided doses) is indicated for suppression of severe motor and phonic tics in patients with Gilles de la Tourette's syndrome. Pimozide's mechanism of action in Gilles de la Tourette's syndrome is unknown. It is thought to exert its effects by postsynaptic and/or presynaptic blockade of CNS dopamine receptors, thus inhibiting dopamine-mediated effects. Pimozide also has anticholinergic, antiemetic, and anxiolytic effects and produces alpha blockade.

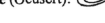

Pilocarpine (Ocusert):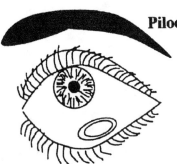

* causes miosis

* reduces intraocular
  pressure

* used in glaucoma

FIGURE 70 **Pilocarpine** is a naturally occurring cholinomimetic agent possessing both muscarinic and nicotinic properties. It causes miosis, reduces intraocular pressure, and is used in the treatment of wide-angle glaucoma. In addition, it may be applied topically in the eye in the form of a drug reservoir (Ocusert).

Because pimozide has anticholinergic properties, it is contraindicated in patients with arrhythmias because the drug may cause ventricular arrhythmias or aggravate existing arrhythmias; in patients with congenital Q-T syndrome because it may cause conduction defects and sudden death; and in comatose states and CNS depression because of the risk of addictive effects.

Concomitant use of pimozide with quinidine, procainamide, disopyramide, and other antiarrhythmics, phenothiazines (other antipsychotics), and antidepressants may further depress cardiac conduction and prolong the Q-T interval, resulting in serious arrhythmias.

Concomitant use with anticonvulsants (phenytoin, carbamazepine, or phenobarbital) may induce seizures, even in patients previously stabilized on anticonvulsants; an anticonvulsant dosage increase may be required.

Concomitant use with amphetamines, methylphenidate, or pemoline may induce Tourette-like tic and may exacerbate existing tics.

Concomitant use with CNS depressants, including alcohol, analgesics, barbiturates, narcotics, anxiolytics, parenteral magnesium sulfate, tranquilizers, and general, spinal, or epidural anesthetics may cause oversedation and respiratory depression because of additive CNS depressant effects.

Clinical signs of overdose include severe extrapyramidal reactions, hypotension, respiratory depression, coma, and ECG abnormalities, including prolongation of Q-T interval, inversion or flattening of T waves, and/or new appearance of U waves.

PINACIDIL

(Pindac)

Pinacidil (12.5 to 25.0 mg daily) appears to be a promising alternative agent for the treatment of moderate to severe hypertension.

Pinacidil is three- and tenfold more potent than hydralazine and minoxidil, respectively. It does not interact with alpha, beta, cholinergic, or histaminergic receptors, and also does not produce vasodilation via an indirect effect that is mediated by adenosine, prostaglandin, or endothelial-derived relaxant factor. Its vasodilating activity does not resemble that brought about by the conventional calcium channel antagonists. Thus, pinacidil-induced vascular relaxation is a direct effect mediated by a novel mechanism.

PINDOLOL
(Visken)

Pindolol, a beta-adrenergic receptor blocking agent (15 to 40 mg daily in three divided doses), is indicated in the management of hypertension. The beta-blocking potency of pindolol is 10 to 40 times that of propranolol, and it is about 10 times more potent that propranolol in its efficacy as an antihypertensive agent. However, its membrane stabilizing activity is lower than that of propranolol. Pindolol is not cardioselective and induces significantly less impairment of bronchial function than propranolol.

As for nearly all beta-antagonists, the main cardiovascular indications for pindolol are hypertension, angina pectoris, and arrhythmias. The usual warnings and precautions for beta-antagonists also apply to pindolol (see also Figure 27).

PIPAZETHATE
(Theratuss)

Noscapine (Nectadon) is a naturally occurring opium alkaloid with a structure and function similar to papaverine's. It is antitussive and has no analgesic or addictive properties.

Diphenhydramine and **chlorcyclizine** are antihistaminic agents that also have antitussive properties. **Dimethoxanate** (Cothera) and **pipazethate** are phenothiazine derivatives without analgesic but with weak antitussive and local anesthetic properties.

PIPECURONIUM BROMIDE
(Arduan)

Pipecuronium, a long-acting nondepolarizing neuromuscular blocking agent, is indicated to provide skeletal muscle relaxation during surgery. Pipecuronium can also be used to provide skeletal muscle relaxation for endotracheal intubation. It is only recommended for procedures anticipated to last 90 minutes or longer. Pipecuronium, like other long-acting neuromuscular blocking agents, displays a great deal of variability in the clinical duration of its effect. For small patients with decreased renal function, the initial dose is <70 to 85 mcg/kg. Pipecuronium competes for cholinergic receptors at the motor end plate, and this action is antagonized by acetylcholinesterase inhibitors such as neostigmine.

Pipecuronium should not be used in patients with myasthenia gravis. Muscle relaxants with short durations of action are more suitable. Aminoglycosides, tetracyclines, bacitracin, polymyxin B, colistin, and sodium colistimethate are apt to prolong the duration of action of pipecuronium. The most frequent side effect of nondepolarizing blocking agents is an extension of the drug's pharmacological action beyond the time period needed for surgery and anesthesia. Clinical signs may vary from skeletal muscle weakness to skeletal muscle paralysis resulting in respiratory insufficiency or apnea (see also Figure 92).

PIPERACILLIN SODIUM
(Pipracil)

Piperacillin (for serious infections 3 to 4 g every 4 to 6 hours as a 20- to 30-minute IV infusion), is indicated for the treatment of:

Intra-abdominal infections (including hepatobiliary and surgical infections), caused by *Escherichia coli, Pseudomonas aeruginosa,* enterococci, *Clostridium sp.,* anaerobic cocci, *Bacteroides sp.* including *B. fragilis*

Urinary tract infections caused by *E. coli, Klebsiella sp., P. aeruginosa, Proteus sp.,* including *P. mirabilis,* and enterococci

Gynecologic infections (including endometritis, pelvic inflammatory disease, pelvic cellulitis), caused by *Bacteroides sp.,* including *B. fragilis,* anaerobic cocci, *Neisseria gonorrhoeae,* enterococci (*Streptococcus faecalis*)

Septicemia (including bacteremia), caused by *E. coli, Klebsiella sp., Enterobacter sp., Serratia sp., P. mirabilis, S. pneumoniae,* enterococci, *P. aeruginosa, Bacteroides sp.,* and anaerobic cocci

Lower respiratory tract infections caused by *E. coli, Klebsiella sp., Enterobacter sp., P. aeruginosa, Serratia sp., Haemophilus influenzae, Bacteroides sp.,* and anaerobic cocci

Skin and skin-structure infections caused by *E. coli, Klebsiella sp., Serratia sp., Acinetobacter sp., Enterobacter sp., P. aeruginosa;* indole-positive *Proteus sp., P. mirabilis, Bacteroides sp.,* including *B. fragilis,* anaerobic cocci, enterococci

Bone and joint infections caused by *P. aeruginosa,* enterococci, *Bacteroides sp.,* and anaerobic cocci

Gonococcal infections, treatment of uncomplicated gonococcal urethritis

Streptococcal infections, infections caused by streptococcus species including group A beta-hemolytic *Streptococcus* and *S. pneumoniae;* however, these infections are ordinarily treated with more narrow spectrum penicillins.

Carbenicillin cures serious infections caused by *Pseudomonas* species and *Proteus* strains resistant to ampicillin. It is not absorbed from the gastrointestinal tract, and therefore must be administered intraperitoneally. **Carbenicillin indanyl** is acid stable and hence can be given orally. **Ticarcillin** is four times more potent than carbenicillin in treating a *Pseudomonas aeruginosa* infection, and **azlocillin** is ten times more potent than carbenicillin against *Pseudomonas.* **Mezlocillin** and **piperacillin** are more active against *Klebsiella* infection than is carbenicillin.

PIPERAZINE CITRATE

(Antepar)

Piperazine (single dose of 3.5 g for two consecutive days) is indicated for the treatment of enterobiasis (pinworm infection) and ascariasis (roundworm infection).

Piperazine blocks the response of Ascaris muscle to acetylcholine, causing flaccid paralysis of the worm. The paralyzed Ascaris are dislodged and expelled via peristalsis. Piperazine affects all stages of the parasite in the gut, but has little effect on larvae in the tissues. Toxic doses of piperazine cause convulsion, hence the drug should be used cautiously in patients with epilepsy.

PIPOBROMAN

(Vercyte)

Pipobroman, an alkylating agent with antineoplastic properties, is indicated in the treatment of polycythemia vera and chronic myelocytic leukemia (see also Figure 2).

PIRBUTEROL ACETATE

(Maxair)

Pirbuterol, a beta-adrenergic agonist with bronchodilating properties (1 to 2 inhalations every 4 to 6 hours), is indicated in the prevention and reversal of bronchospasm and asthma (see also Figure 86).

PIRENZEPINE

Vagal impulses elicit the release of acetylcholine in the parietal cells and in the gastric mucosal cells containing **gastrin**, a peptide hormone. Both the directly released acetylcholine and the indirectly released gastrin then stimulate the parietal cells to secrete hydrogen ions into the gastric lumen.

The most useful anticholinergic drugs are **propantheline** (Pro-Banthine), **pirenzepine**, and **telenzepine**, which antagonize muscarinic cholinergic receptors (M_1 receptors). All three agents depress gastric motility and secretion. The production of pepsin is also reduced. Propantheline may be used as adjunctive therapy with antacids but not as a sole agent. The side effects and contraindications of propantheline use are identical to those of atropine (prostatic hypertrophy, urinary retention, glaucoma, and cardiac arrhythmias).

The **timing** of medication is critical in ulcer therapy. Anticholinergic drugs should be given about 30 minutes before meals, and antacids about 1 hour after meals. A double dose of an antacid is often taken just before bedtime (see also Figure 24).

PIROXICAM
(Feldene)

Piroxicam (25 mg p.o. daily) is indicated in the treatment of osteoarthritis and rheumatoid arthritis. Piroxicam, a nonsteroidal antiinflammatory agent (NSAID) has analgesic and anti-inflammatory properties. It has a long half-life of 50 hours. Piroxicam should be used cautiously in patients with a history of peptic ulcer disease, angioedema, or cardiac disease, because the drug may worsen these conditions; and in patients with decreased renal function because it may cause a further reduction in renal function (see also Table 2).

Patients with known "triad" symptoms (aspirin hypersensitivity, rhinitis/nasal polyps, and asthma) are at high risk of bronchospasm. NSAIDs may mask the signs and symptoms of acute infection, fever, myalgia, erythema.

Concomitant use of piroxicam with anticoagulants and thrombolytic drugs (coumarin derivatives, heparin, streptokinase, or urokinase) may potentiate anticoagulant effects. Bleeding problems may occur if used with other drugs that inhibit platelet aggregation, such as azlocillin, parenteral carbenicillin, dextran, dipyridamole, mezlocillin, piperacillin, sulfin-pyrazone, ticarcillin, valproic acid, cefamandole, cefoperazone, moxalactam, plicamycin, aspirin, or other antiinflammatory agents. Concomitant use with salicylates, antiinflammatory agents, alcohol, corticotropin, or steroids may cause increased GI adverse effects, including ulceration and hemorrhage. Aspirin may decrease the bioavailability of piroxicam. Because of the influence of prostaglandins on glucose metabolism, concomitant use with insulin or oral hypoglycemic agents may potentiate hypoglycemic effects.

Piroxicam may displace highly protein-bound drugs from binding sites. Toxicity may occur with coumarin derivatives, phenytoin, verapamil, or nifedipine. Increased nephrotoxicity may occur with gold compounds, other antiinflammatory agents, or acetaminophen. Piroxicam may decrease the renal clearance of methotrexate and lithium. Piroxicam may decrease the effectiveness of antihypertensive agents and diuretics. Concomitant use with diuretics may increase risk of nephrotoxicity.

PLAGUE VACCINE

This bacterial vaccine is used primarily for immunization and as a booster.

PLASMA PROTEIN FRACTION
(Plasmanate, Plasma-Plex, Plasmatein, Protenate)

Plasma protein fraction, a plasma volume expander, is indicated in hypoproteinemia and shock.

PLATELET-ACTIVATING FACTOR

A platelet-activating factor, 1-0-alkyl-2(R)acetyl-sn-glyceryl-3-phosphocholine, is released in the presence of shock and ischemia. The platelet-activating factor antagonist can protect the heart and brain against ischemic injury.

Advances in medical practice, including the aggressive use of catheters and other invasive equipment, the implantation of prosthetic devices, the administration of chemotherapy to cancer patients, and the administration of immunosuppressive agents and corticosteroids to patients with organ transplants, have increased the risk of sepsis, septic syndrome, and septic-shock.

The initiating event in the sepsis cascade is the **release of endotoxin**, which prompts the release of **tumor necrosis factor alpha, interleukin-1, interleukin-6, interleukin-8**, and **platelet-activating factor** from mononuclear phagocytes and endothelial cells.

Neonates with sepsis are treated with **ampicillin**, which is effective against group B streptococci, *Listeria monocytogenes*, enterococci, and some Gram-negative rods, and **gentamicin**, which provides broader coverage against the Enterobacteriaceae.

PLICAMYCIN
(Formerly Mithramycin — Mithracin)

Plicamycin, an antineoplastic agent with hypocalcemic effect, is used in hypercalcemia and testicular cancer.

PNEUMOCOCCAL VACCINE, POLYVALENT
(Pneumovax 23, Pnu-Imune 23)

This bacterial vaccine is used for pneumococcal immunization.

PODOFILOX
(Condylox)

Podofilox, a keratolytic agent with antimimetic properties (0.5% in 95% alcohol to be applied q. 12 hours for three days), is used in the treatment of external genital warts.

POLIOVIRUS VACCINE, LIVE, ORAL, TRIVALENT
(TOPV, Sabin) (Orimune Trivalent)

This viral vaccine is used for the primary series of poliovirus immunizations.

POLYETHYLENE GLYCOL-ELECTROLYTE SOLUTION
(Peg-ES, Colovage, Colyte, Golytely, NuLytely, OCL)

Polyethylene glycol-electrolyte nonabsorbable solution, with laxative properties, is used for bowel preparation before GI examination.

POLYMYXIN B SULFATE
(Aerosporin)

Polymyxin B, a polypeptide antibiotic (500,000 units in 300 to 500 ml of 5% dextrose in water for continuous IV drip), is used in acute infections caused by susceptible strains of *Pseudomonas aeruginosa*. It may be used topically and subconjunctivally in the treatment of infections of the eye caused by susceptible strains of *P. aeruginosa*.

It may be indicated (when less toxic drugs are ineffective or contraindicated) in serious infections caused by susceptible strains of the following organisms: *Haemophilus influenzae* (meningeal infections); *Escherichia coli* (urinary tract infections); *Enterobacter aerogenes* (bacteremia); *Klebsiella pneumoniae* (bacteremia). In meningeal infections, polymyxin B sulfate must be administered only intrathecally.

The polymyxins consist of: polymyxin B (Aerosporin) and polymyxin E, or colisten (Coly-Mycin). These agents, which are bactericidal, are effective in the management of Gram-negative bacteria infections, especially *Pseudomonas*. Polymyxins are cationic detergent peptides, possessing both lipophilic and lipophobic groups that are able to bind and subsequently damage the bacterial cell membranes. Polymyxins are not absorbed orally and must be **administered parenterally** for the treatment of systemic infections. Reversible **nephrotoxicity** (proteinuria, hematuria, and cyclindruria) can occur with their use, as well as **neurotoxicity**, which is characterized by giddiness, numbness, paresthesia, neuromuscular blockade, confusion, ataxia, and convulsions.

POLYTHIAZIDE
(Renese)

Polythiazide, a thiazide diuretic (2 to 4 mg p.o. daily), is used in the treatment of hypertension.

POTASSIUM CHANNELS

Calcium-activated potassium channels increase their **permeability to potassium ions** in response to increases in the intracellular calcium concentration. These potassium channels couple the membrane potential to the intracellular calcium concentration of calcium, in that a rise in the intracellular calcium levels leads to an efflux of potassium ions and hence hyperpolarization of the membrane.

POTASSIUM IODIDE
(K1, SSK1) (Losat, Pima, Thyro-Block)

Potassium iodide is used as an expectorant, in preoperative thyroidectomy, nuclear radiation protection, and in the management of thyrotoxic crisis.

POTASSIUM SALTS, ORAL

POTASSIUM ACETATE

POTASSIUM BICARBONATE
(Klor-Con, EF, K-Lyte, Quic-K)

POTASSIUM CHLORIDE
(Cena-K, Kalium, Kaochlor, Kaochlor S-F, Kaon-CL, Kato, Kay Ciel, K-Dur, K-Lor, Klor-10%, Klor-Con, Klor-Con/25, Klorvess, Klotrix, K-Lyte/Cl Powder, K-Tab, Micro-K, Potachlor, Potage, Potasalan, Potassine, Rum-K, Slow-K, Ten-K)

POTASSIUM GLUCONATE

Potassium salts are used in hypokalemic states.

POTASSIUM-SPARING DIURETICS

The potassium-sparing diuretics consist of **spironolactone** (Aldactone), which is an aldosterone antagonist, and **triamterene** (Dyrenium) and **amiloride** (Midamor), which exert their effects through a mechanism other than a mineralocorticoid action.

All act in the distal tubule, where the resorption of sodium is accompanied by the transfer of potassium into the lumen contents. When sodium resorption is hindered, potassium excretion is correspondingly reduced, such that more potassium is retained. The potassium-sparing diuretics are not very efficacious, as they affect only 1 to 2% of the filtered load of sodium. All are given orally and eliminated in the urine, mostly by glomerular filtration, though some active tubular secretion may also occur (see Figure 4).

A potassium-sparing diuretic can be given along with a thiazide or a loop diuretic to prevent hypokalemia. Spironolactone can also be beneficial in some patients with severe congestive heart failure or cirrhosis associated with ascites.

The potassium-sparing diuretics should not be used concurrently with potassium supplements, as this combination is likely to produce hyperkalemia. Poor renal function also heightens the risk of hyperkalemia. Gastrointestinal disturbances, rash, drowsiness, or dizziness are all associated with their use. Spironolactone can cause the blood urea nitrogen level to increase and lead to menstrual irregularities (see also Table 25).

PRALIDOXIME CHLORIDE

(2-Pam Chloride, Pyridine-2-Aldoxime Methochloride, Protopam)

Pralidoxime, a quaternary ammonium oxime, is used to antidote poisoning from organophosphate pesticides (see also Figure 71).

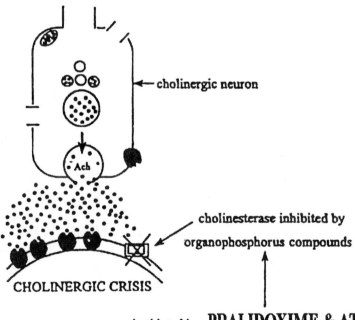

FIGURE 71   The clinical manifestations of acute and severe poisoning from the organophosphorous insecticides include **cholinergic crisis**, resulting from the stimulation of muscarinic cholinergic receptors (**bronchoconstriction, salivation, sweating, lacrimation, bradycardia, hypotension,** and **urinary and fecal incontinence**), from the stimulation of nicotinic cholinergic receptors (muscular fasciculation), and from central nervous system (CNS) effects (with initial restlessness, tremors, ataxia, and convulsions, followed by CNS depression and respiratory and circulatory depression). The treatment of a cholinergic crisis caused by organophosphorous compounds includes the administration of a cholinesterase reactivator such as **pralidoxime (2-PAM) together with atropine**. (Adapted from Ebadi, M., *Pharmacology, An Illustrated Review with Questions and Answers*, 3rd Edition, Lippincott-Raven Press, Philadelphia, 1996.)

PRAMIPEXOLE

Pramipexole, a dopamine receptor agonist with activity at both autoreceptors and postsynaptic receptors, has shown efficacy in animal models of parkinsonism.

PRAVASTATIN

The hypolipidemic agent pravastatin differs from other HMG-CoA reductase inhibitors (e.g., lovastatin and simvastatin) because it has greater hydrophilicity as a result of the hydroxyl group attached to its decalin ring. The hydrophilic nature of pravastatin accounts for its minimal penetration into the intracellular space of nonhepatic tissues, including an apparent inability to cross the blood-brain barrier. The drug is also well tolerated because it is rapidly absorbed and excreted, and does not accumulate in plasma even with repeated administration (see also Figure 25).

PRAVASTATIN SODIUM

(Pravachol)

Pravastatin, an inhibitor of HMG-CoA reductase (5 to 10 mg daily), is used for reduction of low-density lipoprotein and total cholesterol levels in patients with primary hypercholesterolemia (types IIa and IIb) (see also Figure 25).

PRAZEPAM

(Centrax)

Prazepam, a benzodiazepine derivative (30 mg p.o. daily), is used in anxiety (see also Figure 40 and Table 8).

Prazepam, a benzodiazepine derivative (30 mg p.o. daily in divided doses), is indicated for the management of anxiety disorders and for the short-term relief of the symptoms of anxiety. Prazepam depresses the CNS at the limbic and subcortical levels of the brain. It produces an antianxiety effect by enhancing the effect of the neurotransmitter gamma-aminobutyric acid (GABA) on its receptor in the ascending reticular activating system, which increases inhibition and blocks both cortical and limbic arousal.

Prazepam is metabolized to desmethyldiazepam and oxazepam, which is a pharmacologically short-acting anxiety agent. The half-life of demethyldiazepam ranges from 30 to 200 hours, and that of oxazepam ranges from 5 to 15 hours.

Prazepam potentiates the CNS depressant effects of phenothiazines, narcotics, antihistamines, monoamine oxidase inhibitors, barbiturates, alcohol, general anesthetics, and antidepressants.

Concomitant use with cimetidine and possibly disulfiram causes diminished hepatic metabolism of prazepam, which increases its plasma concentration.

Heavy smoking accelerates prazepam's metabolism, thus lowering its clinical effectiveness.

Antacids may delay the absorption of prazepam. Prazepam may antagonize levodopa's therapeutic effects. Clinical manifestations of overdose include somnolence, convulsion, coma, hypoactive reflexes, dyspnea, labored breathing, hypotension, bradycardia, slurred speech, and unsteady gait or impaired coordination (see also Table 8).

PRAZIQUANTEL

(Biltricide)

Praziquantel (three doses of 20 mg/kg as one day treatment only) is indicated for the treatment of infections due to *Schistosoma mekongi, S. japonicum, S. mansoni,* and *S. hematobium;* and for infections due to liver flukes, *Clonorchis sinensis/Opisthorchis viverrini.*

Praziquantel increases membrane permeability in susceptible worms, resulting in a loss of intracellular calcium, massive contractions and paralysis of their musculature. The drug further results in vacuolization and disintegration of the schistosome tegument. This effect is followed by attachment of phagocytes to the parasite and death.

PRAZOSIN
(Minipress)

Prazosin, (1 mg t.i.d.) alone or in combination with other drugs such as a diuretic, is indicated in the management of moderate hypertension. It is a direct vasodilator and is used for long-term therapy. Its side effects are sedation, postural hypotension, and headache (due to vasodilation). As much as 97% of prazosin is bound to plasma protein. When used for the first time or in larger than recommended doses, prazosin may cause pronounced hypotension, faintness, dizziness, and palpitations. These effects, which have been labeled **first-dose phenomena**, are seen especially in salt- and water-depleted patients. Therefore, the initial dose of prazosin is small, and it is given at bedtime.

PREDNISOLONE

Prednisone, a glucocorticoid, is inactive and must be metabolized to prednisolone, which is available in the following preparations (see also Table 10):

Nonproprietary and Proprietary Names	Oral Forms	Injectable Forms
Methylprednisolone (Medrol)	2–32 mg	—
Methylprednisolone acetate		
(Depo-Medrol, Medrol Acetate)	—	20–80 mg/ml (susp.)
Prednisolone (Delta-Cortef)	5 mg	—
Prednisolone acetate		
(Econopred)	3 mg/ml (syrup)	—
Prednisolone sodium phosphate		
(Hydeltra-T.B.A.)	1 mg/ml (liquid)	20 mg/ml (susp.)
Prednisone	1–50 mg	—
(Deltasone)	1 mg/ml (syrup)	—
	1,5 mg/ml (soln)	
	1–8 mg	

The administration of glucocorticoids to human subjects brings about lymphocytopenia, monocytopenia, and eosinopenia. In addition, glucocorticoids block a number of lymphocytic functions.

Although considered to be immunosuppressive, therapeutic doses of glucocorticoids do not significantly decrease the concentration of antibodies in the circulation. Furthermore, during glucocorticoid therapy, patients exhibit a nearly normal antibody response to antigenic challenge. Glucocorticoids are extensively used in medicine, and some of them are outlined in Table 10. For example, in bronchial asthma, **prednisone** is available in oral form, and **beclamethasone** may be used as an aerosol, especially in children. The corticosteroids may exert their effects through multiple mechanisms, including relaxing bronchospasm, decreasing mucus secretion, potentiating beta-adrenergic receptors, antagonizing cholinergic actions, stabilizing lysosomes possessing antiinflammatory properties, inhibiting antibody formation, and antagonizing histamine actions.

Corticosteroids do not inhibit the release of mediators from mast cells or block the early response to allergens, but they do block the late response and the subsequent bronchial hyperresponsiveness (see also Figure 29).

Steroids such as **beclomethasone dipropionate, budesonide, triamcinolone acetonide**, and **flunisolide** are active when given topically, and can control asthma without causing systemic effects or adrenal suppression. However, orally administered steroids such as **prednisone, prednisolone,** or **methylprednisolone** are still needed by some patients.

The **side effects** of high-dose inhalational steroids include oropharyngeal candidiasis and dysphonia. The orally administered steroids may produce osteoporosis, weight gain, hypertension, diabetes, myopathy, psychiatric disturbances, skin fragility, or cataracts.

PREDNISOLONE (SYSTEMIC)
(Cortalone, Delta-Cortef, Prelone)

PREDNISOLONE ACETATE
(Articulose, Key-Pred, Predaject, Predate, Predcor)

PREDNISOLONE ACETATE AND PREDNISOLONE SODIUM PHOSPHATE

PREDNISOLONE SODIUM PHOSPHATE
(Hydeltrasol, Key-Pred SP, PediaPred, Predate-S)

PREDNISOLONE TERBUTATE
(Hydeltra-T.B.A., Metalone T.B.A., Norpred T.B.A., Predate T.B.A., Predcor T.B.A., Predisol T.B.A.)

Prednisolone, a glucocorticoid–mineralocorticoid with antiinflammatory and immunosuppressant properties, is used for severe inflammation or immunosuppression (see also Tables 10 and 13).

PREDNISOLONE ACETATE (OPHTHALMIC)
(Ak-Tate, Econopred Ophthalmic, I-Prednicet, Ocu-Pred-A, Predair-A, Pred Forte, Pred Mild Ophthalmic)

PREDNISOLONE SODIUM PHOSPHATE
(Ak Pred, Inflamase, Inflamase Mild Ophthalmic, Inflamase Forte, I-Pred, Metreton, Ocu-Pred, Predair)

Prednisolone, a corticosteroid with ophthalmic antiinflammatory properties, is used in inflammation of the palpebral and bulbar conjunctiva, cornea, and the anterior segment of the globe.

PREDNISONE
(Meticorten, Orasone, Panasol, Prednicen-M, SK-Prednisone)

Prednisone, an adrenocorticoid with antiinflammatory and immunosuppressant properties, is used in severe inflammation or immunosuppression, and in acute exacerbations of multiple sclerosis. In addition, prednisone has been used as an adjunct to antiinfective therapy in the treatment of moderate to severe *Pneumocystis carinii* pneumonia.

PREPARATHYROID HORMONE
Parathyroid hormone is a single-chain polypeptide composed of 84 amino acids. It has a molecular weight of 9,500 and lacks an intrachain disulfide linkage. Parathyroid hormone is

produced by means of two sequential enzymic cleavages from a larger precursor polypeptide, **preparathyroid hormone**.

The organs principally responsible for the peripheral metabolism of parathyroid hormone are the kidney and liver, and possibly bone (see Figure 66).

PRILOCAINE HYDROCHLORIDE
(Citanest)

Prilocaine, a local anesthetic (4% with 1:200,000 epinephrine in 1 to 8 ml dental cartridge), is indicated for local anesthesia by nerve block or infiltration in dental procedures.

Prilocaine, which is equal in potency to lidocaine, has a longer duration of action. It is metabolized to o-toluidine, which in toxic doses may cause methemoglobinemia.

PRIMAQUINE PHOSPHATE

Primaquine, an 8 aminoquinoline (26.3 mg daily for 14 days), is recommended only for the radical cure of vivax malaria, the prevention of relapse in vivax malaria, or following the termination of chloroquine phosphate suppressive therapy in an area where vivax malaria is endemic.

Primaquine may disrupt the parasite's mitochondria and bind to native DNA. The resulting structural changes create a major disruption in the metabolic process. The gametocyte and exoerythrocyte forms are inhibited. Some gametocytes are destroyed, while others are rendered incapable of undergoing maturation division in the mosquito gut. By eliminating tissue (exoerythrocyte) infection, primaquine prevents development of blood (erythrocytic) forms responsible for relapses in vivax malaria.

Primaquine is rapidly metabolized to a carboxylic acid derivative and then to further metabolites which have varying degrees of activity; elimination half-life is around 4 hours. Approximately 1% is excreted unchanged in the urine. Primaquine may cause hemolytic anemia, especially in patients who are deficient in glucose 6-phosphate dehydrogenase.

PRIMIDONE
(Mysoline)

Primidone, an anticonvulsant, is given at an initial dose of 100 to 125 mg/day at bedtime, increasing gradually to a maintenance dose of 125 to 250 mg three times daily. The most frequent side effect of primidone is heavy sedation, which seems to be due to primidone itself and not to its metabolite phenobarbital. Tolerance develops to this sedation within a few days or weeks of continuous administration.

Primidone is a nonbarbiturate compound that is structurally related to phenobarbital. Primidone is absorbed well and does not bind to plasma proteins extensively. It is probably not advisable to administer this agent to subjects with a history of adverse reaction to **phenobarbital**.

Primidone is indicated for control of grand mal, psychomotor, or focal epileptic seizures, either alone or with other anticonvulsants. It may control grand mal seizures refractory to other anticonvulsants. Primidone raises electroshock or chemoshock seizure thresholds or alters seizure patterns. The mechanism of antiepileptic action is not known.

Primidone and its two metabolites, phenobarbital and phenylethyl-malonamide (PEMA), have anticonvulsant activity. In addition, PEMA potentiates the activity of phenobarbital. Abrupt withdrawal of primidone may cause status epilepticus. Acetazolamide, succinimides, and carbamazepine reduce the plasma level of primidone, whereas the coadministration of hydantoin, isoniazid, or nicotinamide increases it (see also Figure 68).

PROBENECID
(Benemid)

Probenecid, a uricosuric agent (initially 0.25 g t.i.d. for one week), is indicated in the treatment of hyperuricemia associated with gout and gouty arthritis. In addition, probenecid is used as an adjunct to therapy with penicillins or cephalosporins, and for elevation and prolongation of plasma levels of these antibiotics.

A uricosuric and renal tubular blocking agent, probenecid inhibits the tubular resorption of urate, thus increasing the urinary excretion of uric acid and decreasing serum uric acid levels. Effective uricosuria reduces the miscible urate pool, retards urate deposition, and promotes resorption of urate deposits.

Probenecid also inhibits the tubular secretion of most penicillins and cephalosporins and usually increases plasma levels by any route the antibiotic is given. A twofold to fourfold plasma elevation has been demonstrated.

The most commonly used uricosuric agents are **probenecid** and **sulfinpyrazone** (Anturane). In low doses, these agents block tubular secretion, but, at higher doses, they also block the tubular resorption of uric acid. Because the solubility of uric acid is increased in alkaline urine, the administration of sodium bicarbonate may at times be advantageous for offsetting this condition. In addition, probenecid and sulfinpyrazone inhibit the excretion of agents such as aspirin, penicillin, ampicillin, and indomethacin. Although probenecid and sulfinpyrazone may be coadministered, neither should be given with aspirin, as their uricosuric effects will then be nullified.

On the other hand, probenecid increases the plasma level of acyclovir, allopurinol, barbiturate, benzodiazepines, clofibrate, dapsone, dyphylline, methotrexate, NSAIDs, penicillamine, sulfonylureas, and zidovudine.

PROBUCOL
(Lorelco)

Probucol, an antihyperlipidemic agent (500 mg twice daily with meals), is indicated for reduction of elevated serum cholesterol in patients with primary hypercholesterolemia (elevated LDL) who have not responded to diet, weight reduction, and control of diabetes mellitus. It may be useful to lower elevated cholesterol that occurs with combined hypercholesterolemia and hypertriglyceridemia, but it is not indicated when hypertriglyceridemia is the major concern.

Probucol lowers serum cholesterol with relatively little effect on serum triglycerides. Patients responding to probucol exhibit a decrease in low density lipoprotein (LDL) cholesterol. Cholesterol is reduced not only in the LDL fraction, but also in some high density lipoprotein (HDL) fractions with proportionately greater effect on the HDL portion in some patients. Epidemiological studies have shown that low HDL cholesterol and high LDL cholesterol are independent risk factors for coronary heart disease. The risk of lowering HDL cholesterol while lowering LDL cholesterol is unknown. Little or no effect is reported on very low density lipoprotein (VLDL).

Probucol increases the fractional rate of LDL catabolism. This effect may be linked to the increased excretion of fecal bile acids. Probucol also inhibits early stages of cholesterol synthesis and slightly inhibits absorption of dietary cholesterol. There is no increase in the cyclic precursors of cholesterol; hence, probucol does not appear to affect later stages of cholesterol biosynthesis.

Prolongation of the QT interval can occur in patients on probucol, predisposing to ventricular tachycardia (see also Figure 25).

PROCAINAMIDE HYDROCHLORIDE
(Pronestyl)

Procainamide (an initial total daily oral dose up to 50 mg/kg) is indicated for the treatment of documented ventricular arrhythmias, such as sustained ventricular tachycardia that is judged to be life threatening. Because procainamide has the potential to produce serious hematologic disorders, particularly leukopenia or agranulocytosis, its use should be reserved for patients in whom the benefits of treatment clearly outweigh the risks.

Quinidine and procainamide decrease automaticity by reducing the **rate of phase 4 diastolic depolarization**, which is probably mediated by a diminished membrane permeability to sodium, and decrease conduction velocity throughout the conducting system. They produce an indirect (vagolytic) effect that sometimes counteracts the direct effect at the AV node, producing a paradoxical tachycardia in some cases of atrial flutter or fibrillation. These agents terminate re-entry arrhythmias by producing a bidirectional block in infarcted conducting tissues. They directly depress contractility, leading to a decline in cardiac output (see also Figure 76).

These agents are **potent vasodilators**, especially when given intravenously. This effect is so great that quinidine is rarely given parenterally and great care must be taken when it is given by this route. They depress blood pressure by means of their dual effects on cardiac output and peripheral resistance.

These agents produce widening of the QRS complex (by depressing ventricular conduction) and lengthening of the PR interval (by slowing AV conduction). A 25 to 30% widening of the QRS complex is considered the therapeutic limit with these agents. They are excreted up to 50% unmetabolized in the urine. They commonly cause **gastrointestinal disturbances**, and these constitute their major side effect. **Emboli** may be liberated from the atria during conversion of atrial flutter or fibrillation. **Toxicity** is manifested by a profound fall in blood pressure that leads to a shock-like state accompanied by a variety of arrhythmias.

Quinidine and procainamide may also provoke some unique but uncommon side effects. Quinidine may produce **cinchonism** (tinnitus, dizziness, visual disturbances, and vertigo) and **cutaneous hypersensitivity reactions.** Procainamide may produce **agranulocytosis** during long-term therapy, and a dose-dependent (>2 gm/day) **lupus erythematosus-like syndrome**. These agents are mainly used in the management of atrial (supraventricular) arrhythmias, although procainamide is also of value in treating premature ventricular contractions and ventricular tachycardia. If either drug is used to convert atrial flutter or fibrillation, digitalis must be given first to protect against paradoxical tachycardia.

PROCAINE HYDROCHLORIDE
(Novocain)

Procaine is indicated for infiltration anesthesia (0.25 to 0.50% solution), peripheral nerve block (0.5 to 2% solution), and spinal anesthesia (10% solution). Procaine, which has a pK_a of 8.9, is highly ionized at the physiologic pH and has a short duration of action. Because it causes vasodilation, a vasoconstricting substance is added to the procaine solution to delay

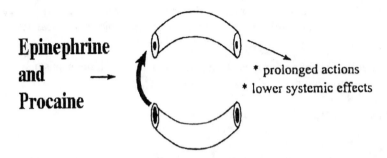

Epinephrine and Procaine →

* prolonged actions
* lower systemic effects

FIGURE 72   Procaine has a short duration of action. Because it causes vasodilation, a vasoconstricting substance is added to the procaine solution to delay systemic absorption. (Adapted from Ebadi, M., *Pharmacology, An Illustrated Review with Questions and Answers*, 3rd Edition, Lippincott-Raven Press, Philadelphia, 1996.)

systemic absorption (see Figure 72). **Procainamide**, a congener of procaine, is an effective oral antiarrhythmic agent. Procaine may prolong the effect of **succinylcholine**, since both drugs are metabolized by the same enzyme. Cholinesterase inhibitors alter procaine's metabolism.

PROCARBAZINE HYDROCHLORIDE

(Matulane)

Procarbazine, an antineoplastic agent (2 to 4 mg/kg/day for the first week) in combination with other antineoplastic agents (MOPP regimen — nitrogen mustard, vincristine, procarbazine, prednisone), is indicated for treatment of Stage III and IV Hodgkin's disease. Procarbazine inhibits the synthesis of protein (ribonucleic acid (RNA) and deoxyribonucleic acid (DNA) (see also Figure 2).

Procarbazine may inhibit transmethylation of methyl groups of methionine into tRNA. The absence of functional tRNA could cause the cessation of protein synthesis and consequently DNA and RNA synthesis. In addition, procarbazine may directly damage DNA. Hydrogen peroxide, formed during the auto-oxidation of the drug, may attack protein sulfhydryl groups contained in residual protein which is tightly bound to DNA.

Procarbazine is rapidly and completely absorbed from the GI tract and quickly equilibrates between plasma and cerebrospinal fluid (CSF). Peak CSF levels occur in 30 to 90 minutes. Following oral administration, maximum peak plasma concentrations occur within 60 minutes.

The drug is metabolized in the liver to cytotoxic products. The major portion of drug is excreted in the urine as N-isopropylterephthalamic acid (approximately 70% within 24 hours following oral and IV administration). Less than 5% is excreted in urine unchanged.

After IV injection, the plasma half-life is approximately 10 minutes. Procarbazine crosses the blood-brain barrier.

The most frequent adverse reactions of procarbazine are nausea, vomiting, leukopenia, anemia, and thrombocytopenia.

PROCHLORPERAZINE

(Compazine)

Prochlorperazine, an antiemetic and antipsychotic agent, is indicated for controlling preoperative nausea (5 to 10 mg IM 1 to 2 hours before induction of anesthesia and severe nausea and vomiting (5 to 10 mg p.o. t.i.d.) associated with circulating physical agents (radiation

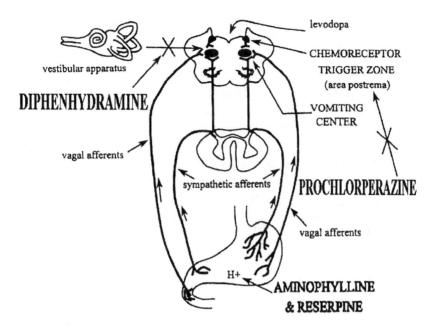

FIGURE 73 Phenothiazine derivatives such as chlorpromazine, perphenazine, **prochlorperazine**, promethazine, triethylperazine, and triflupromazine, exert their antiemetic effects by blocking the dopamine receptors in the **area postrema**.

therapy and virus particles) and chemical agents (toxins and cancer chemotherapeutic agents) (see Figure 73).

Prochlorperazine is thought to exert its antipsychotic effects by postsynaptic blockade of CNS dopamine receptors, thus inhibiting dopamine-mediated effects. Its antiemetic effects are attributed to dopamine receptor blockade in the medullary chemoreceptor trigger zone (Figure 73).

Prochlorperazine causes sedation, has weak anticholinergic properties, and produces a high incidence of movement disorders.

Concomitant use of prochlorperazine with sympathomimetics, including epinephrine, phenylephrine, phenylpropranolamine, and ephedrine (often found in nasal sprays), and with appetite suppressants may decrease their stimulatory and pressor effects and may cause epinephrine reversal (hypotensive response to epinephrine).

Prochlorperazine may inhibit blood pressure response to centrally acting antihypertensive drugs, such as guanethidine, guanabenz, guanadrel, clonidine, methyldopa, and reserpine. Additive effects are likely after concomitant use of prochlorperazine with CNS depressants, including alcohol, analgesics, barbiturates, narcotics, tranquilizers, and anesthetics (general, spinal, or epidural), and parenteral magnesium sulfate (oversedation, respiratory depression, and hypotension); antiarrhythmic agents, quinidine, disopyramide, and procainamide (increased incidence of cardiac arrhythmias and conduction defects); atropine and other anticholinergic drugs, including antidepressants, monoamine oxidase inhibitors, phenothiazines, antihistamines, meperidine, and antiparkinsonian agents (oversedation, paralytic ileus, visual changes, and severe constipation); nitrates (hypotension); and metrizamide (increased risk of convulsions).

Beta-blocking agents may inhibit prochlorperazine metabolism, increasing plasma levels and toxicity.

Concomitant use with propylthiouracil increases risk of agranulocytosis; concomitant use with lithium may result in severe neurologic toxicity with an encephalitis-like syndrome, and in decreased therapeutic response to prochlorperazine.

Pharmacokinetic alterations and subsequent decreased therapeutic response to prochlorperazine may follow concomitant use with phenobarbital (enhanced renal excretion); aluminum- and magnesium-containing antacids and antidiarrheals (decreased absorption); caffeine, or heavy smoking (increased metabolism).

Prochlorperazine may antagonize the therapeutic effect of bromocriptine on prolactin secretion; it also may decrease the vasoconstricting effects of high-dose dopamine and may decrease effectiveness and increase toxicity of levodopa (by dopamine blockade). Prochlorperazine may inhibit metabolism and increase toxicity of phenytoin.

PROCHLORPERAZINE EDISYLATE
(Compazine)

PROCHLORPERAZINE MALEATE
(Chlorazine, Compazine, Compazine Spansule)

Prochlorperazine, a phenothiazine derivative with antiemetic properties, is used to control preoperative nausea and severe nausea and vomiting.

PROCYCLIDINE HYDROCHLORIDE
(Kemadrin)

Procyclidine (2.5 mg t.i.d. with meals) is indicated in the treatment of Parkinson's disease at its early stage. In addition, it is effective in relieving the neuroleptic-induced extrapyramidal symptoms. Procycline is an anticholinergic agent, which by blocking central cholinergic receptors, helps to re-establish the proper cholinergic-dopaminergic transmission in the basal ganglion.

Procyclidine is contraindicated in patients with narrow-angle glaucoma, because drug-induced cycloplegia and mydriasis may increase intraocular pressure. Procyclidine should be administered cautiously in patients with tachycardia, because the drug may block vagal inhibition of the sinoatrial node pacemaker, thus exacerbating tachycardia, and in patients with urinary retention or prostatic hypertrophy, because the drug may exacerbate these conditions.

Procyclidine may reduce the antipsychotic effectiveness of haloperidol and phenothiazines, possibly by direct CNS antagonism related to its anticholinergic properties. Haloperidol and phenothiazine exert their effects in part by blocking the hyperactivity of dopaminergic transmission in the mesocortical and mesolimbic systems. Concomitant use with phenothiazine derivatives, especially thioridazine having pronounced anticholinergic effects also increases the risk of anticholinergic adverse effects. Paralytic ileus may result from concomitant use with phenothiazines or tricyclic antidepressants. Concomitant use with alcohol and other CNS depressants increases procyclidine's sedative effects.

Antacids and antidiarrheals may decrease procyclidine's absorption, thus reducing its effectiveness.

Clinical symptoms of overdosage with procycline which result primarily from its anticholinergic effects, include central stimulation followed by depression, and such psychotic symptoms as disorientation, confusion, hallucinations, delusions, anxiety, agitation, and restlessness.

Peripheral effects may include dilated, nonreactive pupils, blurred vision, flushed, hot, dry skin, dry mucus membranes, dysphagia, decreased or absent bowel sounds, urinary retention, hyperthermia, tachycardia, hypertension, and increased respiration.

PROGESTERONE

(Bay Progest, Femotrone, Gesertol 50, Progestaject-50, Progestasert, Progesteronaq-LA)

Progesterone is synthesized in the ovaries, the adrenal glands, and the placenta. In a non-pregnant woman, it is produced by the **corpus luteum** during the latter part of the menstrual cycle under the influence of luteinizing and luteotropic hormones. In a pregnant woman, it is produced initially by the corpus luteum under the influence of chorionic gonadotropins and is synthesized by the **placenta** after failure of the corpus luteum.

Progesterone is not only an important **progestin**, but is also an important precursor for androgen. It is synthesized according to the following scheme:

Acetate → cholesterol → pregnenolone → progesterone → testosterone → estradiol

Progesterone is absorbed rapidly when given orally and has a plasma half-life of 5 minutes. It is completely metabolized in the liver and is cleared completely during first passage through the liver.

Progesterone initially prepares the uterus for **implantation** of the fertilized egg and prevents uterine contraction that would expel the fetus. Progesterone has been used in the past to prevent threatened abortion. In addition, progesterone exerts effects on the secretory cells of the mammary glands. Progesterone competes with aldosterone and causes a decrease in sodium resorption; therefore it antagonizes aldosterone-induced sodium retention. Progesterone increases the body temperature and decreases the plasma level of many amino acids.

In the treatment of progesterone-related disorders, progesterone, which must be injected and has a short duration of action, has been replaced by the progestins. These newer synthetic derivatives of progesterone are effective orally and have a longer duration of action. Unlike progesterone, some of these agents have androgenic, estrogenic, and even glucocorticoid-like effects.

Progestins are used as **antifertility agents** and in the treatment of **dysfunctional uterine bleeding**, which may occur as a result of insufficient estrogen or because of continued estrogen secretion in the absence of progesterone.

Progestins such as medroxyprogesterone are useful in the diagnosis and treatment of amenorrhea.

Because prostaglandin F_{2a} is capable of inducing contraction in the uterus, agents that are able to block the synthesis of prostaglandin, such as aspirin or aspirin-like substances, have been shown to be effective in easing dysmenorrhea. For sexually active women, oral contraceptives have been found to be effective in relieving dysmenorrhea.

Endometriosis, which was formerly treated by surgical removal of the ovaries and uterus, is now treated with the continuous administration of progestin, or with progestin combined with estrogen. In addition, progestin may be useful in the management of endometrial carcinoma.

Estrogen, progesterone, and bromocriptine (a dopamine receptor agonist) are all effective in suppressing postpartum lactation.

PROMAZINE HYDROCHLORIDE

(Sparine)

Promazine (initially 50 to 150 mg IM) is indicated for the management of psychotic disorders. In addition, it has antiemetic and antivertigo properties and possesses antihistaminic actions and hence may be used pre- or postoperatively (25 to 50 mg IM). The antiemetic effects of promazine may be due to its anticholinergic actions. Furthermore, promazine inhibits the medullary chemoreceptor trigger zone for emesis. The antipsychotic effects of promazine may be due in part to blockade of hyperactive dopaminergic transmission in the mesocortical and mesolimbic systems.

Like other antihistamines, promethazine has significant anticholinergic effects; it should be used with caution in patients with narrow-angle glaucoma, peptic ulcer, or pyloroduodenal obstruction or urinary bladder obstruction from prostatic hypertrophy or narrowing of the bladder neck. It also should be used with caution in patients with cardiovascular disease or hypertension because of the risk of palpitations with acute or chronic respiratory dysfunction (especially children) because promazine may depress the cough reflex.

Clinical manifestations of overdose may include either CNS depression (sedation, reduction in mental alertness, apnea, and cardiovascular collapse) or CNS stimulation (insomnia, hallucinations, tremors, or convulsions). Atropine-like symptoms, such as dry-mouth, flushed skin, fixed and dilated pupils, and GI symptoms are common, especially in children.

PROMETHAZINE HYDROCHLORIDE

(Phenergan)

Promethazine (25 mg one hour before travel) is indicated for acute and prophylactic treatment of motion sickness, and for prevention and control of nausea and vomiting associated with anesthesia and surgery.

Promethazine competes with histamine for the H_1-receptor, thereby suppressing allergic rhinitis and urticaria; the drug does not prevent the release of histamine.

The central anticholinergic and antihistaminic effects of promethazine causing inhibition of the medullary chemoreceptor trigger zone for emesis is responsible for its antiemetic and antivertigo effects (see also Figure 73).

Promethazine causes sedation by reducing stimuli to the brain stem reticular system. Like other antihistamines, promethazine has significant anticholinergic effects; it should be used with caution in patients with narrow-angle glaucoma, peptic ulcer, or pyloroduodenal obstruction or urinary bladder obstruction from prostatic hypertrophy or narrowing of the bladder neck. It also should be used with caution in patients with cardiovascular disease or hypertension because of the risk of palpitations with acute or chronic respiratory dysfunction (especially children) because promazine may depress the cough reflex.

Concurrent administration of drugs such as promethazine or chlorpromazine may greatly enhance meperidine-induced sedation without slowing clearance of the drug.

Clinical manifestations of overdose may include either CNS depression (sedation, reduced mental alertness, apnea, and cardiovascular collapse) or CNS stimulation (insomnia, hallucinations, tremors, or convulsions). Atropine-like symptoms, such as dry mouth, flushed skin, fixed and dilated pupils, and GI symptoms are common, especially in children.

PROPAFENONE HYDROCHLORIDE
(Rythmol)

Propafenone (150 mg every 8 hours) is indicated in the treatment of documented life-threatening ventricular arrhythmias, such as sustained ventricular tachycardia. In addition, propafenone appears to be effective in the treatment of supraventricular tachycardias including atrial fibrillation and flutter and arrhythmias associated with Wolff-Parkinson-White syndrome.

Propafenone is a Class 1C antiarrhythmic drug with local anesthetic effects and a direct stabilizing action on myocardial membranes. The electrophysiological effect of propafenone manifests itself in a reduction of upstroke velocity (Phase O) of the monophasic action potential. In Purkinje fibers, and to a lesser extent myocardial fibers, propafenone reduces the fast inward current carried by sodium ions. The diastolic excitability threshold is increased and the effective refractory period prolonged. Propafenone reduces spontaneous automaticity and depresses triggered activity.

Propafenone, which has a weak beta-adrenergic blocking effect (1/40 that of propranolol) causes a dose-related decrease in the rate of single and multiple PVCs and can suppress recurrence of ventricular tachycardia. Additionally, like other Class 1C antiarrhythmic drugs, propafenone exerts a negative inotropic effect on the myocardium.

Propafenone is completely absorbed after oral administration, exhibits an extensive first-pass metabolism, and its clearance is reduced and the elimination half-life increased in patients with significant hepatic dysfunction.

Propafenone is metabolized into two active metabolites: 5-hydroxypropafenone and N-depropylpropafenone. Propafenone is contraindicated in congestive heart failure, cardiogenic shock, sinoatrial, AV, and intraventricular disorders of impulse generation or conduction (e.g., sick sinus node syndrome, AV block) in the absence of an artificial pacemaker; as well as in bradycardia, marked hypotension, bronchospastic disorders, and manifest electrolyte imbalance.

Cimetidine and quinidine increase and rifampin decreases the serum level of propafenone. Propafenone increases the plasma levels and hence the actions of anticoagulants, beta adrenergic receptor blocking agents, cyclosporine, and digoxin. The adverse reactions occurring most often are headaches, dizziness, unusual taste, first-degree AV block, intraventricular conduction delay, nausea or vomiting, and constipation.

Symptoms of overdosage which are usually most severe within 3 hours of ingestion may include hypotension, somnolence, bradycardia, intra-atrial and intraventricular conduction disturbances, and rarely convulsions and high-grade ventricular arrhythmias.

PROPANIDID

Propanidid is a nonbarbiturate ultra short-acting anesthetic agent that may cause hypotension and tachycardia. Unlike thiopental, which is redistributed, propanidid is metabolized rapidly by pseudocholinesterases.

PROPANTHELINE BROMIDE
(Pro-Banthine)

Propantheline (50 to 100 mg every six hours) is indicated as an adjunctive therapy in the treatment of peptic ulcer. In addition, it has been advocated for its antisecretory and antispasmodic effects for use in irritable bowel syndrome and other GI disorders and to reduce duodenal motility during diagnostic radiologic procedures (see also Figure 24).

Propantheline, a muscarinic cholinergic receptor antagonist, competitively blocks acetylcholine's actions at cholinergic neuroeffector sites, decreasing GI motility and inhibiting gastric acid secretion.

Like other anticholinergic agents, propantheline is contraindicated in patients with narrow-angle glaucoma, because drug-induced cycloplegia and mydriasis may increase intraocular pressure; in patients with obstructive uropathy and obstructive GI tract disease, severe ulcerative colitis, myasthenia gravis, paralytic ileus, intestinal atony, or toxic megacolon, because the drug may exacerbate these conditions.

It should be administered cautiously in patients with autonomic neuropathy, hyperthyroidism, coronary artery disease, cardiac arrhythmias, congestive heart failure, or ulcerative colitis, because the drug may exacerbate symptoms of these disorders; in patients with hepatic or renal disease, because toxic accumulation may occur; in patients over age 40, because the drug increases glaucoma risk; in patients with hiatal hernia associated with reflux esophagitis, because the drug may decrease lower esophageal sphincter tone; and in hot or humid environments, because the drug may predispose the patient to heatstroke.

Overdosage with propantheline may cause curare-like symptoms and such peripheral effects as headache, dilated, nonreactive pupils, blurred vision, flushed, hot, dry skin, dryness of mucus membranes, dysphagia, decreased or absent bowel sounds, urinary retention, hyperthermia, tachycardia, hypertension, and increased respiration.

PROPARACAINE HYDROCHLORIDE

(Ak-Taine, Alcaine, Ophthaine Hydrochloride, Opthetic Sterile Ophthalmic Solution)

Proparacaine, a local anesthetic (ophthalmic solution 0.5%), is used in anesthesia for tonometry, anesthesia for the removal of foreign bodies or sutures from the eye, and anesthesia for cataract extraction and glaucoma surgery.

PROPOFOL

(Diprivan)

Propofol, a rapidly acting IV anesthetic agent, is indicated for induction or maintenance of anesthesia as part of a balanced anesthetic technique for inpatient and outpatient surgery in adults and children 3 years of age or under. Propofol can be used to initiate and maintain monitored anesthesia care (MAC) sedation during diagnostic procedures in adults, and it may also be used for MAC sedation in conjunction with local/regional anesthesia in patients undergoing surgical procedures (see Figure 74).

When nitrous oxide, oxygen, and propofol are used for maintenance of general anesthesia, supplementation with analgesics and neuromuscular blocking agents is usually required.

Induction of anesthesia with propofol is frequently associated with apnea. If spontaneous ventilation is maintained, a major cardiovascular effect is arterial hypotension.

Propofol is chiefly eliminated by hepatic conjugation to inactive metabolites which are excreted by the kidney. A glucuronide conjugate accounts for about 50% of the administered dose. Following an IV bolus dose, plasma levels initially decline rapidly due to both high metabolic clearance and rapid drug distribution into tissues. Distribution accounts for about half of this decline following a bolus of propofol.

CNS depressants (e.g., hypnotics/sedatives, inhalational anesthetics, narcotics) can increase the CNS depression induced by propofol. Morphine premedication with nitrous oxide decreases the necessary propofol maintenance infusion rate and therapeutic blood concentrations when compared to non-narcotic (e.g., lorazepam) premedication. In addition, the induction dose

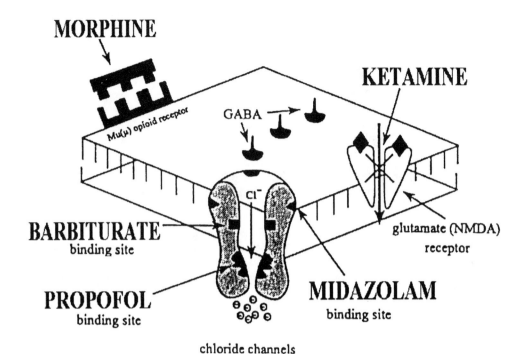

FIGURE 74   Propofol, like thiopental, induces anesthesia rapidly, but the maintenance of anesthesia may require nitrous oxide, inhalational anesthetics, and opioids. Propofol does not impair hepatic or renal functions. (Adapted from Ebadi, M., *Pharmacology, An Illustrated Review with Questions and Answers,* 3rd Edition, Lippincott-Raven Press, Philadelphia, 1996.)

requirements of propofol may be reduced in patients with IM or IV premedication, particularly with narcotics alone or in combination with sedatives. These agents may increase the anesthetic effects of propofol and may also result in more pronounced decreases in systolic, diastolic, and mean arterial pressures and cardiac output.

PROPOXYPHENE HYDROCHLORIDE
(Dextropropoxyphene, Darvon)

Propoxyphene (65 mg every 4 hours as needed) is indicated for the relief of mild to moderate pain. Propoxyphene is structurally very similar to methadone and possesses four stereoisomers. Dextropropoxyphene is an analgesic with a potency two thirds that of codeine. Levopropoxyphene is an antitussive but lacks analgesic properties.

Adverse reactions to dextropropoxyphene include nausea, vomiting, sedation, dizziness, constipation, and skin rash, with a frequency of incidence somewhat less than that seen with codeine use. Although respiratory depression is a cardinal sign of acute dextropropoxyphene poisoning, the drug apparently does not affect respiration in the usual therapeutic doses of 32 to 65 mg.

The symptoms of overdosage are usually somnolent but may be stuporous or comatose and convulsing. Respiratory depression is characteristic; ventilatory rate or tidal volume is decreased, resulting in cyanosis and hypoxia. Pupils, initially pinpoint, may dilate as hypoxia increases. Cheyne-Stokes respiration and apnea may occur. Blood pressure falls and cardiac performance deteriorates, resulting in pulmonary edema and circulatory collapse, unless corrected promptly. Cardiac arrhythmias and conduction delay may be present. A combined respiratory-metabolic acidosis occurs due to hypercapnia and lactic acid formation. Death may occur. Naloxone (0.4 to 2 mg IV) reverses the propoxyphene-induced respiratory depression.

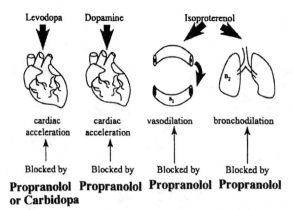

FIGURE 75   Therapeutic doses of levodopa produce cardiac stimulation by activating the beta$_1$ receptor site in the heart. The cardiac stimulation is blocked by **propranolol**, a beta-adrenergic receptor-blocking agent, or carbidopa, a peripheral dopa decarboxylase inhibitor. (Adapted from Ebadi, M., *Pharmacology, An Illustrated Review with Questions and Answers*, 3rd Edition, Lippincott-Raven Press, Philadelphia, 1996.)

PROPRANOLOL

(Inderal)

Propranolol, a noncardioselective beta-adrenoreceptor blocker (80 to 480 mg/day p.o.) is approved for more indications than any other beta-adrenergic receptor blocking drug. The three major areas of use in cardiovascular medicine are the management of coronary artery disease, the treatment of hypertension, and the treatment and prophylaxis of supraventricular and ventricular arrhythmias. In addition, propranolol has many other uses and has had a major impact on areas of medicine remote from cardiology and hypertension (see Figure 75).

Propranolol has an oxypropanolamine side chain attached to the 1 position of naphthalene. All beta-adrenergic blocking drugs, including propranolol, have asymmetric centers at the beta-carbon to which the –OH is attached (see Figure 57).

The major effect of propranolol is to antagonize the action of norepinephrine and epinephrine at all beta-adrenergic receptors. However, propranolol does not distinguish between receptor subtypes and is therefore called a nonselective beta-adrenergic blocker. The beta-adrenergic receptor antagonism produced by propranolol is competitive in that it binds reversibly with high affinity to the beta-adrenergic receptor, but it can be displaced by a sufficiently high concentration of agonist. Although propranolol binds to the same site on the receptor as the agonists, the antagonist does not trigger any response, indicating that it does not have any agonist or intrinsic sympathomimetic activity.

Propranolol is converted to a large number of metabolites resulting from oxidation or conjugation of the aromatic ring, the side chain, or both. One metabolite, 4-hydroxypropranolol, is an active beta-adrenergic blocker having nearly the same activity as the parent compound and is formed in substantial quantities only after oral dosing. However, the metabolite has a half-life that is shorter than that of propranolol and thus accumulates less than the parent drug during multiple-dose therapy. For this reason, the metabolite does not make a substantial contribution to the beta-adrenergic blockade that is present during chronic therapy.

When given intravenously, propranolol is extracted approximately 90% from the blood on a single passage through the liver, resulting in a clearance of 1.0 to 1.2 L/min, which is close to hepatic blood flow.

TABLE 24
Drugs Used in the Treatment of Chronic Postural Hypotension

Drugs	Routes	Doses	Likely Duration of Action (hr)
Mineralocorticoids			
Fludrocortisone acetate	Oral	0.1–1 mg	12–24
Prostaglandin synthetase inhibitors			
Indomethacin	Oral	25–50 mg	8–12
Flurbiprofen	Oral	50–200 mg	8–12
Beta-adrenergic receptor agonists/antagonists			
Propranolol	Oral	10–80 mg	8–12
Pindolol	Oral	5–15 mg	8–12
Xamoterol	Oral	200 mg	12
Alpha-adrenergic receptor agonists/antagonists			
Phenylpropanolamine	Oral	25–75 mg	2–3
Phenylephrine	Oral	30 mg	4–6
Ephedrine	Oral	30 mg	4–6
Clonidine	Oral	0.2–0.4 mg	6–8
Yohimbine	Oral	5 mg	8–12
Monoamine-oxidase inhibitors			
Tranylcypromine	Oral	10–20 mg	8–12
Phenelzine	Oral	15 mg	8
Vasopressors			
Dihydroergotamine	SC	10 mcg/kg	8–12
Ergotamine	Oral	1–4 mg	4–6
Desmopressin	Nasal	5–40 mcg	8–24
	IM	2–4 mcg	8–24
Somatostatin	SC	0.2–0.4 mcg/kg	12–24
Dopamine antagonists			
Domperidone	Oral	10 mg	8–12

SC = subcutaneous; IM = intramuscular

Because of the high hepatic extraction of propranolol, changes in hepatic blood flow can alter the delivery of propranolol to the liver and affect the drug's clearance. Because beta-adrenergic blockade with propranolol reduces cardiac output and hepatic blood flow, the drug reduces its own clearance. This effect accounts for the fact that (+)-propranolol, which does not produce beta-adrenergic blockade, has a higher clearance than racemic propranolol, which reduces hepatic blood flow.

After the first dose of propranolol, cardiac output and heart rate are reduced with a reflex rise in peripheral vascular resistance, such that arterial pressure is little changed. When given acutely, propranolol reduces renal blood flow because of the reduction in cardiac output and the reflex rise in vascular resistance. When given chronically, propranolol may continue to produce small reductions in renal blood flow and glomerular filtration rate. These effects are usually of no clinical consequence (see Figure 14 and Table 24).

Propranolol gains ready access to the brain because of its lipophilicity, and it can produce side effects attributable to central nervous system (CNS) function. The genesis of these side effects is unclear. Do they occur because propranolol interacts with beta-adrenergic receptors in the brain, or are they related to nonspecific effects of the drug? It seems unlikely that propranolol dissolved in brain lipid would produce abnormalities in neuronal function, but it is conceivable that the drug could reach high enough concentrations to produce membrane-stabilizing effects. However, beta-adrenergic receptor blocking drugs that are less lipid soluble and do not have membrane-stabilizing effects also can produce symptoms attributable to action in the CNS, suggesting that blockade of beta-adrenergic receptors in the brain is likely to account for some of the side effects. Water-soluble drugs are claimed to have fewer side effects attributable to CNS dysfunction. However, it has been suggested recently that the magnitude of the CNS effects of the lipophilic and hydrophilic drugs is similar but the time course of these effects varies.

Propranolol has spermicidal effects at high concentrations. Such concentrations are not achieved in sperm or seminal fluid but may be achieved in cervical mucus in women taking the drug. The clinical importance of this observation is unknown, but it should be kept in mind as a potential explanation for infertility in women receiving propranolol.

Stimulation of the beta$_2$-adrenergic receptors on skeletal muscle will cause a tremor that can be blocked by propranolol.

Propranolol has been shown to be effective in the management of angina pectoris, myocardial infarction, ventricular and supraventricular arrhythmias, hypertension, aortic dissection, hypertrophic cardiomyopathy, mitral valve prolapse, thyrotoxicosis, migraine, tremor, and performance anxiety (stage fright).

Patients with compensated heart failure often have increased sympathetic nervous activity as a compensatory mechanism. Propranolol can precipitate acute exacerbation of congestive heart failure in such patients.

Propranolol effectively blocks the beta$_2$-adrenergic receptors that mediate bronchodilation. Patients with bronchospastic pulmonary disease may develop exacerbations when given propranolol, and such attacks are resistant to therapy with beta-adrenergic receptor agonists. Thus, propranolol should never be given to an asthmatic patient. Patients with bronchospastic pulmonary disease in remission also should not receive propranolol; however, if a beta-adrenergic receptor blocker is required, a beta$_1$-selective drug should be chosen.

Hepatic dysfunction can decrease the clearance of propranolol because of reduced metabolic enzyme activity and reduced hepatic blood flow.

PROPYLTHIOURACIL
(PTU)

Propylthiouracil, a thyroid hormone antagonist, is used in hyperthyroidism, in thyrotoxic crisis, and in preparation for thyroidectomy (see also Figure 56).

PROTAMINE SULFATE

Protamine sulfate, a heparin antagonist, is used in heparin overdose (see also Table 16).

PROTEASE INHIBITORS

Cellular proteases are required for processing many protein antigens. Protease inhibitors with specificities for cathepsin-like enzymes, such as **leupeptin**, block the presentation of protein antigens by antigen-presenting cells (APC). The function of proteases is to cleave native protein antigens into small peptides. These proteases also probably act on the invariant chain, promoting its dissociation from Class II MHC (major histocompatability complex) molecules. Many cellular proteases function optimally at acid pH, and this is probably the reason antigen processing occurs best in acidic compartments.

Novel cysteine protease and serine protease inhibitors are being developed for respiratory and cardiovascular applications, for cancer and inflammation, and for viral targets. **Indinovir** and **ritonavir** are potent HIV inhibitors.

HIV-1 encodes an aspartate protease consisting, in its active form, of two symmetric subunits. This enzyme is required for cleavage of polypeptide precursors that generate the structural proteins and enzymes of the virus, including reverse transcriptase, integrase, and the protease itself.

Other inhibitors interact with catalytic residues and displace a structural water molecule. These protease inhibitors block viral maturation and are therefore active in both acutely and chronically infected cells. Resistance to these agents develops *in vitro* and in patients treated over a period of months and may limit the usefulness of monotherapy. However, viruses with reduced susceptibility to structurally similar compounds may retain susceptibility to others. Some of these protease inhibitors lack *in vivo* activity because of high plasma protein binding, particularly to alpha-1 acid glycoprotein, low oral bioavailability, and/or short plasma elimination half-lives. Most peptidomimetic inhibitors are cleared through cytochrome P450 metabolism in the liver and gastrointestinal tract. However, **saquinavir** (600 mg three times a day) has been well tolerated and associated with antiretroviral effects despite low oral bioavailability (approximately 4%). About 50% of patients have emergence of resistance, generally of moderate degree (three- to tenfold) after 1 year.

PROTRIPTYLINE HYDROCHLORIDE
(Triptil, Vivactil)

Protriptyline, a tricyclic antidepressant (15 to 40 mg p.o. daily), is used in the treatment of depression (see also Tables 3 through 5).

PSEUDOEPHEDRINE HYDROCHLORIDE

PSEUDOEPHEDRINE SULFATE
(Afrinol, Cenafed, Decofed, Dorcol, Efidac 24, Myfedrine, NeoFed, Novafed, PediaCare, Pseudogest, Sudafed, Sinufed)

Pseudoephedrine, a sympathomimetic agent with decongestant properties (60 mg p.o. q. 4 to 6 hours), is used in nasal and eustachian tube decongestion.

PSYCHIATRIC SYMPTOMS CAUSED BY DRUGS	
Drugs	**Reactions**
Acyclovir	Hallucinations, fearfulness, confusion, insomnia, hyperacusis, paranoia, depression
Albuterol	Hallucinations, paranoia
Alprazolam	See Benzodiazepines
Amantadine	Visual hallucinations, paranoid delusions, nightmares, mania, exacerbation of schizophrenia
Aminocaproic acid	Acute delirium, hallucinations
Amiodarone (*Cordarone*)	Delirium, hallucinations
Amitriptyline	See Antidepressants
Amphetamine-like drugs	Bizarre behavior, hallucinations, paranoia, agitation, anxiety, manic symptoms, depression
Amphotericin B	Delirium

Drugs	Reactions
Anabolic steroids	Aggression, mania, depression, psychosis
Anticholinergics and atropine	Confusion, memory loss, disorientation, depersonalization, delirium, auditory and visual hallucinations, fear, paranoia, agitation, bizarre behavior
	Sudden incoherent speech, delirium with high fever, flushed dry skin, hallucinations, retrograde amnesia
Anticonvulsants	Agitation, confusion, delirium, depression, psychosis, aggression, mania, toxic encephalopathy
Antidepressants, tricyclic	Mania or hypomania, delirium, hallucinations, paranoia
Antihistamines	Hallucinations
Asparaginase	Confusion, depression, paranoia
Atenolol	See Beta-adrenergic blockers
Atropine	See Anticholinergics and atropine
Baclofen	Hallucinations, paranoia, nightmares, mania, depression, anxiety, confusion
Barbiturates	Excitement, hyperactivity, visual hallucinations, depression, delirium-tremens-like syndrome
Belladonna alkaloids	See Atropine and Anticholinergics
Benzodiazepines	Rage, hostility, paranoia, hallucinations, delirium, depression, nightmares, anterograde amnesia, mania
Beta-adrenergic blockers	Depression, confusion, nightmares, hallucinations, paranoia, delusions, mania, hyperactivity
Betaxolol	See Beta-adrenergic blockers
Biperiden	See Anticholinergics and Atropine
Bromocriptine	Mania, delusions, hallucinations, paranoia, aggressive behavior, schizophrenic relapse, depression, anxiety
Desipramine	See Antidepressants, tricyclic
Diazepam	See Benzodiazepines
Diethylpropion	See Amphetamine-like drugs
Digitalis glycosides	Nightmares, confusion, paranoia, depression, visual hallucinations
Diltiazem	Depression, suicidal thoughts
Disopyramide	Hallucinations, paranoia, panic, depression
Disulfiram	Catatonia, delirium, depression, psychosis
Dronabinol	Anxiety, disorientation, psychosis
Enalapril	Agitation, depression, panic, hallucinations
Ephedrine	Hallucinations, paranoia
Ethchlorvynol	Agitation, hallucinations, paranoia
Ethionamide	Depression, hallucinations
Ethosuximide	See Anticonvulsants
Etretinate	Severe depression
Famotidine	See Histamine H_2-receptor antagonists
Fenfluramine	See Amphetamine-like drugs
Flecainide	Visual hallucinations
Fluoxetine	Mania, hypomania, depersonalization
Flurbiprofen	See Nonsteroidal antiinflammatory drugs
Fluvoxamine	Mania, hypomania

Drugs	Reactions
Ganciclovir	Hallucinations, delirium, confusion, agitation
Gentamicin	Confusion, disorientation, hallucinations
Histamine H_2-receptor antagonists	Hallucinations, paranoia, bizarre behavior, delirium, disorientation, depression, mania
Hydroxychloroquine	Irritability, difficulty concentrating, psychosis
Ibuprofen	See Nonsteroidal antiinflammatory drugs
Imipramine	See Antidepressants, tricyclic
Indomethacin	See Nonsteroidal antiinflammatory drugs
Iohexol	Confusion, disorientation
Iopamidol	Confusion, disorientation
Isocarboxazid	Mania, insomnia, anxiety, paranoid delusions
Isoniazid	Depression, agitation, hallucinations, paranoia
Isosorbide dinitrate	Hallucinations, depression, suicidal thoughts
Isotretinoin	Depression
Ketamine	Nightmares, hallucinations, crying, delirium
Ketoconazole	Hallucinations
Levodopa	Delirium, depression, agitation, hypomania, nightmares, night terrors, hallucinations, paranoia
Lidocaine	See Procaine
Loperamide	Delirium
Lorazepam	See Benzodiazepines
Lovastatin	Depression
Loxapine	Mania
Maprotiline	Hallucinations, agitation, disorientation
Mefloquine	Psychosis, panic attacks, depression
Methandrostenolone	See Anabolic steroids
Meperidine	See Narcotics
Methadone	See Narcotics
Methyldopa	Depression, amnesia, nightmares, psychosis
Methylphenidate	Hallucinations, paranoia
Methyltestosterone	See Anabolic steroids
Methysergide	Depersonalization, hallucinations, agitation
Metoclopramide	Mania, severe depression, crying, delirium
Metrizamide	Confusion, hallucinations, depression, anxiety
Metronidazole	Depression, agitation, uncontrollable crying, disorientation, hallucinations
Midazolam	See Benzodiazepines
Misoprostol	Delirium
Morphine	See Narcotics
Nalidixic acid	Confusion, depression, hallucinations
Nalorphine	See Narcotics
Naloxone	Violent behavior
Naproxen	See Nonsteroidal antiinflammatory drugs

Drugs	Reactions
Narcotics	Nightmares, anxiety, agitation, euphoria, dysphoria, depression, paranoia, hallucinations
Nifedipine	Irritability, agitation, panic, belligerence, depression
Niridazole	Confusion, hallucinations, mania, suicide
Nonsteroidal antiinflammatory drugs	Paranoia, depression, anxiety, disorientation, hallucinations
Norfloxacin	Depression, anxiety
Nortriptyline	See Antidepressants
Ofloxacin	Delirium, depression and mania, catatonia
Oxandrolone	See Anabolic steroids
Oxymetazoline	Hallucinations
Oxymetholone	See Anabolic steroids
Pargyline	Manic psychosis
Penicillin G procaine	See Procaine derivatives
Pentazocine	See Narcotics
Pergolide	Hallucinations, paranoia, confusion, anxiety, depression
Phenelzine	Paranoia, delusions, fear, mania, rage
Phenmetrazine	See Amphetamine-like drugs
Phentermine	See Amphetamine-like drugs
Phenylephrine	Depression, hallucinations, paranoia, delusions
Phenylpropanolamine	See Amphetamine-like drugs
Phenytoin	See Anticonvulsants
Podophyllin	Delirium, paranoia, bizarre behavior
Polythiazide	See Thiazides
Pravastatin	Depression
Prazosin	Hallucinations, depression, paranoia
Primidone	See Anticonvulsants
Procainamide	See Procaine derivatives
Procaine derivatives	Confusion, "doom" anxiety, psychosis, agitation, bizarre behavior, depression, panic
Procarbazine	Mania
Promethazine	Hallucinations, terror
Propafenone	Agitation, delusions, disorientation, mania, paranoia
Propoxyphene	See Narcotics
Propranolol	See Beta-adrenergic blockers
Pseudoephedrine	Hallucinations, paranoia
Quinacrine	Mania, paranoia, anxiety, hallucinations, delirium
Quinidine	Confusion, agitation, psychosis
Ranitidine	See Histamine H_2-receptor antagonists
Reserpine	Depression, nightmares
Salicylates	Agitation, confusion, hallucinations, paranoia
Scopolamine	See Atropine and Anticholinergics
Selegiline	Hallucinations, mania, nightmares

Drugs	Reactions
Simvastatin	Depression
Sulfonamides	Confusion, disorientation, depression, euphoria, hallucinations
Sulindac	See Nonsteroidal antiinflammatory drugs
Tamoxifen	Delusions
Theophylline	Withdrawal, mutism, hyperactivity, anxiety, mania
Thiabendazole	Psychosis
Thiazides	Depression, suicidal ideation
Thyroid hormones	Mania, depression, hallucinations, paranoia
Timolol	See Beta-adrenergic blockers
Tobramycin	Delirium, hallucinations, agitation
Tocainide	See Procaine derivatives
Tranylcypromine	Mania or hypomania
Trazodone	Delirium, hallucinations, paranoia, mania
Triazolam	See Benzodiazepines
Trichlormethiazide	See Thiazides
Trihexyphenidyl	See Atropine and Anticholinergics
Trimethoprim-sulfamethoxazole	Psychosis, depression, disorientation, hallucinations, delusions
Valproic acid	See Anticonvulsants
Verapamil	Auditory, visual, and tactile hallucinations
Vincristine	Hallucinations
Zidovudine	Mania, paranoia, hallucinations

The drug-induced psychiatric symptoms are dose-dependent, of idiosyncratic nature, and reversible.

PSYCHOTROPIC MEDICATIONS: SIDE EFFECTS OF

ACETOPHENAZINE, see Phenothiazines, Piperazine

ALPRAZOLAM, see Benzodiazepines

AMITRIPTYLINE, see Tricyclic antidepressants

AMOXAPINE, see Tricyclic antidepressants

BENZODIAZEPINES (alprazolam, chlordiazepoxide, clorazepate, diazepam, halazepam, lorazepam, oxazepam, prazepam, temazepam)

Frequent: Drowsiness; ataxia

Occasional: Confusion; amnesia; disinhibition; paradoxical excitement; depression; dizziness; withdrawal symptoms, including convulsions, on abrupt discontinuance (withdrawal may be especially difficult with alprazolam); rebound insomnia or excitement

Rare: Hypotension; blood dyscrasias; jaundice; allergic reactions; paradoxical rage reactions; stuttering with alprazolam

BUPROPION, Anxiety; agitation; insomnia; tremor; anorexia

BUSPIRONE, Dizziness; headache; nausea; paresthesias; diarrhea

CHLORDIAZEPOXIDE, see Benzodiazepines

CHLORPROMAZINE, see Phenothiazines, aliphatic

CHLORPROTHIXENE, similar to Phenothiazines

CLOMIPRAMINE, see Tricyclic antidepressants

CLORAZEPATE, see Benzodiazepines

CLOZAPINE

Frequent: Drowsiness; anticholinergic effects; postural hypotension; increase in body temperature; increased salivation; EKG changes

Occasional: Constipation; hypertension; granulocytopenia; agranulocytosis in 1% to 2%; seizures

DESIPRAMINE, see Tricyclic antidepressants

DIAZEPAM, see Benzodiazepines

DOXEPIN, see Tricyclic antidepressants

FLUOXETINE

Frequent: Nausea; nervousness; headache; insomnia; sexual dysfunction (anorgasmia)

Occasional: Akathisia; rash; fever; arthralgia; mania; aminotransferase elevations; abulia; alopecia

Rare: Extrapyramidal reactions; seizures in patients with pre-existing seizure disorder; leukocytosis; bradycardia with syncope; respiratory distress

FLUPHENAZINE, see Phenothiazines, piperazine

HALAZEPAM, see Benzodiazepines

HALOPERIDOL

Extrapyramidal effects (especially in young patients); blood dyscrasias; postural hypotension; sedation; menstrual changes; galactorrhea; tardive dyskinesia; cholestatic jaundice; photosensitivity; rash; weight gain; convulsions; impotence; neurotoxicity in hyperthyroid patients; neuroleptic malignant syndrome

IMIPRAMINE, see Tricyclic antidepressants

ISOCARBOXAZID, see MAO inhibitors

LITHIUM

At therapeutic serum concentrations (0.6-1.2 mEq/L): Thirst; polyuria; fine tremor; GI irritation; mild diarrhea; weight gain; edema; acne; leukocytosis

At toxic serum concentrations (above 2 mEq/L): Confusion; vomiting; diarrhea; polyuria; muscle weakness; ataxia; lethargy; slurred speech; tinnitus; blurred vision; nystagmus; stupor; coma; convulsions; permanent neurologic impairment

Occasional (at all serum concentrations): Goiter; hypothyroidism; nephrogenic diabetes insipidus; acne; renal tubular acidosis; metallic taste; induction or exacerbation of psoriasis; folliculitis; T-wave changes; nausea; extrapyramidal effects

Rare (at all serum concentrations): Exophthalmos; cardiac arrhythmias; vomiting; acute renal failure; progressive decrease in renal function; Raynaud's phenomenon; hypoglycemia; hair loss; pseudotumor cerebri; hyperthyroidism; hyperparathyroidism; serum concentrations and toxic effects are increased by dehydration, diuretics, sweating, fever, protracted diarrhea, or diminished intake of sodium

LORAZEPAM, see Benzodiazepines

LOXAPINE, see Phenothiazines, piperazine

MAO INHIBITORS (isocarboxazid, phenelzine tranylcypromine)

Hypotension; restlessness; insomnia; daytime sleepiness; mania; urinary retention; tremors; sexual disturbances; paresthesias; dry mouth; nausea; constipation; anorexia; weight gain; edema; rash; hepatitis; tinnitus; muscle spasm; lupus-like reaction; leukopenia; hyperthermia; hypertension; interactions with other drugs or foods may be severe

MAPROTILINE

Similar to tricyclics, but seizures occur more frequently (especially with more than 200 mg/day) and anticholinergic effects may occur less frequently

MESORIDAZINE, see Phenothiazines, piperidine

MOLINDONE

Extrapyramidal effects; akathisia; anticholinergic effects; drowsiness; dystonia; menstrual changes; anorexia; weight loss; rash; tardive dyskinesia; leukopenia; postural hypotension; ECG abnormalities; liver abnormalities; neuroleptic malignant syndrome

NORTRIPTYLINE, see Tricyclic antidepressants

OXAZEPAM, see Benzodiazepines

PERPHENAZINE, see Phenothiazines, piperazine

PHENELZINE, see MAO inhibitors

PHENOTHIAZINES, ALIPHATIC (chlorpromazine, triflupromazine)

Frequent: Drowsiness; anticholinergic effects; postural hypotension

Occasional: Extrapyramidal effects; galactorrhea; photosensitivity; menstrual changes; cholestatic jaundice; rashes; skin pigmentation; convulsions; ECG changes; tardive dyskinesia; weight gain; lenticular deposits and opacities; blood dyscrasias; gastritis, nausea and vomiting, dizziness and tremulousness following withdrawal of high-dose therapy; disturbed temperature regulation; lupus-like syndrome; neuroleptic malignant syndrome

PHENOTHIAZINES, PIPERAZINE (acetophenazine, fluphenazine, loxapine, perphenazine, prochlorperazine, trifluoperazine)

Frequent: Extrapyramidal effects

Occasional: Anticholinergic effects; photosensitivity; galactorrhea; menstrual changes; drowsiness; postural hypotension; anorexia; rash; tardive dyskinesia; weight gain

Rare: Cholestatic jaundice; blood dyscrasias; lenticular deposits and opacities; ECG abnormalities; convulsions; gastritis; neuroleptic malignant syndrome; nausea and vomiting, dizziness and tremulousness following withdrawal of high-dose therapy; disturbed temperature regulation

PHENOTHIAZINES, PIPERIDINE (mesoridazine, thioridazine)

Frequent: Drowsiness; anticholinergic effects; postural hypotension; weight gain; inhibition of ejaculation

Occasional: Extrapyramidal effects (but less than with aliphatic phenothiazines); menstrual changes; photosensitivity reactions; ECG abnormalities; galactorrhea; tardive dyskinesia

Rare: Pigmentary retinopathy (thioridazine has an 800 mg/day upper limit on recommended dosage because of a high incidence of pigmentary retinopathy); cholestatic jaundice; blood dyscrasias; dystonia; convulsions; rash; gastritis, nausea and vomiting, dizziness and tremulousness following withdrawal of high-dose therapy; disturbed temperature regulation; neuroleptic malignant syndrome; torsade de pointes; ventricular arrhythmia with thioridazine

PRAZEPAM, see Benzodiazepines

PROCHLORPERAZINE, see Phenothiazines, piperazine

PROTRIPTYLINE, see Tricyclic antidepressants

TEMAZEPAM, see Benzodiazepines

THIORIDAZINE, see Phenothiazines, piperidine

THIOTHIXENE

Frequent: Extrapyramidal effects; anticholinergic effects

Occasional: Galactorrhea; menstrual changes; drowsiness; postural hypotension; anorexia; rash; tardive dyskinesia

Rare: Blood dyscrasias; lenticular deposits and opacities (with long-term high dosage); ECG abnormalities; convulsions; neuroleptic malignant syndrome

TRANYLCYPROMINE, see MAO inhibitors

TRAZODONE

Frequent: Drowsiness; headaches; gastrointestinal upset

Occasional: Ventricular arrhythmias; peripheral edema

Rare: Priapism in men; increased libido

TRICYCLIC ANTIDEPRESSANTS (amitriptyline, amoxapine, clomipramine, desipramine, doxepin, imipramine, nortriptyline, protriptyline, trimipramine)

Frequent: Anticholinergic effects; hypotension (less with nortriptyline); drowsiness; weight gain; tachycardia

Occasional: Mania; psychosis; tremor; first-degree heart block; other ECG abnormalities; rash; sweating; confusion; insomnia; sexual disturbances, especially with clomipramine; increase in dental caries; gingivitis

Rare: Hepatic toxicity; tinnitus; bone marrow depression, including agranulocytosis; seizures; peripheral neuropathy; severe cardiovascular effects in patients with cardiac disease; photosensitivity; dysarthria;

stuttering; withdrawal symptoms; nausea, tremor, anorgasmia and seizures may be more common with clomipramine; tardive dyskinesia and neuroleptic malignant syndrome with amoxapine; renal failure with overdosage of amoxapine

TRIFLUOPERAZINE, see Phenothiazines, piperazine

TRIFLUPROMAZINE, see Phenothiazines, aliphatic

TRIMIPRAMINE, see Tricyclic antidepressants

PSYLLIUM

(e.g., Metamucil)

(Wafers: approximately 1.7 g psyllium mucilloid, 18 g carbohydrate, 18 mg sodium, 4.5 g fat, 96 calories per dose).

Psyllium, lignin, and pectin bind bile acids, reducing their intestinal reabsorption and promoting their excretion. The consequent enhancement of hepatic synthesis of bile acids from cholesterol may reduce plasma cholesterol in low-density lipoproteins. With several months of use, bulk-forming agents reduce intraluminal rectosigmoid pressure and relieve symptoms in patients with irritable bowel syndrome and diverticular disease of the colon. The capacity of these agents to absorb water makes them useful in relieving the symptoms of mild diarrhea and for the regulation of effluent in patients with ileostomy or colostomy.

Irritable bowel syndrome is a functional bowel disorder exhibiting the following characteristics: abdominal pain, symptoms of disturbed defecation (urgency, straining, and feeling of incomplete evacuation), altered stool consistency, and altered stool frequency and timing. There are also symptoms of bloatedness (distention).

If **diarrhea** is the chief complaint, it is treated with **loperamide** or **cholestyramine. Pain** is treated with **dicyclomine, amitriptyline,** and **peppermint oil. Bran** and **psyllium** are used to treat the **constipation** that may occur in irritable bowel syndrome. **Flatulence** is treated with **simethicone.**

PULMONARY TOXICITY: DRUG-INDUCED	
Drugs	**Reactions**
Amiodarone	Acute pneumonitis, fibrosis, hypersensitivity pneumonitis
Aspirin	see Salicylates
Atracurium	see Neuromuscular blockers
Azathioprine	Hypersensitivity pneumonitis
Beta-adrenergic blockers	Bronchospasm
Bleomycin	Acute pneumonitis, fibrosis, bronchiolitis obliterans, hypersensitivity pneumonitis
Bromocriptine	Pleuritis, fibrosis
Busulfan	Fibrosis
Captopril	Cough
Carbamazepine	Hypersensitivity pneumonitis
Carmustine	Acute pneumonitis, fibrosis
Chlorambucil	Acute pneumonitis, fibrosis
Cocaine	Edema, hemorrhage
Cyclophosphamide	Hypersensitivity pneumonitis, edema, fibrosis
Cytarabine	Edema

Drugs	Reactions
Dantrolene	Pleuritis, pneumonitis
Diclofenac	see NSAIDs
Enalapril	Cough
Ethchlorvynol	Edema
Gold salts	Hypersensitivity pneumonitis, fibrosis, bronchiolitis obliterans
Hydrochlorothiazide	Edema
Ibuprofen	see NSAIDs
Indomethacin	see NSAIDs
Interleukin-2 (Proleukin)	Edema
Lidocaine	Edema
Lisinopril	Cough
Lomustine	Fibrosis
Melphalan	Fibrosis
Methadone	see Opiates
Methotrexate	Pleuritis, hypersensitivity pneumonitis, edema, fibrosis
Methysergide	Pleuritis
Mitomycin	Acute pneumonitis, fibrosis
Naloxone	Edema
Naproxen	see NSAIDs
Neuromuscular blockers	Bronchospasm
Nitrofurantoin	Hypersensitivity pneumonitis, fibrosis
NSAIDs	Bronchospasm, hypersensitivity pneumonitis, edema, fibrosis
Opiates	Edema
Pancuronium	see Neuromuscular blockers
Penicillamine	Bronchiolitis obliterans, hypersensitivity pneumonitis, fibrosis, pulmonary-renal syndrome
Phenylbutazone	see NSAIDs
Phenytoin	Hypersensitivity pneumonitis
Pilocarpine	Bronchospasm
Pindolol	see Beta-adrenergic blockers
Piroxicam	see NSAIDs
Procarbazine	Hypersensitivity pneumonitis
Propafenone	Bronchospasm
Propoxyphene	see Opiates
Propranolol	see Beta-adrenergic blockers
Protamine	Edema
Pyrimethamine-chloroquine	Hypersensitivity pneumonitis
Pyrimethamine-dapsone	Hypersensitivity pneumonitis
Pyrimethamine-sulfadoxine	Hypersensitivity pneumonitis
Salicylates	Edema, bronchospasm
Semustine	Fibrosis
Sulfasalazine	Hypersensitivity pneumonitis, bronchiolitis obliterans, fibrosis

Drugs	Reactions
Sulindac	see NSAIDs
Suxamethonium	see Neuromuscular blockers
Terbutaline	Edema
Timolol	see Beta-adrenergic blockers
Tocainide	Pneumonitis, fibrosis
Ritodrine	Edema
Tryptophan	Pneumonitis
Tubocurarine	see Neuromuscular blockers
Vecuronium	see Neuromuscular blockers
Vinblastine	Acute pneumonitis, bronchospasm
Vindesine	Acute pneumonitis, bronchospasm

PYRANTEL PAMOATE
(Antiminth)

Pyrantel, a pyrimidine derivative with antihelmintic properties (single dose of 11 mg/kg p.o.), is used in the treatment of roundworm and pinworm infections.

PYRIDOSTIGMINE BROMIDE
(Mestinon, Regonol)

Pyridostigmine, a cholinesterase inhibitor, is used as an antagonist for curariform paralysis and in myasthenia gravis.

PYRIDOXINE HYDROCHLORIDE
(Vitamin B$_6$) (Beesix, Hexa-Betalin, Nestrex)

Pyridoxine, a water-soluble vitamin, is used in dietary vitamin B$_6$ deficiency, seizures related to vitamin B$_6$ deficiency or dependency, vitamin B$_6$-responsive anemias or dependency syndrome (inborn errors of metabolism), prevention of vitamin B$_6$ deficiency during isoniazid therapy, and treatment of vitamin B$_6$ deficiency secondary to isoniazid.

PYRILAMINE MALEATE
(Nisaval)

Pyrilamine, an ethylenediamine antihistaminic substance, has mild sedative and antihistaminic properties with no anticholinergic and antiemetic actions. Pyrilamine (25 to 50 mg p.o. t.i.d.) is indicated for relief of symptoms associated with perennial and seasonal allergic rhinitis, vasomotor rhinitis, allergic conjunctivitis, temporary relief of runny nose and sneezing due to the common cold, allergic and nonallergic pruritic symptoms, mild, uncomplicated urticaria and angioedema, amelioration of allergic reactions to blood or plasma, dermatographism, and adjunctive therapy in anaphylactic reactions.

Pyrilamine competitively antagonizes histamine at the H$_1$ receptor site, but does not bind with histamine to inactivate it. Terfenadine and astemizole, the most specific H$_1$ antagonists available, bind preferentially to peripheral rather than central H$_1$ receptors. Antihistamines do not block histamine release, antibody production, or antigen–antibody interactions. They antagonize in varying degrees most of the pharmacological effects of histamine (see Figure 49).

PYRIMETHAMINE

(Daraprim)

Pyrimethamine (25 mg once weekly) is indicated for chemoprophylaxis of malaria due to susceptible strains of plasmodia. Fast-acting schizonticides (chloroquine or quinine) are preferable for treatment of acute attacks. However, concurrent pyrimethamine will initiate transmission control and suppressive cure.

In addition, sulfadoxine and pyrimethamine (Fansidar) are indicated for prophylaxis of malaria in individuals traveling to areas where chloroquine-resistant *P. falciparum* malaria is endemic. However, resistant strains may be encountered. Regardless of the prophylactic regimen used, it is still possible to contract malaria. Moreover, this combination has been used as a prophylactic agent for the prevention of *Pneumocystis carinii* pneumonia in patients with AIDS.

Pyrimethamine is a folic acid antagonist; its therapeutic action is based on differential requirements between host and parasite for nucleic acid precursors involved in growth as it selectively inhibits plasmodial dihydrofolate reductase. Pyrimethamine inhibits the enzyme dihydrofolate reductase which catalyzes the reduction of dihydrofolate to tetrahydrofolate. This activity is highly selective against plasmodia and *Toxoplasma gondii*. It does not destroy gametocytes but arrests sporogony in the mosquito. Pyrimethamine possesses a blood schizonticidal, and some tissue schizonticidal activity may be slower than that of 4-aminoquinoline compounds.

Overdose effects of pyrimethamine may include abdominal pain, nausea, and severe and repeated vomiting, possibly including hematemesis. CNS toxicity may be manifest by initial excitability, generalized and prolonged convulsions which may be followed by respiratory depression, circulatory collapse, and death within a few hours. Neurological symptoms, including convulsive seizures, appear rapidly (30 min to 2 hours after drug ingestion), suggesting that in gross overdosage, pyrimethamine has a direct toxic effect on the CNS.

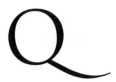

QUAZEPAM

(Doral)

Quazepam, a benzodiazepine derivative with hypnotic-sedative properties (15 mg p.o.), is used in the treatment of insomnia (see also Table 8).

QUINAPRIL HYDROCHLORIDE

(Accupril)

Quinapril, an angiotensin-converting enzyme (ACE) inhibitor with antihypertensive properties, is used in hypertension and in hypertension in patients receiving diuretics (see also Figure 21).

QUINESTROL

(Estrovis)

Quinestrol (100 mcg daily for 7 days), which mimics the action of endogenous estrogen, is indicated for the treatment of moderate to severe vasomotor symptoms associated with menopause, atrophic vaginitis, kraurosis vulvae, female hypogonadism, female castration, and primary ovarian failures. Quinestrol is stored in body fat, slowly released over several days, and metabolized to ethinyl estradiol.

Quinestrol is contraindicated in patients with thrombophlebitis or thromboembolism because it may induce thromboembolic disease; in patients with estrogen-responsive carcinoma (breast or genital tract cancer), because it may increase tumor growth; in patients with undiagnosed abnormal genital bleeding; and in pregnant or breast-feeding women.

Quinestrol should be administered cautiously to patients with disorders that may be aggravated by fluid and electrolyte accumulation, such as asthma, seizure disorders, migraine, or cardiac, renal, or hepatic dysfunction. Carefully monitor female patients who have breast nodules, fibrocystic breast disease, or a family history of breast cancer. Because of the risk of thromboembolism, therapy with this drug should be discontinued at least one week before elective surgical procedures associated with an increased incidence of thromboembolism.

Concomitant administration of drugs that induce hepatic metabolism, such as rifampin, barbiturates, pyrimidone, carbamazepine, and phenytoin, may result in decreased estrogenic effects from a given dose. These drugs are known to accelerate the rate of metabolism of certain other agents.

In patients with diabetes, this agent increases blood glucose levels, necessitating dosage adjustment of insulin or oral hypoglycemic drugs.

Quinestrol has the potential to decrease the effects of warfarin-type anticoagulants. Patients receiving this drug concurrently with an adrenocorticosteroid or adrenocorticotropic hormone are at greater risk for fluid and electrolyte accumulation.

QUINETHAZONE

(Hydromox)

Quinethazone, a quinazoline derivative with diuretic and antihypertensive properties (50 to 100 mg p.o. daily), is used in edema.

QUINIDINE GLUCONATE
(Duraquin, Quinaglute Dura-Tabs, Quinalan, Quinate)

QUINIDINE POLYGALACTURONATE
(Cardioquin)

QUINIDINE SULFATE
(Cin-Quin, Novoquinidin, Quinidex Extentabs, Quinora)

Quinidine (200 to 600 mg t.i.d.), a cinchona alkaloid with antiarrhythmic properties, is indicated for premature atrial, AV junctional, and ventricular contractions; paroxysmal atrial (supraventricular) tachycardia; paroxysmal AV junctional rhythm; atrial flutter; paroxysmal and chronic atrial fibrillation; established atrial fibrillation when therapy is appropriate; paroxysmal ventricular tachycardia not associated with complete heart block; and mainte-nance therapy after electrical conversion of atrial fibrillation or flutter (see Figure 76).

Quinidine, a Class 1A antiarrhythmic, depresses myocardial excitability, conduction velocity, and contractility. Therapeutically, it prolongs the effective refractory period and increases conduction time, thereby preventing the reentry phenomenon. In addition, quinidine exerts an indirect anticholinergic effect; it decreases vagal tone and may facilitate conduction in the atrioventricular junction.

Quinidine and procainamide decrease automaticity by reducing the **rate of phase 4 diastolic depolarization**, which is probably mediated by a diminished membrane permeability to sodium, and they decrease conduction velocity throughout the conducting system (Figure 76). They produce an indirect (vagolytic) effect that sometimes counteracts the direct effect at the AV node, producing a paradoxical tachycardia in some cases of atrial flutter or fibrillation. These agents terminate reentry arrhythmias by producing a bidirectional block in infarcted conducting tissues. They directly depress contractility, leading to a decline in cardiac output.

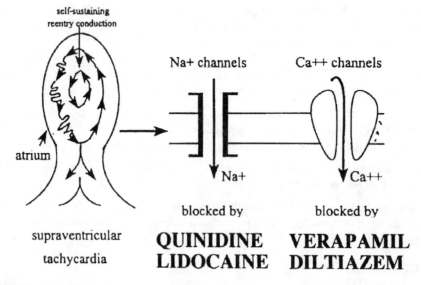

FIGURE 76   As antiarrhythmic drugs, quinidine and procainamide decrease automaticity by reducing the **rate of phase 4 diastolic depolarization**, which is probably mediated by a diminished membrane permeability to sodium, and they decrease **conduction velocity** throughout the conducting system. (Adapted from Ebadi, M., *Pharmacology, An Illustrated Review with Questions and Answers*, 3rd Edition, Lippincott-Raven Press, Philadelphia, 1996.)

These agents are **potent vasodilators**, especially when given intravenously. This effect is so great that quinidine is rarely given parenterally, and great care must be taken when it is given by this route. They depress blood pressure by means of their dual effects on cardiac output and peripheral resistance.

These agents produce widening of the QRS complex (by depressing ventricular conduction) and lengthening of the PR interval (by slowing AV conduction). A 25 to 30% widening of the QRS complex is considered the therapeutic limit with these agents. They are excreted up to 50% unmetabolized in the urine. They commonly cause **gastrointestinal disturbances**, and these constitute their major side effect. **Emboli** may be liberated from the atria during conversion of atrial flutter or fibrillation. **Toxicity** is manifested by a profound fall in blood pressure that leads to a shock-like state accompanied by a variety of arrhythmias.

Quinidine and procainamide may also provoke some unique but uncommon side effects. Quinidine may produce **cinchonism** (tinnitus, dizziness, visual disturbances, and vertigo) and **cutaneous hypersensitivity reactions.** Procainamide may produce **agranulocytosis** during long-term therapy, and dose-dependent (>2 gm/day) **lupus erythematosus-like syndrome.** These agents are mainly used in the management of atrial (supraventricular) arrhythmias, although procainamide is also of value in treating premature ventricular contractions and ventricular tachycardia. If either drug is used to convert atrial flutter or fibrillation, **digitalis** must be given first to protect against paradoxical tachycardia.

QUININE SULFATE

(Quinora)

Quinine (650 mg every 8 hours for 5 to 7 days) is indicated for the treatment of chloroquine-resistant falciparum malaria, either alone, with **pyrimethamine** and a **sulfonamide** or with a **tetracycline**. It is also considered as an alternative therapy for chloroquine-sensitive strains of *P. falciparum, P. malariae, P. ovale,* and *P. vivax.* **Mefloquine** and **clindamycin** may also be used with quinine depending on the geographical location in which the malaria was acquired.

Quinine, a cinchona alkaloid, acts primarily as a blood schizonticide. Quinine's antimalarial action is unclear. It was once believed to be due to the intercalation of the quinoline moiety into the DNA of the parasite, thereby reducing the effectiveness of DNA to act as a template, as well as depression of the oxygen uptake and carbohydrate metabolism of the plasmodia. Recently it has been thought that quinine's pH elevation in the intracellular organelles of the parasites plays a role in the mechanism.

Quinine has a skeletal muscle relaxant effect, increasing the refractory period by direct action on the muscle fiber, decreasing the excitability of the motor end plate by a curariform action, and affecting the distribution of calcium within the muscle fiber. It also has analgesic, antipyretic, and oxytocic effects.

Quinine is contraindicated in patients with glucose-6-phosphate dehydrogenase (G-6-PD) deficiency, optic neuritis, tinnitus, or a history of blackwater fever and thrombocytopenia purpura. The symptoms of overdosage are tinnitus, dizziness, skin rash, and GI disturbance (intestinal cramping). With higher doses, cardiovascular and CNS effects may occur, including headache, fever, vomiting, apprehension, confusion, and convulsions.

Aluminum-containing antacids may decrease the absorption of quinine. Quinine may depress the hepatic enzyme system that synthesizes the vitamin-K-dependent clotting factors and thus may enhance the action of warfarin and other oral anticoagulants. **Cimetidine** may reduce quinine's oral clearance and increase its elimination half-life. **Digoxin** serum concentrations may be increased by concurrent quinine.

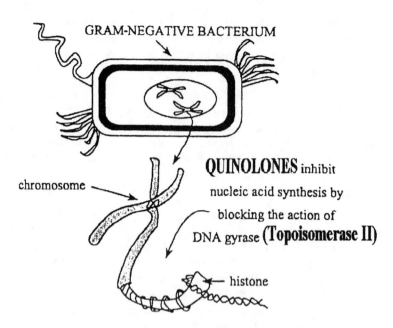

FIGURE 77   The quinolones include **nalidixic acid** (NegGram), **cinoxacin** (Cinobac), **norfloxacin** (Noroxin), and **ciprofloxacin** (Cipro). Other members of the quinolone family are **pefloxacin, ofloxacin, enoxacin,** and **fleroxacin.** (Adapted from Ebadi, M., *Pharmacology, An Illustrated Review with Questions and Answers*, 3rd Edition, Lippincott-Raven Press, Philadelphia, 1996.)

Quinine may potentiate the actions of neuromuscular blocking agents causing respiratory depression.

QUINOLONE AND FLUOROQUINOLONE ANTIBIOTICS		
Amifloxacin	Lomefloxacin	Ofloxacin
Cinoxacin	Nalidixic acid	Pefloxacin
Ciprofloxacin	Norfloxacin	Sparfloxacin
Fleroxacin		

QUINOLONE ANTIBIOTICS

The quinolones include **nalidixic acid** (NegGram), **cinoxacin** (Cinobac), **norfloxacin** (Noroxin), and **ciprofloxacin** (Cipro). Other members of the quinolone family are **pefloxacin, ofloxacin, enoxacin,** and **fleroxacin.** The bacterial enzyme **DNA gyrase** is responsible for the continuous introduction of negative supercoils into DNA, and the quinolones inhibit this gyrase-mediated DNA supercoiling (see Figure 77).

Nalidixic acid and **cinoxacin** are bactericidal against Gram-negative organisms that cause urinary tract infections. The **fluoroquinolones** are bactericidal and considerably more potent against *Escherichia coli* and various species of *Salmonella, Shigella, Enterobacter, Campylobacter,* and *Neisseria.* **Ciprofloxacin** also has good activity against staphylococci, including methicillin-resistant strains.

The quinolones and fluoroquinolones may produce arthropathy, and hence should not be used in prepubertal children or pregnant women.

Nalidixic acid and **cinoxacin** are useful only for treating urinary tract infections. **Ciprofloxacin** is useful for both urinary tract infections and prostatitis.

R

RABIES IMMUNE GLOBULIN, HUMAN
(RIG)

This rabies prophylaxis agent is used in rabies exposure.

RABIES VACCINE, HUMAN DIPLOID CELL
(HDCV)

This viral vaccine is used as a preexposure prophylaxis immunization for persons in high-risk groups.

RADIOACTIVE IODINE
(Sodium Iodide)

^{131}I

(Iodotope Therapeutic, Sodium Iodide ^{131}I Therapeutic)

Radioactive iodine, a thyroid hormone antagonist, is used in hyperthyroidism and in thyroid cancer (see also Table 19).

RADIOPAQUE AGENTS	
Oral Cholecystographic Agents Containing Iodine	
Iocetamic acid (62% iodine)	(Cholebrine)
Iopanoic acid (66.68% iodine)	(Telepaque)
Ipodate calcium (61.7% iodine)	(Oragrafin Calcium)
Ipodate sodium (61.4% iodine)	(Bilivist, Oragrafin Sodium)
Tyropanoate sodium (57.4% iodine)	(Bilopaque)
GI Contrast Agents Containing Iodine	
Diatrizoate sodium 41.66% (24.9% iodine)	(Hypaque Sodium)
Diatrizoate sodium (59.87% iodine)	(Hypaque Sodium)
Diatrizoate meglumine 66% and diatrizoate sodium 10% (37% iodine)	(Gastrografin, MD-Gastroview)
GI Contrast Agents Containing Barium	
Barium sulfate	(Baro-cat, Prepcat, Enecat, Tomocat, Entrobar, Liquid Barosperse, HD 85, Barobag, Liquipake, Flo-Coat, Epi-C, Barium Sulfate, USP, Baroflave, Tonopaque, Baricon, HD 200 Plus, Barosperse, Anatrast)
GI Contrast Agents (Miscellaneous)	
Radiopaque polyvinyl chloride	(Sitzmarks)
Sodium bicarbonate	(Baros)
Radiopaque Agents Administered Parenterally	
Diatrizoate meglumine 30% (14.1% iodine)	(Hypaque Meglumine 30%, Reno-M-Dip, Urovist Meglumine DIU/CT)

Diatrizoate meglumine 60% (28% iodine)	(Angiovist 282, Hypaque Meglumine 60%, Reno-M-60)
Diatrizoate meglumine 76% (35.8% iodine)	(Diatrizoate Meglumine 76%)
Diatrizoate sodium 25% (15% iodine)	(Hypaque Sodium 25%)
Diatrizoate sodium 50% (30% iodine)	(Hypaque Sodium 50%)
Gadopentetate dimeglumine 46.9%	(Magnevist)
Iodamide meglumine 24% (11.1% iodine)	(Renovue-Dip)
Iodamide meglumine 65% (30% iodine)	(Renovue-65)
Iodipamide meglumine 10.3% (5.1% iodine)	(Cholografin Meglumine)
Iodipamide meglumine 52% (25.7% iodine)	(Cholografin Meglumine)
Iohexol (46.36% iodine)	(Omnipaque)
Iopamidol 26% (12.8% iodine)	(Isovue-128)
Iopamidol 41% (20% iodine)	(Isovue-200)
Iopamidol 61% (30% iodine)	(Isovue-300)
Iopamidol 76% (37% iodine)	(Isovue-370)
Iothalamate meglumine 30% (14.1% iodine)	(Conray 30)
Iothalamate meglumine 43% (20.2% iodine)	(Conray 43)
Iothalamate meglumine 60% (28.2% iodine)	(Conray)
Iothalamate sodium 54.3% (32.5% iodine)	(Conray 325)
Iothalamate sodium 66.8% (40% iodine)	(Conray 400)
Iothalamate sodium 80% (48% iodine)	(Angio Conray)
Ioversol 34% (16% iodine)	(Optiray 160)
Ioversol 51% (24% iodine)	(Optiray 240)
Ioversol 68% (32% iodine)	(Optiray 320)
Ioversol 74% (35% iodine)	(Optiray 350)
Metrizamide (48.25% iodine)	(Amipaque)
Diatrizoate meglumine 28.5% and diatrizoate sodium 29.1% (31% iodine)	(Renovist II)
Diatrizoate meglumine 34.3% and diatrizoate sodium 35% (37% iodine)	(Renovist)
Diatrizoate meglumine 50% and diatrizoate sodium 25% (38.5% iodine)	(Hypaque-M, 75%)
Diatrizoate meglumine 52% and diatrizoate sodium 8% (29.3% iodine)	(Angiovist 292, MD-60, Renografin-60)
Diatrizoate meglumine 60% and diatrizoate sodium 30% (46.2% iodine)	(Hypaque-M, 90%)
Diatrizoate meglumine 66% and diatrizoate sodium 10% (37% iodine)	(Angiovist 370, Hypaque-76, MD-76, Renografin-76)
Iothalamate meglumine 52% and iothalamate sodium 26% (40% iodine)	(Vascoray)
Ioxaglate meglumine 39.3% and ioxaglate sodium 19.6% (32% iodine)	(Hexabrix)

Radiographic contrast media (radiopaques) increase the absorption of X-rays as they pass through the body and are used for delineating body structures. Magnetic resonance contrast agents enhance the images obtained from the absorption of radio waves by atomic nuclei.

RADIOSENSITIZERS

Malignant neoplastic diseases may be treated by various approaches: surgery, radiation therapy, immunotherapy, chemotherapy, or a combination of these. The extent of a malignant disease (staging) should be ascertained in order to plan an effective therapeutic intervention. Surgery is effective for eliminating localized tumors but is ineffective for metastasized or disseminated tumors. Often the treatment regimen for this type of tumor combines surgery with radiotherapy or chemotherapy. For example, soft-tissue sarcomas are initially treated by local excision, high-dose radiation, and adjuvant chemotherapy with **doxorubicin, cyclophosphamide,** or **methotrexate**. Radiation therapy is an effective alternative to surgery and is used for the locoregional, but not widely disseminated, treatment of a malignancy. Rapidly dividing malignant cells are especially sensitive to radiation. The beneficial effects of radiation therapy stem from its ability to cause the formation of ion pairs or reactive oxygen metabolites such as superoxide, H_2O_2, or hydroxyl radicals. These have the ability to cause breaks in the cancer cell DNA, which, if not repaired, will lead to cell death. **Radiosensitizers** such as **metronidazole** and **bromodeoxyuridine** are agents that enhance the effect of radiation; **radioprotectors** are designed to protect normal cells.

RAMIPRIL

(Altace)

Ramipril, an angiotensin-converting enzyme (ACE) inhibitor with antihypertensive properties (2 to 5 mg p.o. daily), is used in the treatment of hypertension either alone or in combination with thiazide diuretics (see also Figure 21).

Ramipril is a long-acting nonsulfhydryl angiotensin-converting enzyme (ACE) inhibitor. Ramipril is a prodrug that undergoes de-esterification in the liver to form **ramiprilat,** its active metabolite. No clinically significant pharmacokinetic interactions between ramipril and other drugs have been reported. The drug has been generally well tolerated, with the most prevalent adverse effects being dizziness, headache, weakness, and nausea. Ramipril is an effective and well-tolerated drug for the treatment of hypertension and congestive heart failure in all patients, including those with renal or hepatic dysfunction, and in the elderly (see also Figure 21).

RANITIDINE

(Zantac)

Ranitidine, a histamine$_2$ receptor antagonist (150 to 400 mg p.o. daily as a single or divided dose), is indicated for the treatment of duodenal ulcer, benign gastric ulcer, pathological hypersecretory conditions, gastroesophageal reflux disease, and erosive esophagitis. Ranitidine competitively inhibits histamine's action at H_2-receptors in gastric and parietal cells. This reduces basal and nocturnal gastric acid secretion, as well as that caused by histamine, food, amino acids, insulin, and pentagastrin. Antacids reduce the absorption of ranitidine and should not be administered concomitantly (see also Table 9 and Figures 24 and 63).

RAUWOLFIA

(Raudixin, Rauval, Rauverid, Wolfina)

Rauwolfia alkaloid, a peripherally acting adrenergic blocking agent (200 to 400 mg p.o. daily), is used in the treatment of mild to moderate hypertension.

RESCINNAMINE
(Moderil)

Rescinnamine, a rauwolfia alkaloid with peripherally acting adrenergic blocking effects (1 mg p.o. daily), is used in mild to moderate hypertension.

RESERPINE
(Sandril, Serpalan, Serpanray, Serpasil, Serpate, Zepine)

Reserpine, a rauwolfia alkaloid with peripherally acting anti-adrenergic effects (0.5 mg p.o.), is used in mild to moderate essential hypertension. In addition, reserpine (0.1 to 1 mg p.o. daily) has been used as an antipsychotic (see also Figure 27).

RESTACORIN

Restacorin, a novel Class 1C antiarrhythmic drug, exerts a concentration-related negative inotropic effect. It has hemodynamic effects similar to other Class 1 antiarrhythmic drugs.

RESTLESS LEGS SYNDROME: TREATMENT OF

Restless legs syndrome is characterized by an unpleasant creeping discomfort that is perceived as arising deep within the legs and occasionally in the arms as well. Such symptoms tend to occur when patients are relaxed, especially while lying down or sitting, and lead to a need to move about. They are often particularly troublesome at night and may delay the onset of sleep. A sleep disorder associated with periodic movements during sleep may also occur and can be documented by polysonographic recording. The cause is unknown, although the disorder seems especially common among pregnant women and is not uncommon among uremic or diabetic patients with neuropathy. Most patients, however, have no obvious predisposing cause. Symptoms sometimes resolve following correction of coexisting iron-deficiency anemia, and they may respond to treatment with drugs such as levodopa, bromocriptine, diazepam, clonazepam, or opiates. When opiates are required, those with long half-lives or low addictive potential should be used.

RETINOIDS

The retinoids comprise a family of polyisoprenoid lipids that includes **vitamin A** (retinol) and structurally related compounds. The biological activity of retinoids can be modified, for example, by changes in the molecules' state of oxidation and *cis/trans* isomerization. Their activity is also dependent on the levels of specific types of retinoid-binding proteins which exist in extracellular, cytosolic, and nuclear compartments. The role of retinoids in gene expression represents an important biological function for this family of molecules. Retinoid-dependent modulation of gene expression is critical for normal cell and tissue function in mature as well as developing animals.

RETINOIDS
First Generation
Retinol
Tretinoin
Isotretinoin
Second Generation
Etretinate
Acitretin
Third Generation
Arotinoid

Rh_O (D) IMMUNE GLOBULIN, HUMAN
(Gamulin Rh, HypRh$_o$-D, Rhesonativ, Rh$_o$Gam)

Rh_O (D) IMMUNE GLOBULIN, MICRODOSE
(HypRh$_o$-D, Mini-Dose, MICRh$_o$GAM, Mini-Gamulin Rh)

This immune serum is used in Rh-positive exposure (full-term pregnancy or termination of pregnancy beyond 13 weeks of gestation); in transfusion accidents; in termination of pregnancy (spontaneous or induced abortion or ectopic pregnancy) up to 13 weeks of gestation; and in amniocentesis or abdominal trauma during pregnancy.

RIBAVIRIN
(Virazole)

Ribavirin is indicated for the treatment of carefully selected hospitalized infants and young children with severe lower respiratory tract infections due to respiratory syncytial virus (RSV). In addition, ribavirin (600 to 1800 mg/day for 10 to 14 days) has shown effectiveness in acute and chronic hepatitis, herpes genitalis, measles, and Lassa fever.

Ribavirin has antiviral inhibitory activity *in vitro* against respiratory syncytial virus, influenza virus, and herpes simplex virus.

The antiviral mechanism of action of ribavirin relates to alteration of cellular nucleotide pools and inhibition of viral messenger RNA synthesis. Intracellular phosphorylation to the mono-, di-, and triphosphate derivatives is mediated by host cell enzymes. In both uninfected and RSV-infected cells, the predominant derivative (>80%) is the triphosphate, which has an intracellular $t_{1/2}$ of elimination of less than 2 hours.

Ribavirin monophosphate competitively inhibits cellular inosine-5′-phosphate dehydrogenase and interferes with the synthesis of guanosine triphosphate (GTP) and, thus, nucleic acid synthesis in general. Ribavirin triphosphate also competitively inhibits the GTP-dependent 5′-capping of viral messenger RNA and, specifically, influenza virus transcriptase activity. Ribavirin appears to have multiple sites of action, and some of these (e.g., inhibition of GTP synthesis) may potentiate others (e.g., inhibition of GTP-dependent enzymes).

Ribavirin, which is teratogenic, gonadotoxic, embryotoxic, and oncogenic, has caused malformation of skull, palate, eye, jaw, skeleton, and GI tract, and hence is contraindicated in female subjects who are or intend to become pregnant during exposure to the drug.

Aerosolized ribavirin has been well tolerated but may cause mild conjunctival irritation, rash, transient wheezing, and occasional reversible deterioration in pulmonary function. When used in conjunction with mechanical ventilation, equipment modifications and frequent monitoring are required to prevent plugging of ventilator valves and tubing with ribavirin.

Systemic ribavirin causes dose-related anemia due to extravascular hemolysis and dose-related suppression of bone marrow. Reversible increases of serum bilirubin, serum iron, and uric acid concentrations occur during short-term oral administration. Bolus intravenous infusion may cause rigors. In HIV-infected patients, chronic oral therapy is also associated with dose-related lymphopenia and gastrointestinal and CNS complaints, including headache, lethargy, insomnia, and mood alteration.

RIBOFLAVIN
(Vitamin B$_2$)

Riboflavin, a water-soluble vitamin (5 to 30 mg daily), is indicated in riboflavin deficiency or as an adjunct to thiamine treatment for polyneuritis or cheilosis secondary to pellagra.

RIFABUTIN
(Mycobutin)

Rifabutin is a newly marketed, semisynthetic antimycobacterial agent similar to rifampicin (rifampin) in structure and activity. However, rifabutin has important pharmacokinetic differences compared with rifampicin. The clinical effectiveness of rifabutin for prophylaxis of disseminated *Mycobacterium avium* complex infections has recently been demonstrated in HIV-positive patients with low CD4 counts.

RIFAMPIN
(Rifadin)

Rifampin (600 mg once daily) is indicated for the treatment of all forms of tuberculosis in conjunction with at least one other antituberculous drug. Frequently used regimens include: **isoniazid** and rifampin; **ethambutol** and rifampin; or isoniazid, ethambutol, and rifampin; or isoniazid, **pyrazinamide**, and rifampin. In addition, it is used in the treatment of asymptomatic carriers of *Neisseria* meningitis in order to eliminate meningococci from the nasopharynx. It is not indicated for treatment of meningococcal infection.

Rifampin inhibits DNA-dependent RNA polymerase of mycobacteria and other microorganisms by forming a stable drug–enzyme complex, leading to suppression of initiation of chain formation (but not chain elongation) in RNA synthesis. More specifically, the beta subunit of this complex enzyme is the site of action of the drug, although rifampin binds only to the holoenzyme. Nuclear RNA polymerase from a variety of eukaryotic cells does not bind rifampin, and RNA synthesis is correspondingly unaffected. While rifampin can inhibit RNA synthesis in the mammalian mitochondria, considerably higher concentrations of the drug are required than for the inhibition of the bacterial enzyme. High concentrations of rifampin antibiotics also inhibit viral DNA-dependent RNA polymerases and reverse transcriptases. Rifampin is bactericidal for both intracellular and extracellular microorganisms.

Rifampin is absorbed well orally and is bound to plasma proteins to the extent of 80%. It penetrates and concentrates in many body tissues, including the cerebrospinal fluid, and is metabolized in the liver by deacetylation, which is active against *Mycobacterium* tuberculosis.

Rifampin induces the activity of the hepatic microsomal enzyme, metabolizing numerous drugs including acetaminophen, anticoagulants, barbiturates, benzodiazepines, beta-blockers, chloramphenicol, clofibrate, contraceptives, corticosteroids, cyclosporine, digitoxin, disopyramide, estrogens, hydantoins, methadone, mexiletine, quinidine, sulfones, sulfonylureas, theophyllines, tocainide, and verapamil. The plasma levels and effectiveness of these agents may be decreased.

Rifampin is generally well tolerated. When given in usual doses, fewer than 4% of patients with tuberculosis have significant adverse reactions; the most common are rash (0.8%), fever (0.5%), and nausea and vomiting (1.5%). The most notable problem is the development of jaundice.

Hepatitis from rifampin rarely occurs in patients with normal hepatic function; likewise, the combination of isoniazid and rifampin appears generally safe in such patients. However, chronic liver disease, alcoholism, and old age appear to increase the incidence of severe hepatic problems when rifampin is given alone or concurrently with isoniazid.

RIMANTADINE HYDROCHLORIDE
(Flumadine)

Rimantadine (100 mg t.i.d.) and amantadine are indicated for prophylaxis and treatment of illness caused by various strains of influenza A virus. Amantadine and rimantadine share two mechanisms of antiviral action. They inhibit an early step in viral replication, probably viral uncoating; for some strains, they have an effect on a late step in viral assembly probably mediated through altering hemagglutinin processing. The primary locus of action is the influenza A virus M2 protein, an integral membrane protein that functions as an ion channel. By interfering with this function of the M2 protein, the drugs inhibit the acid-mediated dissociation of the ribonucleoprotein complex early in replication and potentiate acidic pH-induced conformational changes in the hemagglutinin during its intracellular transport later in replication (see also Figure 6).

Resistant variants are selected readily by virus passage in the presence of drug and have been recovered from treated persons. Resistance with over 100-fold increases in inhibitory concentrations has been associated with single nucleotide changes leading to amino acid substitutions in the transmembrane region of M2. Amantadine and rimantadine share cross-susceptibility and resistance (see Figure 6).

Following oral administration, rimantadine is extensively metabolized in the liver, with <25% of the dose excreted in the urine as unchanged drug. Three hydroxylated metabolites have been found in plasma. These metabolites, an additional conjugated metabolite, and parent drug account for 74% of a single 200 mg dose excreted in urine over 72 hours. Acetaminophen and aspirin reduce, whereas cimetidine increases, the plasma level of rimantadine.

The most common side effects related to amantadine and rimantadine are minor dose-related gastrointestinal and central nervous system (CNS) complaints. These include nervousness, lightheadedness, difficulty concentrating, insomnia, and loss of appetite or nausea. CNS side effects occur in approximately 5 to 33% of patients treated with amantadine at doses of 200 mg/day, but are significantly less frequent with rimantadine. Amantadine dose reductions are required in older adults (100 mg/day) because of decreased renal function, but 20 to 40% of infirm elderly patients will experience side effects even at this lower dose.

High amantadine plasma concentrations (1.0 to 5.0 microgram/ml) have been associated with serious neurotoxic reactions, including delirium, hallucinosis, seizures or coma, and cardiac arrhythmias. Exacerbations of pre-existing seizure disorders and psychiatric symptoms may occur with amantadine and possibly with rimantadine.

RINGER'S INJECTION
Ringer's solution is used in fluid and electrolyte replacement.

RISPERIDONE
(Risperidal)

Risperidone, a benzisoxazole derivative causing few movement disorders (1 mg p.o. b.i.d.), is used in psychosis (see also Table 23).

RITODRINE HYDROCHLORIDE
(Yutopar)

Ritodrine (0.1 mg/min IV and 10 mg orally 30 min before termination of IV therapy) is indicated in the management of preterm labor. Ritodrine is a $beta_2$-adrenergic receptor agonist influencing the uterine smooth muscle. Stimulation of the $beta_2$ receptors inhibits contractility of the uterine smooth muscle by stimulation of adenyl cyclase, which increases intracellular cyclic adenosine $3'$-$5'$-monophosphate (cAMP); this leads to altering cellular calcium balance that affects smooth muscle contractility. In addition, ritodrine may directly affect the interaction between the actin and myosin of muscle through inhibition of myosin light-chain kinase.

Ritodrine is contraindicated in antepartum hemorrhage which demands immediate delivery; eclampsia and severe preeclampsia; intrauterine fetal death; chorioamnionitis; maternal cardiac disease; pulmonary hypertension; maternal hyperthyroidism; uncontrolled maternal diabetes mellitus. Overdosage with ritodrine may cause tachycardia (maternal and fetal), palpitations, cardiac arrhythmia, hypotension, dyspnea, nervousness, tremor, nausea, and vomiting.

RITONAVIR
(Norvir)

Ritonavir is an inhibitor of the human immunodeficiency virus (HIV) protease, which in combination with nucleoside analogs (600 mg/b.i.d. p.o.) is indicated for the treatment of HIV infection. Ritonavir is a peptidomimetic inhibitor of both the HIV-1 and HIV-2 proteases. Inhibition of HIV protease renders the enzyme incapable of processing the gag-pol polyprotein precursor, which leads to production of noninfectious immature HIV particles.

Ritonavir exhibits additive to synergistic effects against HIV when used in combination with reverse transcriptase inhibitors such as **zidovudine** or **zalcitabine**. Ritonavir produces a large increase in plasma concentration of amiodarone, astemizole, bepridil, bupropion, cisapride, clozapine, encainide, flecainide, meperidine, peroxicam, propafenone, propoxyphene, quinidine, rifabutin, and terfenadine.

ROCURONIUM BROMIDE
(Zemuron)

Rocuronium, a nondepolarizing neuromuscular blocking agent (0.6 mg/kg IV bolus), is used as an adjunct to general anesthesia, facilitation of endotracheal intubation, or skeletal muscle relaxation during surgery or mechanical ventilation (see also Figure 92).

ROPINIROLE

Ropinirole is an efficacious and highly selective nonergoline D_2 agonist. It has no significant alpha or beta-adrenergic nor serotoninergic activity. Ropinirole has beneficial adjuvant effects in parkinsonian patients with moderate motor disability and motor fluctuations (see also Figures 23 and 79).

RUBELLA AND MUMPS VIRUS VACCINE, LIVE
(Biavax II)

This viral vaccine is used in rubella (German measles) and mumps immunization.

RUBELLA VIRUS VACCINE, LIVE, ATTENUATED
(Meruvax II)

This viral vaccine is used in rubella (German measles) immunization.

S

SACCHARIDE IRON OXIDE

Extensive numbers of oral preparations are available for the treatment of iron deficiency anemias. In general, the **ferrous salts** (ferrous sulfate, ferrous gluconate, and ferrous fumarate) are better absorbed than the **ferric salts** (ferric sulfate). Ferrous calcium citrate is used mostly in patients during pregnancy to provide iron as well as calcium.

The parenteral iron medications available include **iron-dextran** (ferric hydroxide and high-molecular-weight dextran) for intramuscular use, **dextriferron** (a complex of ferric hydroxide and partially hydrolyzed dextran) for intravenous use, and **saccharated iron oxide** (a complex of ferric hydroxide and sucrose) for intravenous use. These preparations are reserved for those cases in which oral preparations are not tolerated, absorbed, or rapid enough in their onset of action, or are otherwise not suitable for noncompliant patients.

SALICYCLATES AND ALLIED MEDICATIONS

Salicylates and allied compounds have **analgesic, antipyretic, uricosuric,** and **antiinflammatory** properties. Their mechanisms of action differ from those of the antiinflammatory steroids and the opioid analgesics. They are classified into the following categories (see Table 2):

Salicylate derivatives
  Acetylsalicylic acid (aspirin)
  Diflunisal (Dolobid)
  Salsalate (Arthra-G, Disalcid, Mono-Gesic)
Pyrazolone derivatives
  Phenylbutazone (Butazolidin)
  Oxyphenbutazone (Oxalid, Tandearil)
  Sulfinpyrazone (Anturane)
Paraaminophenol derivatives
  Acetaminophen (Tylenol, Datril)
  Phenacetin (Acetophenetidin)
Propionic acid derivatives
  Ibuprofen (Motrin)
  Naproxen (Naprosyn)
  Fenoprofen (Nalfon)
  Flurbiprofen (Ansaid)
  Ketoprofen (Orudis)
Others
  Indomethacin (Indocin)
  Suldindac (Clinoril)
  Mefenamic acid (Ponstel)
  Tolmetin (Tolectin)
  Piroxicam (Feldene)
  Diclofenac sodium (Voltaren)
  Etodolac
  Nabumetone

Unlike the narcotic analgesics such as morphine, salicylates do not depress respiration, are relatively nontoxic, and lack addiction liability. They are weak or mild analgesics effective in ameliorating short, intermittent types of pain such as neuralgia, myalgia, and toothache.

They do not have the efficacy of morphine and cannot relieve the severe, prolonged, and lancinating types of pain associated with trauma such as burns or fractures. Like morphine, they produce analgesia by raising the pain threshold in the thalamus, but, unlike morphine, they do not alter the patient's reactions to pain. Because they do not cause hypnosis or euphoria, their sites of action have been postulated to be subcortical. In addition to **raising the pain threshold,** the antiinflammatory effects of salicylates may contribute to their analgesic actions. However, no direct association between the antiinflammatory and analgesic effects of these compounds should be expected. For example, aspirin has both analgesic and antiinflammatory properties, whereas acetaminophen has analgesic but not antiinflammatory properties. Furthermore, potent antiinflammatory agents such as phenylbutazone have only weak analgesic effects.

Salicylates, including aspirin, do not alter the normal body temperature, which is maintained by a balance between heat production and dissipation. In a fever associated with infection, increased oxidative processes enhance heat production.

Salicylates act by causing cutaneous vasodilation, which prompts perspiration and enhances heat dissipation. This effect is mediated via the hypothalamic nuclei, as proved by the fact that a lesion in the preoptic area suppresses the mechanism through which aspirin exerts its antipyretic effects. The antipyretic effects of aspirin and other salicylates may be due to their inhibition of hypothalamic prostaglandin synthesis. Although aspirin-induced diaphoresis contributes to its antipyretic effects, it is not an absolutely necessary process, since antipyresis takes place in the presence of atropine.

Salicylates, including aspirin, have an **antiinflammatory** action as well as **antirheumatic** and **antiarthritic** effects, and may therefore be used in the treatment of rheumatic fever. However, they cannot alter the cardiac lesion and other visceral effects of the disease. Aspirin is extremely effective in managing rheumatoid arthritic and allied diseases involving the joints, such as ankylosing spondylitis and osteoarthritis. It is thought that aspirin and indomethacin exert their antiinflammatory effects by inhibiting **prostaglandin** synthesis through the inhibition of **cyclooxygenase.** The presynthesized prostaglandins are released during a tissue injury that fosters inflammation and pain. Furthermore, aspirin reduces the formation of prostaglandin in the platelets and leukocytes, which is responsible for the reported hematologic effects associated with aspirin (see Figures 11 and 12).

SALMETEROL XINOFOATE

(Serevent)

Salmeterol, a sympathomimetic (25 mcg salmeterol base/actuation t.i.d.), is indicated in the prevention of bronchospasm and in the maintenance treatment of those with obstructive airway disease including patients with symptoms of nocturnal asthma. In addition, salmeterol may be used in the prevention of exercise-induced bronchospasm.

The selective beta$_2$-adrenergic stimulants cause bronchodilation without cardiac acceleration. **Metaproterenol** and **terbutaline** are available in tablet form, and terbutaline is also available for subcutaneous injection. Metaproterenol and **albuterol** are available in metered-dose inhalers. Inhaled selective beta$_2$-adrenergic receptor agonists (**albuterol, terbutaline, fenoterol,** and **bitolterol**) have a rapid onset of action and are effective for 3 to 6 hours. **Formoterol** and **salmeterol** are longer-acting agents (12 hours) and may prove useful in treating nocturnal symptoms. The **side effects** of beta-adrenergic receptor agonists are tremor, tachycardia, and palpitations (see also Figure 86).

SALSALATE
(Athra-G, Disalcid, Mono-Gesic)

Salsalate, a non-narcotic analgesic, antipyretic, and antiinflammatory agent (3 g p.o. daily divided q.i.d. p.r.n.), is indicated for minor pain associated with arthritis. Unlike the narcotic analgesics such as morphine, salsalate does not depress respiration, is relatively nontoxic, and lacks addiction liability. It is a weak or mild analgesic that is effective for ameliorating short, intermittent types of pain such as neuralgia, myalgia, toothache, and minor pain associated with arthritis and related disorders. Salsalate does not have the efficacy of morphine and cannot relieve the severe, prolonged, and lancinating types of pain associated with trauma such as burns or fractures. Like morphine, it produces analgesia by raising the pain threshold in the thalamus, but, unlike morphine, it does not alter the patient's reactions to pain. Because salsalate does not cause hypnosis or euphoria, its sites of action have been postulated to be subcortical. In addition to **raising the pain threshold,** the antiinflammatory effects of salsalate may contribute to its analgesic actions. However, no direct association between the antiinflammatory and analgesic effects of salicylate should be expected. For example, aspirin has both analgesic and antiinflammatory properties, whereas acetaminophen has analgesic but not antiinflammatory properties. Furthermore, potent antiinflammatory agents such as phenylbutazone have only weak analgesic effects.

Salicylates including aspirin do not alter the normal body temperature, which is maintained by a balance between heat production and dissipation. In a fever associated with infection, increased oxidative processes enhance heat production.

Salicylates act by causing cutaneous vasodilation, which prompts perspiration and enhances heat dissipation. This effect is mediated via the hypothalamic nuclei, as proved by the fact that a lesion in the preoptic area suppresses the mechanism through which aspirin exerts its antipyretic effects. The antipyretic effects of aspirin and other salicylates may be due to their inhibition of hypothalamic prostaglandin synthesis. Although aspirin-induced diaphoresis contributes to its antipyretic effects, it is not an absolutely necessary process, since antipyresis takes place in the presence of atropine.

Salicylates including aspirin have an **antiinflammatory** action as well as **antirheumatic** and **antiarthritic** effects, and may therefore be used in the treatment of rheumatic fever. However, they cannot alter the cardiac lesion and other visceral effects of the disease. Aspirin is extremely effective in managing rheumatoid arthritis and allied diseases involving the joints, such as ankylosing spondylitis and osteoarthritis. It is thought that aspirin and indomethacin exert their antiinflammatory effects by inhibiting **prostaglandin** synthesis through the inhibition of **cyclooxygenase.** The presynthesized prostaglandins are released during a tissue injury that fosters inflammation and pain. Furthermore, aspirin reduces the formation of prostaglandin in the platelets and leukocytes, which is responsible for the reported hematologic effects associated with aspirin (see also Figures 11 and 12).

Salsalate is contraindicated in patients with known hypersensitivity to aspirin or other nonsteroidal antiinflammatory drugs (NSAIDs) and in the presence of GI ulcer or GI bleeding, because the drug may irritate the GI tract. It should be used cautiously in patients with hypothrombobinemia, vitamin K deficiency, and bleeding disorders, because of the potential for bleeding problems.

Patients with known "triad" symptoms (aspirin hypersensitivity, rhinitis/nasal polyps, and asthma) are at high risk of cross-sensitivity to salicylates with precipitation of bronchospasm.

Concomitant use of salsalate with drugs that are highly protein-bound (phenytoin, sulfonylureas, warfarin) may cause displacement of either drug, and adverse effects. Therapy must be monitored closely for both drugs. Concomitant use with other GI-irritating drugs (steroids, antibiotics, other NSAIDs) may potentiate adverse GI effects of salsalate.

Ammonium chloride and other urine acidifiers, as well as probenecid and sulfinpyrazone, increase salsalate blood levels. Antacids in high doses and other urine alkalizers decrease salsalate blood levels. Corticosteroids enhance salsalate elimination. Food and antacids delay and decrease absorption of salsalate.

Overdosage of salicylate causes metabolic acidosis with respiratory alkalosis; hyperpnea and tachypnea are caused by increased CO_2 production and direct stimulation of the respiratory center.

SARAFOTOXIN

The endothelins belong to a family of potent vasoconstrictor peptides that were originally isolated from the supernatant of cultured aortic endothelial cells. Endothelins bear striking structural similarities to the sarafotoxins, which are potent cardiotoxic peptides isolated from the venom of the burrowing asp *Atractaspis engadensis*. Four endothelins and four sarafotoxin isopeptides, having different receptor subtypes, have been identified (see also Figure 34).

SARGRAMOSTIM
(Granulocyte Macrophage-Colony Stimulating Factor (GM-CSF) (Leukine, Prokine)

Sargramostim, a colony-stimulating factor, is used for acceleration of hematopoietic reconstitution after autologous bone marrow transplantation in patients with non-Hodgkin's lymphoma, acute lymphoblastic leukemia, or Hodgkin's disease undergoing autologous bone marrow transplantation (BMT); and for bone marrow transplantation failure or engraftment delay (see also **Cytokines**).

SAQUINAVIR MESYLATE
(Invirase)

Saquinavir is an inhibitor of the human immunodeficiency virus (HIV) protease, which in combination with nucleoside analogs (three 200 mg capsules t.i.d.) is indicated for the treatment of HIV infection. HIV protease cleaves viral polyprotein precursors to generate functional proteins in HIV-infected cells. The cleavage of viral polyprotein precursors is essential for maturation of infectious virus. Saquinavir mesylate is a synthetic peptide-like substrate analog that inhibits the activity of HIV protease and prevents the cleavage of viral polyproteins. Saquinavir inhibits HIV activity in both acutely and chronically infected cells. Moreover, saquinavir exhibits additive to synergistic effects against HIV in double and triple combination regimens with reverse transcriptase inhibitors **zidovudine, zalcitabine,** and **didanosine** without enhanced cytotoxicity.

Rifampin, phenobarbital, phenytoin, or carbamazepine reduce the plasma concentration of saquinavir. On the other hand, agents which inhibit the activity of the cytochrome P450 3A pathway, such as terfenadine, astemizole, or cisapride, elevate the plasma concentration of saquinavir. The long-term adverse effects of saquinavir remain to be established. However, the low incidences of side effects of saquinavir are diarrhea (3.8%), abdominal discomfort, nausea, abdominal pain, buccal mucosal ulceration, headache, paresthesia, asthenia, rash, and musculoskeletal pain (0.6%).

SCOPOLAMINE
(Transderm Scop)

SCOPOLAMINE HYDROBROMIDE
(Isopto Hyoscine, Triptone)

Scopolamine, an anticholinergic agent, is used as an adjunct to anesthesia. In addition, scopolamine is indicated for cycloplegia and mydriasis in diagnostic procedures for preoperative and postoperative states in the treatment of iridocyclitis. For uveitis, 1 or 2 drops of 0.25% solution is instilled into the eye(s) up to 4 times daily. For refraction, 1 or 2 drops is instilled into the eye(s) one hour before refraction.

Scopolamine (0.32 to 0.65 mg SC, IM, or IV) is indicated for producing preanesthetic sedation and obstetric amnesia in conjunction with analgesics. It may be used for calming delirium and for motion sickness.

Atropine and **scopolamine**, which are obtained from belladonna alkaloids, as well as other synthetic anticholinergic drugs, inhibit the actions of acetylcholine and cholinomimetic drugs at muscarinic receptors in smooth muscles, heart, and exocrine glands. In addition to these peripheral effects, anticholinergic drugs, by blocking the acetylcholine receptor sites in the CNS, have pronounced CNS effects such as restlessness, irritability, excitement, and hallucinations. Scopolamine, on the other hand, depresses the CNS and, in therapeutic doses, produces fatigue, hypnosis, and amnesia. Therefore, it is used extensively in numerous medications, often in combination with antihistamines (see also Figure 18).

The ability of scopolamine to prevent motion-induced nausea is believed to be associated with inhibition of vestibular input to the CNS, which results in inhibition of the vomiting reflex. In addition, scopolamine may have a direct action on the vomiting center within the reticular formation of the brain stem (see also Figure 73).

The transdermal system is a 0.2-mm-thick film with four layers. It is 2.5 cm^2 in area and contains 1.5 mg scopolamine, which is gradually released from an adhesive matrix of mineral oil and polyisobutylene following application to the postauricular skin. An initial priming dose released from the system's adhesive layer saturates the skin binding site for scopolamine and rapidly brings the plasma concentration to the required steady-state level. A continuous controlled release of scopolamine flows from the drug reservoir through the rate-controlling membrane to maintain a constant plasma level. Antiemetic protection is produced within several hours following application behind the ear.

The most common adverse reactions of scopolamine are dry mouth, drowsiness, transient impairment of accommodation including mydriasis and blurred vision. The infrequent adverse reactions of scopolamine, especially in higher than therapeutic doses, include disorientation, memory disturbances, dizziness, restlessness, hallucinations, confusion, difficulty urinating, rashes or erythema, acute narrow-angle glaucoma, and dry, itchy, or red eyes.

SECOBARBITAL
(Seconal)

Secobarbital, a barbiturate sedative-hypnotic and anticonvulsant (200 to 300 mg 1 to 2 hours before surgery), is used to cause preoperative sedation; secobarbital (100 to 200 mg p.o.) is used for short-term treatment of insomnia since it appears to lose its effectiveness after two weeks; secobarbital (5.5 mg/kg IM or slow IV) is indicated for treating acute tetanus convulsions; and secobarbital (50 mg/min IV) is indicated for treating acute psychotic agitation.

Secobarbital acts throughout the CNS as a nonselective depressant with a rapid onset of action and short duration of action. Particularly sensitive to this drug is the reticular activating system, which controls CNS arousal. Secobarbital decreases both presynaptic and postsynaptic membrane excitability by facilitating the action of gamma-aminobutyric acid (GABA) (see also Figure 40).

After oral administration, 90% of secobarbital is absorbed rapidly. After rectal administration, secobarbital is nearly 100% absorbed. Peak serum concentration after oral or rectal administration occurs between 2 and 4 hours. The onset of action is rapid, occurring within 15 minutes when administered orally. Peak effects are seen 15 to 30 minutes after oral and rectal administration, 7 to 10 minutes after IM administration, and 1 to 3 minutes after IV administration.

Secobarbital is distributed rapidly throughout body tissues and fluids; approximately 30 to 45% is protein bound. It is oxidized in the liver to inactive metabolites. Duration of action is 3 to 4 hours; 90% of a secobarbital dose is eliminated as glucuronide conjugates and other metabolites in urine. Secobarbital has an elimination half-life of about 30 hours.

Secobarbital is contraindicated in patients with bronchopneumonia, status asthmaticus, or other severe respiratory distress because of the potential for respiratory depression. Secobarbital should not be used in patients who are depressed or have suicidal ideation because the drug can worsen depression; in patients with uncontrolled acute or chronic pain, because exacerbation of pain and paradoxical excitement can occur; and in patients with porphyria, because this drug can trigger symptoms of this disease.

Secobarbital should be used cautiously in patients who must perform hazardous tasks requiring mental alertness, because this drug causes drowsiness.

Clinical manifestations of overdose with secobarbital include unsteady gait, slurred speech, sustained nystagmus, somnolence, confusion, respiratory depression, pulmonary edema, areflexia, and coma. Typical shock syndrome with tachycardia and hypotension, jaundice, hypothermia, followed by fever, and oliguria may occur.

SEDATIVE-HYPNOTICS

Sedatives, hypnotics, and alcohol are depressants of the central nervous system (CNS). The degree of this reversible depression depends on the amount of drug ingested, producing effects according to the following scheme:

$$\text{Sedation} \rightleftarrows \text{Hypnosis} \rightleftarrows \text{Anesthesia} \rightarrow \text{Death}$$

Sedation is defined as the act of calming or reducing the activity or excitement of an individual. **Hypnosis** represents a condition of artificially produced sleep or a trance resembling sleep. **Anesthesia** constitutes a loss of feeling or sensation.

The degree of CNS depression, including the loss of consciousness, may be assessed according to the response to painful stimuli, and is graded according to the following criteria.

   Drowsy but response to vocal command
   Unconscious but response to minimal stimuli
   Unconscious and response only to maximal painful stimuli
   Unconscious and no response is evident

Contrary to the general belief, the size and activity of the pupils and the limb reflexes are too variable to be useful indices of the degree of CNS depression. However, **absent bowel sounds**, when noted on auscultation of the abdomen, are often associated with pronounced CNS depression.

Sedatives and hypnotics may be divided into two categories: barbiturates and nonbarbiturates (see Table 8).

In the past, barbiturates were used extensively as hypnotic-sedatives but have been replaced by the much safer benzodiazepine derivatives. They do continue to be used as anesthetics and as anticonvulsants. The primary mechanism of action of barbiturates is to increase inhibition of neurons through the **gamma-aminobutyric acid (GABA)** system. Anesthetic barbiturates also decrease excitation via a decrease in calcium conductance (see also Figure 40).

The most commonly used barbiturates are:

   Thiopental (Pentothal)
   Methohexital (Brevital)

Secobarbital (Seconal)
Pentobarbital (Nembutal)
Amobarbital (Amytal)
Phenobarbital (Luminal)

Barbiturates are classified according to their **duration of action**. These are: **ultra short-acting** (thiopental and methohexital), **short- to intermediate-acting** (pentobarbital, secobarbital, and amobarbital), and **long-acting** (phenobarbital).

In general, the more **lipid soluble** a barbiturate derivative is, the greater its plasma- and tissue-binding capacity, the extent of its metabolism, and its storage in adipose tissues. In addition, very lipid-soluble substances have a faster onset of action and a shorter duration of action.

Barbiturates do not raise the **pain threshold** and have no **analgesic** property. In anesthetic doses, they depress all areas of the CNS, including the hypothalamic thermoregulatory system, respiratory center, and vasomotor centers, as well as the **polysynaptic pathways** in the spinal column. In addition, some, such as phenobarbital, but not all are anticonvulsants. In toxic doses, barbiturates cause oliguria.

Barbiturates are absorbed orally and distributed widely throughout the body. They are metabolized in the liver by aliphatic oxygenation, aromatic oxygenation, and N-dealkylation.

The inactive metabolites are excreted in the urine. The administration of **bicarbonate** enhances the urinary excretion of barbiturates that have a pK_a of 7.4 (phenobarbital and thiopental). This generalization is not true of other barbiturates. The long-term administration of barbiturates activates the cytochrome P450 drug metabolizing system.

Acute barbiturate toxicity is characterized by **automatism**, or a state of drug-induced confusion, in which patients lose track of how much medication they have taken and take more. Death results from **respiratory failure**. The treatment of poisoning consists of supporting the respiration, preventing hypotension, diuresis, hemodialysis, and in the event of phenobarbital poisoning, administering **sodium bicarbonate**. Tolerance does not develop to lethal doses.

The abrupt withdrawal from barbiturates may cause tremors, restlessness, anxiety, weakness, nausea and vomiting, seizures, delirium, and cardiac arrest.

The selection of a barbiturate is in part determined by the duration of action desired and by the clinical problems at hand. An ultra short-acting drug is used for inducing anesthesia. For treating epilepsy, a long-acting drug is used, whereas in a sleep disorder, a short-acting or an intermediate-type drug is used, depending on whether patients have difficulty falling asleep or if they have difficulty staying asleep.

Flurazepam (Dalmane), **temazepam** (Restoril), and **triazolam** (Halcion) are all marketed as hypnotic agents, but other benzodiazepine derivatives are also effective hypnotic agents (see Table 8).

Chloral Hydrate
Chloral hydrate (Noctec and Somnos) lacks analgesic effects. It also has no effect on respiration or circulation when given in therapeutic doses. In toxic doses (10 gm), it causes hypotension and respiratory depression. **Chloral hydrate** is reduced to **trichlorethanol**.

Ethchlorvynol
Ethchlorvynol has a rapid onset and short duration of action. It has sedative, hypnotic, muscle relaxant, and anticonvulsant properties. It has a mint-like aftertaste and causes **facial numbness**.

Paraldehyde
The therapeutic uses of paraldehyde (Paral) resemble those of chloral hydrate.

Glutethimide
Glutethimide (Doriden) is used to cause daytime or preoperative sedation, or for the treatment of simple insomnia. Furthermore, it is useful in patients who cannot tolerate barbiturates.

Methaqualone
Methaqualone (Quaalude and Sopor) is used for daytime sedation and in patients with simple insomnia. It is useful for patients who cannot tolerate barbiturates.

Methyprylon
Methyprylon (Nodular) is used for the treatment of simple insomnia and is also useful in patients who cannot tolerate barbiturates.

SEIZURES: TREATMENT OF	
Seizure Disorders	**Drugs**
Primary Generalized Tonic-clonic (Grand Mal)	
Drugs of Choice:	Carbamazepine or Phenytoin or Valproate
Alternatives:	Phenobarbital Primidone
Partial, Including Secondarily Generalized	
Drugs of Choice:	Carbamazepine or Phenytoin
Alternatives:	Phenobarbital Primidone
Absence (Petit Mal)	
Drugs of Choice:	Ethosuximide or Valproate
Alternative:	Clonazepam
Atypical Absence, Myoclonic, Atonic	
Drug of Choice:	Valproate
Alternative:	Clonazepam
Status Epilepticus	
Drugs of Choice: (adults and children)	Diazepam, IV Phenytoin, IV Phenobarbital, IV

SELECTINS
There is a variety of adhesion molecules which facilitate the adherence of formed elements in the blood (for example, platelets and leukocytes) to the vascular endothelium. These leukocyte-endothelial adhesion molecules belong to one of three major families of molecules: (1) the integrins, (2) the immunoglobulin superfamily, and (3) the selectin family. The adhesion molecules appear to act in concert in attracting leukocytes to the reperfused coronary endothelium and in promoting adherence, transendothelial migration, and activation of the

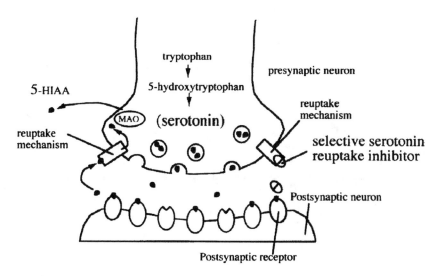

FIGURE 78   Selective serotonin reuptake inhibitors (SSRIS) such as citalopram, fluoxetin, fluvox-amine, paroxetine, and sertraline, are antidepressants with equivalent or superior efficacy to the tricyclic antidepressants (see Tables 3 through 5, and Figures 7, 31, and 41).

leukocytes. One important property of selectins is that they appear to be the initial adhesion molecules to influence the properties of leukocytes at the start of the inflammatory process and hence in ischemia–reperfusion injury.

SELECTIVE SEROTONIN/NORADRENALINE REUPTAKE INHIBITORS

(SNRIs)

In recent years, potential new antidepressants have been developed that inhibit serotonin (5-hydroxytryptamine; 5-HT) and noradrenaline (norepinephrine) reuptake in a selective manner. Examples of these serotonin/noradrenaline reuptake inhibitors (SNRIs) are **dulox-etine, milnacipran,** and **venlafaxine.** Controlled studies in depressed patients have shown an efficacy superior or comparable to tricyclic antidepressants (see Tables 3 through 5 and Figures 41 and 78).

SELEGILINE HYDROCHLORIDE

(L-Deprenyl, Eldepryl)

Selegiline, a monoamine oxidase B inhibitor (5 to 10 mg in divided doses), is indicated as an adjunct in the management of parkinsonian patients being treated with levodopa/carbidopa who exhibit deterioration in the quality of their response to this therapy. Selegiline is effective in the treatment of parkinsonism because it inhibits the catabolism of dopamine. Monoamine oxidase inhibitors are classified into A and B types. **Monoamine oxidase A** preferentially uses serotonin and norepinephrine as substrates and is inhibited by **chlorgyline** and harmaline. **Monoamine oxidase B** preferentially uses dopamine and is inhibited by **selegiline** (Figure 79). Clinical evidence indicates that 10 mg of selegiline in combination with levodopa and carbidopa is superior to levodopa-carbidopa therapy alone. There are indications that selegiline alone can slow the progression of the disease. Although the factors responsible for the loss of nigrostriatal dopaminergic neurons in Parkinson's disease are not understood, the

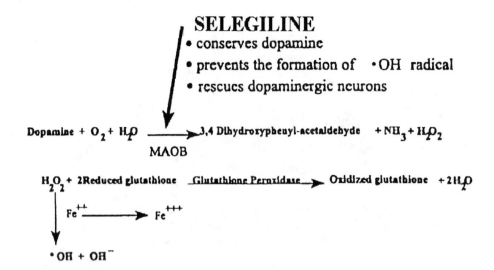

FIGURE 79   **Monoamine oxidase B** preferentially uses dopamine and is inhibited by **selegiline**. Clinical evidence indicates that 10 mg of selegiline in combination with levodopa and carbidopa is superior to levodopa-carbidopa therapy alone. There are indications that selegiline alone can slow the progression of Parkinson's disease, when taken in the early stages of the disease.

findings from neurochemical studies have suggested that the surviving striatal dopamine neurons accelerate the synthesis of dopamine, thus enhancing the formation of H_2O_2 according to the scheme depicted in Figure 79.

The evidence suggesting that **oxidative reactions** may contribute to the pathogenesis of Parkinson's disease includes the following: In patients with Parkinson's disease, the **iron** content is increased in the substantia nigra; the **ferritin** level is decreased in the brain; and the **glutathione** concentration is decreased in the substantia nigra. Furthermore, although 1-methyl-4-phenyl-1,2,3,6-tetrahydropyridine (**MPTP**) is not in itself toxic, when oxidized by monoamine oxidase B to the methylphenylpyridium ion, it becomes a select nigral toxin that interferes with mitochondrial respiratory mechanisms. The toxicity of MPTP may be prevented by pretreatment with a monoamine oxidase B inhibitor such as selegiline. Therefore, it is thought that selegiline, by conserving dopamine and preventing the formation of ·OH radicals, rescues dopaminergic neurons.

SEMILENTE INSULIN

Insulin preparations are fast-, intermediate-, or long-acting, as summarized in Table 18. **Crystalline** (regular) **insulin** may be used as a supplemental injection or for instituting corrective measures in the management of infection and trauma, for postoperative stabilization, and for the rehabilitation of patients recovering from ketoacidosis and coma. In addition, NPH contains regular insulin. **Ultralente** or **semilente insulin** is used to eliminate nocturnal and early morning hyperglycemia (see also Table 18).

SEMUSTINE

(Methy-CCNU)

The alkyl sulfonate busulfan (Myleran) is metabolized to an alkylating agent. Because it produces selective myelosuppression, it is used in cases of chronic myelocytic leukemia. It causes pronounced hyperuricemia stemming from the catabolism of purine.

SENNA

(Black Draught, Fletcher's Castoria, Genna, Gentlax-B, Gentle Nature, Nytilax, Senexon, Senokot, Senolax, X-Prep)

Senna, an anthraquinone derivative with laxative properties, is used in acute constipation and preparation for bowel examination.

SERMORELIN ACETATE

(Geref)

Sermorelin, a growth hormone releasing hormone, is used as a diagnostic aid to determine the pituitary gland's ability to secrete growth hormone.

SEROTONIN

5-Hydroxytryptamine (serotonin) is metabolized according to the following scheme:

Tryptophan

$\downarrow$ Tryptophan 5-hydroxylase

5-Hydroxytryptophan

$\downarrow$ Aromatic *L*-amino acid decarboxylase

5-Hydroxytryptamine (serotonin)

$\downarrow$ Monoamine oxidase

5-Hydroxyindoleactaldehyde

$\downarrow$ Aldehyde dehydrogenase

5-Hyroxyindoleacetic acid

A large amount of 5-hydroxyindoleacetic acid is excreted by patients with **malignant carcinoid**.

Extensive ligand-binding studies and molecular biologic examination of membrane preparations have revealed that there are at least fourteen types of serotonin receptors, including $5\text{-}HT_{1A}$, $5\text{-}HT_{1B}$, $5\text{-}HT_{1D}$, $5\text{-}HT_3$, and $5\text{-}HT_4$.

Serotonin possesses many actions. It:

Is involved in the neural network that regulates intestinal motility.
Is released by a carcinoid.
Is released by platelets (also ADP) during aggregation.
Causes vasoconstriction by stimulating $5\text{-}HT_2$ receptors, and this effect is blocked by
  ketanserine.
Causes vasodilation by stimulating $5\text{-}HT_1$ receptors.
Causes positive inotropic and chronotropic effects by interacting with both $5\text{-}HT_1$ and
  $5\text{-}HT_3$ receptors.
Increases the motility of the stomach as well as small and large intestines.
Causes uterine contractions.
Causes bronchial contractions.

Following are the serotonin receptor agonist-antagonists:

Ketanserine, a $5\text{-}HT_2$ and alpha$_1$-adrenergic receptor antagonist, lowers blood pressure.

Methysergide, a 5-HT_{1C} antagonist, has been used for the prophylactic treatment of migraine and other vascular headache, including Horton's syndrome. Calcium entry blockers such as **flunarizine** have been shown to be effective in treating migraine.

Cyproheptadine, a serotonin and histamine$_1$ receptor- and muscarinic cholinergic receptor-blocking agent, has been used in the treatment of the postgastrectomy dumping syndrome and the intestinal hypermotility seen with carcinoid.

Sumatriptan, an agonist of the 5-HT_1-like receptor, is highly effective in the treatment of migraine (see Figure 85).

Ondansetron, granisetron, tropisetron, and batanopride are antagonists of the 5-HT_3 receptor and are considered effective in controlling cancer chemotherapy-induced emesis (see Figure 64).

Clozapine, an effective antipsychotic agent with little or no extrapyramidal side effects, blocks the 5-HT_2 receptor (see also Table 23).

SEROTONIN RECEPTOR SUBTYPES		
Subtypes	**Drugs**	**Disorders**
5-HT_{1A}	Buspirone, ipsaperone	Anxiety, depression
5-HT_{1B}		
5-HT_{1D}	Sumatriptan	Migraine
5-HT_{1E}		
5-HT_{1F}		
5-HT_{2A}	Ketanserin	Hypertension
5-HT_{2B}	Methysergide, risperidone	Migraine, depression, schizophrenia
5-HT_{2C}		
5-HT_3	Ondansetron	Chemotherapy-induced emesis
5-HT_4	Cisapride	Gastrointestinal disorders
5-HT_{5A}		
5-HT_{5B}		
5-HT_6		
5-HT_7		
5-HT transporter	Fluoxetine, sertraline	Depression, obsessive-compulsive disorder
Buspirone, ipsaperone, sumatriptan, and cisapride are agonists; whereas methysergide, risperidone, ketanserin, and ondansetron are antagonists at serotonin receptors.		

SERTRALINE HYDROCHLORIDE
(Zoloft)

Sertraline (50 mg p.o. daily) is a nontricyclic, potent, and selective serotonin reuptake inhibitor (SSRI) which is currently approved for the treatment of depression. The role of serotonin in the etiology of obsessive compulsive disorder (OCD) has been established through considerable indirect evidence. The strongest evidence comes from the fact that drugs known to be SSRIs have been found to be useful in the pharmacotherapy of OCD (see also Figure 78 and Tables 3 through 5).

SEXUAL DYSFUNCTIONS CAUSED BY DRUGS	
Drugs	**Adverse Effects**
Acetazolamide	Loss of libido; decreased potency
Alprazolam	Inhibition of orgasm; delayed or no ejaculation; decreased libido
Amiloride	Impotence; decreased libido
Amiodarone	Decreased libido
Amitriptyline	Loss of libido; impotence; no ejaculation
Amoxapine	Loss of libido; impotence; ejaculatory problems
Amphetamines and related anorexic drugs	Chronic abuse; impotence; delayed or no ejaculation in men; no orgasm in women
Anticholinergics	Impotence
Atenolol	Impotence
Baclofen	Impotence; inability to ejaculate
Barbiturates	Decreased libido; impotence
Bromocriptine	Painful clitoral tumescence; impotence
Buserelin	Loss of libido; impotence
Buspirone	Priapism
Carbamazepine	Impotence
Chlorpromazine	Decreased libido; impotence; no ejaculation; priapism
Chlorprothixene	Inhibition of ejaculation
Chlorthalidone	Decreased libido; impotence
Cimetidine	Decreased libido; impotence
Clofibrate	Decreased libido; impotence
Clomipramine	Decreased libido; impotence; retarded or no ejaculation or orgasm; orgasm precipitated by yawning; painful ejaculation
Clonidine	Impotence; delayed or retrograde ejaculation; decreased libido
Clozapine	Priapism
Cocaine	Priapism
Danazol	Increased or decreased libido
Desipramine	Decreased libido; impotence; painful orgasm
Diazepam	Decreased libido; delayed ejaculation; retarded or no orgasms in women; erection difficulties
Dichlorphenamide	Decreased libido; impotence
Digoxin	Decreased libido; impotence
Disopyramide	Impotence
Disulfiram	Impotence
Doxepin	Decreased libido; ejaculatory dysfunction
Ethosuximide	Increased libido
Ethoxzolamide	Decreased libido
Etretinate	Erection difficulties
Famotidine	Impotence
Fenfluramine	Loss of libido with large doses or long-term use; impotence
Fluoxetine	Anorgasmia; delayed orgasm; spontaneous orgasm; ejaculation difficulties; penile anesthesia; decreased libido

Drugs	Adverse Effects
Fluphenazine	Changes in libido; erection difficulties; inhibition of ejaculation; priapism
Gemfibrozil	Impotence; loss of libido
Guanabenz	Impotence
Guanadrel	Decreased libido; delayed or retrograde ejaculation; impotence
Guanethidine	Decreased libido; impotence; delayed, retrograde, or no ejaculation
Guanfacine	Impotence
Haloperidol	Impotence; painful ejaculation
Hydralazine	Impotence; priapism
Imipramine	Decreased libido; impotence; painful, delayed ejaculation; delayed orgasm in women
Indapamide	Decreased libido; impotence
Indomethacin	Sexual dysfunction; impotence; decreased libido
Interferon alfa	Decreased libido; impotence
Isocarboxazid	Impotence; delayed ejaculation; no orgasm in women
Ketoconazole	Impotence; decreased libido
Labetalol	Priapism; impotence; delayed or no ejaculation; decreased libido
Leuprolide	Impotence
Levodopa	Increased libido
Lithium	Decreased libido; impotence
Lorazepam	Loss of libido
Maprotiline	Impotence; decreased libido
Mazindol	Impotence; spontaneous ejaculation; painful testes
Mecamylamine	Impotence; decreased libido
Mepenzolate bromide	Impotence
Mesoridazine	No ejaculation; impotence; priapism
Methadone	Decreased libido; impotence; no orgasm (men and women); retarded ejaculation
Methandrostenolone	Decreased libido
Methantheline bromide	Impotence
Methazolamide	Decreased libido; impotence
Methotrexate	Impotence; erection difficulties
Methyldopa	Decreased libido; impotence; delayed or no ejaculation or orgasm
Metoclopramide	Impotence; decreased libido
Metoprolol	Impotence
Metyrosine	Impotence; failure of ejaculation
Mexiletine	Impotence; decreased libido
Molindone	Priapism
Nafarelin	Impotence; loss of libido
Naltrexone	Delayed ejaculation; decreased potency
Naproxen	Impotence; no ejaculation
Nifedipine	Priapism
Nizatidine	Impotence
Norethandrolone	Decreased libido; impotence

Drugs	Adverse Effects
Nortriptyline	Impotence; decreased libido
Omeprazole	Painful nocturnal erections
Papaverine	Priapism, especially with neurological disorders
Pargyline	No ejaculation; impotence
Pergolide	Hypersexuality; priapism; spontaneous ejaculation
Perphenazine	Decreased or no ejaculation
Phenelzine	Impotence; retarded or no ejaculation; delayed or no orgasm; priapism
Phenytoin	Decreased libido; impotence; priapism
Pimozide	Impotence; no ejaculation; decreased libido
Prazosin	Impotence; priapism
Primidone	Decreased libido; impotence
Propantheline bromide	Impotence
Propofol	Sexual disinhibition
Propranolol	Loss of libido; impotence
Protriptyline	Loss of libido; impotence; painful ejaculation
Ranitidine	Impotence; loss of libido
Reserpine	Decreased libido; impotence; decreased or no ejaculation
Sertraline	Sexual dysfunction
Spironolactone	Decreased libido; impotence
Sulfasalazine	Impotence
Tamoxifen	Priapism
Testosterone	Priapism
Thiazide diuretics	Impotence
Thioridazine	Impotence; priapism; delayed, decreased, painful, retrograde, or no ejaculation; anorgasmia
Thiothixene	Spontaneous ejaculations; impotence; priapism
Timolol	Decreased libido; impotence
Tranylcypromine	Impotence; painful ejaculation; retarded ejaculation
Trazodone	Priapism; clitoral priapism; increased libido; retrograde or no ejaculation; anorgasmia
Trifluperazine	Painful ejaculation; spontaneous ejaculations
Verapamil	Impotence

Drugs cause sexual dysfunctions by diversified mechanisms such as having peripheral sympatholytic actions (guanadrel), central sympatholytic actions (clonidine), anticholinergic actions (imipramine), or enhancing the concentration of prolactin (amoxapine). Drug-induced sexual dysfunctions are usually reversible with dose reduction or discontinuation of drugs.

SEXUALLY TRANSMITTED DISEASES: TREATMENT OF		
Diseases	**First Drug of Choice**	**Alternate Drug(s)**
Chlamydia Trachomatis		
Urethritis, cervicitis, conjunctivitis, or proctitis	Azithromycin **or** Doxycycline	Ofloxacin Erythromycin

Diseases	First Drug of Choice	Alternate Drug(s)
Infection in Pregnancy	Erythromycin	Amoxicillin Azithromycin
Neonatal		
Ophthalmia	Erythromycin	Sulfisoxazole
Pneumonia	Erythromycin	
Lymphogranuloma venereum	Doxycycline	Erythromycin
Gonorrhea		
Urethral, cervical, rectal, or pharyngeal	Ceftriaxone	Cefixime Ciprofloxacin Ofloxacin Spectinomycin
Ophthalmia	Ceftriaxone	
Bacteremia, arthritis, and disseminated	Ceftriaxone	Ceftizoxime or Cefotaxime
Neonatal		
Ophthalmia	Cefotaxime **or** Ceftriaxone	Penicillin G
Bacteremia, arthritis, and disseminated	Cefotaxime	Penicillin G
Children		
Urogenital, rectal, and pharyngeal	Ceftriaxone	Spectinomycin Amoxicillin **plus** Probenecid
Bacteremia, arthritis, and disseminated	Ceftriaxone **or** Cefotaxime	Penicillin G
Sexually Acquired Epididymitis		
	Ofloxacin	Ceftriaxone **followed by** Doxycycline
Pelvic Inflammatory Disease		
Hospitalized patients	Cefoxitin **or** Cefotetan **either one plus** Doxycycline **followed by** Doxycycline	Clindamycin **plus** Gentamicin **followed by** Gentamicin **followed by** Doxycycline
Outpatients	Cefoxitin **plus** Probenecid **or** Cetriaxone **either one** **followed by** Doxycycline	Ofloxacin **plus** Metronidazole **or** Clindamycin
Vaginal Infection		
Trichomoniasis	Metronidazole	Metronidazole
Bacterial vaginosis	Metronidazole **or** Clindamycin	Metronidazole Clindamycin

Diseases	First Drug of Choice	Alternate Drug(s)
Vulvovaginal candidiasis	Topical butoconazole, clotrimazole, miconazole, terconazole, **or** tioconazole	Fluconazole
Syphilis		
Early	Penicillin G benzathine	Doxycycline
Late	Penicillin G benzathine	Doxycycline
Neurosyphilis	Penicillin G	Penicillin G procaine **plus** Probenecid
Congenital	Penicillin G **or** Penicillin G procaine	
Chancroid	Erythromycin **or** Ceftriaxone **or** Azithromycin	Ciprofloxacin
Herpes Simplex		
First Episode Genital	Acyclovir	Acyclovir
First Episode Proctitis	Acyclovir	Acyclovir
Recurrent	Acyclovir	
Severe (hospitalized patients)	Acyclovir	
Prevention of Recurrence	Acyclovir	Acyclovir

SHINGLES: TREATMENT OF

Varicella zoster virus (VZV) is responsible for a primary infection (varicella) followed by a latency, eventually resulting in herpes zoster (shingles).

Treatment of herpes zoster primarily relies upon antiviral drugs and incidentally on immunomodulating agents, specific immunoglobulins, antimicrobial agents, antiviral enzymes, and corticosteroids. Drugs with a clinically relevant activity against varicella zoster virus infections include acyclovir, adenosine monophosphate, bromodeoxyuridine, descyclovir, fiacitabine, idoxuridine, interferon-α, and vidarabine. Among them, acyclovir appears to be a first-line agent. Its efficacy has been well established by many clinical studies. Promising drugs for the future include **famciclovir, pencyclovir, valacyclovir,** and other molecules currently under investigation.

SIBUTRAMINE

Sibutramine, a novel pharmacologic agent, is a specific reuptake inhibitor for norepinephrine and serotonin. Sibutramine and its two metabolites reduce food intake and hence show promise as antiobesity medications (see also Figure 78).

SILVER NITRATE, SILVER NITRATE 1%

(Dey Drops Silver Nitrate)

Silver nitrate, an ophthalmic antiseptic and topical cauterizing agent, is used for prevention of gonorrheal ophthalmia neonatorum; and to treat indolent wounds, destroy exuberant granulations, freshen the edges of ulcers and fissures, provide styptic action, and treat vesicular bullous or aphthous lesions.

SILVER SULFADIAZINE
(SSD Cream, Silvadene Cream, SSD AF, Thermazene)

Silver sulfadiazine, a synthetic topical antibacterial agent (1% cream), is used as an adjunct in the prevention and treatment of wound infection for second- and third-degree burns.

SIMVASTATIN
(Zocor)

Simvastatin, an HMG-CO reductase inhibitor with antilipemic activity (5 to 10 mg daily), is used for reduction of low-density lipoprotein (LDL) and total cholesterol levels in patients with primary hypercholesterolemia (types IIa and IIb) (see also Figure 25).

SINUSITIS: TREATMENT OF
Normal physiological functioning of the sinuses depends on ostial patency, mucociliary function, and the quantity and quality of secretions. Retention of sinus secretions may result if ostial diameter is compromised; if cilia are damaged, impairing mucociliary clearance of secretions; or if increased viscosity or volume of secretions exceeds the clearing capacity of the sinus mucociliary drainage system.

Factors predisposing to the development of sinusitis are:

Adenoidal hypertrophy	Dysmotile cilia syndrome
Allergic rhinitis	Immune deficiency
Barotrauma	Nasal polyps
Bone spurs	Overuse of topical decongestants
Bronchiectasis	Swimming and diving
Cigarette smoke	Tumors
Deviated nasal septum	Upper respiratory infection

The goal in treatment of sinusitis is eradication of infection with clearance of the infected material from the sinuses. While the use of an appropriate antibiotic is necessary, the use of ancillary therapy is also of utmost importance. Steam and nasal saline, decongestants, topical corticosteroids, and mucoevacuants are given in an attempt to reduce nasal obstruction, increase sinus ostia size, promote improved mucociliary function, decrease mucosal inflammation, and thin secretions. In selected patients who fail to respond to aggressive medical therapy, functional endoscopic surgery can often provide relief. In patients with poorly controlled asthma, treatment of underlying sinusitis has been shown to dramatically improve the asthmatic state.

SODIUM BENZOATE-SODIUM PHENYLACETATE
(Ucephan)

Sodium benzoate sodium phenylacetate (25 mg/kg p.o. daily) is used as an adjunctive therapy for the prevention of hyperammonemia in patients with urea cycle enzymopathy.

SODIUM BICARBONATE
(Neut, Soda Mint)

Sodium bicarbonate, an alkalinizing agent (1 mEq/kg IV bolus), is used as an adjunct to advanced cardiac life support in metabolic acidosis, as a urinary alkalinization, and as an antacid.

SODIUM CELLULOSE PHOSPHATE
(Calcibind)

Sodium cellulose phosphate, an ion exchange resin with antiurolithic properties (15 g p.o. daily), is used for absorptive hypercalciuria Type I and prophylaxis of calcium renal calculi.

SODIUM CHLORIDE

(Slo-Salt, Thermotab)

Sodium chloride is used for water and electrolyte replacement in hyponatremia from electrolyte loss or severe sodium chloride depletion.

SODIUM FLUORIDE

(Act, Fluorigard, Fluorinse, Fluoritabs, Flura, Flura-Drops, Flura-Loz, Gel II, Karidium, Karigel, Karigel-N, Listermint with Fluoride, Luride, Luride Lozi-Tabs, Luride-SF Lozi Tabs, Pediaflor, Phos-Flur, Point Two, PreviDent, Thera-Flur, Thera-Flur-N)

Fluoride, a trace mineral, is used as an aid in the prevention of dental caries.

SODIUM LACTATE

Sodium lactate, an alkalinizing agent, is used to alkalinize urine and as treatment in mild to moderate metabolic acidosis.

SODIUM POLYSTYRENE SULFONATE

(Kayexalate, SPS)

Sodium polystyrene sulfonate, a cation exchange resin removing potassium (15 g p.o. daily), is used in hyperkalemia.

SODIUM SALICYLATE

(Uracel)

Sodium salicylate, a non-narcotic analgesic, antipyretic, and antiinflammatory agent, is used in minor pain or fever, and in rheumatoid arthritis, osteoarthritis, or other inflammatory conditions (see also Table 2).

SODIUM THIOSALICYLATE

(Arthrolate, Asproject, Rexolate, Thiocyl, Thiosal, Tusal)

Sodium thiosalicylate, a non-narcotic analgesic, antipyretic, and antiinflammatory agent, is indicated for mild pain, in the treatment of rheumatic fever, or acute gouty arthritis (see also Table 2).

SOMATOSTATIN

Somatostatin, a cyclic tetradecapeptide with a disulfide bond between the third and fourteenth amino acid residues, has the following structure:

H-Ala-Gly-Cys-Lys-Asn-Phe-Phe-Tryp-Lys-Thr-Phe-Thr-Ser-Cys-OH

The administration of somatostatin inhibits the secretion of a variety of peptides, including:

Hypothalamic hormones
Growth hormone releasing hormone (GHRH) (see also Table 14)
Anterior pituitary hormones
Growth hormone (GH)
Thyrotropin
Pancreatic hormones
Insulin
Glucagon

Gastrin
Cholecystokinin
Secretin
Pepsin
Motilin
Pancreatic polypeptide
Gastrointestinal peptide
Vasoactive intestinal polypeptide
Kidney hormones
Renin

Octreotide (Sandostatin), a long-acting somatostatin analog, has been approved for the management of secretory carcinoid tumors and vasoactive intestinal peptide-secreting tumors.

SOMATREM

(Protropin)

Somatrem, an anterior pituitary hormone, is used for long-term treatment of growth failure from lack of adequate endogenous growth hormone secretion.

SOTALOL HYDROCHLORIDE

(Betapace)

Sotalol (80 mg t.i.d.) is indicated in the treatment of documented ventricular arrhythmias, such as sustained ventricular tachycardia.

Sotalol is a nonselective beta-adrenergic blocker that depresses sinus heart rate, slows AV conduction, increases AV nodal refractoriness, prolongs the refractory period of atrial and ventricular muscle and AV accessory pathways in both anterograde and retrograde directions, decreases cardiac output, and lowers systolic and diastolic blood pressure.

Sotalol is well absorbed after oral administration with a bioavailability of 90 to 100%. Peak plasma concentrations are reached in 2.5 to 4 hours, and steady-state plasma concentrations are attained in 2 to 3 days. Sotalol does not bind to plasma proteins and crosses the blood-brain barrier poorly. Sotalol is not metabolized and is excreted primarily in the urine and in unchanged form.

Sotalol is contraindicated in patients with bronchial asthma, sinus bradycardia, second- and third-degree AV block (unless a functioning pacemaker is present), congenital or acquired long QT syndromes, cardiogenic shock, or uncontrolled congestive heart failure.

Sotalol should be used cautiously in pregnant patients and patients with renal failure or diabetes mellitus. Sotalol should be used with extreme caution in patients with sick sinus syndrome associated with symptomatic arrhythmias, because the drug can cause sinus bradycardia, sinus pauses, or sinus arrest.

Catecholamine-depleting drugs, such as **reserpine** and **guanethidine**, enhance the hypotensive effects of sotalol. Calcium channel antagonists enhance myocardial depression and should not be given concomitantly with sotalol. Sotalol may enhance the rebound hypertensive effect seen after withdrawal of **clonidine**.

Sotalol may require dosage adjustments with insulin or oral antidiabetic agents because it may increase blood glucose. It also may mask symptoms of hypoglycemia.

Overdosage of sotalol may cause bradycardia, congestive heart failure, hypotension, hypoglycemia, and bronchospasm.

Because of the lack of protein binding, hemodialysis is useful in reducing sotalol plasma concentrations. Patients should be carefully observed until QT intervals are normalized.

In addition, **atropine**, another anticholinergic drug, a beta-adrenergic agonist, or transvenous cardiac pacing may be used to treat bradycardia; transvenous cardiac pacing may be employed to treat second- or third-degree heart block; epinephrine can be used to treat hypotension (depending on associated factors); aminophylline or an aerosol beta$_2$-receptor stimulant can be used to treat bronchospasm; and DC cardioversion, transvenous cardiac pacing, epinephrine, or magnesium sulfate can be used to treat torsades de pointes.

SPARFLOXACIN

Sparfloxacin is a recently developed fluoroquinolone. The drug has shown potent antimicrobial activity against a wide range of Gram-positive and Gram-negative bacteria, glucose nonfermenters, anaerobes, *Legionella spp.*, *Mycoplasma spp.*, *Chlamydia spp.*, and *Mycobacterium spp.* Methicillin-resistant *Staphylococcus aureus* is also susceptible to sparfloxacin (see also Figure 77).

SPIRAMYCIN

Spiramycin is a macrolide antibiotic. However, in contrast to other macrolide derivatives such as erythromycin salts, ototoxicity, neurosensorial disorders, and cardiac rhythm disorders do not appear to have been described after spiramycin. Reported adverse effects of spiramycin include gastrointestinal disorders, immune-allergic reactions, and liver injury (see also Figure 80).

SPIRONOLACTONE

(Aldactone)

The potassium-sparing diuretics consist of spironolactone, which is an aldosterone antagonist, and **triamterene** (Dyrenium) and **amiloride** (Midamor), which exert their effects through a mechanism other than a mineralocorticoid action (see also Figure 4).

All act in the distal tubule, where the resorption of sodium is accompanied by the transfer of potassium into the lumen contents (see also Figure 4). When sodium resorption is hindered, potassium excretion is correspondingly reduced, such that more potassium is retained. The potassium-sparing diuretics are not very efficacious, as they affect only 1 to 2% of the filtered load of sodium. All are given orally and eliminated in the urine, mostly by glomerular filtration, though some active tubular secretion may also occur.

A potassium-sparing diuretic can be given along with a thiazide or a loop diuretic to prevent hypokalemia. Spironolactone can also be beneficial in some patients with severe congestive heart failure or cirrhosis associated with ascites.

The potassium-sparing diuretics should not be used concurrently with potassium supplements, as this combination is likely to produce hyperkalemia. Poor renal function also heightens the risk of hyperkalemia. Gastrointestinal disturbances, rash, drowsiness, or dizziness are all associated with their use. Spironolactone can cause the blood urea nitrogen level to increase and lead to menstrual irregularities.

SPECTINOMYCIN

(Trobicin)

Spectinomycin (2 g IM into the upper outer quadrant of the gluteus) is indicated in the treatment of acute gonorrheal urethritis and proctitis in the male and acute gonorrheal cervicitis and proctitis in the female due to susceptible strains of *Neisseria gonorrhoeae*. The injection may be painful. A single injection of 2 g produces an average peak serum concentration of 160 mcg/ml at 2 hours.

Spectinomycin is not effective in the treatment of syphilis. Antibiotics used to treat gonorrhea may mask or delay the symptoms of incubating syphilis. All patients with gonorrhea should have a serologic test for syphilis at the time of diagnosis and a follow-up test after 3 months.

Spectinomycin is not effective in pharyngeal infections due to *N. gonorrhoeae*.

Spectinomycin selectively inhibits protein synthesis in Gram-negative bacteria. The antibiotic binds to and acts on the 30S ribosomal subunit (see also Figure 80). Its action has similarities to that of the aminoglycosides; however, spectinomycin is not bactericidal and does not cause misreading of polyribonucleotides. A high degree of bacterial resistance may develop as a result of mutation.

Spectinomycin, when given as a single intramuscular injection, produces few significant untoward effects. Urticaria, chills, and fever have been noted after single doses, as have dizziness, nausea, and insomnia. The injection may be painful.

STANOZOLOL
(Winstrol)

Stanozolol, an anabolic steroid (2 mg t.i.d.), is indicated as a prophylactic measure in reducing the frequency and severity of hereditary angioedema (see also Table 6).

Stanozolol increases the concentration of C1 esterase inhibitor in patients with hereditary angioedema. This leads to an increased level of the C4 component of complement, which may be deficient in these patients, thus decreasing the number and severity of attacks of this disorder.

Stanozolol is contraindicated in patients with severe renal or cardiac disease, which may be worsened by the fluid and electrolyte retention that this drug may cause; in patients with hepatic disease because impaired elimination may cause toxic accumulation of the drug; in female patients with breast cancer, in male patients with benign prostatic hypertrophy with obstruction, or undiagnosed abnormal genital bleeding because this drug can stimulate the growth of cancerous breast or prostate tissues; and in pregnant women because studies have shown that administration of anabolic steroids during pregnancy causes masculinization of the fetus. Because of its hypercholesterolemic effects, stanozolol should be administered cautiously in patients with a history of coronary artery disease. In patients with diabetes, decreased blood glucose levels require adjustment of insulin or oral hypoglycemic drug dosage.

Stanozolol may potentiate the effects of warfarin-type anticoagulants, prolonging prothrombin time. The adverse reactions to stanozolol in female subjects include deepening of voice, clitoral enlargement, and changes in libido. The adverse effects in prepubertal male subjects include premature epiphyseal closure, priapism, phallic enlargement; in postpubertal males: testicular atrophy, oligospermia, decreased ejaculatory volume, impotence, gynecomastia, and epididymitis.

STAVUDINE
(d4T) (Zerit)

Stavudine, a synthetic thymidine nucleoside analog, is used in the treatment of patients with advanced HIV infection who are intolerant of or unresponsive to other antiviral therapies.

STREPTOKINASE

(Kabikinase, Streptase)

Streptokinase (1,500,000 IU within 60 minutes by IV infusion) is indicated for lysis of **coronary artery thrombosis** after acute myocardial infarction; streptokinase (250,000 IU by IV infusion pump into each occluded limb of the cannula over 25 to 35 minutes) is indicated in **arteriovenous cannula occlusion**; and streptokinase (250,000 IU IV infusion over 30 minutes) is indicated in the treatment of **venous thrombosis, pulmonary embolism**, and **arterial thrombosis** and **embolism**.

Streptokinase is a 47-kDa protein produced by beta-hemolytic streptococci. It has no intrinsic enzymatic activity, but it forms a stable, noncovalent 1:1 complex with plasminogen. This produces a conformational change that exposes the active site on plasminogen that cleaves arginine 560 on free plasminogen molecules to form free plasmin.

A loading dose of streptokinase (250,000 U; 2.5 mg) must be given intravenously to overcome plasma antibodies that are directed against the protein. These inactivating antibodies result from prior streptococcal infections. The half-life of streptokinase (once antibodies are depleted) is about 40 to 80 minutes. The streptokinase-plasminogen complex is not inhibited by alpha$_2$-antiplasmin. Levels of antibodies differ greatly among individuals, but this variable probably is of little clinical significance when streptokinase is given in the large doses currently used for coronary thrombolysis.

Plasminogen activation begins promptly after infusion or instillation of streptokinase; adequate activation of the fibrinolytic system occurs in 3 to 4 hours. Streptokinase does not cross the placenta, but its antibodies do.

Streptokinase is removed from circulation by antibodies and the reticuloendothelial system. Half-life is biphasic: Initially it is 18 minutes (from antibody action) and then extends up to 83 minutes. Anticoagulant effect may persist for 12 to 24 hours after infusion is discontinued.

Concomitant use with anticoagulants may cause hemorrhage. It may also be necessary to reverse effects of oral anticoagulants before beginning therapy. Concomitant use with aspirin, indomethacin, phenylbutazone, or other drugs affecting platelet activity increases the risk of bleeding.

Streptokinase is contraindicated in patients with ulcerative wounds, active internal bleeding, recent trauma with possible internal injuries, visceral or intracranial malignancy, ulcerative colitis, diverticulitis, severe hypertension, acute or chronic hepatic or renal insufficiency, uncontrolled hypocoagulation, chronic pulmonary disease with cavitation, subacute bacterial endocarditis or rheumatic valvular disease, recent cerebral embolism, thrombosis, or hemorrhage, and diabetic hemorrhagic retinopathy, because excessive bleeding may occur.

Epsilon-aminocaproic acid inhibits the activator-mediated formation of plasmin and hence may be used as an antidote to streptokinase–urokinase, or in a defibrination syndrome when bleeding from a mucus membrane occurs (Figure 35).

STREPTOMYCIN SULFATE

Streptomycin, an aminoglycoside antibiotic (1 g IM q 12 hours for two weeks; then 500 mg IM q 12 hours for four weeks with penicillin), is indicated for primary and adjunctive treatment in **tuberculosis**, for enterococcal endocarditis, and for tularemia. Streptomycin and penicillin produce a synergistic bactericidal effect against strains of enterococci, group D streptococci, and the various oral streptococci of the viridans group.

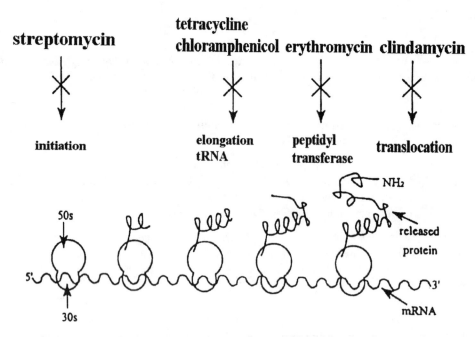

PROTEIN SYNTHESIS IN GRAM-POSITIVE BACTERIA

FIGURE 80   Streptomycin and other aminoglycosides are bactericidal and **inhibit protein synthesis** in susceptible microorganisms. They exert this effect by (1) interfering with the initiation complex of peptide formation, (2) inducing misreading of the code on the messenger RNA template, which causes the incorporation of inappropriate amino acid into peptide, and (3) rupturing the polysomes into monosomes, which become nonfunctional. (Adapted from Ebadi, M., *Pharmacology, An Illustrated Review with Questions and Answers*, 3rd Edition, Lippincott-Raven Press, Philadelphia, 1996.)

However, gentamicin has almost entirely replaced streptomycin for treatment of endocarditis caused by these microorganisms. Penicillin G alone is ineffective in the therapy of enterococcal endocarditis, and either streptomycin (500 mg twice daily) or gentamicin (1 mg/kg three times daily) must also be given to ensure cure. Gentamicin is preferred when the strain is resistant to streptomycin. Both penicillin G and the aminoglycoside are administered for 4 to 6 weeks.

Aminoglycosides are bactericidal and **inhibit protein synthesis** in susceptible microorganisms (see Figure 80). They exert this effect by (1) interfering with the initiation complex of peptide formation, (2) inducing misreading of the code on the messenger RNA template, which causes the incorporation of inappropriate amino acid into peptide, and (3) rupturing the polysomes into monosomes, which become nonfunctional (see Figure 80).

Resistance to aminoglycosides may be due to one or a combination of the following mechanisms:

Interference with the transport of aminoglycoside into bacterial cells.
Deletion of receptors on the 30S ribosomal subunit, thus preventing the functioning of aminoglycosides.
The bacterial biotransformation of aminoglycosides to inactive forms.

In addition, because the initial transport of aminoglycosides into bacterial cells is an **oxygen-dependent process**, microorganisms that are able to grow under **anaerobic conditions** show or develop resistance.

The aminoglycosides are poorly absorbed from the gastrointestinal tract, and, for this reason, they are administered intramuscularly. Furthermore, since they do not penetrate into the central nervous system, they may have to be given intrathecally or intraventricularly in the treatment of meningitis. Aminoglycosides are excreted by glomerular filtration, which is greatly reduced in the presence of renal impairment, thus leading to toxic blood levels.

The most serious toxic reactions following aminoglycoside therapy are cochlear damage and vestibular impairment, which lead to vertigo and disturb the ability to maintain postural equilibrium. Aminoglycosides given during pregnancy cause deafness in the newborn. Nephrotoxicity and reversible neuromuscular blockade causing respiratory paralysis have also been seen following the use of high doses.

STREPTOZOCIN
(Zanosar)

Streptozocin, a naturally occurring nitrosourea antibiotic derived from *Streptomyces acromogenes* (500 mg/m^2 IV for 5 consecutive days q 4 to 6 weeks until maximum benefit or toxicity is observed), is indicated for metastatic islet cell carcinoma of the pancreas. Streptozocin is nephrotoxic causing azotemia, glycosuria and renal tubular acidosis, and mild proteinuria.

Streptozocin exerts its cytotoxic activity by selectively inhibiting DNA synthesis. The drug also causes crosslinking of DNA strands through an alkylation mechanism.

Streptozocin is not active orally; it must be given intravenously.

After an IV dose, streptozocin and its metabolites distribute mainly into the liver, kidneys, intestines, and pancreas. The drug has not been shown to cross the blood-brain barrier; however, its metabolites achieve concentrations in the cerebrospinal fluid equivalent to the concentration in the plasma.

Streptozocin is extensively metabolized in the liver and kidneys.

The elimination of streptozocin from the plasma is biphasic, with an initial half-life of 35 to 40 minutes. The plasma half-life of the metabolites is longer than that of the parent drug. The drug and its metabolites are excreted primarily in urine. A small amount of a dose may also be excreted in expired air.

When used concomitantly, other nephrotoxic drugs may potentiate the nephrotoxicity caused by streptozocin. Concomitant use with doxorubicin prolongs the elimination half-life of doxorubicin and requires a reduced dosage of doxorubicin. Concurrent use with phenytoin may decrease the effects of streptozocin on the pancreas.

Toxicity of streptozocin includes nausea, which is a frequent side effect. Renal or hepatic toxicity occurs in approximately two thirds of cases; although usually reversible, renal toxicity may be fatal, and proximal tubular damage is the most important toxic effect. Serial determinations of urinary protein are most valuable in detecting early renal effects. Hematological toxicity — anemia, leukopenia, or thrombocytopenia — occurs in 20% of patients.

STRONTIUM-89 CHLORIDE
(Metastron)

Strontium-89, a radioisotope, is used in the relief of metastatic bone pain.

STRYCHNINE

Strychnine, a neurotoxin, is the chief alkaloid present in *nux vomica,* which is derived from special species of *Strychnos*, particularly *Strychnos nux vomica* and *Strychnos ignatia*. Strychnine is found chiefly in the seeds of these plants, accompanied usually by **brucine**. Strychnine poisoning causes muscular stiffness, increased reflex reactions, tremors, involuntary twitches, sudden convulsions, and opisthotonus (see Figure 81).

STUTTERING: TREATMENT OF

Stuttering is increasingly being recognized as a neurodevelopmental disorder. This has stimulated new interest in pharmacological approaches to the treatment of the condition. Psychosocial factors are also regarded as important to the course of the condition. Therefore, psychosocial interventions, such as psychotherapy and speech retraining, are important components of a comprehensive treatment program. A wide range of pharmacological agents are effective in reducing stuttering in selected patients. These include haloperidol, verapamil, bethanechol and some antidepressants. The agents are presumed to work through different mechanisms. Unilateral injection of botulinum toxin directly into the vocal folds is another promising treatment.

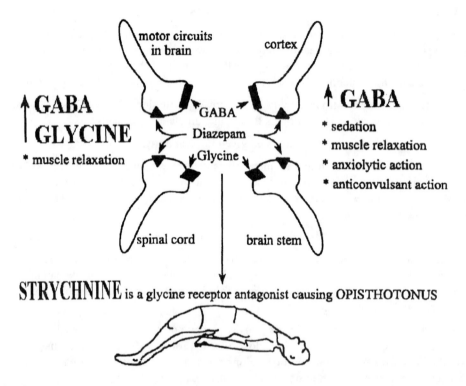

FIGURE 81 Strychnine is the chief alkaloid present in *nux vomica*. In cases of poisoning, it causes convulsions which are accompanied by strong contraction of the face muscles. The respiratory muscles are involved in the general paroxysm and the blood rapidly becomes deoxygenated. (Adapted from Ebadi, M., *Pharmacology, An Illustrated Review with Questions and Answers*, 3rd Edition, Lippincott-Raven Press, Philadelphia, 1996.)

SUCCIMER

(Chemet)

Succimer, a heavy metal chelating agent, is used in the treatment of lead poisoning in children with blood levels about 45 mcg/dl.

SUCCINYLCHOLINE CHLORIDE, SUXAMETHONIUM CHLORIDE

(Anectine, Anectine Flo-Pack, Quelicin, Sucostrin)

Succinylcholine, a depolarizing neuromuscular blocking agent (0.3 to 1.1 mg/kg IV over 10 to 30 seconds), is used to induce skeletal muscle relaxation; to facilitate intubation, ventilation, or orthopedic manipulations; and to lessen muscular contraction in convulsions induced by physicians. A peripheral nerve stimulator may be used to monitor effects and degree of blockade.

Succinylcholine, like **acetylcholine**, interacts with the cholinergic receptors at the end-plate region of the muscle, resulting in depolarization of the chemically excitable membrane. This, in turn, creates local **action potentials**, spreading them to and depolarizing the adjacent excitable membranes, finally culminating in a **muscle contraction**, or **fasciculation**, which is an uncoordinated muscle contraction. However, unlike acetylcholine, succinylcholine is not metabolized by acetylcholinesterase, and hence causes persistent depolarization of the end plate. The continuous presence of succinylcholine leads to inexcitability of the membrane adjacent to the end plate, resulting in neuromuscular blockade, which is not reversed by the administration of cholinesterase inhibitors. In fact, agents such as **neostigmine** may even prolong neuromuscular blockade.

Agents such as **tubocurarine** and **pancuronium** compete with acetylcholine for the cholinergic receptors at the end plate. They combine with the receptors but do not activate them. Competitive or nondepolarizing agents are antagonized by neostigmine (see also Figure 92).

Succinylcholine is an ultra short-acting depolarizing skeletal muscle relaxant. Paralysis usually appears in the following muscles consecutively: levator muscles of the eyelids, muscles of mastication, limb muscles, abdominal muscles, muscles of the glottis, and finally, the intercostals, the diaphragm, and all other skeletal muscles. Recovery of normal muscle tone follows the reverse order.

Succinylcholine has no effect on consciousness, pain threshold, or cerebration. While it has no direct effect upon the myocardium, changes in rhythm may result from vagal stimulation resulting from surgical procedures, or from potassium-mediated alterations in electrical conductivity. These effects are enhanced by halogenated anesthetics. Succinylcholine slightly increases intraocular pressure, which may persist after the onset of complete paralysis. Tachyphylaxis occurs with repeated doses. It has no direct effect on the uterus or other smooth muscles. Because the drug is highly ionized and has a low lipid solubility, it does not readily cross the placenta.

Succinylcholine is metabolized according to the following scheme:

$$\text{Succinylcholine} \xrightarrow{\text{Plasma cholinesterase}} \text{Succinylmonocholine}$$

$$\text{Succinylmonocholine} \xrightarrow[\text{Liver}]{} \text{Succinate and choline}$$

Because cholinesterase is synthesized in the liver, succinylcholine's duration of action is elevated in the presence of liver disease. Cholinesterase inhibitors dramatically increase succinylcholine's duration of action. In patients with **atypical cholinesterase**, the intensity and duration of succinylcholine's effects are enhanced.

Succinylcholine is contraindicated in patients with genetic disorders of plasma pseudocholinesterase because of the potential for impaired metabolism; in patients with personal or family history of malignant hyperthermia because the drug may induce the disorder; with myopathies associated with elevated serum creatine kinase values because the drug may exacerbate the damage associated with the disease; and in patients with narrow-angle glaucoma or penetrating eye injuries because the drug elevates intraocular pressure.

Succinylcholine should be used with extreme caution in patients with low plasma pseudocholinesterase and in those recovering from severe trauma. It also should be used with caution in patients with electrolyte imbalances; in those receiving quinidine or cardiac glycosides, in patients with preexisting hyperkalemia, paraplegia, extensive or severe burns, or extensive denervation of skeletal muscle from disease because the drug may raise potassium levels; and during ocular surgery, because the drug increases intraocular pressure.

Concomitant use of succinylcholine with aminoglycoside antibiotics (including amikacin, gentamicin, kanamycin, neomycin, streptomycin), polymyxin antibiotics (polymyxin B sulfate, colistin), clindamycin, lincomycin, general anesthetics, local anesthetics, antimalarial agents, cholinesterase inhibitors (echothiophate, demecarium, isoflurophate), cyclophosphamide, oral contraceptives, nondepolarizing neuromuscular blocking agents, parenteral magnesium salts, lithium, phenelzine, hexafluorenium, quinidine, quinine, pancuronium, phenothiazines, thiotepa, and exposure to neurotoxic insecticides enhance or prolong succinylcholine's neuromuscular blocking effects.

Clinical manifestations of overdose include apnea or prolonged muscle paralysis, which may be treated with controlled respiration.

SUCRALFATE
(Carafate)

Sucralfate, a pepsin inhibitor with antiulcer effects, is used for short-term (up to 8 weeks) treatment of duodenal ulcer, and for maintenance therapy of duodenal ulcer.

SUFENTANIL CITRATE
(Sufenta)

Sufentanil, an opioid analgesic (8 mcg/kg IV administered with nitrous oxide and oxygen), is indicated in patients undergoing major surgical procedures, such as cardiovascular surgery or neurosurgical procedures in the sitting position, in order to provide favorable myocardial and cerebral oxygen balance or when extended postoperative ventilation is anticipated.

Alfentanil and sufentanil are newer and more potent opioid analgesics than either morphine or fentanyl. The potency of alfentanil (Alfenta) is one third to one fourth that of fentanyl, and its duration of action is about one-half as long, even after administration of large doses. These drugs can induce profound analgesia and, in sufficient doses, anesthesia; cardiovascular stability is impressive, and the desirability of reducing the duration of mechanical ventilation following cardiac surgery has led to an increasing use of these agents. All may be associated with increased intracranial pressure during spontaneous ventilation, so caution is necessary with head trauma. **Remifentanil** is a potent opioid selective for opioid receptors that produces intense analgesia very rapidly. It shares with other opioids respiratory depression, bradycardia, skeletal muscle rigidity, and reversibility by **naloxone**. In contrast to other short-acting opioids, remifentanil contains an ester linkage, and so it is metabolized by circulating and tissue-nonspecific esterases. As a result, recovery time from remifentanil is rapid and almost independent of dose or duration of infusion (see also Figure 58).

Sufentanil is contraindicated in patients with known hypersensitivity to phenylpiperidine opiates including alfentanil, diphenoxylate, fentanyl, or meperidine.

Sufentanil should be administered carefully to patients with supraventricular arrhythmias, recent head injuries or increased intracranial pressure, or pulmonary disease such as asthma.

Concomitant use with other CNS depressants (narcotic analgesics, general anesthetics, antihistamines, phenothiazines, barbiturates, benzodiazepines, sedative-hypnotics, tricyclic antidepressants, alcohol, and muscle relaxants) potentiates respiratory and CNS depression, sedation, and hypotensive effects.

SUICIDE: PREVENTION OF

The assessment and management of suicidal patients are important issues that may be faced by any physician. Risk factors for suicidal behavior which have been identified are:

- Psychiatric diagnosis
- Psychosocial and environmental factors
- Personality disorders and traits
- Genetic and family variables
- Biochemical factors

Psychopharmacological agents such as antidepressants, antipsychotics (in patients with personality disorders) and lithium (in patients with bipolar disorders) have been shown to be effective in preventing suicidal behavior. The efficacy of electroconvulsive therapy (ECT) is more controversial. Another equally important aspect of the optimal clinical management of suicidal patients is the quality of the doctor–patient relationship.

SULCONAZOLE NITRATE
(Exelderm)

Sulconazole, an imidazole derivative with antifungal effectiveness, is used in the treatment of tinea cruris, tinea corporis, and tinea pedis caused by *Trichophyton mentagrophytes, Epidermophyton floccosum,* and *Microsporum canis.* It is also used for treatment of tinea versicolor caused by *Malassezia furfur.*

SULFACETAMIDE SODIUM
(Ak-Sulf Forte, Ak-Sulf Ointment, Bleph-10 S.O.P., Cetamide, Isopto Cetamide, Sodium Sulamyd 10%, Sodium Sulamyd 30%, Sulamyd, Sulf-10, Sulfair 15, Sulten-10)

Sulfacetamide, a sulfonamide antibiotic (instill 1 to 2 drops of 10% solution into lower conjunctival sac), is used in inclusion conjunctivitis, corneal ulcers, trachoma, and prophylaxis for ocular infection.

SULFADIAZINE
(Microsulfon)

Sulfadiazine, a sulfonamide antibiotic, is used in rheumatic fever prophylaxis, as an alternative to penicillin, as an adjunctive regimen in treatment of toxoplasmosis, and in uncomplicated attacks of malaria (see also Figure 82).

SULFADOXINE AND PYRIMETHAMINE
(Fansidar)

Sulfadoxine (1500 mg) and pyrimethamine (75 mg) orally as a single dosage is indicated for the treatment of *Plasmodium falciparum* malaria in patients in whom chloroquine resistance is suspected. However, chloroquine remains the drug of choice for travelers to malarious areas. In addition, sulfadoxine-pyrimethamine has been used as a prophylactic agent for the prevention of *Pneumocystis carinii* pneumonia in patients with AIDS, usually as a second-line agent.

Sulfadoxine/pyrimethamine is an antimalarial agent which acts by reciprocal potentiation of its components, achieved by a sequential blockade of two enzymes involved in the biosynthesis

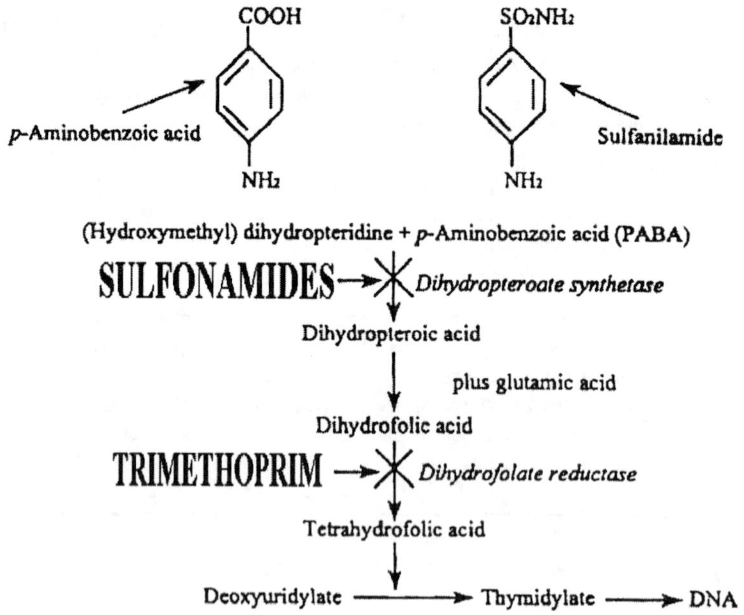

COOH

p-Aminobenzoic acid

NH₂

SO₂NH₂

Sulfanilamide

NH₂

(Hydroxymethyl) dihydropteridine + *p*-Aminobenzoic acid (PABA)

SULFONAMIDES ⟶✕ *Dihydropteroate synthetase*

Dihydropteroic acid

plus glutamic acid

Dihydrofolic acid

TRIMETHOPRIM ⟶✕ *Dihydrofolate reductase*

Tetrahydrofolic acid

Deoxyuridylate ⟶ Thymidylate ⟶ DNA

FIGURE 82   In acute and chronic urinary tract infection, the combination of **trimethoprim** and **sulfamethoxazole** exerts a truly synergistic effect on bacteria. The sulfonamide inhibits the utilization of **p-amino-benzoic acid** in the synthesis of folic acid, while trimethoprim, by inhibiting dihydrofolic acid reductase, blocks the conversion of dihydrofolic acid to **tetrahydrofolic acid**, which is essential to bacteria in the *de novo* synthesis of purines, pyrimidines, and certain amino acids. (Adapted from Ebadi, M., *Pharmacology, An Illustrated Review with Questions and Answers*, 3rd Edition, Lippincott-Raven Press, Philadelphia, 1996.)

of folinic acid within the parasites (see Figure 82). The bacteriostatic action of sulfonamides occurs through competitive antagonism of para-aminobenzoic acid, an essential component in folic acid synthesis. Pyrimethamine inhibits the enzyme dihydrofolate reductase, which catalyzes the reduction of dihydrofolate to tetrahydrofolate and is important to cellular biosynthesis of purines, pyrimidines, and some amino acids.

Antifolic acid medications such as **methotrexate** should not be used in patients receiving sulfadoxine and pyrimethamine. The adverse reactions reported in susceptible patients taking sulfadoxine and pyrimethamine are headache, peripheral neuritis, mental depression, convulsions, ataxia, hallucinations, tinnitus, vertigo, insomnia, apathy, fatigue, muscle weakness, nervousness, glossitis, stomatitis, nausea, emesis, abdominal pains, hepatitis, hepatocellular necrosis, diarrhea, pancreatitis, agranulocytosis, aplastic, megaloblastic, or hemolytic anemia, thrombocytopenia, leukopenia, eosinophilia, purpura, hypoprothrombinemia, and methemoglobulinemia.

SULFAMETHOXAZOLE

(Gantanol)

Sulfamethoxazole (initially 2 g p.o.) is indicated for urinary tract and systemic infections, and for lymphogranuloma venereum (genital, inguinal, or anorectal infection) (1 g p.o. b.i.d. for 21 days).

Sulfamethoxazole like other sulfonamides is bacteriostatic. It acts by inhibiting formation of tetrahydrofolic acid from para-aminobenzoic acid (PABA), thus preventing bacterial cell synthesis of folic acid (see Figure 82).

Sulfamethoxazole's spectrum of action includes some Gram-positive bacteria: *Chlamydia trachomatis*, many Enterobacteriaceae, and some strains of *Toxoplasma* and *Plasmodium*.

Sulfamethoxazole is absorbed from the GI tract after oral administration, and is metabolized partially in the liver; peak serum levels occur at 3 to 4 hours.

Sulfamethoxazole is distributed widely into most body tissues and fluids, including cerebrospinal, synovial, pleural, amniotic, prostatic, peritoneal, and seminal fluids. Sulfamethoxazole crosses the placenta; it is 50 to 70% protein-bound.

Both unchanged drug and metabolites are excreted primarily in urine by glomerular filtration and, to a lesser extent, renal tubular secretion; some drug is excreted in breast milk. Urinary solubility of unchanged drug increases as urine pH increases. Plasma half-life in patients with normal renal function is 7 to 12 hours.

Sulfamethoxazole may inhibit hepatic metabolism of oral anticoagulants, displacing them from binding sites and enhancing anticoagulant effects. Concomitant use with PABA antagonizes sulfonamide effects. With oral hypoglycemics (sulfonylureas), the drug enhances their hypoglycemic effects, probably by displacing sulfonylureas from protein-binding sites; and with either trimethoprim or pyrimethamine (folic acid antagonists with different mechanisms of action), the drug results in synergistic antibacterial effects and delays or prevents bacterial resistance.

The sulfonamides are structurally related to **p-aminobenzoic acid**. The presence of a free **p-amino group** is essential for the antibacterial action. Succinylsulfathiazole (sulfasuxidine) and phthalysulfathiazole (sulfathalidine) are agents with a substituted p-amino group. These intestinal antiseptics are slowly hydrolyzed in the intestine, releasing **sulfathiazole**, which exerts antiseptic effects against the coliform and clostridial organisms (see Figure 82).

SULFASALAZINE
(Azulfidine, Azulfidine En-tabs)

Sulfasalazine, a sulfonamide antibiotic (3 to 4 g p.o. daily in divided dosage), is indicated in the treatment of ulcerative colitis.

Sulfasalazine is cleaved in the colon by intestinal bacteria to form **sulfapyridine** and **mesalamine** (5-aminosalicylic acid; 5-ASA), both of which may act locally within the gut. Mesalamine, which is different from aminosalicylates used to treat tuberculosis, is thought to be the major active moiety. Mucosal production of arachidonic acid metabolites, both through the cyclooxygenase and the lipoxygenase pathways, is increased in patients with inflammatory bowel disease. Mesalamine appears to diminish inflammation by inhibiting cyclooxygenase and lipoxygenase, thereby decreasing the production of prostaglandins, and leukotrienes and hydroxyeicosatetraenoic acids (HETEs), respectively. It is also believed that mesalamine acts as a scavenger of oxygen-derived free radicals, which are produced in greater numbers in patients with inflammatory bowel disease.

Sulfasalazine is absorbed poorly from the GI tract after oral administration: 70 to 90% is transported to the colon where intestinal flora metabolize the drug to its active ingredients, sulfapyridine (antibacterial) and 5-aminosalicylic acid (antiinflammatory), which exert their effects locally. Sulfapyridine is absorbed from the colon, but only a small portion of 5-aminosalicylic acid is absorbed.

Systemically absorbed sulfasalazine is excreted chiefly in urine; some parent drug and metabolites are excreted in breast milk. Plasma half-life is about 6 to 8 hours.

Like all sulfonamides, sulfasalazine is contraindicated in patients with known hypersensitivity to other drugs containing sulfur (thiazides, furosemide, or oral sulfonylureas), in patients with known hypersensitivity to salicylates, in patients with severe renal or hepatic dysfunction,

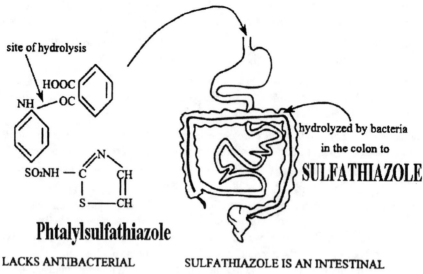

site of hydrolysis

Phtalylsulfathiazole

LACKS ANTIBACTERIAL
ACTIVITY IN VITRO

hydrolyzed by bacteria

in the colon to

SULFATHIAZOLE

SULFATHIAZOLE IS AN INTESTINAL
ANTISEPTIC WITHOUT BEING ABSORBED

FIGURE 83 Sulfonamides that are **poorly absorbed** include succinylsulfathiazole, phthalylsulfathi-azole, and sulfasalazine and are used as **intestinal antiseptics**.

or porphyria, during pregnancy, and during lactation, and in infants and children under age 2. Sulfasalazine is also contraindicated in patients with intestinal or urinary tract obstructions because of the risk of local GI irritation and of crystalluria.

Sulfasalazine may inhibit hepatic metabolism of oral anticoagulants, displacing them from binding sites and enhancing anticoagulant effects.

Concomitant use with oral hypoglycemics (sulfonylureas) enhances hypoglycemic effects, probably by displacing sulfonylureas from protein-binding sites.

Sulfasalazine may reduce GI absorption of digoxin and folic acid.

Concomitant use of urine acidifying agents (ammonium chloride, ascorbic acid) decreases urine pH and sulfonamide solubility, thus increasing risk of crystalluria. Concomitant use with antibiotics that alter intestinal flora may interfere with conversion of sulfasalazine to sulfapyridine and 5-aminosalicylic acid, decreasing its effectiveness.

Concomitant use of antacids may cause premature dissolution of enteric-coated tablets designed to dissolve in the intestines, thus increasing systemic absorption and hazard of toxicity.

SULFINPYRAZONE

(Anturane)

Sulfinpyrazone (200 to 400 mg daily in two divided doses) is indicated in the treatment of chronic and intermittent gouty arthritis (see also Table 2).

Sulfinpyrazone, a pyrazolidine derivative, is a potent uricosuric agent which also has anti-thrombotic and platelet inhibitory effects (see Figure 84). It lacks antiinflammatory and analgesic properties. Sulfinpyrazone inhibits renal tubular reabsorption of uric acid. It reduces renal tubular secretion of other organic anions, e.g., paraaminohippuric acid and salicylic

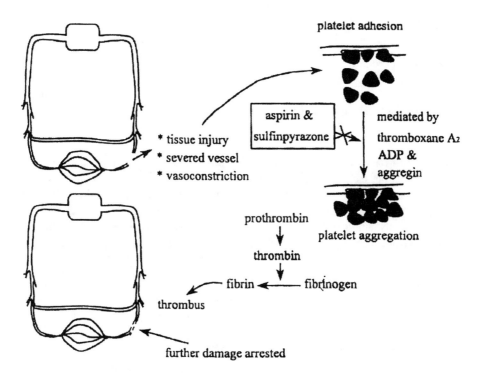

FIGURE 84   As an inhibitor of platelet aggregation, sulfinpyrazone is used in the prophylaxis of thromboembolic disorders.

acid, and displaces other organic anions bound extensively to plasma proteins (e.g., sulfona-mides, salicylates). It is not intended for the relief of an acute attack of gout.

Sulfinpyrazone competitively inhibits prostaglandin synthesis which prevents platelet aggre-gation (Figure 84). It is well absorbed after oral administration; 98 to 99% is bound to plasma proteins. The plasma half-life is about 2.2 to 3 hours. Approximately one half of the admin-istered oral dose appears in the urine unchanged.

Gastrointestinal irritation occurs in 10 to 15% of all patients receiving sulfinpyrazone, and occasionally a patient may require discontinuance of its use. Gastric distress is lessened when the drug is taken in divided doses with meals. Sulfinpyrazone should be given cautiously to patients with a history of peptic ulcer. Hypersensitivity reactions, usually a rash with fever, do occur, but less frequently than with probenecid. The severe blood dyscrasias and salt and water retention, hazards of phenylbutazone therapy, have not been observed during sulfin-pyrazone therapy. However, depression of hematopoiesis has been demonstrated, and periodic blood-cell counts should be examined during prolonged therapy.

Because it is a potent uricosuric agent, sulfinpyrazone may precipitate acute gouty arthritis, urolithiasis, and renal colic, especially in initial stages of therapy. Therefore, adequate fluid intake and alkalinization of the urine are recommended.

Sulfinpyrazone increases the effectiveness of anticoagulants (with a potential to cause hem-orrhage) and of tolbutamide (with a potential to cause hypoglycemia). It increases the plasma clearance of theophylline and verapamil, hence decreasing their effectiveness.

SULFISOXAZOLE

(Gantrisin)

SULFISOXAZOLE DIOLAMINE

(Gantrisin Ophthalmic Ointment, Gantrisin Ophthalmic Solution)

Sulfisoxazole is used in urinary tract and systemic infections; in lymphogranuloma venereum (genital, inguinal, or anorectal infections); in uncomplicated urethral, endocervical, or rectal infections caused by *C. trachomatis*; in conjunctivitis, corneal ulcer, superficial ocular infections; and as an adjunct in systemic treatment of trachoma.

SULFONAMIDES

The **sulfonamides** are structurally related to **p-aminobenzoic acid**. Substances that resemble the sulfonamides but lack antibacterial activities are some of the **oral hypoglycemic agents (tolbutamide)** and some of the **carbonic anhydrase inhibitors (acetazolamide)**. The presence of a free **p-amino group** is essential for the antibacterial action. Succinylsulfathiazole (Sulfasuxide) and phthalylsulfathiazole (Sulfathalidine) are agents with a substituted p-amino group. These intestinal antiseptics are slowly hydrolyzed in the intestine, releasing sulfathiazole, which exerts antiseptic effects against the coliform and clostridial organisms (see Figure 83).

As bacteriostatic agents, the sulfonamides are active against both Gram-positive and Gram-negative bacteria, including streptococci, Gram-negative bacilli, *Chlamydia, Nocardia,* and *Actinomyces.* Sulfonamides alone or in combination with trimethoprim are the drugs of choice in the management of urinary tract infections, nocardiosis, and toxoplasmosis (see Figure 82). Sulfonamides are also used topically in the treatment of burns.

By competing with p-aminobenzoic acid (PABA), the sulfonamides inhibit the synthesis of folic acid, which is essential for the production of purines by bacteria and their ultimate synthesis of nucleic acids. They are also incorporated into folic acid.

The widespread use of sulfonamides against gonococci, meningococci, hemolytic streptococci, and coliform organisms has resulted in the emergence of resistant strains. In general, organisms that are either impermeable to sulfonamides or produce large amounts of p-aminobenzoic acid are resistant to sulfonamides. Furthermore, resistance in a previously sensitive organism may arise as a result of **mutation** and cause either **overproduction of p-aminobenzoic acid** or an alteration in the **folic acid-synthesizing enzymes.**

Except for those sulfonamides that exert their local effects in the bowel, most sulfonamides are absorbed orally, become bound to plasma proteins, are distributed widely throughout the body including the cerebrospinal fluid, pass readily through the placenta to reach the fetal circulation, and become metabolized in the liver by acetylation. The acetylated metabolites, which have no bacteriostatic activity, retain the toxic property of the parent compounds. The **free sulfonamides** undergo glomerular filtration and are not readily absorbed and excreted. The urinary concentration of acetylated derivatives is higher than the plasma level. The **urinary solubility** of the sulfonamides decreases when the pH of the urine decreases. Therefore, there is a tendency for crystalluria to increase in the presence of acidic pHs. Conversely, the solubility of the sulfonamides increases greatly when the pH is alkaline. The recently introduced sulfonamides are more soluble at the usual urinary pH. The incidence of crystalluria can be diminished by the following measures: enhancing fluid intake, alkalization of the urine, and taking a mixture of sulfonamides.

Based on their pharmacokinetic characteristics, the sulfonamides can be classified into four separate categories:

1. Sulfonamides with a **rapid rate of absorption and elimination**. These consist of sulfisoxazole (Gantrisin), sulfamethoxazole (Gantanol), sulfacytine (Renoquid), and sulfamethiazole (Thiosulfil). The highly soluble and recently introduced sulfonamides

have shown excellent antibacterial activity and lack, or show a minimal, renal toxicity, which is a problem with the older sulfonamides. In addition, sulfisoxazole acetyl is tasteless and hence is preferred for oral use in children.

2. Sulfonamides with a **rapid rate of absorption but a slow rate of elimination**. These relatively toxic agents, which are no longer used in the United States, include sulfamethoxypyridazine and sulfadimethoxine.

3. Sulfonamides that are **poorly absorbed**. These agents include: succinylsulfathiazole (Sulfasuxide), phthalylsulfathiazole (Sulfathalidine), and sulfasalazine (Azulfidine); they are used as intestinal antiseptics. Sulfasalazine is used especially in the therapy of regional enteritis and ulcerative colitis.

4. Sulfonamides that are used **topically**. These consist of sulfacetamide (Sulamyd and Isopto Cetamide), which is used in ophthalmic infections, and sulfamylon (Mafenide) and silver sulfadiazine (Silvadene), which are used in infections associated with burns.

Many of the adverse reactions seen with sulfonamides are due to **hypersensitivity reactions**, which include dermatitis, leukopenia, hemolytic anemia, and drug fever. **Stevens-Johnson syndrome** is a very severe, but rare hypersensitivity reaction that occurs only with some of the long-acting sulfonamide preparations.

Renal lesions may be due to the precipitation of sulfonamides and their acetyl derivatives in the urinary tract. **Renal damage** may also be attributable to a direct toxic effect of sulfonamides on the kidney tubules.

Sulfonamides may also cause **jaundice** and **kernicterus** in newborns. This is due to the displacement of bilirubin from protein-binding sites. Therefore, sulfonamides should not be used during pregnancy.

The combination of trimethoprim and sulfamethoxazole (usually five parts sulfamethoxazole to one part trimethoprim) interferes with the **synthesis of active folic acid** by means of two separate reactions. In the first, sulfonamides compete with p-aminobenzoic acid and prevent its conversion to dihydrofolic acid. In the second, trimethoprim, by inhibiting the activity of **dihydrofolic acid reductase**, prevents the conversion of dihydrofolic acid into tetrahydrofolic acid, which is necessary for the synthesis of DNA. These reactions are summarized in Figure 82.

These drug combinations have the following **therapeutic advantages**:

They cause synergistic antibacterial effects.
They have bactericidal activity.
The emergence of bacterial resistance is decreased.
The spectrum of antibacterial activity is enhanced.
Toxicity is reduced.

Folic acid deficiency may occur either following prolonged usage of **methotrexate** or in patients with preexisting folic acid deficiency. **Folinic acid** may be administered to overcome the folic-acid deficiency-related megaloblastic anemia.

Orally administered trimethoprim is used in the treatment of chronic recurring urinary tract infection. Oral forms of trimethoprim-sulfamethoxazole are used in *Shigella* and some *Salmonella* infections, particularly when they are resistant to ampicillin and chloramphenicol. High doses of oral trimethoprim-sulfamethoxazole are used in *Pneumocystis* pneumonia. This combination, along with polymyxin, has been shown to be effective in treating sepsis caused by *Serratia* or *Pseudomonas* organisms.

Intravenously administered trimethoprim-sulfamethoxazole is indicated in severe cases of *Pneumocystis carinii* pneumonia, Gram-negative bacterial sepsis, and shigellosis.

Oral trimethoprim in combination with sulfonamide has been used in the treatment of leishmaniasis, toxoplasmosis, and falciparum malaria.

SULFONAMIDES	
Sulfacetamide	Sulfamethoxine
Sulfadiazine	Sulfamethoxypyrazine
Sulfaguanidine	Sulfamethoxypyridazine
Sulfamerazine	Sulfanilamide
Sulfamethazine	Sulfisomidine
Sulfamethizole	Sulfisoxazole
Sulfamethoxazole	Sulformethoxine

SULFONES

Agents such as primaquine destroy exoerythrocytic tissue schizonts such as those developing in the liver.

Other pharmacologic agents are sometimes used in combination with the antimalarial agents for greater effect. These include:

Sulfonamides — Sulfadoxine or sulfadiazine is used with pyrimethamine.
Sulfones — Dapsone (DDS) is used in place of or in addition to the sulfonamides and pyrimethamine.
Acridines — Quinacrine (Atabrine) has an action similar to chloroquine's.
Biguanides — Chlorguanide (Proguanil and Paludrine) has suppressive as well as prophylactic actions.

SULFONYLUREAS

Oral hypoglycemic agents have advantages over insulin, because, by releasing insulin and by decreasing the release of glucagon, they mimic physiologic processes and cause fewer allergic reactions. Furthermore, they are effective in an oral form, thus eliminating the need for daily injections. The properties of these agents are described in Table 1.

The mechanisms that underlie the hypoglycemic actions of **sulfonylureas** are:

Pancreatic
  Improved insulin secretion
  Reduced glucagon secretion
Extrapancreatic
  Improved tissue sensitivity to insulin
  Direct
    Increased receptor binding
    Improved post-binding action
  Indirect
    Reduced hyperglycemia
    Decreased plasma free fatty-acid concentrations
    Reduced hepatic insulin extraction

Sulfonylureas such as **glyburide** and **glipizide** bind to sulfonylurea receptors located on the surface of beta cells and trigger insulin releases at nanomolar concentrations (Figure 44). Sulfonylureas bind to ATP-sensitive potassium channels and inhibit potassium efflux through these channels. The inhibition of ATP-sensitive potassium channels then leads to depolarization of the beta cell.

SULFOXONE SODIUM

Leprosy (Hansen's disease) is a chronic granulomatous disease that attacks superficial tissues such as the skin, nasal mucosa, and peripheral nerves. There are two types of leprosy: **lepromatous** and **tuberculoid**. The **sulfones**, which are derivatives of 4,4'-diamino-diphenylsulfone, are bacteriostatic. **Dapsone** (DDS) and **sulfoxone** sodium are the most useful and effective agents currently available. They should be given in low doses initially, and then the dosage should be gradually increased until a full dose of 300 to 400 mg per week is reached. During this period, the patient must be monitored carefully. With adequate precautions and appropriate doses, sulfones may be used safely for years. Nevertheless, side effects such as anorexia, nervousness, insomnia, blurred vision, paresthesia, and peripheral neuropathy do occur. **Hemolysis** is common, especially in patients with glucose 6-phosphate dehydrogenase deficiency. A fatal exacerbation of lepromatous leprosy and an infectious mononucleosis-like syndrome rarely occur. **Clofazimine** (Lamprene) may be effective in patients who show resistance to the sulfones and may also dramatically reduce an exacerbation of leprosy. Red discoloration of the skin and eosinophilic enteritis have occurred following clofazime therapy.

Not all mycobacterial infections are caused by *Mycobacterium tuberculosis* or *Mycobacterium leprae*. These atypical mycobacteria require treatment with secondary medications as well as other chemotherapeutic agents. For example, *Mycobacterium maninum* causes skin granulomas, and effective drugs in the treatment of such infections are **rifampin** or **minocycline.** *Mycobacterium fortuitum* cause skin ulcers, and the medications recommended for treatment are **ethambutol, cycloserine,** and **rifampin** in combination with **amikacin.**

SULINDAC

(Clinoril)

Sulindac, a nonsteroidal antiinflammatory agent, is used in osteoarthritis, rheumatoid arthritis, ankylosing spondylitis, acute subacromial bursitis or supraspinatus tendinitis, and acute gouty arthritis (see also Table 2).

SUMATRIPTAN SUCCINATE

(Imitrex)

Sumatriptan, a selective serotonin (5-HT_1) receptor agonist (6 mg SC), is used in acute migraine attack with or without aura (see Figure 85).

SURAMIN

(Naphuride)

Trypanosomiasis is produced by protozoa of the genus *Trypanosoma* and leads to Gambian or mid-African sleeping sickness (*T. gambiense*), Rhodesian or East African sleeping sickness (*T. rhodesiense*), and Chagas' disease, which is seen in the populations of Central and South America (*T. cruzi*).

Agents effective in the treatment of trypanosomiasis are the aromatic **diamidines** (pentamidine, stilbamidine, and propamidine). **Pentamidine** is the preferred drug for the prevention and early treatment of *T. gambiense* infections; however, it cannot penetrate the central nervous system. **Melarsoprol** is the drug recommended for *T. gambiense* infections that do not respond to pentamidine or for managing the late meningoencephalitic stages of infection. It does reach the central nervous system either. **Nifurtimox** (Lampit) is the drug of choice for treating the acute form of Chagas' disease. **Suramin** (Naphuride) is effective only as therapy for African sleeping sickness.

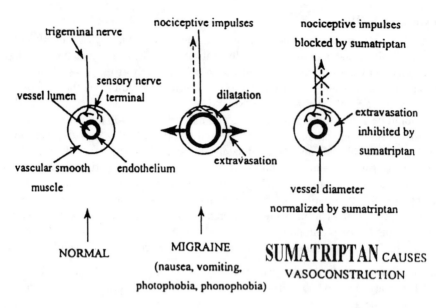

FIGURE 85   **Sumatriptan**, an agonist of the $5HT_1$-like receptor, is highly effective in the treatment of **migraine**.

SUTILAINS

(Travase)

Sutilains, a topical proteolytic enzyme, is used in debridement of major burns, decubitus ulcers, ulcers in peripheral vascular disease, and incisional, traumatic, and pyrogenic wounds.

SYPHILIS: TREATMENT OF	
Stage/type of Syphilis	**Medications**
Primary, secondary, or latent syphilis of less than 1 year's duration	Benzathine penicillin G 2.4 million units IM in a single dose
Syphilis of more than 1 year's duration (except neurosyphilis)	Benzathine penicillin G 2.4 million units IM once a week for three successive weeks
Neurosyphilis	Aqueous crystalline penicillin G 12-24 million units IV (2-4 million units every 4 hours) for 10-14 days, followed by benzathine penicillin G 2.4 million units IM weekly for three doses **or**
	Aqueous procaine penicillin G 2.4 million units IM daily plus probenecid 500 mg PO four times daily, both for 10–14 days, followed by benzathine penicillin G 2.4 million units IM weekly for three doses
Congenital syphilis	Aqueous crystalline penicillin G 50,000 units/kg IV every 8–12 hours for 10-14 days **or**
	Aqueous procaine penicillin G 50,000 U/kg IM daily for 10-14 days
Penicillin-allergic patients	
Primary, secondary, or latent syphilis of less than 1 year's duration	Doxycycline 100 mg PO two times a day for 2 weeks **or** Tetracycline 500 mg PO four times daily for 2 weeks **or** Erythromycin 500 mg PO four times daily for 2 weeks
Syphilis of more than 1 year's duration (except neurosyphilis)	Tetracycline 500 mg PO four times daily for 4 weeks **or** Doxycycline 100 mg PO two times a day for 4 weeks

SYRUP OF IPECAC

Ipecac is a mixture of the alcohol-soluble alkaloid which is obtained from the South American plant *Cephaelis ipecacuanha*, and is used solely in the form of **syrup of ipecac. Apomorphine hydrochloride** and **copper sulfate** are also emetics.

Syrup of ipecac and copper sulfate cause emesis by locally irritating the stomach, whereas apomorphine stimulates the **chemoreceptor trigger zone for emesis** located in the caudal portion of the fourth ventricle (area postrema), which in turn stimulates the vomiting center in the lateral reticular formation of the medulla (see also Figure 73).

T

TACRINE HYDROCHLORIDE
(Cognex)

Tacrine (initially 10 mg p.o. q.i.d.) is indicated in the treatment of mild to moderate dementia of the Alzheimer's type. While many neuronal systems are affected in Alzheimer's disease, the decline in central cholinergic activity is one of the most pronounced neurotransmitter deficits. Tacrine's primary effect is the reversible inhibition of cholinesterase — butyrylcholinesterase more than acetylcholinesterase. This inhibition increases the level of acetylcholine in the central nervous system. In fact, increased levels of acetylcholine have been detected in the cerebrospinal fluid of patients receiving tacrine (see also Figure 18).

Tacrine may also block potassium channels, increasing the duration of the action potential and augmenting acetylcholine release from cholinergic neurons.

In addition, tacrine may moderate cholinergic activity by acting as a partial agonist through direct binding to nicotinic receptors and, with greater affinity, to muscarine receptors.

Additionally, tacrine inhibits monoamine oxidase (MAO) — MAO-A to a greater extent than MAO-B. Tacrine may also inhibit the reuptake of norepinephrine, serotonin, and dopamine.

Because of its mechanism of action, tacrine has the potential to interfere with the activity of anticholinergic medications. A synergistic effect is expected when tacrine is given concurrently with succinylcholine, cholinesterase inhibitors, or cholinergic agonists, such as **bethanecol**. Coadministration of tacrine with **theophylline** increases theophylline elimination half-life and average plasma concentrations.

Overdosage with cholinesterase inhibitors can cause a cholinergic crisis characterized by severe nausea, vomiting, salivation, sweating, bradycardia, hypotension, and seizures. Increasing muscle weakness may occur and can result in death if respiratory muscles are involved. Tertiary anticholinergics, such as atropine, may be used as an antidote for tacrine overdosage.

TACROLIMUS
[FK506] (Prograf)

Tacrolimus, a novel macrocyclic lactone with potent immunosuppressive properties, is currently available as an intravenous formulation and as a capsule for oral use.

Tacrolimus (0.05 to 0.1 mg/kg/day) is used in organ liver rejection prophylaxis.

TAMOXIFEN CITRATE
(Nolvadex)

Tamoxifen (10 to 20 mg morning and evening) is indicated for treatment of axillary node-negative breast cancer in women following total mastectomy or segmental mastectomy, axillary dissection, and breast irradiation; for treatment of node-positive breast cancer in postmenopausal women following total mastectomy or segmental mastectomy, axillary dissection, and breast irradiation; and for the treatment of metastatic breast cancer in men and women.

In addition, tamoxifen has been used in the treatment of mastalgia (10 mg/day for 4 months) and for decreasing the size and pain of gynecomastia.

Tamoxifen is a competitive inhibitor of estradiol binding to the estrogen receptors. When bound to estrogen receptor, tamoxifen induces a change in the three-dimensional shape of the receptor, inhibiting its binding to the estrogen-responsive element on DNA. Under normal physiological conditions, estrogen stimulation increases tumor cell production of transforming growth factor beta (TGF-beta), an autocrine inhibitor of tumor cell growth. By blocking these pathways, the net effect of tamoxifen treatment is to decrease the autocrine stimulation of breast cancer growth, capturing the cell in G_1. In addition, tamoxifen decreases the local production of insulin-like growth factor 1(IGF-1) by surrounding tissues; IGF-1 is a paracrine growth factor for the breast cancer cell (see also Figure 2).

Tamoxifen is metabolized mostly to N-desmethyl tamoxifen, which is an active metabolite, and to a small extent to 4-hydroxytamoxifen. The hypoprothrombinemic effects of anticoagulants may be increased by concomitant administration of tamoxifen.

Bromocriptine may elevate serum tamoxifen and N-desmethyl tamoxifen.

Adverse reactions to tamoxifen are relatively mild and rarely require discontinuation of therapy. If adverse reactions are severe, it is sometimes possible to control severe adverse reactions by dosage reduction without losing control of the disease.

The most frequently occurring side effects of tamoxifen are hot flashes, nausea, and vomiting (up to 25%, rarely severe). The less often occurring side effects of tamoxifen are vaginal bleeding, vaginal discharge, menstrual irregularities, and skin rash.

Hypercalcemia, peripheral edema, food distaste, pruritus vulvae, depression, dizziness, lightheadedness, headache, retinopathy, thrombocytopenia, leukopenia, and hair thinning have been reported on rare occasions.

TELENZEPINE

Vagal impulses elicit the release of acetylcholine in the parietal cells and in the gastric mucosal cells containing **gastrin**, a peptide hormone. Both the directly released acetylcholine and the indirectly released gastrin then stimulate the parietal cells to secrete hydrogen ions into the gastric lumen.

The most useful anticholinergic drugs are **propantheline** (Pro-Banthine), **pirenzepine,** and **telenzepine**, which antagonize muscarinic cholinergic receptors (M_1 receptors). All three agents depress gastric motility and secretion. The production of pepsin is also reduced. Propantheline may be used as adjunctive therapy with antacids but not as a sole agent. The side effects and contraindications of propantheline use are identical to those of atropine (prostatic hypertrophy, urinary retention, glaucoma, and cardiac arrhythmias). The **timing** of medication is critical in ulcer therapy. Anticholinergic drugs should be given about 30 minutes before meals, and antacids about 1 hour after meals. A double dose of an antacid is often taken just before bedtime (see Figure 24).

TEMAZEPAM
(Razepam, Restoril, Temaz)

Temazepam (15 to 30 mg p.o. 30 minutes before bedtime) is indicated in the treatment of insomnia.

Temazepam depresses the CNS at the limbic and subcortical levels of the brain. It produces a sedative-hypnotic effect by potentiating the effect of the neurotransmitter gamma-aminobutyric acid (GABA) on its receptor in the ascending reticular activating system, which increases inhibition and blocks both cortical and limbic arousal (see Table 8 and Figure 40).

Temazepam is metabolized principally by conjugation, though a minor metabolic pathway involves its N-demethylation to **oxazepam**. The absorption of temazepam is complete but may depend greatly on the pharmaceutical preparation used. Protein binding with temazepam is 96 to 98%, and the elimination half-life varies between 8 and 13 hours.

Temazepam potentiates the CNS depressant effects of phenothiazines, narcotics, antihistamines, monoamine oxidase inhibitors, barbiturates, alcohol, general anesthetics, and antidepressants.

Heavy smoking accelerates temazepam metabolism, thus lowering clinical effectiveness. Benzodiazepines block the therapeutic effects of levodopa. Temazepam may decrease plasma levels of haloperidol.

Clinical manifestations of overdose include somnolence, confusion, hypoactivity or absent reflexes, dyspnea, labored breathing, hypotension, bradycardia, slurred speech, unsteady gait or impaired coordination, and ultimately, coma.

Flumazenil, a specific benzodiazepine antagonist, may be useful.

TENIPOSIDE
(VM-26)

Teniposide, a podophyllotoxin with antineoplastic properties, is indicated in acute lymphocytic leukemia in childhood.

TERAZOSIN HYDROCHLORIDE
(Hytrin)

Terazosin (initially 1 mg at bedtime) alone or in combination with other antihypertensive agents such as diuretics or beta-adrenergic receptor blocking agents is indicated in the management of hypertension.

In addition, terazosin is used in the symptomatic treatment of benign prostatic hyperplasia. It improves urinary flow.

Terazosin has a peripheral post-synaptic alpha$_1$-adrenergic blocking action, which is thought to account primarily for its effects (see Figure 27).

Terazosin produces vasodilation and reduces peripheral resistance but generally has little effect on cardiac output. Antihypertensive effect with chronic dosing is usually not accompanied by reflex tachycardia. There is little or no effect on renal blood flow or glomerular filtration rate.

Relaxation of smooth muscle in the bladder neck, prostate, and prostate capsule produced by alpha$_1$-adrenergic blockade results in a reduction in urethral resistance and pressure, bladder outlet resistance, and urinary symptoms.

Terazosin may affect serum lipids. The most consistent changes observed are a decrease in levels of serum total cholesterol and low density lipoprotein (LDL) cholesterol plus very low density lipoprotein (VLDL) cholesterol fraction.

A "first-dose orthostatic hypotensive reaction" sometimes occurs, most frequently 30 minutes to 2 hours after the initial dose of terazosin, and may be severe. Syncope or other postural symptoms, such as dizziness, may occur. Subsequent occurrence with dosage increases is also possible. Incidence appears to be dose-related; thus, it is important that therapy be initiated with a 1 mg dose given at bedtime. Patients who are volume-depleted or sodium-restricted may be more sensitive to the orthostatic hypotensive effects of terazosin, and the effect may be exaggerated after exercise.

TERBUTALINE SULFATE
(Brethine)

Terbutaline, a bronchodilator (5 mg given p.o. at 6 hour intervals 3 times during waking hours), is indicated for relief of bronchospasm in patients with reversible obstructive airway disease (see Figure 86); and terbutaline, a tocolytic agent (10 mcg/minutes IV), is also used in managing premature labor.

Terbutaline acts directly on beta$_2$-adrenergic receptors to relax bronchial smooth muscle, relieving bronchospasm and reducing airway resistance. Cardiac and CNS stimulation may occur with high doses.

When used in premature labor, it relaxes uterine smooth muscle, which in turn inhibits uterine contractions.

Terbutaline is contraindicated in patients with diabetes, hypertension, hyperthyroidism, or cardiac disease (especially when associated with arrhythmias).

When used concomitantly with other sympathomimetics, terbutaline may potentiate the adverse cardiovascular effects of the other drugs; however, as an aerosol bronchodilator (adrenergic-stimulator type), concomitant use may relieve acute bronchospasm in patients on long-term oral terbutaline therapy.

Beta blockers may antagonize the bronchodilating effects of terbutaline. Use of monoamine oxidase inhibitors within 14 days of terbutaline or the concomitant use of tricyclic antidepressants may potentiate terbutaline's effects on the vascular system.

TERCONAZOLE/BUTOCONAZOLE
(Femstat, Terazol 3, Terazol 7)

Terconazole and butoconazole nitrate (Femstat) are available as a 2% vaginal cream for local treatment of vulvovaginal candidiasis (moniliasis). These drugs are used at bedtime for 3 days in nonpregnant females. There is a slower response during pregnancy, which requires a 6-day course of treatment.

TERFENADINE
(Seldane)

Terfenadine, an H$_1$ histamine receptor antagonist (60 mg p.o. q 8 to 12 hours), is indicated for the treatment of rhinitis and symptoms associated with allergy.

Terfenadine, astemizole, loratadine, and **cetirizine** are **second-generation** antihistaminic agents that are relatively **nonsedating.** Other H$_1$ receptor antagonists currently undergoing clinical trials are **azelastine, ebastine**, and **levocabastine**.

Terfenadine, like other antihistamines, compete with histamine for histamine H$_1$-receptor sites on the smooth muscle of the bronchi, GI tract, uterus, and large blood vessels. By binding to cellular receptors, they prevent access of histamine and suppress histamine-induced allergic symptoms, even though they do not prevent its release.

TERBUTALINE   CHOLINOMIMETICS

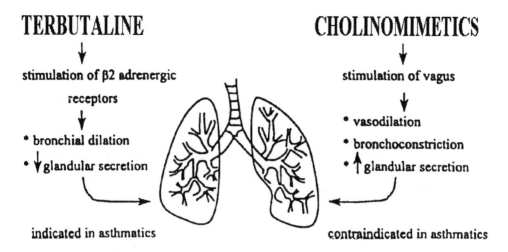

↓   ↓

stimulation of β2 adrenergic   stimulation of vagus

receptors   ↓

↓   * vasodilation

* bronchial dilation   * bronchoconstriction

* ↓ glandular secretion   * ↑ glandular secretion

indicated in asthmatics   contraindicated in asthmatics

FIGURE 86   The selective beta$_2$-adrenergic stimulants cause bronchodilation without cardiac acceleration. **Metaproterenol** and **terbutaline** are available in tablet form, and terbutaline is also available for subcutaneous injection. Metaproterenol and albuterol are available in metered-dose inhalers.

Inhaled selective beta$_2$-adrenergic receptor agonists (**albuterol, terbutaline, fenoterol,** and **bitolterol**) have a rapid onset of action and are effective for 3 to 6 hours. **Formoterol** and **salmeterol** are longer-acting agents (12 hours) and may prove useful in treating nocturnal symptoms.

Terfenadine is absorbed well from the GI tract, distributed mainly into the lungs, liver, GI tract, spleen, and bile; lower concentrations have been detected in the blood, kidneys, and heart. Terfenadine does not cross the blood-brain barrier and hence causes no sedation. It becomes bound to plasma proteins to the extent of 97%, is metabolized in the liver, and the metabolites are excreted in the feces (60%) and urine (40%).

Terfenadine is contraindicated in patients with impaired hepatic function (for example, alcoholic cirrhosis, hepatitis) or in those who take drugs such as ketoconazole, itraconazole, clarithromycin, erythromycin, troleandomycin, or other potent inhibitors of the hepatic cytochrome P450 isoenzyme. Terfenadine should not be given to patients with electrolyte abnormalities such as hypokalemia or hypomagnesemia, who take diuretics with potential for inducing electrolyte abnormalities, or who have congenital QT syndrome.

It should be used with caution in patients with asthma or other lower respiratory diseases, because its mild anticholinergic effects might aggravate these conditions. It should also be used with caution in patients with underlying cardiac disease because of the potential development of ventricular tachyarrhythmia while taking terfenadine.

Unlike other antihistamines, terfenadine has minimal anticholinergic activity and does not potentiate the CNS effects of alcohol, antianxiety agents, or other CNS depressants.

TERPIN HYDRATE

Terpin hydrate, an aliphatic alcohol with expectorant properties (5 to 10 ml of elixir p.o. q 4 to 6 hours), is used in excessive bronchial secretions.

TESTOLACTONE

(Teslac)

Testolactone, an androgen with antineoplastic effectiveness (250 mg p.o. q.i.d.), is used in advanced postmenopausal breast cancer.

TESTOSTERONE

(Aandro 100, Andronaq-50, Histerone, Testaqua, Testoject-50)

TESTOSTERONE CYPIONATE

(Andro-Cyp 100, Andro-Cyp 200, Andronate, dep Andro 100, dep Andro 200, Depo-Testosterone, Duratest 100, Testa-C, Testoject-LA)

TESTOSTERONE ENANTHATE

(Andro L.A. 200, Andryl, Delatestryl, Everone, Testone L.A., Testrin-P.A.)

TESTOSTERONE PROPIONATE

(Testex)

Testosterone, an androgen, is used in male hypogonadism, delayed puberty in males, postpartum breast pain and engorgement, and in inoperable breast cancer (see also Table 6 and Figure 87).

TESTOSTERONE TRANSDERMAL SYSTEM

(Testoderm)

Testosterone transdermal system (4 mg/day) is used in primary or hypogonadotropic hypogonadism in men age 18 and older.

Testosterone (25 to 100 mg/ml) is available in suspension, and testosterone cypionate, testosterone enanthate, and testosterone propionate are supplied in oil.

Testosterone is indicated in male hypogonadism, in delayed puberty in males, in postpartum breast pain and engorgement, and in inoperable breast cancer.

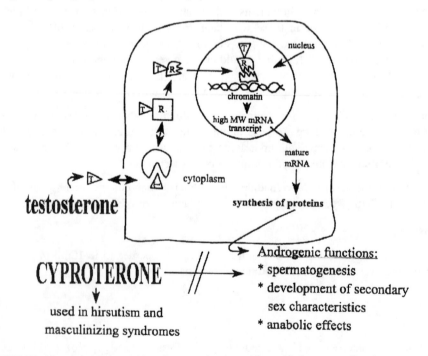

FIGURE 87 Testosterone is used in primary or hypogonadotrophic hypogonadism in men age 18 and older.

At many sites of action, testosterone is not the active form of the hormone. It is converted by steroid 5*a*-reductases in target tissues to the more active dihydrotestosterone. Steroid 5*a*-reductase 1 is located largely in nongenital skin and liver, and steroid 5*a*-reductase 2 is present principally in the urogenital tract of the male and in the genital skin of both sexes.

Testosterone or dihydrotestosterone binds to an intracellular protein receptor, and the hormone-receptor complex is attached in the nucleus to specific hormone regulatory elements on the chromosomes and acts to increase the synthesis of specific RNAs and proteins. The human androgen receptor is a typical member of the superfamily of steroid and thyroid hormone receptors. It is encoded by a gene on the X chromosome and contains androgen-binding, DNA-binding, and functional domains (see Figure 87).

Testosterone, the male sex hormone, is responsible for the development and maintenance of the **male sex organs** (the penis, prostate gland, seminal vesicle, and vas deferens) and **secondary sex characteristics**. In addition, testosterone has **anabolic effects**. Similar to progesterone, testosterone is metabolized very rapidly by the liver by the first-pass mechanism, and hence requires **structural modifications** in order to be effective. For example, the 17–OH group of testosterone may be modified by the addition of propionic acid, which yields testosterone propionate, cyclopentylpropionic acid, which yields testosterone cypionate, or enanthate, which yields testosterone enanthate. In addition, the 17 position may be methylated to yield methyltestosterone, or a fluorine and a methyl group may be inserted to yield fluoxymesterone. In general, these agents are more effective when given orally and have a longer duration of action than testosterone itself (see also Table 6).

Testosterone and its derivatives are used in the treatment of hypogonadism (eunuchoidism), hypopituitarism, accelerated growth, aging in men, osteoporosis, anemia, endometriosis, promotion of anabolism, suppression of lactation, and breast carcinoma.

Hormonal therapy with testosterone should be reserved primarily for patients with **hypogonadal disorders**. There are two important warnings about the indiscriminate use of intramuscular testosterone in patients with serum testosterone levels in the normal range. First, many impotent patients are older and may have adenocarcinoma of the prostate, thus exogenous testosterone may accelerate the growth of the neoplasm. Second, although testosterone may induce a marked increase in libido, patients may still be unable to achieve adequate erection.

Although hypogonadism and sexual dysfunction are common in alcoholic cirrhotic males, currently there are no effective medications to treat the sexual dysfunction. Vitamin A therapy has not proved effective.

One of the side effects of testosterone compounds is **masculinization in women** (such as hirsutism, acne, depression of menses, and clitoral enlargement) and of their female offspring. Therefore, androgens are contraindicated in pregnant women. **Prostatic hypertrophy** may occur in males, which leads to urinary retention. Therefore, androgens are contraindicated in men with prostatic carcinoma.

Cyproterone inhibits the action of androgens (see Figure 87), and **gossypol** prevents spermatogenesis without altering the other endocrine functions of the testis (see Figure 47).

TETANUS IMMUNE GLOBULIN, HUMAN
(TIG) (Hyper-Tet)

Tetanus immune globulin, an immune serum with tetanus prophylaxis effectiveness, is used in tetanus exposure and tetanus treatment.

TETANUS TOXOID, ABSORBED

TETANUS TOXOID, FLUID

This tetanus prophylaxis agent is used in primary immunization (absorbed formulation), primary immunization (fluid formulation), and tetanus prophylaxis in wound management.

TETRACYCLINES

Tetracyclines, which are bacteriostatic, have the broadest spectrum of activity and are effective against infections with Gram-positive and Gram-negative bacteria: *Rickettsia*, mycoplasma, amoeba, and *Chlamydia*. These agents consist of:

Tetracycline (Achromycin and Panmycin)
Chlortetracycline (Aureomycin)
Oxytetracycline (Terramycin)
Demeclocycline (Declomycin)
Doxycycline (Vibramycin)
Minocycline (Minocin and Vectrin)
Methacycline (Rondomycin) (see Figure 88)

Tetracyclines enter bacterial cells by both passive diffusion and active transport, and then accumulate intracellularly. This does not occur in mammalian cells. The tetracyclines bind to the 30S subunit of the bacterial ribosome in such a way that the binding of the aminoacyl-transfer RNA to the acceptor site on the messenger RNA ribosome complex is blocked (see Figure 80).

The resistant mutant bacteria do not transport or accumulate tetracycline. This plasmid-controlled resistance is transmitted by transduction or by conjugation.

The absorption of tetracyclines from the gastrointestinal tract is **nonuniform**. Up to 30% of chlortetracycline is absorbed. The absorption for tetracycline, oxytetracycline, and demeclo-cycline ranges between 60 and 80%, whereas as much as 90 to 100% of doxycycline and minocycline is absorbed. The unabsorbed tetracycline may modify the intestinal flora. The

Structural Formulas of the Tetracyclines

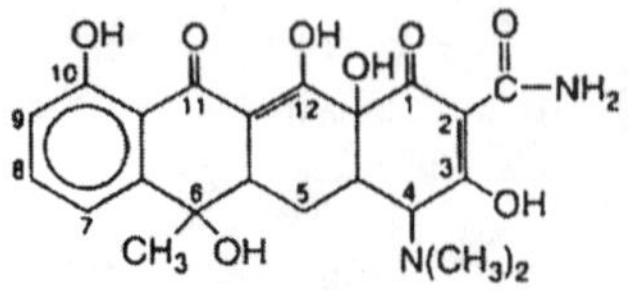

TETRACYCLINE

CONGENERS	SUBSTITUENT(S)	POSITION(S)
Chlortetrcycline	—Cl	(7)
Oxytetracycline	—OH,—H	(5)
Demeclocycline	—OH,—H; —Cl	(6; 7)
Methacycline	—OH,—H; =CH₂	(5; 6)
Doxycycline	—OH,—H; —CH₃,—H	(5; 6)
Minocycline	—H,—H; —N(CH₃)₂	(6; 7)

FIGURE 88 Tetracyclines, which are bacteriostatic, have the broadest spectrum of activity and are effective against infections with Gram-positive and Gram-negative bacteria, *Rickettsia*, mycoplasma, amoeba, and *Chlamydia*.

absorption of tetracyclines is impaired by **divalent cations** (calcium, magnesium, and ferrous iron), by aluminum, and by extremely alkaline pHs. Tetracyclines are distributed widely throughout the body fluid, cross the placental barrier, and can accumulate in growing bones. The concentrations of chlortetracycline in spinal fluid are only one-fourth of those in plasma. Minocycline, a more lipid-soluble tetracycline, reaches a high concentration in tears and saliva and can eradicate the meningococcal carrier state. The tetracyclines are metabolized in the liver and excreted mainly by the bile and urine. The concentrations of tetracyclines in the bile are ten times higher than those in serum.

Tetracyclines are effective in the treatment of Rocky Mountain spotted fever, murine typhus, recrudescent epidemic typhus, scrub typhus, Q fever, lymphogranuloma venereum, psittacosis, tularemia, brucellosis, gonorrhea, certain urinary tract infections, granuloma inguinale, chancroid, syphilis, and disease due to *Bacteroides* and *Clostridium.*

Tetracyclines in general cause toxic and hypersensitivity reactions. These consist commonly of gastrointestinal irritations that are disabling and may necessitate discontinuation of the medications. With continuous usage, tetracyclines may alter the normal flora, allowing the growth of *Pseudomonas, Proteus,* staphylococci-resistant coliforms, *Clostridium*, and *Candida* organisms. These superinfections should be recognized and treated appropriately with vancomycin (see Figure 93) and other drugs.

Tetracyclines have been known to cause hepatic necrosis, especially when given in large intravenous doses or when taken by pregnant women or patients with preexisting liver impairment.

Tetracycline preparations whose potency has expired can cause **renal tubular acidosis**. With the exception of doxycycline, tetracyclines accumulate in patients with renal impairment. Tetracyclines also produce **nitrogen retention**, especially when given with diuretics.

The systemic administration of demeclocycline elicits photosensitization to ultraviolet light or sunlight. Minocycline causes vertigo and dizziness. The intravenous administration of tetracyclines has been observed to cause venous thrombosis.

Tetracyclines bind to calcium and then become deposited in bone, causing damage to developing bone and teeth.

TETRACYCLINES	
Chlortetracycline	Minocycline
Demeclocycline	Oxytetracycline
Doxycycline	Tetracycline
Methacycline	

TETRAHYDROZOLINE HYDROCHLORIDE
(Collyrium Fresh, Murine Plus, Ocu-Drop, Soothe, Tyzine Pediatric, Visine)

Tetrahydrozoline, a sympathomimetic agent with vasoconstrictor properties, is used in nasal congestion and conjunctival congestion.

TETRANDRINE

Tetrandrine, a traditional medicinal alkaloid, has been used in China for the treatment of hypertension, cardiac arrhythmia, and angina pectoris. Recently, it has been shown that tetrandrine blocks voltage activated L-type Ca^{++} channels in a variety of excitable cells including cardiac tissue (see Figures 76 and 95). The binding site of tetrandrine is located at the benzothiazepine receptor on the a_1-subunit of the channel. It is clear that tetrandrine's actions in the treatment of cardiovascular diseases, including hypertension and supraventricular arrhythmia, are due primarily to its blocking of voltage activated L-type and T-type Ca^{++} channels.

THEOPHYLLINE

(Aerolate, Bronkodyl, Constant-T, Elixophylin, Slo-bid, Slo-Phyllin, Somophyllin-T, Sustaire, Theobid, Theoclear, Theo-Dur, Theolair, Theophyl, Theospan-SR, Theo-24, Theovent, Uniphyl)

THEOPHYLLINE SODIUM GLYCINATE

(Synophylate)

Theophylline, a bronchodilator, is indicated for the symptomatic relief of bronchospasm in patients not currently receiving theophylline who require rapid relief of acute symptoms and for prophylaxis of bronchial asthma, bronchospasm of chronic bronchitis, and emphysema (see also Figure 86).

The methylxanthines consist of **aminophylline, dyphylline, enprofylline,** and **pentoxifylline.** Aminophylline (theophylline ethylenediamine) is the most widely used of the soluble theophyllines. Its main therapeutic effect is bronchodilation. In addition, it causes central nervous system stimulation, cardiac acceleration, diuresis, and gastric secretion. Aminophylline is available in an oral, rectal (pediatric), or intravenous solution, which is used in the treatment of status asthmaticus. Although aminophylline is a less effective bronchodilator than beta-adrenergic agonists, it is particularly useful in preventing nocturnal asthma.

Mechanisms of xanthine-induced physiologic and pharmacological effects have included (1) inhibition of phosphodiesterases, thereby increasing intracellular cyclic AMP, (2) direct effects on intracellular calcium concentration, (3) indirect effects on intracellular calcium concentrations via cell membrane hyperpolarization, (4) uncoupling of intracellular calcium increased with muscle contractile elements, and (5) antagonism of adenosine receptors. A large body of evidence suggests that adenosine receptor antagonism is the most important factor responsible for the most pharmacological effects of methylxanthines in doses that are administered therapeutically or consumed in xanthine-containing beverages.

Xanthines are biotransformed in the liver (85 to 90%) to 1,3-dimethyluric acid, 3-methylxanthine, and 1-methyluric acid; 3-methylxanthine accumulates in concentrations approximately 25% of those of theophylline.

Dyphilline, a chemical derivative of theophylline, is not a theophylline salt as are the other agents. It is about one tenth as potent as theophylline. Following oral administration, dyphylline is 68 to 82% bioavailable.

Aminoglutethimide, rifampin, barbiturates, charcoal, ketoconazole, smoking (cigarettes and marijuana), sulfinpyrazone, sympathomimetics (beta-agonists), all decrease the plasma levels of theophylline, whereas allopurinol, beta blockers (nonselective), calcium channel blockers, cimetidine, contraceptives, corticosteroids, disulfiram, ephedrine, interferon, macrolides, mexiletine, quinolones, thiabendazole, all increase the plasma levels of theophylline.

When used concomitantly, theophylline increases the excretion of lithium. Also, cimetidine, allopurinol (high dose), propranolol, erythromycin, and troleandomycin may cause an increase in serum concentrations of theophylline by decreasing the hepatic clearance. Barbiturates and phenytoin enhance hepatic clearance and hepatic metabolism of theophylline, decreasing plasma levels. Beta-adrenergic blockers exert an antagonistic pharmacologic effect.

THIABENDAZOLE

(Mintezol)

Thiabendazole, an anthelmintic (22 mg/kg t.i.d. after meals), is indicated for the treatment of strongyloidiasis (threadworm infection), cutaneous larva migrans (creeping eruption), and visceral larva migrans.

Thiabendazole is vermicidal or vermifugal against *Enterobius vermicularis* (pinworm), *Ascaris lumbricoides* (roundworm), *Strongyloides stercoralis* (threadworm), *Necator americanus* and *Ancylostoma duodenale* (hookworm), *Trichuris trichiura* (whipworm), *Ancylostoma braziliense* (dog and cat hookworm), and *Toxocara canis* and *Toxocara cati* (ascarids).

Thiabendazole's effect on larvae of *Trichinella spiralis* that have migrated to muscle is questionable. It suppresses egg and larval production and may inhibit the subsequent development of those eggs or larvae which are passed in the feces. While the exact mechanism is unknown, the drug inhibits the helminth-specific enzyme fumarate reductase. The anthelmintic activity against *Trichuris trichiura* (whipworm) is least predictable.

Thiabendazole is absorbed rapidly from the gastrointestinal tract. It is metabolized by hydroxylation and conjugation with glucuronic acid. The commonly occurring side effects are anorexia, nausea, and dizziness. It should be used with caution in patients with decreased hepatic function.

THIAMINE HYDROCHLORIDE

(Vitamin B$_1$) (Biamine)

Thiamine, a water-soluble vitamin, is indicated in beriberi, anemia secondary to thiamine deficiency, polyneuritis secondary to alcoholism, pregnancy or pellagra, Wernicke's encephalopathy, and "wet beri-beri" with myocardial failure.

THIAZIDE DIURETICS

The thiazide diuretics, also called *sulfonamide* or *benzothiadiazide diuretics*, vary in their actions. For instance, the potency of **hydrochlorothiazide** (Hydro-Diuril and Esidrix) is ten times greater than that of **chlorothiazide** (Diuril), but the drugs have equal efficacy. The duration of action of hydrochlorothiazide, which is 6 to 12 hours, equals that of chlorothiazide. On the other hand, **chlorthalidone** (Hygroton) has a duration of action lasting 48 hours. Some thiazide derivatives inhibit carbonic anhydrase, which is unrelated to their diuretic activity. Those that are active in this respect may, at sufficient doses, have the same effect on bicarbonate excretion as does acetazolamide. They cause a moderate loss of sodium (5 to 10% of the filtered load), chloride, and water, and the clearance of free water is impaired. They may cause **metabolic alkalosis** (resorption of bicarbonate and loss of hydrogen ions), **hyperuricemia** (enhanced resorption of uric acid), or **hyperglycemia** (due to directly inhibited insulin release and to **hypokalemia**).

Thiazide diuretics are used in the treatment of edema of cardiac and gastrointestinal origin and bring about a state of intravascular volume depletion. Because this depleted intravascular volume is replenished from the interstitial (edematous) sites, the thiazide diuretics should not be administered too frequently. For example, hydrochlorothiazide is given every other day and chlorthalidone is given once every 2 to 3 days (Table 25).

In small doses, thiazide diuretics are extremely effective in controlling essential hypertension. They exert their effects initially by bringing about volume depletion, then they reduce the peripheral resistance and sensitivity of vascular receptor sites to catecholamine. Thiazide diuretics are also used in conjunction with antihypertensive medications (see Figure 89).

TABLE 25
Sites of Action of Diuretics

Drugs	Sites of Action
Sulfonamide diuretics	
Hydrochlorothiazide	Thick ascending limb (cortical) of the loop of Henle
Chlorthalidone	or distal tubule
Loop diuretics	
Furosemide	Thick ascending limb (medullary)
Ethacrynic acid	of the loop of Henle
Potassium-sparing diuretics	
Spironolactone (Aldactone)	Distal tubules
Triamterene	
Amiloride	
Uricosuric diuretics	
Tienilic acid	Thick ascending limb (cortical) of the loop of Henle
Osmotic diuretics	
Urea	Proximal tubules, descending limb of the loop of
Mannitol	Henle, and collecting tubule
Carbonic anhydrase inhibitors	
Acetazolamide	Proximal tubules
Ethoxzolamide	
Dichlorphenamide	(See Figure 4)

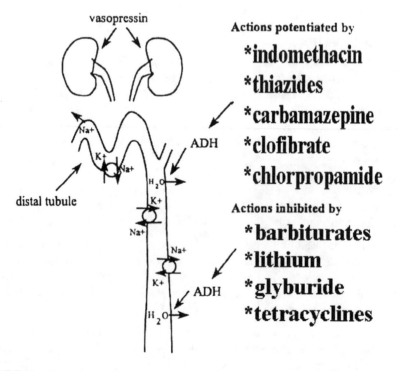

FIGURE 89   Many agents alter the secretion and/or actions of antidiuretic hormone (ADH).

The thiazides decrease the urinary calcium concentration by diminishing glomerular filtration and also enhance the urinary magnesium level.

The thiazide diuretics can reduce free water formation in patients with diabetes insipidus, in whom large amounts of free water are eliminated.

The loss of potassium can produce **hypokalemia**, which is particularly dangerous in patients receiving **digitalis** because it increases the risk of **arrhythmias**. Hypokalemia can be offset either by giving a potassium supplement (potassium chloride), or by the concurrent use of a potassium-sparing diuretic. However, not both measures should be adopted because **hyperkalemia** will result. **Hyperglycemia** is a potential hazard for patients with **diabetes mellitus**. **Hyperuricemia** can precipitate an acute attack of **gout**, but usually only in those patients who either have already had gout or have the propensity for it. Since thiazides can cause a decrease in the GFR, they should not be used in patients whose renal function is less than one third of normal. The risk of thiazide-induced **hypercalcemia** should be kept in mind in patients with conditions such as **malignancies** or **hyperparathyroidism** that are associated with hypercalcemia (see Table 25).

THIAZOLIDINEDIONE DERIVATIVES

Thiazolidinedione derivatives, namely **ciglitazone, englitazone, pioglitazone,** and **troglitazone**, which lower blood glucose by improving peripheral insulin resistance, are a newly developed group of oral antihyperglycemic agents that are completely different from sulfonylurea compounds. This class of drugs shows promise for use in clinical practice for treatment of patients, especially older patients, with noninsulin-dependent diabetes mellitus (see also Tables 1 and 18).

THIETHYLPERAZINE

(Vesprin)

Thiethylperazine (10 to 30 mg daily in divided doses) is indicated for relief of nausea and vomiting, especially emesis associated with surgery, cancer chemotherapy, radiation therapy, and toxins.

The physiologic purpose of **nausea** is to discourage food intake, and **vomiting** is meant to expel food or other toxic substances present in the upper part of the gastrointestinal tract. **Protracted vomiting** may not only cause electrolyte imbalance, dehydration, or a malnutrition syndrome, but may also lead to mucosal laceration and upper gastrointestinal hemorrhage (**Mallory-Weiss syndrome**).

Nausea and vomiting may occur when the stomach is overly irritated, stimulated, or distended (from overeating). In addition, nausea and vomiting may occur when the **chemoreceptor trigger zone for emesis** or the **vomiting center**, or both, are directly stimulated (see Figure 73).

Pharmacologic agents such as aspirin and levodopa may cause vomiting by directly irritating the stomach. Agents such as aminophylline, isoniazid, reserpine, antiinflammatory steroids, and caffeine may also elicit vomiting in susceptible individuals by causing the release of hydrochloric acid. This drug-induced emesis may be avoided by having patients take the drugs with meals. Antiemetics are not effective in rectifying these conditions and their use is not justified.

In addition to agents that stimulate or irritate the stomach, many other factors may be responsible for inducing emesis centrally. The central control of vomiting is vested in two areas:

1. The **vomiting center**, which is located in the lateral reticular formation in the midst of a group of cells governing such activities as salivation and respiration.
2. The **chemoreceptor trigger zone**, which is a narrow strip along the floor of the fourth ventricle located close to the vomiting center.

The functions of these two areas are distinct but interdependent.

The vomiting center is activated by impulses that originate from the gastrointestinal tract and other peripheral structures. In addition, there are unidentified tracts that extend from the cerebral cortex to the vomiting center, such that emotional trauma and unpleasant olfactory and visual stimuli may cause nausea and vomiting.

Stimulation of the **vestibular apparatus** that responds to movements of the head, neck, and eye muscles may also cause nausea and vomiting by stimulating the vomiting center. On the other hand, circulating chemicals, toxins, virus, and ions may provoke nausea and vomiting by first stimulating the **chemoreceptor zone for emesis**, which in turn stimulates the vomiting center.

The nausea and vomiting associated with circulating physical agents (radiation therapy and virus particles) and chemical agents (toxins and cancer chemotherapeutic agents) are treated with phenothiazine derivatives such as chlorpromazine, perphenazine, prochlorperazine, promethazine, triethylperazine, and triflupromazine. These agents block the dopamine receptors in the **area postrema** (see Figure 73).

THIOGUANINE

(6-Thioguanine, 6-TG, Thioguanine Tabloid)

Thioguanine, a purine antimetabolite (2 mg/kg daily p.o.), is indicated in the treatment of acute lymphoblastic and myelogenous leukemia, and chronic granulocytic leukemia.

Thioguanine is not effective in chronic lymphocytic leukemia, Hodgkin's lymphoma, multiple myeloma, or solid tumors. Although thioguanine is one of several agents with activity in the treatment of the chronic phase of chronic myelogenous leukemia, more objective responses are observed with **busulfan**; therefore, busulfan is usually regarded as the preferred drug.

6-Mercaptopurine (6MP) and 6-thioguanine are analogs of the purines, hypoxanthine and guanine, which must be activated by nucleotide formation according to the following scheme:

$$6-MP + \text{phosphoribosylpyrophosphate (PRPP)} \xrightarrow{\substack{\text{Hypoxanthine-guanine} \\ \text{phosphoribosyl} \\ \text{transferase}}} 6 \text{ ThioIMP}$$
$$6TG + PRPP \longrightarrow 6 \text{ ThioGMP}$$

Thioguanine competes with hypoxanthine and guanine for the enzyme hypoxanthine-guanine phosphoribosyltransferase (HGPTRase) and is converted to 6-thioguanylic acid (TGMP). TGMP interferes at several points with the synthesis of guanine nucleotides; it inhibits *de novo* purine biosynthesis by inhibiting glutamine-6-phosphoribosylpyro-phosphate amidotransferase. Thioguanine nucleotides are incorporated into both RNA and DNA by phosphodiester linkages, and incorporation of such fraudulent bases may contribute to the cytotoxicity of thioguanine.

Thioguanine has multiple metabolic effects. Its tumor inhibitory properties may be due to one or more of its effects on feedback inhibition of *de novo* purine synthesis: inhibition of purine nucleotide interconversions; or incorporation into DNA and RNA. The net consequence of its actions is a sequential blockade of the synthesis and utilization of the purine nucleotides.

Resistance may result from the loss of HGPRTase activity (inability to convert thioguanine to TGMP) or increased catabolism of TGMP by a nonspecific phosphatase. Although it is variable, cross-resistance with mercaptopurine usually occurs.

The adverse reactions of thioguanine are nausea, vomiting, anorexia, and stomatitis. The rapid cell lysis causes hyperuricemia which should be minimized by taking allopurinol, a xanthine oxidase inhibitor which prevents the formation of uric acid.

Myelosuppression is the most frequent adverse reaction to thioguanine.

THIOPENTAL SODIUM
(Pentothal)

Thiopental, an ultra short-acting barbiturate, is indicated for induction of anesthesia in short surgical procedures, for supplementing the actions of other anesthetic agents, and for creating a hypnotic state. Thiopental may be used to control convulsive states and in neurosurgical patients with increased intracranial pressure. In addition, it has been used rectally as a suspension to cause narcosis to take care of minor procedures where muscular relaxation and analgesia are not required. The onset of action is 10 minutes.

The ultra short-acting barbiturates, thiopental, thiamylal, and methohexital, quickly cross the blood-brain barrier but are rapidly redistributed from the brain to other body tissues, first to highly perfused visceral organs (liver, kidneys, heart) and muscle, and later to fatty tissues.

These agents produce anesthesia within one minute. Recovery after a small dose is rapid, with somnolence and retrograde amnesia. Muscle relaxation occurs at the onset of anesthesia. The duration of anesthetic activity following a single IV dose is 20 to 30 minutes for thiopental and thiamylal, and somewhat shorter for methohexital.

THIORIDAZINE
(Mellaril)

Thioridazine (50 to 100 mg p.o. t.i.d.) is indicated in psychosis. Thioridazine has potent anticholinergic properties and causes heavy sedation. However, it produces a very low incidence of extrapyramidal reactions such as akathisia, dystonia, parkinsonism, tardive dyskinesia, and neuroleptic malignant syndrome. Thioridazine is metabolized to **mesoridazine**, which is an active antipsychotic (see Table 23).

Because of its potent anticholinergic properties, thioridazine should be used cautiously in patients with cardiac diseases such as congestive heart failure, arrhythmias, angina pectoris, or heart block; in encephalitis, Reye's syndrome, head injury, respiratory disease, epilepsy and other seizure disorders, glaucoma, prostatic hypertrophy, urinary retention, Parkinson's disease, and pheochromocytoma because the drug may exacerbate these conditions; and in hypocalcemia because it increases the risk of extrapyramidal reactions.

Concomitant use of thioridazine with sympathomimetics, including epinephrine, phenylephrine, phenylpropranolamine, and ephedrine (often found in nasal sprays), and with appetite suppressants may decrease their stimulatory and pressor effects. Thioridazine, having alpha-adrenergic receptor blocking effects, may cause epinephrine reversal, where the administration of epinephrine would cause only hypotension.

Thioridazine may inhibit blood pressure response to centrally acting antihypertensive drugs, such as guanethidine, guanabenz, guanadrel, clonidine, methyldopa, and reserpine. Additive effects are likely after concomitant use of thioridazine with CNS depressants, including alcohol, analgesics, barbiturates, narcotics, tranquilizers, anesthetics (general, spinal, or epidural), and parenteral magnesium sulfate (oversedation, respiratory depression, and hypotension), antiarrhythmic agents, including quinidine, disopyramide, and procainamide (increased incidence of cardiac arrhythmias and conduction defects); atropine and other anticholinergic drugs, including antidepressants, MAO inhibitors, antihistamines, meperidine, and antiparkinsonian agents (oversedation, paralytic ileus, visual changes, and severe constipation); nitrates (hypotension) and metrizamide (increased risk of seizures).

Beta-blocking agents may inhibit thioridazine metabolism, increasing plasma levels and toxicity.

Concomitant use with propylthiouracil increases risk of agranulocytosis; concomitant use with lithium may result in severe neurologic toxicity with an encephalitis-like syndrome and in decreased therapeutic response to thioridazine.

Thioridazine may antagonize the therapeutic effect of bromocriptine on prolactin secretion; it also may decrease the vasoconstricting effects of high-dose dopamine and may decrease effectiveness and increase toxicity of levodopa (by dopamine blockade). Thioridazine may inhibit metabolism and increase toxicity of phenytoin.

Overdose of thioridazine causes CNS depression characterized by deep, unarousable sleep and possible coma, hypotension or hypertension, extrapyramidal symptoms, abnormal involuntary muscle movements, agitation, seizures; arrhythmias, ECG changes, hypothermia or hyperthermia, and autonomic nervous system dysfunction.

THIOTEPA

Thiotepa, an alkylating agent with antineoplastic properties, is indicated in breast, lung, and ovarian cancer, Hodgkin's disease, lymphomas, and in bladder tumor and neoplastic effusions.

THIOTHIXENE HYDROCHLORIDE

(Intensol)

Thiothixene (2 mg t.i.d. in mild cases) is indicated in the management of psychotic disorders. Thiothixene and chlorprothixene are thioxanthene antipsychotics. Their select pharmacological properties are compared with chlorpromazine and haloperidol and are shown in Table 23.

THROMBIN

(Thrombinar, Thrombogen, Thrombostat)

Thrombin, a topical hemostatic, is indicated in bleeding from parenchymatous tissue, cancellous bone, dental sockets, during nasal and laryngeal surgery, and in plastic surgery and skin-grafting procedures.

THROMBOLYTIC AGENTS: A NEED FOR IMPROVEMENT

Cardiovascular diseases, comprising acute myocardial infarction, stroke, and venous thromboembolism, have, as their immediate underlying cause, thrombosis of critically situated blood vessels with loss of blood flow to vital organs. One approach to the treatment of thrombosis consists of pharmacologic dissolution of the blood clot via the intravenous infusion of plasminogen activators, which activate the blood fibrinolytic system.

Despite their widespread use in patients with acute myocardial infarction, all currently available thrombolytic agents suffer from a number of significant limitations, including resistance to reperfusion, the occurrence of acute coronary reocclusion, and bleeding complications. Therefore, the quest continues for thrombolytic agents with a higher thrombolytic potency, specific thrombolytic activity, and/or a better fibrin-selectivity.

The fibrinolytic system comprises an inactive proenzyme, plasminogen, which is converted by plasminogen activators to the active enzyme, plasmin, which degrades fibrin. Two immunologically distinct plasminogen activators have been identified: tissue-type plasminogen activator (t-PA) and urokinase-type plasminogen activator (u-PA). Plasminogen activation is regulated by specific molecular interactions between its main components, as well as by controlled synthesis and release of plasminogen activator inhibitors, primarily from endothelial cells. The observed association between abnormal fibrinolysis and a tendency toward bleeding or thrombosis demonstrates the (patho)physiological importance of the fibrinolytic system. Transgenic animals are a suitable experimental model in which to examine the *in vivo* impact of fibrinolytic components in thrombosis and thrombolysis. Inactivation, by homologous recombination, of the tissue-type plasminogen activator genes in mice impairs thrombolysis in a significant manner, whereas inactivation of the plasminogen activator-1 gene enhances the rate of spontaneous lysis.

Several lines of research toward improvement of thrombolytic agents are being explored, including the construction of mutants and variants of plasminogen activators, chimeric plasminogen activators, conjugates of plasminogen activators with monoclonal antibodies, or plasminogen activators from animal or bacterial origin.

THYROGLOBULIN

(Proloid)

In the treatment of hypothyroidism, levothyroxine (Levothroid and Synthroid Sodium; 2 to 25 microgram/kg) is given for replacement therapy in patients with hypothyroidism. Following are other **thyroid preparations:**

Thyroglobulin (Proloid), purified from hog thyroid gland and standardized to yield a T_4 to T_3 ratio of 2.5 to 1.

Liothyronine (Cytomel and Cytomine) has a short half-life and hence is used diagnostically in the T_3 suppression test.

Liotrix (Euthyroid, Thyrolar) is a combination of T_4 and T_3, and is standardized to yield a T_4 to T_3 ratio of 4 to 1.

THYROID USP (DESICCATED)

(Armour Thyroid, Dathroid, Delcoid, S-P-T, Thermoloid, Thyrar, Thyrocrine, Thyroid Strong, Thyro-teric)

Thyroid hormone is used in adult hypothyroidism, in adult myxedema, and in cretinism and juvenile hypothyroidism.

Thyroid USP affects protein and carbohydrate metabolism, promotes gluconeogenesis, increases the utilization and mobilization of glycogen stores, stimulates protein synthesis, and regulates cell growth and differentiation. The major effect of thyroid is to increase the metabolic rate of tissue.

THYROID PREPARATIONS	
Thyroid, USP Armour Thyroid, $^1/_4$, $^1/_2$, $1^1/_2$, 2, 3, 4, and 5 grain tablets	Desiccated hog, beef, or sheep thyroid gland
Thyroglobulin 32 mg ($^1/_2$ grain), 65 mg (1 grain), 100 mg ($1^1/_2$ grain), 130 mg (2 grain), and 200 mg (3 grain)	Partially purified hog thyroglobulin
L-Thyroxine Synthroid, Levothroid, 25, 50, 75, 100, 125, 150, 175, 200, and 300 µg tablets; 100 µg/mL, 5 mL	Synthetic T_4
Liothyronine Cytomel, 5, 25, and 50 µg tablets	Synthetic T_3
Liotrix Euthyroid, Thyrolar, $^1/_4$, $^1/_2$, 1, 2, and 3 strength tablets	Synthetic T_4:T_3 in 4:1 ratio

Thyroid USP is contraindicated in patients with thyrotoxicosis, acute myocardial infarction, or uncorrected adrenal insufficiency (see Figure 56).

Thyroid USP should be used cautiously in patients with angina or other cardiovascular disease because of the risk of increased metabolic demands.

Concomitant use of thyroid USP with adrenocorticoids or corticotropin causes changes in thyroid status, and changes in thyroid dosages may require adrenocorticoid or corticotropin dosage changes as well. Concomitant use with anticoagulants may alter anticoagulant effect; an increased thyroid USP dosage may necessitate a lower anticoagulant dose.

Use with tricyclic antidepressants or sympathomimetics may increase the effects of these medications or of thyroid USP, possibly leading to coronary insufficiency or cardiac arrhythmias. Use with oral antidiabetic agents or insulin may affect dosage requirements of these agents. Estrogens, which increase serum thyroxine-binding globulin levels, raise thyroid USP requirements.

Hepatic enzyme inducers (for example, phenytoin) may increase hepatic degradation of levothyroxine, causing increased dosage requirements of levothyroxine. Concomitant use with somatrem may accelerate epiphyseal maturation. Intravenous phenytoin may release free **thyroid** from thyroglobulin. Cholestyramine and colestipol may decrease absorption.

Overdosage with thyroid USP causes exaggerated signs and symptoms of hyperthyroidism, including weight loss, increased appetite, palpitations, nervousness, diarrhea, abdominal cramps, sweating, tachycardia, increased pulse and blood pressure, angina, cardiac arrhythmias, tremor, headache, insomnia, heat intolerance, fever, and menstrual irregularities.

THYROTROPIN

(Thyroid-Stimulating Hormone, or TSH) (Thytropar)

Thyrotropin is indicated in diagnosis of thyroid cancer remnant with ^{131}I after surgery (see Table 19); in the differential diagnosis of primary and secondary hypothyroidism; in protein-bound iodine or ^{131}I uptake determinations for differential diagnosis of subclinical hypothyroidism or low thyroid reserve; as therapy for thyroid carcinoma (local or metastatic) with ^{131}I; and to determine the thyroid status of patients receiving thyroid therapy (see Figure 91).

THYROTROPIN-RELEASING HORMONE
(TRH)

The production of thyroid hormones is regulated in two ways: (1) by **thyrotropin** and (2) by a variety of nutritional, hormonal, and illness-related factors. The secretion of thyrotropin is regulated by the circulating levels of T_4 and by thyrotropin-releasing hormone (TRH), as shown in Figure 90.

Thyrotropin is synthesized by **thyrotrophs** located in the anterior pituitary gland and consists of two peptide subunits, the **alpha subunit** (see also **Luteinizing hormone, Follicle-stimulating hormone,** and **Chorionic gonadotropin**), and the **beta subunit**, which determines the biologic activities of thyrotrophs. T_3 and T_4 inhibit both the synthesis and release of thyrotropin.

The concentration of TSH increases rapidly following the administration of TRH. In hyperthyroidism, the high levels of T_3 and T_4 inhibit the action of TSH and cause a lack of response to TRH.

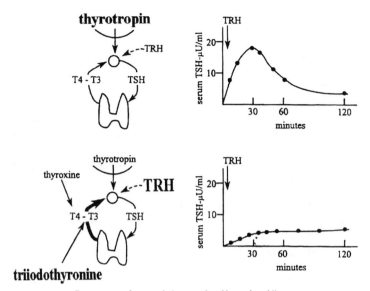

Responses to thyrotropin in normal and hyperthyroidism states

FIGURE 90   The production of thyroid hormones is regulated in two ways: (1) by **thyrotropin**, and (2) by a variety of nutritional, hormonal, and illness-related factors.

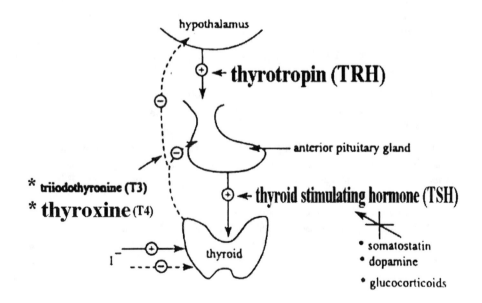

THE REGULATION OF THYROID HORMONE PRODUCTION

FIGURE 91   The secretion of thyrotropin is regulated by the circulating levels of T_4 and by thyrotropin-releasing hormone (TRH).

THYROXINE (T$_4$)

The ingested iodide (100 to 150 microgram/day) is actively transported to (**iodide trapping**) and then accumulates in the thyroid gland. Following this, the trapped iodide is oxidized by a peroxidase system to active iodine, which iodinates the tyrosine residue of glycoprotein to yield **monoiodotyrosine** (MIT) and **diiodotyrosine** (DIT). This process is called **iodide organification**. The MIT and DIT combine to form T$_3$, whereas two molecules of DIT combine to form T$_4$. T$_3$ and T$_4$ are released from thyroglobulin through the actions of pinocytosis and the proteolysis of thyroglobulin by lysosomal enzymes. In the circulation, 75% of T$_4$ is bound to **thyroxine-binding globulin** (TBG), and the remainder is bound mostly to **thyroxine-binding prealbumin** (TBPA). Approximately 0.05% of T$_4$ remains free. T$_3$ is similarly bound to TBG, allowing only 0.5% of it to remain in the free form.

T$_4$ may undergo deamination, decarboxylation, and glucuronic acid conjugation. However, it is mostly deiodinated in one of two ways: it may either be deiodinated to 3,5,3'-triiodothyronine, which is more efficacious than T$_4$, or it may be deiodinated to the pharmacologically inactive 3,3',5'-triiodothyronine (**reverse T$_3$**) (see Figure 56).

TICARCILLIN DISODIUM

(Ticar)

Ticarcillin, extended-spectrum penicillin, alpha-carboxypenicillin, is indicated for the treatment of bacterial septicemia, skin and soft-tissue infections, acute and chronic respiratory tract infections caused by susceptible strains of *Pseudomonas aeruginosa, Proteus* species (both indole-positive and indole-negative), and *Escherichia coli*; and for genitourinary tract infections (complicated and uncomplicated) due to susceptible strains of *P. aeruginosa, Proteus* species (both indole-positive and indole-negative), *E. coli, Enterobacter,* and *Streptococcus faecalis* (enterococcus).

Ticarcillin disodium/clavulanate potassium (**Timentin**) is an extended-spectrum penicillin and inhibits beta-lactamase.

Ampicillin, amoxicillin, carbenicillin, ticarcillin, piperacillin, mezlocillin, and azlocillin differ from penicillin G in having greater activity against Gram-negative bacteria, but they are inactivated by beta-lactamases (see also Table 22).

Carbenicillin resembles ampicillin but has more activity against *Pseudomonas* and *Proteus* organisms, though *Klebsiella* species are usually resistant. In susceptible populations of *Pseudomonas*, resistance to carbenicillin may emerge rapidly. Therefore, in *Pseudomonas* sepsis (e.g., burns, immunosuppressed patients), carbenicillin, 12 to 30 g/d intravenously (300 to 500 mg/kg/d), is usually combined with an aminoglycoside, e.g., gentamicin, 5 to 7 mg/kg/d intramuscularly, to delay emergence of resistance and perhaps to obtain synergistic effects. Carbenicillin contains Na$^+$, 4.7 mEq/g. Carbenicillin indanyl sodium is acid-stable and can be given orally in urinary tract infections. Ticarcillin resembles carbenicillin in single and combined activity, but the dose may be lower, e.g., 200 to 300 mg/kg/d intravenously. Piperacillin, mezlocillin, azlocillin, and others resemble ticarcillin and claim special effectiveness against Gram-negative aerobic rods, including *Pseudomonas*. However, in serious *Pseudomonas* infections, they should be used in combination with an aminoglycoside.

Ampicillin, amoxicillin, ticarcillin, and others in this group can be protected from destruction by beta-lactamases if they are administered together with beta-lactamase inhibitors such as **clavulanic acid, sulbactam,** or **tazobactam.** Such mixtures have been employed against lactamase-producing *H. influenzae* or coliform organisms.

Ticarcillin is excreted primarily (80 to 93%) in urine by renal tubular secretion and glomerular filtration; it is also excreted in bile and in breast milk. Therefore, it should be used cautiously in patients with renal impairment because it is excreted in urine.

Aminoglycoside and ticarcillin are physically and chemically incompatible and are inactivated when mixed or given together.

The clinical signs of overdosage with ticarcillin include neuromuscular hypersensitivity or seizures resulting from CNS irritation by high drug concentrations.

TICARCILLIN DISODIUM/CLAVULANATE POTASSIUM
(Timentin)

Ticarcillin, an extended-spectrum penicillin, which inhibits beta lactamase, is indicated in infections of the lower respiratory tract, urinary tract, bones and joints, skin and skin structures, and septicemia when caused by susceptible organisms.

TICLOPIDINE HYDROCHLORIDE
(Ticlid)

Ticlopidine, a platelet aggregation inhibitor possessing antithrombotic effects (250 mg p.o. b.i.d.), is used to reduce the risk of thrombotic stroke in patients with a history of stroke or who have experienced stroke precursors (see also Figures 12 and 84). Ticlopidine, a thienopyridine derivative, and a new antiplatelet agent for secondary prevention of stroke, causes potent inhibition of adenosine diphosphate (ADP)-induced platelet aggregation and moderate inhibition of aggregation induced by collagen, epinephrine, thrombin, and platelet-activating factor.

TICNILIC ACID
(Ticrynafen)

Ticnilic acid, which is a uricosuric diuretic, is chemically related to ethacrynic acid, but pharmacologically it resembles the thiazide diuretics. Ticnilic acid is as efficacious as hydrochlorothiazide, but it is superior in enhancing uric acid excretion, which is a problem with most effective diuretics. The usefulness of this agent in medicine awaits confirmation.

TIMOLOL MALEATE
(Timoptic-XE) Timolol Maleate (Biocarden)

Timolol (10 mg t.i.d.) alone or in combination with other antihypertensive agents, such as thiazide diuretics, is used in the management of hypertension. Timolol is indicated for the treatment of myocardial infarction and prophylaxis of migraine headaches. Timolol (1 drop of 0.25% solution twice daily) is effective in lowering intraocular pressure in patients with chronic open-angle glaucoma.

Timolol's beta-blocking action decreases the production of aqueous humor, thereby decreasing intraocular pressure.

Timolol is a nonselective beta-adrenergic blocking agent; the affinity to beta$_1$- and beta$_2$-receptors is almost equal. In currently recommended dosages, it has no membrane-stabilizing and only negligible partial agonist activity. In humans, it is 8 to 10 times more potent than propranolol in reducing resting heart rate and 14 times more potent in suppressing tachycardia induced by isoproterenol infusion.

When timolol tablets are administered orally, 90 to 100% of the drug is rapidly absorbed, uninfluenced by food ingestion. Between 5 and 10% is excreted unchanged in the urine; the rest is broken down into several inactive metabolites that are subsequently excreted through the kidneys. Plasma half-life is not influenced by a moderate degree of renal failure.

Timolol is an effective antihypertensive agent. It improves exercise tolerance in patients with angina pectoris. It substantially reduces the long-term risk of sudden death and reinfarction in patients surviving acute myocardial infarction. It has been shown to reduce the size of an acute myocardial infarction when given intravenously within 4 hours after the onset of symptoms. Timolol is effective in the treatment of supraventricular arrhythmias and in certain cases of recurrent ventricular tachycardia.

Similar to other beta-adrenergic blocking agents, timolol reduces systemic blood pressure mainly through a decrease in cardiac output. In hypertensive patients with normal cardiac function, the stroke index remains largely unaffected. Maximum blood pressure reductions usually occur after several days of therapy, when the initial rise in total peripheral resistance begins to fall toward pretreatment levels.

Similar to other nonselective beta-adrenergic blocking agents, timolol causes a decrease in plasma renin activity.

In hypertension, timolol may be used either alone or in combination with most other antihypertensive agents. The combination with angiotensin-converting enzyme inhibitors is probably less useful because both agents exert part of their effect by diminishing the activity of the renin-angiotensin system. Combination with verapamil should be avoided because of the effect on AV nodal conduction.

In angina pectoris, doses of 5 mg b.i.d. may prove sufficient for optimal increase of exercise tolerance, especially in elderly patients.

Timolol seems particularly indicated in patients with hypertension, angina, or both after acute myocardial infarction because of the drug's combined effect on those conditions. It also has a well-documented protective effect in diabetic patients who have had myocardial infarction.

Timolol is contraindicated in patients with unstabilized cardiac failure or bronchial obstruction, AV conduction disturbances of the second and third grade, unstable insulin-dependent diabetes, and severe peripheral arterial obstruction. The most common side effects are muscular fatigue, cold hands and feet, symptomatic hypotension, and bradycardia.

TIOCONAZOLE
(Vagistat-1)

Tioconazole, an imidazole derivative with antifungal activity (vaginal ointment 6.5%), is used in the treatment of vulvovaginal candidiasis.

TIOPRONIN
(Thiola)

Tiopronin, a thiol compound which stabilizes the cystine moiety, is used in prevention of urinary cystine stone formation in patients with severe homozygous cystinuria (urinary cystine excretion exceeding 500 mg daily) unresponsive to other therapies.

TIZANIDINE

Tizanidine is a clonidine derivative which has been introduced recently for treatment of spasticity. It is more effective than buclofen. It is a centrally acting myorelaxant with predominantly alpha$_2$-adrenergic properties. Tizanidine is an imidazole derivative that exhibits central muscle relaxant activity that principally affects spinal polysynaptic reflexes. This action arises from agonistic activity of the compound at noradrenergic alpha$_2$ receptors resulting in both direct impairment of excitatory amino acid release from spinal interneurons and a concomitant inhibition of facilitatory coeruleospinal pathways. Tizanidine has received widespread acceptance in the treatment of spasticity and rheumatological conditions associated with painful muscle spasm (see also Figures 27 and 81).

TOBRAMYCIN SULFATE

(Nebcin)

Tobramycin is available in ophthalmic ointments and solutions. Tobramycin (1 mg/kg initially, to be adjusted thereafter) is indicated in the treatment of:

> Serious infections caused by susceptible strains of *Pseudomonas aeruginosa, Escherichia coli, Proteus sp.* (indole-positive and indole-negative) including *P. mirabilis, Morganella morganii* and *P. vulgaris, Providencia sp.* including *P. rettgeri,* the *Klebsiella-Enterobacter-Serratia* group, *Citrobacter sp.* and staphylococci, including *S. aureus* (coagulase-positive and coagulase-negative)
>
> Septicemia (neonates, children, and adults) caused by *P. aeruginosa, E. coli,* and *Klebsiella sp.*
>
> Lower respiratory tract infections caused by *P. aeruginosa, Klebsiella sp., Enterobacter sp., Serratia sp., E. coli,* and *S. aureus* (penicillinase- and nonpenicillinase-producing strains)
>
> Serious CNS infections (meningitis) caused by susceptible organisms
>
> Intra-abdominal infections, including peritonitis, caused by *E. coli, Klebsiella sp.,* and *Enterobacter sp.*
>
> Skin, bone, and skin structure infections caused by *P. aeruginosa, Proteus sp., E. coli, Klebsiella sp., Enterobacter sp.,* and *S. aureus*
>
> Complicated and recurrent urinary tract infections (UTIs) caused by *P. aeruginosa, Proteus sp.* (indole-positive and indole-negative), *E. coli, Klebsiella sp., Enterobacter sp., Serratia sp., S. aureus, Providencia sp.,* and *Citrobacter sp.* The drug is not indicated in uncomplicated initial episodes of UTIs unless the organisms are not susceptible to less toxic antibiotics.

The antimicrobial activity and pharmacokinetic properties of **tobramycin** are very similar to those of **gentamicin.** Tobramycin may be given either intramuscularly or intravenously. Dosages are identical to those for gentamicin. When doses of 1.5 mg/kg are given intravenously every 8 hours, peak concentrations in plasma are typically 5 to 8 microgram/ml, and minimal concentrations are 1 to 2 microgram/ml. Toxicity is most common at minimal (trough) concentrations that exceed 2 microgram/ml for a prolonged period. The latter observation usually requires reduction of dosage.

Tobramycin, like other aminoglycosides, causes both nephrotoxicity and ototoxicity. However, tobramycin may be less toxic to hair cells in the cochlear and vestibular end organs and cause less renal tubular damage than does gentamicin.

TOCAINIDE HYDROCHLORIDE

(Tonocard)

Tocainide, an antiarrhythmic (initially 400 mg t.i.d.), is indicated in the treatment of life-threatening ventricular arrhythmias.

Tocainide may be beneficial in the treatment of myotonic dystrophy (800 to 1200 mg/day) and trigeminal neuralgia (20 mg/kg/day in 3 divided doses). Tocainide is a Class 1B antiarrhythmic with electrophysiologic properties similar to those of lidocaine (see Figure 76). In patients with cardiac disease, tocainide produces no clinically significant changes in sinus nodal function, effective refractory periods, or intracardiac conduction times. Tocainide does not prolong QRS duration or QT intervals. Theoretically, it may be useful for ventricular arrhythmias associated with a prolonged QT interval.

Tocainide produces a small degree of depression on left ventricular function and left ventricular end diastolic pressure.

Tocainide does not change heart rate or blood pressure. Tocainide is contraindicated in patients with second- or third-degree AV block in the absence of an artificial ventricular pacemaker.

Cimetidine (but not ranitidine) or rifampin reduces the plasmic level of tocainide, whereas metoprolol has added effects with tocainide on wedge pressure and cardiac index.

The most frequent adverse reactions following tocainide are dizziness, vertigo, nausea, paresthesia, and tremor. However, fatal agranulocytosis, bone marrow depression, leukopenia, neutropenia, aplastic/hypoplastic anemia, thrombocytopenia, interstitial pneumonitis, fibrosing alveolitis, pulmonary edema, and pneumonia have occurred in patients receiving tocainide.

TOLAZAMIDE

(Tolinase)

Tolazamide, a sulfonylurea oral hypoglycemic agent (100 mg p.o. daily with breakfast), is indicated as an adjunct to diet to lower blood glucose levels in patients with noninsulin-dependent diabetes mellitus (Type II); and it is indicated as a medication for switching patients from insulin to oral therapy (see Table 1).

Oral hypoglycemic agents have advantages over insulin because, by releasing insulin and decreasing the release of glucagon, they mimic physiologic processes and cause fewer allergic reactions. Furthermore, they are effective in an oral form, thus eliminating the need for daily injections.

The mechanisms that underlie the hypoglycemic actions of sulfonylureas are:

Pancreatic
>   Improved insulin secretion
>   Reduced glucagon secretion

Extrapancreatic
>   Improved tissue sensitivity to insulin
>   Direct
>>   Increased receptor binding
>>   Improved post-binding action
>   Indirect
>>   Reduced hyperglycemia
>>   Decreased plasma free fatty-acid concentrations
>>   Reduced hepatic insulin extraction

Tolazamide is five times more potent than tolbutamide but is considerably weaker than glipizide and glyburide.

Tolazamide is metabolized by the liver and is excreted by the kidneys. It has diuretic effects but possesses no disulfiram-like properties.

Tolazamide should not be used in patients with burns, acidosis, diabetic coma, severe infection, ketosis, or severe trauma, or in those who are undergoing major surgery, because such conditions of severe physiologic stress require insulin for adequate blood glucose control.

Concomitant use with anticoagulants may increase plasma levels of both drugs and, after continued therapy, may reduce the plasma levels of anticoagulant effects. Use with chloramphenicol, guanethidine, insulin, monoamine oxidase inhibitors, probenecid, salicylates, or sulfonamides may enhance the hypoglycemic effect by displacing tolazamide from its protein-binding sites.

Concomitant use with beta-adrenergic blocking agents may increase the risk of hypoglycemia, mask its symptoms (rising pulse rate and blood pressure), and prolong it by blocking gluconeogenesis. Use with drugs that may increase blood glucose levels (adrenocorticoids, glucocorticoids, amphetamines, baclofen, corticotropin, epinephrine, ethacrynic acid, furosemide, phenytoin, thiazide diuretics, triamterene, and thyroid hormones) may require dosage adjustments.

Because smoking increases corticosteroid release, smokers may require higher doses of tolazamide.

Clinical manifestation of overdosage with tolazamide includes low blood glucose levels, tingling of lips and tongue, hunger, nausea, decreased cerebral function (lethargy, yawning, confusion, agitation, nervousness), increased sympathetic activity (tachycardia, sweating, tremor), and ultimately, seizures, stupor, and coma.

TOLAZOLINE HYDROCHLORIDE
(Priscoline)

Tolazoline, an alpha-adrenergic receptor blocking agent with vasodilating properties (1 to 2 mg/kg IV via a scalp vein over 10 minutes), is indicated in persistent pulmonary vasoconstriction and hypertension of the newborn (persistent fetal circulation) (see also Figure 27).

TOLBUTAMIDE
(Oramide, Orinase, SK-Tolbutamide)

Tolbutamide, a sulfonylurea antidiabetic agent (1 to 2 g p.o. daily), is indicated in stable, maturity-onset nonketotic diabetes mellitus uncontrolled by diet alone and previously untreated (see Figure 44 and Table 1).

TOLFENAMIC ACID

Tolfenamic acid is an effective nonsteroidal antiinflammatory drug which belongs to the fenamate group. Tolfenamic acid possesses analgesic, antipyretic, and antiinflammatory properties (see Table 2), and tolfenamic acid inhibits cyclic AMP- and cyclic GMP phosphodiesterase. It inhibits cyclooxygenase, reducing the formation of prostaglandin; and inhibits lipoxygenase, leading to formation of leukotriene (see also Figure 11).

TOLMETIN SODIUM
(Tolectin)

Tolmetin (400 mg t.i.d.) is indicated in the treatment of acute flares and long-term management of rheumatoid arthritis and osteoarthritis. In addition, it is effective in the treatment of juvenile rheumatic arthritis (see also Table 2).

Tolmetin has analgesic, antipyretic, and antiinflammatory properties.

Tolmetin is rapidly and completely absorbed after oral administration. Peak concentrations are achieved 20 to 60 minutes after oral administration, and the half-life in plasma is about 5 hours. Accumulation of the drug in synovial fluid begins within 2 hours and persists for up to 8 hours after a single oral dose.

After absorption, tolmetin is extensively (99%) bound to plasma proteins. Virtually all of the drug can be recovered in the urine after 24 hours; some is unchanged, but most is conjugated or otherwise metabolized. The major metabolic transformation involves oxidation of the para-methyl group to a carboxylic acid.

The most common side effects of tolmetin are gastrointestinal side effects consisting of epigastric pain, dyspepsia, nausea, and vomiting. Tolmetin is able to cause gastric erosion and to prolong bleeding time.

Tolmetin is contraindicated in patients in whom aspirin or other nonsteroidal antiinflammatory drugs (NSAIDs) induce symptoms of asthma, urticaria, or rhinitis.

Serious GI toxicity, especially ulceration or hemorrhage, can occur at any time in patients on chronic NSAID therapy. Tolmetin should be used cautiously in patients with a history of GI bleeding or GI ulcer because the drug may irritate the GI tract; in patients with renal disease because the drug may be nephrotoxic; or in patients with cardiac disease because it may cause peripheral edema, sodium retention, and hypertension.

Patients with known "triad" symptoms (aspirin hypersensitivity, rhinitis/nasal polyps, and asthma) are at high risk of cross-sensitivity to tolmetin with precipitation of bronchospasm.

The signs and symptoms of acute infection (fever, myalgias, erythema) may be masked by the use of tolmetin.

The actions of anticoagulants and thrombolytic drugs may be potentiated by the platelet-inhibiting effect of tolmetin. Concomitant use of tolmetin with highly protein-bound drugs (for example, phenytoin, sulfonylureas, warfarin) may cause displacement of either drug and adverse effects. Concomitant use with other GI-irritating drugs (such as steroids, antibiotics, NSAIDs) may potentiate the adverse GI effects of tolmetin.

Antacids and food can delay and decrease the absorption of tolmetin. NSAIDS are known to decrease renal clearance of lithium carbonate, thus increasing lithium serum levels and risks of adverse effects. Concomitant use of tolmetin and aspirin may decrease plasma levels of tolmetin.

TOLNAFTATE

(Tinactin, Aftate)

Tolnaftate (1% cream, solution and gel) is indicated for treatment of tinea pedis (athlete's foot), t. cruris (jock itch), or t. corporis (ringworm) due to infection with *Trichophyton rubrum, T. mentagrophytes, T. tonsurans, Microsporum canis, M. audouini,* and *Epidermophyton floccosum,* and as treatment for tinea versicolor due to *Malassezia furfur.*

In onychomycosis, in chronic scalp infections in which fungi are numerous and widely distributed in skin and hair follicles, where kerion has formed, and in fungus infections of palms and soles, tolnaftate may be used concurrently for adjunctive local benefit in these lesions.

TOPIRAMATE

Topiramate is a novel antiepileptic drug which inhibits amygdala-induced seizures.

TRACE MINERALS ESSENTIAL FOR HEALTH	
Elements	Sign of Deficiency
Zinc	Dermatitis, hypogeusia, alopecia, diarrhea, apathy, depression
Copper	Neutropenia, hypochromic anemia, osteoporosis, decreased hair and skin pigmentation, dermatitis, anorexia, diarrhea
Chromium	Glucose intolerance, peripheral neuropathy, increased free fatty acid levels, low respiratory quotient
Manganese	Nausea, vomiting, dermatitis, color changes in hair, hypocholesterolemia, growth retardation
Selenium	Muscle weakness and pain, cardiomyopathy
Molybdenum	Tachycardia, tachypnea, altered mental status, visual changes, headache, nausea, vomiting
Iodine	Hyperthyroid goiter, hypothyroidism

TORSEMIDE
(Demadex)

Torsemide, a loop diuretic (10 to 20 mg p.o.), is used to cause diuresis in patients with congestive heart failure (CHF); diuresis in patients with chronic renal failure; and diuresis in patients with hepatic cirrhosis (see also Table 25).

TRANYLCYPROMINE SULFATE
(Parnate)

Tranylcypromine, a monoamine oxidase alpha inhibitor (30 mg/day in divided doses), is indicated for the treatment of depression.

Monoamine oxidase can metabolize monoamines by oxidative deamination and convert them to inactive acidic derivatives. Monoamine oxidase inhibitors seem to compete with physiologically active monoamine for the active site of the enzyme. In general, not only do these agents inhibit the oxidase that metabolizes amines, but they also inhibit the oxidase that metabolizes drugs and essential nutrients. Hence, the incidence of drug–drug and drug–food interactions is extremely high with these agents. Monoamine oxidases have various applications. They may be used as a local **anesthetic** (cocaine), an **antihistaminic** (diphenylhydramine), or an **antidepressant** (tranylcypromine). Monoamine oxidase inhibitors have been used in the treatment of hypertension (direct blockade of sympathetic ganglion), angina pectoris (coronary dilation), narcolepsy (stimulating the reticular activating system), and depression (increasing the brain's norepinephrine pool). Needless to say, these agents should be used with extreme caution in conjunction with sympathomimetic amines, ganglionic blocking agents, procaine, and anesthetic agents. They are contraindicated in patients with hyperthyroidism and in combination with tricyclic antidepressants. In the event of poisoning, adrenergic blocking agents such as phentolamine may be effective for combating the hypertensive crisis.

The high incidence of drug–food and drug–drug interactions rules out monoamine oxidase inhibitors as antidepressants of first choice. However, there are circumstances in which these agents may be used effectively and successfully. These are:

When a patient has not responded to a tricyclic antidepressant for an adequate trial period and with an appropriate dosage.

When a patient has developed allergic reactions to tricyclics.

When a patient has had previous depressive episodes that responded well to monoamine oxidase inhibitors.

TRAVELER'S DIARRHEA: PREVENTION OF

Diarrhea is by far the most common medical problem among people traveling to the tropical and semitropical areas of Latin America, parts of the Caribbean, such as Haiti and the Dominican Republic, southern Asia, and North, East, and West Africa.

Bacterial enteropathogens cause as least 80% of traveler's diarrhea, which explains the prophylactic and therapeutic effects of antibacterial drugs. Although different organisms predominate in different regions, the principal agents in most of the high-risk areas are, in decreasing order of importance, enterotoxigenic *Escherichia coli, Shigella* species, *Campylobacter jejuni, Aeromonas* species, *Plesiomonas shigelloides, salmonella* species, and noncholera *Vibrios*. Doxycycline and trimethoprim-sulfamethoxazole may be used for prophylaxis.

Other approaches to the prevention of traveler's diarrhea are the use of lactobacillus preparations or bismuth subsalicylate. Lactobacilli are bacteria that metabolize dietary carbohydrate to lactic acid and other organic acids, reducing the intraluminal pH and inhibiting the growth of enteropathogens.

Bismuth subsalicylate has short-term intraluminal antimicrobial action, but it must be given four times daily, with meals and at bedtime.

Drugs	Dose
Bismuth subsalicylate	tablets chewed four times a day
Fluoroquinolone antibiotics	
Norfloxacin	400 mg daily
Ciprofloxacin	500 mg daily
Ofloxacin	300 mg daily
Fleroxacin	400 mg daily
Trimethoprim- sulfamethoxazole	160 mg of trimethoprim and 800 mg of sulfamethoxazole once daily
Doxycycline	100 mg daily

TRAZODONE HYDROCHLORIDE

(Desyrel)

Trazodone (150 mg/day) is indicated in the treatment of depression. Trazodone selectively inhibits serotonin reuptake in the brain, causes beta-receptor subsensitivity, and induces significant changes in serotonin-receptor binding with only a slight effect on alpha-adrenergic receptors. Also, trazodone potentiates the action of 5-hydroxytryptophan, the precursor of serotonin (see also Tables 3 through 5).

Trazodone is perhaps the most sedative antidepressant available, being more sedative than amitriptyline, trimipramine, doxepan, or imipramine. Therefore, death has occurred in patients taking trazodone with alcohol, chloral hydrate, diazepam, chlordiazepoxide, meprobamate, or amobarbital.

The most severe reactions reported with overdose of trazodone alone have been priapism, respiratory arrest, seizures, and ECG changes.

TREFOIL PEPTIDES

Trefoil peptides constitute a rapidly growing family of peptides containing one or more characteristic trefoil domains. A trefoil domain is defined as a sequence of 38 or 39 amino acid residues in which 6 cysteine residues are disulfide-linked in the configuration 1-5, 2-4 and 3-6 when the cysteines are numbered from the N-terminal end of the peptide. The amino acid sequence together with the disulfide bonds thus forms a distinctive three-leafed structure giving the peptide family its name.

Although trefoil peptides have been cloned or isolated from a series of different organs and tissues from several species, recent evidence indicates that trefoil peptides may have their main function in association with the mucous layer of the gastrointestinal tract. Trefoil peptides have thus been suggested as possible naturally occurring **healing factors for peptic ulcers, inflammatory bowel disease,** and other diseases in the gastrointestinal tract involving mucosal injury.

TRETINOIN
(Retin-A)

Tretinoin, a vitamin A derivative possessing antiacne properties (cream, gel, and solution 0.01 to 0.05%), is used in acne vulgaris (especially grades I, II, and III). In addition, tretinoin has been used in the treatment of photodamaged and wrinkled skin.

TRIAMCINOLONE (SYSTEMIC)
(Aristocort, Kenacort)

TRIAMCINOLONE ACETONIDE
(Kenalog, Kenalone, Triam-A)

TRIAMCINOLONE ACETONIDE (ORAL INHALANT)
(Azmacort)

Triamcinolone (2 inhalations t.i.d.) is indicated in the treatment of steroid-dependent asthma.

TRIAMCINOLONE ACETONIDE (TOPICAL)
(Aristocort, Flutex, Kenalog, Kenalog in Orabase, Triacet)

Topical triamcinolone (cream, lotion, aerosol, and paste 0.025 to 0.5%) is indicated in the treatment of inflammation of corticosteroid-responsive dermatoses.

TRIAMCINOLONE DIACETATE
(Amcort, Aristocort, Aristocort Forte, Aristocort Intralesional, Articulose LA, Cenocort Forte, Cinalone, Kenacort, Triam-Forte, Triamolone, Tristoject)

TRIAMCINOLONE HEXACETONIDE
(Aristospan Intra-Articular, Aristospan Intralesional)

Triamcinolone, a glucocorticoid (4 to 12 mg p.o. daily), is indicated in adrenal insufficiency; and triamcinolone (4 to 60 mg p.o. daily) is indicated for severe inflammation and immunosuppression.

The glucocorticoids possess a plethora of physiologic actions, including a role in **differentiation** and **development**. They are vital in the treatment of adrenal insufficiency and are used extensively in large pharmacologic doses as antiinflammatory and immunosuppressive agents. Some of the nonendocrine conditions for which they may be used include arthritis, tenosynovitis, systemic lupus erythematosus, acute rheumatic carditis, bronchial asthma, organ transplantation, ulcerative colitis, cerebral edema, and myasthenia gravis.

The relative antiinflammatory potency and sodium-retaining properties of several steroids are listed in Tables 10 and 13.

Glucocorticoids have an anti-insulin effect and aggravate the pathologic consequences of diabetes mellitus. They increase gluconeogenesis, inhibit the peripheral utilization of glucose, and cause hyperglycemia and glucosuria. Cortisol's effect, for example, is opposite to that of insulin's.

Glucocorticoids promote the breakdown of proteins and inhibit protein synthesis. This leads to muscle wasting in the quadriceps-femoris groups, and muscular activities may become difficult as a result.

The effects of glucocorticoids on glycogen accumulation appear to be predominantly, although not exclusively, insulin dependent, since glycogen accumulation is markedly reduced in pancreatectomized animals. Glucocorticoid-stimulated increases in insulin secretion promote further glycogen accumulation.

Glucocorticoids cause the abnormal deposition of a fat pad called "buffalo hump." Glucocorticoids cause hypernatremia, hypokalemia, and hypercalciurea. Glucocorticoids cause hyperuricemia by suppressing the renal tubular resorption of uric acid. Glucocorticoids promote the production of gastric hydrochloric acid, and, like epinephrine, they augment the coagulability of blood.

Glucocorticoids exert their antiinflammatory effects in part by blocking the release and action of histamine. In addition, they decrease the migration of polymorphonuclear leukocytes.

Glucocorticoids produce eosinophilia and cause the involution of lymphoid tissues. They bring about lymphocytopenia, monocytopenia, and eosinopenia. In addition, glucocorticoids block a number of lymphocytic functions.

Although considered to be immunosuppressive, therapeutic doses of glucocorticoids do not significantly decrease the concentration of antibodies in the circulation. Furthermore, during glucocorticoid therapy, patients exhibit a nearly normal antibody response to antigenic challenge.

Glucocorticoids, which do penetrate the blood-brain barrier, affect behavior, mood, and neural activity, and are able to regulate the permeability of the blood-brain barrier to other substances. Hence they are used to treat brain edema. Both glucocorticoid deficiency and excess may cause mood swings and rarely psychosis. Patients receiving glucocorticoids have a feeling of well-being. On the other hand, patients with spontaneously evolving **Cushing's syndrome**, which involves the overproduction of glucocorticoids, are commonly depressed. Patients with **Addison's disease**, which is caused by a deficiency of cortisol and aldosterone, tend to be depressed, negativistic, irritable, seclusive, and apathetic. Patients with Addison's disease also suffer from anorexia, whereas a glucocorticoid excess stimulates the appetite. In addition, high doses of glucocorticoids can affect sleep, with a trend toward increased wakefulness, a reduction in rapid-eye-movement (REM) sleep, increase in stage II sleep, and an increase in the time to the first REM sleep.

Glucocorticoids affect bone metabolism in a variety of ways. Mild hyperkalemia can occur in Addison's disease. Conversely, glucocorticoids are used to treat certain hypercalcemias — largely granulomatous conditions such as sarcoidosis, in which the steroid blocks the formation of 1-alpha,25-dihydroxycholecalciferol [1-alpha,25-$(OH)_2D_3$] by the granulomatous tissues. However, most hypercalcemias are not glucocorticoid responsive and, in general, glucocorticoid excess does not result in lower serum calcium levels. Serum phosphate levels are lowered and urinary calcium and phosphorous concentrations are elevated in glucocorticoid excess states. Glucocorticoid excess ultimately leads to **osteoporosis**, the major limitation to their long-term use.

Besides the adverse effects just described, glucocorticoid therapy is contraindicated under the following circumstances: diabetes mellitus, digitalis therapy, glaucoma, hypertension, infection, osteoporosis, peptic ulcer, tuberculosis, and viral infection.

TRIAMTERENE
(Dyrenium)

Triamterene, a potassium-sparing diuretic (100 mg p.o. b.i.d.), is used to cause diuresis.

TRIAZOLAM
(Halcion)

Triazolam, a benzodiazepine derivative (0.125 to 0.25 mg p.o.), is indicated in insomnia.

Triazolam, a short-acting hypnotic sedative, depresses the CNS at the limbic and subcortical levels of the brain. It produces a sedative-hypnotic effect by potentiating the effect of the neurotransmitter gamma-aminobutyric acid (GABA) on its receptor in the ascending reticular activating system, which increases inhibition and blocks both cortical and limbic arousal (Table 8).

Triazolam is absorbed well orally, exerts its sedative effects in 15 minutes, is distributed widely in the body, is bound to plasma proteins to the extent of 90%, is metabolized to 6-hydroxytriazolam which is subsequently conjugated with glucuronic acid, and is excreted in the urine.

Triazolam is contraindicated in patients in coma, because the drug's hypnotic or hypotensive effect may be prolonged or intensified; in pregnant patients, because it may be fetotoxic; and in patients with acute alcohol intoxication who have depressed vital signs, because the drug will worsen CNS depression.

Triazolam should be used cautiously in patients with impaired hepatic function, which prolongs elimination of the drug; in elderly or debilitated patients, who are usually more sensitive to the drug's CNS effects; and in individuals prone to addiction or drug abuse.

Triazolam potentiates the CNS depressant effects of phenothiazines, narcotics, antihistamines, MAO inhibitors, barbiturates, alcohol, general anesthetics, and antidepressants. Enhanced amnestic effects have been reported when combined with alcohol (even in small amounts).

Concomitant use with cimetidine and possibly disulfiram causes diminished hepatic metabolism of triazolam, which increases its plasma concentration.

Heavy smoking accelerates triazolam metabolism, thus lowering clinical effectiveness. Benzodiazepines may decrease the therapeutic effects of levodopa. Triazolam may decrease serum levels of haloperidol. Erythromycin decreases clearance of triazolam.

The clinical manifestations of overdosage with triazolam are somnolence, confusion, hypoactive reflexes, dyspnea, labored breathing, hypotension, bradycardia, slurred speech, unsteady gait, or impaired coordination, and, ultimately, coma.

Flumazenil, a specific benzodiazepine receptor antagonist will antidote and reverse the deleterious effects of triazolam (see Figure 40).

TRICHLORMETHIAZIDE
(Diurese, Metahydrin, Naqua, Trichlorex)

Trichlormethiazide, a thiazide diuretic (1 to 4 mg p.o. daily), is used in hypertension.

TRIENTINE HYDROCHLORIDE
(Cuprid, Syprine)

Trientine, a heavy metal chelating agent (750 to 1250 mg in divided doses), is used in Wilson's disease in patients who are intolerant of **penicillamine.**

TRIETHANOLAMINE POLYPEPTIDE OLEATE-CONDENSATE
(Cerumenex)

Triethanolamine, an oleic acid derivative with cerumenolytic properties, is used in impacted cerumen.

TRIFLUOPERAZINE HYDROCHLORIDE
(Stelazine)

Trifluoperazine, a phenothiazine antipsychotic with antiemetic properties (2 to 5 mg p.o. t.i.d.), is indicated in the management of manifestations of psychotic disorders (see Table 23).

Trifluoperazine exerts its antipsychotic effects by postsynaptic blockade of CNS dopamine receptors, thereby inhibiting the action of dopamine.

Trifluoperazine's antiemetic effects are attributed to dopamine receptor blockade in the medullary chemoreceptor trigger zone (see also Figure 73).

Trifluoperazine exhibits low incidences of sedative and anticholinergic properties, but causes high incidence of extrapyramidal movement disorders including akathisia, dystonia, parkinsonism, tardive dyskinesia, and neuroleptic malignant syndrome.

Concomitant use of trifluoperazine with sympathomimetics, including epinephrine, phenylephrine, phenylpropanolamine, and ephedrine (often found in nasal sprays), and appetite suppressants may decrease their stimulatory and pressor effects. Using epinephrine as a pressor agent in patients taking trifluoperazine may result in epinephrine reversal or further lowering of blood pressure.

Trifluoperazine may inhibit blood pressure response to centrally acting antihypertensive drugs, such as guanethidine, guanabenz, guanadrel, clonidine, methyldopa, and reserpine. Additive effects are likely after concomitant use of trifluoperazine with CNS depressants, including alcohol, analgesics, barbiturates, narcotics, tranquilizers, anesthetics (general, spinal, epidural), and parenteral magnesium sulfate (oversedation, respiratory depression, and hypotension); antiarrhythmic agents, quinidine, disopyramide, and procainamide (increased incidence of cardiac arrhythmias and conduction defects); atropine and other anticholinergic drugs, including antidepressants, monoamine oxidase inhibitors, phenothiazines, antihistamines, meperidine, and antiparkinsonian agents (oversedation, paralytic ileus, visual changes, and severe constipation); nitrates (hypotension); and metrizamide (increased risk of seizures).

The clinical manifestations of overdosage of trifluoperazine include CNS depression characterized by deep, unarousable sleep and possible coma, hypotension or hypertension, extrapyramidal symptoms, dystonia, abnormal involuntary muscle movements, agitation, seizures, arrhythmias, ECG changes, hypothermia or hyperthermia, and autonomic nervous system dysfunction.

TRIFLUPROMAZINE HYDROCHLORIDE
(Vesprin)

Triflupromazine (60 mg IM, up to 150 mg/day) is indicated in the management of manifestations of psychotic disorders; and triflupromazine (5 to 15 mg q. 4 hours) is used to control severe nausea and vomiting.

Triflupromazine causes heavy sedation and has potent anticholinergic properties. It causes a moderate degree of extrapyramidal movement disorders such as akathisia, dystonia, Parkinson's disease, tardive dyskinesia, and neuroleptic malignant syndrome.

Triflupromazine, possessing strong anticholinergic properties, is contraindicated in patients with cardiac diseases such as congestive heart failure, arrhythmias, angina pectoris, and heart block; in encephalitis; Reye's syndrome; head injury; respiratory disease; epilepsy and other seizure disorders; glaucoma; prostatic hypertrophy; urinary retention; Parkinson's disease and pheochromocytoma, because it may exacerbate these conditions; in patients with hypocalcemia, because the drug increases the risk of extrapyramidal reactions; and in patients with hepatic or renal dysfunction (diminished metabolism and excretion cause the drug to accumulate).

Triflupromazine, possessing potent sedative properties, is contraindicated in patients with disorders accompanied by coma, brain damage, CNS depression, circulatory collapse, or cerebrovascular disease (additive CNS depression and adverse blood pressure effects); and in patients taking adrenergic-blocking agents or spinal or epidural anesthetics (excessive respiratory, cardiac, and CNS depression).

As is the case with trifluoperazine, concomitant use of triflupromazine with sympathomimetics, including epinephrine, phenylephrine, phenylpropanolamine, ephedrine (often found in nasal sprays), and appetite suppressants may decrease their stimulatory and pressor effects. Using epinephrine as a pressor agent in patients taking triflupromazine may result in epinephrine reversal or further lowering of blood pressure.

Triflupromazine may inhibit blood pressure response to centrally acting antihypertensive drugs, such as guanethidine, guanabenz, guanadrel, clonidine, methyldopa, and reserpine. Additive effects are likely after concomitant use of triflupromazine with CNS depressants, including alcohol, analgesics, barbiturates, narcotics, tranquilizers, anesthetics (general, spinal, epidural), and parenteral magnesium sulfate (oversedation, respiratory depression, and hypotension); antiarrhythmic agents, quinidine, disopyramide, and procainamide (increased incidence of cardiac arrhythmias and conduction defects); atropine and other anticholinergic drugs, including antidepressants, monoamine oxidase inhibitors, phenothiazines, antihistamines, meperidine, and antiparkinsonian agents (oversedation, paralytic ileus, visual changes, and severe constipation); nitrates (hypotension); and metrizamide (increased risk of seizures) (see Table 23).

The clinical manifestations of overdosage with triflupromazine are characterized by deep, unarousable sleep and possible coma, hypotension and hypertension, extrapyramidal symptoms, dystonia, abnormal involuntary muscle movements, agitation, seizures, arrhythmias, ECG changes, hypothermia or hyperthermia, and autonomic nervous system dysfunction.

TRIFLURIDINE

(Viroptic)

Trifluridine, an antiviral agent (1 drop of 1% solution onto the cornea), is used every 2 hours while awake until the corneal ulcer has re-epithelialized completely. Trifluridine is indicated for primary keratoconjunctivitis and recurrent epithelial keratitis due to herpes simplex virus types 1 and 2. In addition, it is used for epithelial keratitis that has not responded clinically to topical idoxuridine, or when ocular toxicity or hypersensitivity to idoxuridine has occurred.

The antiviral mechanism of action of trifluridine involves inhibition of viral DNA synthesis. Trifluridine monophosphate irreversibly inhibits thymidylate synthetase, and trifluridine triphosphate is a competitive inhibitor of thymidine triphosphate incorporation into DNA by DNA polymerases. Trifluridine is incorporated into viral and cellular DNA. Trifluridine-resistant HSV with altered thymidine kinase substrate specificity can be selected *in vitro*, and resistance in clinical isolates has been described.

The most frequent adverse reactions reported are mild, transient burning or stinging upon instillation and palpebral edema.

TRIHEXYPHENIDYL HYDROCHLORIDE
(Artane)

Trihexyphenidyl, an anticholinergic agent (1 mg p.o. daily), is indicated as an adjunct with other medications in the treatment of Parkinson's disease, and especially in drug-induced parkinsonism.

Belladonna alkaloids, antagonists of muscarinic cholinergic receptors, were initially used in the treatment of Parkinson's disease before the discovery of levodopa. It seems likely that trihexyphenidyl acts within the neostriatum, through the receptors that normally mediate the response to the intrinsic cholinergic innervation of this structure, which arises primarily from cholinergic striatal interneurons. Several muscarinic cholinergic receptors have been cloned, and like the dopamine receptors, these are proteins with seven transmembrane domains that are linked to second-messenger systems by G proteins. Five subtypes of muscarinic receptor have been identified; at least four, and probably all five, subtypes are present in the striatum, although each has a distinct distribution.

Neurochemically, Parkinson's syndrome is considered a **striatal dopamine-deficiency syndrome**, and the main **extrapyramidal symptoms** — tremor, akinesia, and rigidity — correlate positively with the degree of this deficiency. Although eight separate neurotransmitters interact in the nigro-striato-nigral loop, the basic therapeutic problem in parkinsonism has been to find suitable compounds that (1) increase the concentration of dopamine, (2) stimulate the dopamine receptor sites directly, or (3) suppress the activity at cholinergic receptor sites.

Trihexyphenidyl blocks central cholinergic receptors, helping to balance cholinergic activity in the basal ganglia. It may also prolong dopamine's effects by blocking dopamine reuptake and storage at central receptor sites.

Trihexyphenidyl is contraindicated in patients with narrow-angle glaucoma because drug-induced cycloplegia and mydriasis may increase intraocular pressure; in patients with cardiac disorders, arteriosclerosis, renal disorders, hepatic disorders, hypertension, obstructive GI or genitourinary tract disease, or suspected prostatic hypertrophy because the drug may exacerbate these conditions.

Concomitant use with amantadine may amplify trihexyphenidyl's anticholinergic adverse effects, causing confusion and hallucinations. Concomitant use with haloperidol or phenothiazines may decrease the antipsychotic effectiveness of these drugs, possibly from direct CNS antagonism; concomitant phenothiazine use also increases the risk of anticholinergic adverse effects.

Concomitant use with CNS depressants, such as tranquilizers, sedative-hypnotics, and alcohol, increases trihexyphenidyl's sedative effects. When used with levodopa, dosage of both drugs may need adjustment because of synergistic anticholinergic effects and possible enhanced gastrointestinal metabolism of levodopa from reduced gastric motility and delayed gastric emptying. Antacids and antidiarrheals may decrease trihexyphenidyl's absorption.

Overdosage with trihexyphenidyl causes clinical symptoms consisting of central stimulation followed by depression, with such psychotic symptoms as disorientation, confusion, hallucinations, delusions, anxiety, agitation, and restlessness. Peripheral effects may include dilated, nonreactive pupils, blurred vision, flushed, dry, hot skin, dry mucous membranes, dysphagia, decreased or absent bowel sounds, urinary retention, hyperthermia, headache, tachycardia, hypertension, and increased respiration.

TRIIODOTHYRONINE

The steps involved in the synthesis of thyroid hormones are depicted in Figure 56. First the ingested iodide (100 to 150 microgram/day) is actively transported (**iodide trapping**) and then accumulates in the thyroid gland. Following this, the trapped iodide is oxidized by a peroxidase system to active iodine, which iodinates the thyrosine residue of glycoprotein to yield **monoiodotyrosine** (MIT) and **diiodotyrosine** (DIT). This process is called **iodide organification**. The MIT and DIT combine to form triiodothyronine T_3, whereas two molecules of DIT combine to form thyroxine T_4. T_3 and T_4 are released from thyroglobulin through the actions of pinocytosis and the proteolysis of thyroglobulin by lysosomal enzymes. In the circulation, 75% of T_4 is bound to **thyroxine-binding globulin** (TBG), and the remainder is bound mostly to **thyroxine-binding prealbumin** (TBPA). Approximately 0.05% of T_4 remains free. T_3 is similarly bound to TBG, allowing only 0.5% of it to remain in the free form.

T_4 may undergo deamination, decarboxylation, and glucuronic acid conjugation. However, it is mostly deiodinated in one of two ways: it may either be deiodinated to 3,5,3'-triiodothyronine, which is more efficacious than T_4, or it may be deiodinated to the pharmacologically inactive 3,3',5'-triiodothyronine (**reverse T_3**) (see Figure 56).

TRILOSTANE
(Modrastane)

Trilostane, a glucocorticoid suppressant (30 mg p.o. q.i.d.), is used in the treatment of adrenocortical hyperfunction in Cushing's syndrome.

TRIMAZOSIN

The newer selective alpha$_1$-adrenoreceptor-blocking agents, such as **trimazosin, doxasozin,** and **terazosin**, display a pharmacologic profile virtually identical to that of prazosin, but pharmacokinetic differences between the various alpha$_1$-blockers exist.

The bioavailability, plasma half-life (3 hours), and extensive metabolism of trimazosin are similar to those of prazosin. 1-Hydroxytrimazosin, a major metabolite in human beings, may have antihypertensive efficacy, and the delayed onset of the peak hypotensive effect of trimazosin may reflect the rate of formation of this metabolite. Although therapeutic doses of trimazosin are ten- to fifty-fold higher than those of prazosin, the drug is highly selective for alpha$_1$-adrenergic receptors. However, high doses of trimazosin may produce vasodilation directly (see also Figure 27).

TRIMEPRAZINE TARTRATE
(Temaril)

Trimeprazine, a phenothiazine antihistaminic possessing antipruritic activity (25 mg p.o. q.i.d.), is used in pruritis.

TRIMETHADIONE
(Tridione)

Trimethadione (300 mg p.o. t.i.d.) is indicated in the treatment of refractory absence seizures. The oxazolidine derivatives consist of **trimethadione** and **paramethadione** (Paradione).

Trimethadione is rapidly absorbed when given orally, and its binding to plasma proteins is negligible. Trimethadione is demethylated to dimethadione, which is an active anticonvulsant. The rate of conversion of trimethadione to dimethadione is rapid, but its rate of elimination is slow. As a result, the plasma ratio of dimethadione to trimethadione is 20 to 1.

Like ethosuximide, dimethadione inhibits T-type Ca^{2+} currents in dissociated thalamic neurons in therapeutically relevant concentrations. This provides a plausible explanation of the anti-absence seizure effects of trimethadione.

The consequences of trimethadione **toxicity** consist of hematologic side effects (neutropenia, pancytopenia), hemeralopia (day blindness), photophobia, diplopia, dermatologic side effects (rash and erythema multiform), CNS side effects (drowsiness and tolerance), nephrotoxic syndrome (albuminuria), and teratogenic effects such as **fetal trimethadione syndrome**. From this it is apparent that trimethadione is only indicated for the control of absence seizures that are not responsive or have become refractory to treatment with less toxic substances such as ethosuximide or valproic acid.

TRIMETHAPHAN CAMSYLATE
(Arfonad)

Trimethaphan (500 mg/10 ml by IV infusion) is indicated for the production of controlled hypotension during surgery, for the short-term acute control of blood pressure in hypertensive emergencies, and in the emergency treatment of pulmonary edema in patients with pulmonary hypertension associated with systemic hypertension. In addition, trimethaphan has been used in patients with dissecting aortic aneurysm or in ischemic heart disease when other agents could not be used.

Trimethaphan camsylate is a ganglionic-blocking drug that inhibits both sympathetic and parasympathetic autonomic activities. It has a rapid onset and brief duration of action and must be administered by continuous intravenous infusion with constant monitoring of blood pressure. Trimethaphan camsylate is particularly useful in aortic dissection because it can be titrated carefully to permit smooth control of blood pressure and because it decreases cardiac output and left ventricular ejection rate. Tachyphylaxis develops rapidly, making early transition to oral antihypertensive agents mandatory.

Adverse effects including blurred vision, exacerbation of glaucoma due to mydriasis and cycloplegia, dry mouth, respiratory depression, nausea, constipation, fetal meconium ileus, paralytic ileus, impairment of renal blood flow with azotemia, and urinary retention frequently complicate therapy with trimethaphan camsylate. Because of the frequency and severity of the side effects associated with this drug and the availability of more effective agents, it is now rarely used.

TRIMETHOBENZAMIDE HYDROCHLORIDE
(Tigan)

Trimethobenzamide (250 mg t.i.d.) is indicated for controlling nausea and vomiting. The modest antiemetic effects of trimethobenzamide appear to result from blockade of dopamine receptors mediated through the chemoreceptor trigger zone for emesis. The direct impulse to the vomiting center is not inhibited.

Trimethobenzamide is contraindicated in patients with hypersensitivity to benzocaine, or other local anesthetics. The injectable form is contraindicated in neonates and premature infants.

Encephalitis, gastroenteritis, dehydration, electrolyte imbalance and CNS reactions have occurred when used, especially in children and debilitated elderly patients.

The drug's antiemetic effect may mask signs of overdose of toxic agents, intestinal obstruction, brain tumor, or other conditions. Antiemetics should not be the sole therapy of severe emesis. Restoration of fluid and electrolyte balance and relief of the underlying disease process are critical.

Alcohol and other CNS depressants, including tricyclic antidepressants, antihypertensives, phenothiazines, and belladonna alkaloids may increase trimethobenzamide toxicity.

Overdosage with trimethobenzamide may produce clinical symptoms consisting of severe neurologic reactions such as opisthotonos, seizures, coma, and extrapyramidal reactions.

TRIMETHOPRIM
(Proloprim, Trimpex)

Trimethoprim, a synthetic folate antagonist (100 mg p.o. q. 12 hours), is used in the treatment of uncomplicated urinary tract infections and in prophylaxis of chronic and recurrent urinary tract infections.

TRIMETHOPRIM-SULFAMETHOXAZOLE
(Bactrim; Septra)

The combination of trimethoprim and sulfamethoxazole (usually five parts sulfamethoxazole to one part trimethoprim) interferes with the **synthesis of active folic acid** by means of two separate reactions. In the first, sulfonamides compete with p-aminobenzoic acid and prevent its conversion to dihydrofolic acid. In the second, trimethoprim, by inhibiting the activity of dihydrofolic acid reductase, prevents the conversion of dihydrofolic acid into tetrahydrofolic acid, which is necessary for the synthesis of DNA. These reactions are summarized in Figure 82).

These drug combinations have the following **therapeutic advantages:**

They cause synergistic antibacterial effects.
They have bactericidal activity.
The emergence of bacterial resistance is decreased.
The spectrum of antibacterial activity is enhanced.
Toxicity is reduced.

Folic acid deficiency may occur either following prolonged usage of methotrexate or in patients with preexisting folic acid deficiency. **Folinic acid** may be administered to overcome the folic-acid deficiency-related megaloblastic anemia.

Orally administered trimethoprim is used in the treatment of chronic recurring urinary tract infection. Oral forms of trimethoprim-sulfamethoxazole are used in *Shigella* and some *Salmonella* infections, particularly when they are resistant to ampicillin and chloramphenicol. High doses of oral trimethoprim-sulfamethoxazole are used in *Pneumocystis* pneumonia. This combination, along with polymyxin, has been shown to be effective in treating sepsis caused by *Serratia* or *Pseudomonas* organisms.

Intravenously administered trimethoprim-sulfamethoxazole is indicated in severe cases of *Pneumocystis carinii* pneumonia, Gram-negative bacterial sepsis, and shigellosis.

Oral trimethoprim in combination with sulfonamide has been used in the treatment of leishmaniasis, toxoplasmosis, and falciparum malaria.

TRIMETREXATE GLUCURONATE
(Neutrexin)

Trimetrexate, an inhibitor of dihydrofolate reductase, is available for hospital use in treatment of patients with *Pneumocystis carinii* pneumonia and who have exhibited serious (severe or life-threatening) intolerance to both co-trimazole and pentamidine.

TRIMIPRAMINE MALEATE
(Surmontil)

Trimipramine, a tricyclic antidepressant (75 mg/day in divided doses), is indicated in the management of depression and enuresis. Trimipramine exerts its antidepressant effects by equally inhibiting reuptake of norepinephrine and serotonin in CNS nerve terminals, which results in increased concentration and enhanced activity of these neurotransmitters in the synaptic cleft. Trimipramine also has anxiolytic effects and inhibits gastric acid secretion (see Tables 3 through 5).

Trimipramine exhibits moderate affinity for alpha$_1$-adrenergic receptors and muscarinic cholinergic receptors, and a very strong affinity for H$_1$ histamine receptors. Trimipramine causes heavy sedation, has strong anticholinergic properties, and exhibits a moderate degree of orthostatic hypotension.

Trimipramine is contraindicated in patients with known hypersensitivity to tricyclic antidepressants, trazodone, and related compounds; in the acute recovery phase of myocardial infarction (MI), because the drug depresses cardiac function and causes dysrhythmia in patients in coma or severe respiratory depression (additive CNS and respiratory depression); and during or within 14 days of therapy with monoamine oxidase inhibitors.

Trimipramine should be used cautiously in patients with other cardiac disease (arrhythmias, CHF, angina pectoris, valvular disease, or heart block), respiratory disorders, seizure disorders, scheduled electroconvulsive therapy, bipolar disease, glaucoma, hyperthyroidism, and parkinsonism; in patients taking thyroid replacement; in patients with diabetes Types I and II; in patients with prostatic hypertrophy, paralytic ileus, or urinary retention because the drug may worsen these conditions; in patients with hepatic or renal dysfunction because diminished metabolism and excretion causes the drug to accumulate; and in patients undergoing surgery using general anesthesia because the drug may increase cardiac sensitivity to the effects of general anesthetics or pressor agents.

Concomitant use of trimipramine with sympathomimetics, including epinephrine, phenylephrine, phenylpropranolamine, and ephedrine (often found in nasal sprays) may increase blood pressure. Use with warfarin may increase prothrombin time and cause bleeding.

Concomitant use with thyroid medication, pimozole, and antiarrhythmic agents (quinidine, disopyramide, procainamide) may increase incidence of cardiac arrhythmias and conduction defects.

Trimipramine may decrease hypotensive effects of centrally acting antihypertensive drugs, such as guanethidine, guanabenz, quanadrel, clonidine, methyldopa, and reserpine.

Concomitant use with disulfiram or ethchlorvynol may cause delirium and tachycardia.

Additive effects are likely after concomitant use of trimipramine with CNS depressants, including alcohol, analgesics, barbiturates, narcotics, tranquilizers, and anesthetics (oversedation), atropine and other anticholinergic drugs, including phenothiazines, antihistamines, meperidine, and antiparkinsonian agents (oversedation, paralytic ileus, visual changes, and severe constipation), and metrizamide (increased risk of seizures).

Barbiturates and heavy smoking induce trimipramine metabolism and decrease therapeutic efficacy; phenothiazines and haloperidol decrease its metabolism, thus decreasing therapeutic efficacy; methylphenidate, cimetidine, oral contraceptives, propoxyphene, and beta-blockers may inhibit trimipramine metabolism, increasing plasma levels and toxicity.

Overdosage with trimipramine causes CNS stimulation followed by CNS depression. The first 12 hours after acute ingestion are a stimulatory phase characterized by excessive anticholinergic activity (agitation, irritation, confusion, hallucinations, parkinsonian symptoms, seizure, urinary retention, dry mucous membranes, pupillary dilatation, constipation, and ileus). This is followed by CNS depressant effects, including hypothermia, decreased or absent reflexes, sedation, hypotension, cyanosis, and cardiac irregularities (including tachycardia, conduction disturbances, and quinidine-like effects on the ECG).

TRIPELENNAMINE CITRATE
(PBZ)

TRIPELENNAMINE HYDROCHLORIDE
(PBZ, PBZ-SR, Pelamine)

Tripelennamine, an ethylene-diamine-derivative antihistamine (25 to 50 mg p.o. q. 4 to 6 hours), is indicated in rhinitis, allergy symptoms, allergic reactions to blood or plasma, and as an adjunct to epinephrine in anaphylaxis.

In addition, it is used in pruritis, minor burns, insect bites, sunburn, and skin irritations. Tripelennamine competes with histamine for the H_1-receptor, thereby ameliorating histamine effects in target tissues, but does not prevent the release of histamine.

Tripelennamine is contraindicated in patients with known hypersensitivity to similar chemical structures, such as pyrilamine; in neonates, other infants, and breast-feeding women because young children may be more susceptible to the toxic effects of antihistamines; during asthma attacks because it thickens bronchial secretions; and in patients who have taken MAO inhibitors within the preceding two weeks.

Because of the significant anticholinergic effects, tripelennamine should be used with caution in patients with narrow-angle glaucoma; in those with pyloroduodenal obstruction or urinary bladder obstruction from prostatic hypertrophy or narrowing of the bladder neck; and in patients with cardiovascular disease or hypertension because the drug may cause palpitations.

MAO inhibitors interfere with the detoxification of antihistamines and phenothiazines and thus prolong and intensify their central depressant and anticholinergic effects; additive CNS depression and sedation may occur when tripelennamine is administered with other CNS depressants, such as alcohol, barbiturates, tranquilizers, sleeping aids, or antianxiety agents.

Overdosage with tripelennamine may include manifestations such as either CNS depression (sedation, reduced mental alertness, apnea, and cardiovascular collapse) or CNS stimulation (insomnia, hallucinations, tremors, or seizures). Anticholinergic symptoms such as dry mouth, flushed skin, fixed and dilated pupils, and GI symptoms, are common especially in children. Children may also experience fever, excitement, ataxia, and athetosis.

TRIPROLIDINE HYDROCHLORIDE
(Actidil, Myidyl)

Triprolidine, an alkylamine antihistamine, is used in colds and allergy symptoms.

TROLEANDOMYCIN
(TAO)

Troleandomycin, a macrolide antibiotic (250 to 500 mg p.o. q. 6 hours), is used in pneumonia or respiratory tract infection caused by sensitive pneumococci or group A beta-hemolytic streptococci.

TROMETHAMINE
(THAM)

Tromethamine is indicated for prevention and correction of system acidosis such as metabolic acidosis associated with cardiac bypass surgery; correction of acidity of Acid Citrate Dextrose (ACD) blood in cardiac bypass surgery, or cardiac arrest.

Tromethamine, a highly alkaline, sodium-free organic amine, acts as a proton acceptor to prevent or correct acidosis. When administered IV as a $0.3\,M$ solution, it combines with hydrogen ions from carbonic acid to form bicarbonate and a cationic buffer. It also acts as an osmotic diuretic, increasing urine flow, urinary pH, and excretion of fixed acids, carbon dioxide, and electrolytes.

Tromethamine is contraindicated in anuria or uremia.

TROPICAMIDE
(Mydriacyl)

Tropicamide, an anticholinergic agent causing mydriasis and cycloplegia, is used for cycloplegic refractions and fundus examinations.

TUBERCULOSIS: TREATMENT OF	
Drugs	**Main Adverse Effects**
Isoniazid (INH)	Hepatic toxicity, peripheral neuropathy
Rifampin	Hepatic toxicity, flu-like syndrome
Pyrazinamide	Arthralgias, hepatic toxicity, hyperuricemia
Ethambutol	Optic neuritis
Streptomycin	Vestibular toxicity, renal damage
Combinations	
Rifamate (isoniazid 150 mg, rifampin 300 mg) Rifater (isoniazid 50 mg, rifampin 120 mg, pyrazinamide 300 mg)	
Second-line Drugs	
Capreomycin	Auditory and vestibular toxicity, renal damage
Kanamycin	Auditory toxicity, renal damage
Amikacin	Auditory toxicity, renal damage
Cycloserine	Psychiatric symptoms, seizures
Ethionamide	Gastrointestinal and hepatic toxicity, hypothyroidism
Ciprofloxacin	Nausea, abdominal pain, restlessness, confusion
Ofloxacin	Nausea, abdominal pain, restlessness, confusion
Aminosalicylic acid (PAS)	Gastrointestinal disturbance
Tuberculosis continues to be a major problem, particularly in areas of the world where drug resistance is common. Treatment should be continued 12 to 24 months after the culture becomes negative.	

TUBERCULOSIS SKIN TEST ANTIGENS

TUBERCULIN PURIFIED PROTEIN DERIVATIVE (PPD)
(Aplisol, Tubersol)

TUBERCULIN CUTANEOUS MULTIPLE-PUNCTURE DEVICE (APLITEST [PPD]

Mono-vacc Test [Old Tuberculin], Sclavo-Test [PPD], Tine Test [Old Tuberculin], Tine Test [PPD])

This *Mycobacterium tuberculosis* and *Mycobacterium bovis* antigen is used for diagnosis of tuberculosis and evaluation of immunocompetence in patients with cancer or malnutrition.

D-TUBOCURARINE CHLORIDE

(Tubarine)

Tubocurarine (6 to 9 mg IV) is indicated as an adjunct to general anesthesia to induce skeletal muscle relaxation, facilitate intubation, and reduce fractures and dislocations.

Agents such as **tubocurarine** and **pancuronium** compete with acetylcholine for the cholinergic receptors at the end plate. They combine with the receptors but do not activate them. Competitive or nondepolarizing agents are antagonized by neostigmine (see Figure 92).

Neuromuscular blockade takes place in the following sequence: rapidly contracting muscles (eyes, fingers, and toes) followed by slowly contracting muscles (diaphragm, limbs, and trunk). The onset and duration of action of succinylcholine are 1 and 5 minutes, respectively. The onset and duration of action of tubocurarine are 5 and 20 minutes, respectively.

The skeletal muscle relaxants have quaternary ammonium groups, are ionized at the physiologic pH, and are highly water soluble. They have a limited volume of distribution and do

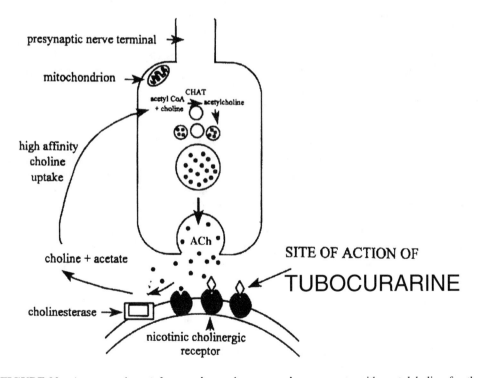

FIGURE 92 Agents such as **tubocurarine** and **pancuronium** compete with acetylcholine for the cholinergic receptors at the end plate. They combine with the receptors but do not activate them. Competitive or nondepolarizing agents are antagonized by neostigmine.

not readily cross the placenta or blood-brain barrier. After intravenous administration, their concentration rises and then falls rapidly.

Antiarrhythmic agents such as quinidine, procainamide, and propranolol have been shown to augment d-tubocurarine-induced blockade. Quinidine has also been reported to unmask or worsen the symptoms of myasthenia gravis and to cause postoperative respiratory depression after the use of muscle relaxants.

Diuretics such as thiazides, ethacrynic acid, and furosemide intensify the effects of nonpolarizing muscle relaxants, possibly because of a diuresis-induced reduction in the volume of distribution and an associated electrolyte imbalance, such as hypokalemia.

The **local anesthetics** procaine and lidocaine enhance the neuromuscular block produced by nonpolarizing and depolarizing muscle relaxants.

Phenytoin has been shown to interfere with neuromuscular transmission, and the drug has been reported to exacerbate **myasthenia gravis. Lithium** augments the effects of both depolarizing and nondepolarizing muscle relaxants and also reportedly unmasks myasthenia gravis.

Chlorpromazine has been shown to potentiate nondepolarizing relaxants The administration of steroids may lead to a transient worsening of symptoms in patients with myasthenia gravis, but the mechanism by which they interfere with neuromuscular transmission is unknown. The antagonism of pancuronium-induced blockade by **hydrocortisone** has also been reported. **d-Penicillamine**, which is used in the treatment of **Wilson's disease**, may cause a myasthenia gravis-like syndrome. These patients have elevated serum levels of antibody to acetylcholine receptors, suggesting that an immunologic mechanism is involved in this drug-induced syndrome. **Azathioprine** antagonizes nondepolarizing neuromuscular blockade, possibly by inhibiting phosphodiesterase.

Calcium ions play an important role in the presynaptic release of acetylcholine, and prolonged neuromuscular blockade has been reported after calcium antagonist administration during anesthesia that includes concurrent nondepolarizing neuromuscular blockade. **Ketamine** potentiates neuromuscular blockade produced by tubocurarine but not that produced by succinylcholine.

All of the inhalational agents augment both the degree and duration of the neuromuscular blockade induced by the nondepolarizing muscle relaxants. Possible mechanisms by which they exert their effect include depression of the central nervous system, presynaptic inhibition of acetylcholine mobilization and release, postsynaptic receptor desensitization, or an action imposed on the muscle at some point distal to the cholinergic receptor.

The generation of **action potentials** by muscle and nerve results from changes in the conductance of their membranes to sodium and potassium, and normal neuromuscular function depends on the maintenance of the correct ratio between intracellular and extracellular ionic concentrations.

An acute decrease in the extracellular **potassium** concentration tends to elevate the **end-plate transmembrane potential**, causing hyperpolarization and an increased resistance to depolarization, together with a greater sensitivity to the nondepolarizing muscle relaxants. Conversely, an increased extracellular potassium concentration lowers the resting end-plate transmembrane potential and thereby partially depolarizes the membrane, which should augment the effects of the depolarizing agents and oppose the action of the nondepolarizing drugs. Diuretic-induced chronic hypokalemia reduces the pancuronium requirements for neuromuscular blockade, and thus more neostigmine is required to achieve antagonism.

The release of **acetylcholine** from the **motor nerve terminal** is also affected by calcium and magnesium ion concentrations, which have opposing effects. **Calcium** increases the quantal release of acetylcholine from the nerve terminal, decreases the sensitivity of the postjunctional membrane to transmitter, and enhances the excitation-contraction coupling mechanisms of muscle. In contrast, **magnesium** decreases acetylcholine release and reduces the sensitivity of the postjunctional membrane to acetylcholine. Consequently, the action of the nondepolarizing muscle relaxants can be accentuated by low calcium and high magnesium levels. In addition, magnesium augments the block produced by depolarizing relaxants. Therefore, the dose of a muscle relaxant should be reduced in patients who have **toxemia** associated with **pregnancy** and are undergoing magnesium replacement therapy.

Respiratory acidosis enhances d-tubocurarine- and pancuronium-induced neuromuscular block and opposes reversal by neostigmine.

Hypothermia prolongs the neuromuscular blockade produced by d-tubocurarine and pancuronium.

The plasma concentrations of d-tubocurarine and pancuronium are increased in patients with impaired liver function because liver disease interferes with the metabolism of pancuronium.

Neonates are more sensitive to nondepolarizing muscle relaxants, and the response of the small infant to some extent resembles that of an adult patient with myasthenia gravis.

Although the main site of action of the neuromuscular blocking agents is the nicotinic receptor of striated muscle, they may act at other cholinergic receptor sites throughout the body, such as the **nicotinic receptors** in the autonomic ganglia and the **muscarinic receptors** in the heart.

Succinylcholine may cause tachycardia, cardiac arrhythmias, and hypertension, which is brought about by stimulation of the sympathetic ganglia. It may also provoke bradycardia, caused by stimulation of muscarinic receptor sites in the sinus node of the heart. This effect is more pronounced following a second dose of succinylcholine. The bradycardia may be blocked by thiopental, atropine, and ganglionic blocking agents.

Succinylcholine increases **intraocular pressure** transiently. It can also cause muscle pain, which may be due to fasciculation and uncoordinated muscle contraction. The prior administration of a competitive blocking agent may prevent both fasciculation and pain.

Patients with **myotonia congenita** and **myotonia dystrophica** respond differently to succinylcholine, in that their muscles are contracted rather than relaxed.

Tubocurarine, metocurine, and **succinylcholine** have all been shown to elicit histamine release in humans. However, histamine release is less common with **pancuronium** and **alcuronium. Vecuronium** does not cause histamine release.

TYPHOID VACCINE

This bacterial vaccine is used for primary immunization (exposure to typhoid carrier or plans to travel to an area endemic for typhoid fever).

U

UNDECYLENIC ACID

(Desenex)

Undecylenic acid is available as a foam, ointment, cream, powder, soap, and liquid, all administered topically. It is indicated as an antifungal and antibacterial agent for tinea pedis (athlete's foot), exclusive of the nails and hairy areas. Also recommended for the relief and prevention of diaper rash, itching, burning and chafing, prickly heat, tinea cruris (jock itch), excessive perspiration, and irritation in the groin area and bromhidrosis.

Zinc undecylenate is marketed in combination with other ingredients. The zinc provides an astringent action that aids in the suppression of inflammation. Compound undecylenic acid ointment contains both undecylenic acid (about 5%) and zinc undecylenate (about 20%). Calcium undecylenate (Caldesene, Cruex) is available as a powder. At best, the clinical "cure" rate is about 50% and is thus much lower than that obtained with the imidazoles, haloprogin, or tolnaftate.

UPPER RESPIRATORY TRACT INFECTION: TREATMENT OF						
		Haemophilus influenzae		Moraxella catarrhalis		Group A β-hemolytic streptococci
	Streptococcus pneumoniae	β-Lactamase		β-Lactamase		
Antibiotic*		Negative	Positive	Negative	Positive	
Ampicillin	+	+	−	+	−	+
Amoxicillin	+	+	−	+	−	+
Erythromycin-sulfisoxazole	+	+	+	+	+	+
Trimethoprim-sulfamethoxazole	+	+	+	+	−	−
Amoxicillin/clavulanate	+	+	+	+	+	+
Cefaclor	+	+	+	+	±	+
Cefixime	+	+	+	+	+	+
Cefuroxime axetil	+	+	+	+	+	+
* Spectrum of activity						

URACIL MUSTARD

Uracil mustard, an alkylating agent with antineoplastic activity (1 to 2 mg p.o. daily for three months), is indicated for the treatment of chronic lymphocytic and myelocytic leukemia; Hodgkin's disease, non-Hodgkin's lymphomas of the histiocytic and lymphocytic types; reticulum cell sarcoma; lymphomas; mycosis fungoides; polycythemia vera; ovarian, cervical, and lung cancer.

URAPIDIL

Urapidil is an alpha$_1$-adrenoreceptor antagonist that also has a central antihypertensive effect. Its plasma half-life is about 5 hours. Urapidil reduces peripheral resistance and has no significant effect on cardiac output; there is no reflex tachycardia. Comparative clinical studies have shown that urapidil (30 to 90 mg/day) and acebutalol (200 to 400 mg/day) were effective in lowering blood pressure by about the same amount, but acebutalol significantly reduced heart rate, while urapidil did not. Urapidil causes arteriolar vasodilation and may have some venous dilator effects. The hypotensive action of urapidil results from blockade of vascular postsynaptic alpha$_1$-adrenoreceptors, and a central hypotensive effect occurs by a mechanism not yet completely elucidated but which appears to be unrelated to alpha-adrenoreceptors. The central mechanism is not the same as that of clonidine and other alpha$_2$-adrenoreceptor antagonists, and appears to be unrelated to activity at central alpha$_2$- or alpha$_1$-adrenoreceptors or at histamine (H$_1$ and H$_2$), dopamine (DA$_2$), muscarine (M$_1$), serotonin (5-HT$_2$), or opioid receptors. It is possible that some central 5-HT$_{1A}$ antagonist activity occurs, but the pharmacologic implications of this are not clear.

UREA

(Carbamide, Ureaphil)

Urea, an osmotic diuretic (1 to 1.5 g/kg as a 30% solution given by slow IV infusion over two hours) is indicated for reducing intracranial or intraocular pressure. The osmotic diuretics and related agents consist of **mannitol** (Osmitrol), **glycerin** (Glycerol, Osmoglyn), and **isosorbide** (Hydronol). Mannitol and urea are nonelectrolytes that are freely filterable and undergo very little or no metabolism or renal tubular resorption. When given in sufficient quantities, these drugs increase the osmolarity of plasma and the amount of both the glomerular filtrate and the renal tubular fluid. The presence of such a drug in the lumen prevents the resorption of much of the water, hence the urine volume is increased. They do not prevent the active resorption of sodium from the tubular fluid, but some additional sodium is excreted as a normal constituent of the increased volume of urine. Osmotic diuretics are not effective in removing the edematous fluid caused by sodium retention, but can maintain the flow of urine even when the GFR is decreased. Osmotic diuretics are given by intravenous infusion in a hypertonic solution, and they are excreted by glomerular filtration.

The osmotic diuretics may be used for any of the following conditions:

- In congestive glaucoma, to reduce intraocular pressure
- In neurosurgery, to reduce the pressure and volume of cerebrospinal fluid and hence decrease the intracranial pressure
- In acute renal failure, to maintain urine flow
- In drug poisoning, to prevent nephrotoxicity

These agents should not be used in edematous states associated with diminished cardiac reserve, because any increase in the extracellular fluid volume constitutes a hazard.

URINARY TRACT INFECTIONS: TREATMENT OF	
ORAL THERAPY	
Sulfonamides	
Trimethoprim-sulfamethoxazole	
Penicillins	
Ampicillin	Amoxicillin-clavulanic acid
Amoxicillin	Carbenicillin indanyl
Cephalosporins	
Cephalexin	Cefadroxil
Cephradine	Cefuroxime
Cefaclor	Cefixime

Tetracyclines	
Tetracycline Doxycycline	Oxytetracycline Minocycline
Quinolones	
Nalidixic acid Oxolinic acid Cinoxacin	Ciprofloxacin Norfloxacin Ofloxacin
Nitrofurantoin	
Methenamine hippurate Methenamine mandelate	
PARENTERAL THERAPY	
Aminoglycosides	
Gentamicin Tobramycin	Amikacin Netilmicin
Penicillins	
Ampicillin Carbenicillin Ticarcillin	Mezlocillin Piperacillin
Cephalosporins	**Imipenem/cilastatin**
First, second, and third generation	Aztreonam

UROKINASE

(Abbokinase)

Urokinase, a thrombolytic enzyme (4,400 IU/kg over 10 minutes following by 4,400 IU/kg hourly), is indicated for lysis of acute massive pulmonary emboli and of pulmonary emboli accompanied by unstable hemodynamics. In addition, urokinase (6,000 IU/minute of urokinase intraarterial via a coronary artery catheter) is indicated for the treatment of coronary artery thrombosis. Urokinase is a two-chain serine protease containing 411 amino acid residues. It is also isolated from cultured human kidney cells. It has a half-life of 15 to 20 minutes and is metabolized by the liver.

Like streptokinase, it lacks fibrin specificity and therefore readily induces a systemic lytic state. **Saruplase** (prourokinase; single-chain urokinase) does display selectivity for clots by binding to fibrin before activation.

Urokinase is contraindicated in patients with ulcerative wounds, active internal bleeding, and recent trauma with possible internal injuries, pregnancy and the first 10 days postpartum, ulcerative colitis, diverticulitis, severe hypertension, acute or chronic hepatic or renal insufficiency, uncontrolled hypocoagulation, chronic pulmonary disease with cavitation, subacute bacterial endocarditis or rheumatic valvular disease and recent cerebral embolism, thrombosis, or hemorrhage, or diabetic hemorrhagic retinopathy, because of the potential for excessive bleeding.

Concomitant use with anticoagulants may cause hemorrhage; heparin must be stopped and its effects allowed to diminish. It may also be necessary to reverse effects of oral anticoagulants before beginning therapy. Concomitant use with aspirin, indomethacin, phenylbutazone, or other drugs affecting platelet activity increases the risk of bleeding.

Aminocaproic acid inhibits urokinase-induced activation of plasminogen (see Figure 35).

URSODIOL

(Ursodeoxycholic Acid) (Actigall)

Ursodiol, a bile acid with gallstone stabilizing properties (8 to 10 mg/kg/day), is used for dissolution of radiolucent gallbladder stones and to increase the flow of bile in patients with bile duct prosthesis or stents.

UVEITIS: MANAGEMENT OF

Inflammation of the uveal tract has many causes and may involve one or all three portions simultaneously, as in sarcoidosis. The most frequent form of uveitis is acute anterior uveitis (iritis), usually unilateral and characterized by a history of pain, photophobia, and blurring of vision; a red eye (circumcorneal flush) without purulent discharge; and a small or irregular pupil.

The treatment of uveitis includes reduction of inflammation, relief of symptoms, and an attempt to restore or preserve vision. Idiopathic uveitis (autoimmune) requires the systemic administration of corticosteroids, cyclosporin, and cytotoxic agents.

The arsenal of immunosuppressive agents available for the treatment of uveitis has expanded recently to include: **tacrolimus, sirolimus** (rapamycin), and **mycophenolate mofetil**.

V

VAGINAL CANDIDIASIS: TREATMENT OF	
Drugs	**Formulations**
Butoconazole	2% cream
Clotrimazole	
Gyne-Lotrimin (OTC)	100 mg vaginal tablet 1% cream
Mycelex-G	100 mg vaginal tablet 500 mg vaginal tablet 1% cream
Miconazole	
Monistat-7	2% cream 100 mg vaginal suppository
Monistat-3	200 mg vaginal suppository
Nystatin	
Mycostatin	100,000 U vaginal tablet
Nilstat	100,000 U vaginal tablet
Terconazole	
Terazol-7	0.4% cream
Terazol-3	80 mg vaginal suppository or 0.8% cream
Tioconazole	
Vagistat	6.5% ointment
All regimens of topical antifungal drugs are safe and effective for most patients with vulvovaginal candidiasis. Burning and itching can occur with all of the topical antifungal drugs used for vaginal candidiasis. Other adverse effects include contact dermatitis, irritation, vulval edema, dysuria, and dyspareunia.	

VALACICLOVIR

Acyclovir was the first antiherpetic agent to selectively inhibit herpes virus replication while maintaining an excellent safety profile, and currently constitutes the standard therapy for the management of herpes virus infections. Research to improve the oral bioavailability of acyclovir has resulted in the development of its L-valyl ester, valaciclovir. Oral valaciclovir is rapidly and extensively converted to acyclovir, substantially increasing acyclovir bioavailability, and thus it has the potential for improved efficacy and more convenient dosing than oral acyclovir (see also Figure 3).

VALPROIC ACID
(Depakote)

Valproic acid, a broad-spectrum anticonvulsant, (initially 15 mg/kg/day p.o.), is indicated as a sole and adjunctive therapy in simple (petit mal) and complex absence seizures. Also, it is used adjunctively in patients with multiple seizure types including absence seizures.

In addition, valproic acid has shown effectiveness against myoclonic and grand mal seizures, and possibly against atonic, complex partial, and infantile spasm seizures. Moreover, it has been used effectively in preventing recurrent febrile seizures in children and in treating rapidly cycling bipolar affective disorders. The mechanism of action of valproic acid has been postulated to be its enhancement of GABAergic transmission (see Figure 96). Valproic acid is rapidly absorbed orally, rapidly distributed, and highly bound (90%) to plasma proteins, primarily albumin. Increases in dose may decrease protein binding. Significantly reduced plasma protein binding has occurred in renal insufficiency, cirrhosis, and acute viral hepatitis. The drug is primarily metabolized in the liver and is excreted as the glucuronide. Elimination of valproic acid and its metabolites occurs principally in the urine. Very little unmetabolized drug is excreted in the urine and feces.

Chlorpromazine, cimetidine, and salicylates decrease the clearance of valproic acid and increase its half-life. Addition of valproic acid to phenobarbital may result in an increased phenobarbital level and an increase in CNS effects.

The side effects of valproic acid are gastrointestinal in nature, consisting of transient and inconsequential nausea and vomiting. In addition, sedation occurs (50%), especially when the drug is taken in combination with phenobarbital. Additional rare side effects include hepatic toxicity, pancreatitis, alopecia, and hematologic problems.

Hepatic failure resulting in fatalities has occurred in patients receiving valproic acid and its derivatives. Children <2 years of age are at considerable increased risk of developing fatal hepatotoxicity, especially those on multiple anticonvulsants, those with congenital metabolic disorders, those with severe seizure disorders accompanied by mental retardation, and those with organic brain disease.

VANADIUM

Vanadium is a transition metal found in relative abundance in nature. It can readily change its oxidation state and take an anionic or a cationic form. Vanadium has insulin-like effects in that it induces a sustained fall in blood glucose level in insulin-dependent animals. Recent short-term trials with vanadium salts seem promising in Type II (noninsulin-dependent) diabetic patients in whom liver and peripheral insulin resistance was attenuated, indicating the therapeutic potential of vanadium salts.

VANCOMYCIN
(Vancocin)

Vancomycin (500 mg IV q. 6 hours) is indicated for the treatment of severe staphylococcal infections, when other antibiotics are ineffective or contraindicated. Vancomycin (125 to 500 mg p.o. q. 6 hours for 7 to 10 days) is indicated for the treatment of antibiotic-associated pseudomembranous and staphylococcal enterocolitis; and vancomycin (1 g IV given slowly over 1 hour, starting 1 hour before procedure) is indicated for endocarditis prophylaxis for dental, GI, biliary, and genitourinary instrumentation procedures; and as surgical prophylaxis in patients allergic to penicillin. It is indicated in the treatment of serious or severe infections not treatable with other antimicrobials, including the penicillins and cephalosporins (see Figure 93).

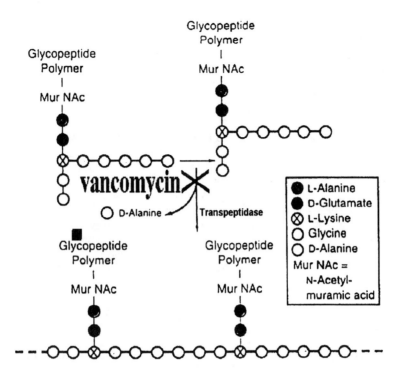

FIGURE 93 Vancomycin, a bactericidal antibiotic, inhibits cell wall synthesis in Gram-positive bacteria. It is effective against methicillin-resistant organisms and as an alternate to semisynthetic penicillins or cephalosporins in patients with severe staphylococcal infections.

Vancomycin is an antibiotic produced by *Streptococcus orientalis,* an actinomycete isolated from soil samples. Other glycopeptide antimicrobial agents, **daptomycin** and **teicoplanin**, are available. Vancomycin is primarily active against Gram-positive bacteria. *Staph. aureus* and *Staph. epidermidis*, including strains resistant to methicillin, are usually inhibited by concentrations of 1.0 to 5.0 microgram/ml. Synergism between vancomycin and gentamicin or tobramycin occurs against *S. aureus*, including methicillin-resistant strains. *Strep. pyogenes, Strep. pneumoniae*, and viridans streptococci are highly susceptible, as are most strains of *Enterococcus* spp. Vancomycin is not generally bactericidal for *Enterococcus* spp., and the addition of a synergistic aminoglycoside is necessary to produce a bactericidal effect. *Corynebacterium* spp. (diphtheroids) are inhibited by less than 0.04 to 3.1 microgram/ml of vancomycin; most species of Actinomyces by 5 to 10 microgram/ml; and *Clostridium* spp. by 0.39 to 6 microgram/ml. Vancomycin inhibits the synthesis of the cell wall in sensitive bacteria by binding with high affinity to the D-alanyl-D-alanine terminus of cell wall precursor units (Figure 93). The drug is rapidly bactericidal for dividing microorganisms.

Vancomycin has caused reversible neutropenia, nephrotoxicity, hypotension (rapid bolus injection), and pseudomembranous colitis (rare). The concomitant use of vancomycin with aminoglycosides increases the risk of nephrotoxicity. Vancomycin potentiates the neuromuscular blocking effects of nondepolarizing skeletal muscle relaxants such as *d*-tubocurarine.

VARICELLA-ZOSTER IMMUNE GLOBULIN
(VZIG)

This immune substance is used for passive immunization of susceptible patients, primarily immunocompromised patients after exposure to varicella (chicken pox or herpes zoster).

TABLE 26
Classification of Vasodilators by Peripheral Site of Action

Sites of Action	Agents
Venodilators	Nitrates/nitroglycerin (low dose)
	Molsidomine
Arterial dilators	Hydralazine, dihydralazine, endralazine
	Minoxidil
	Calcium antagonists
	Phentolamine
	Fenoldopam
Balanced-type vasodilators	Prazosin, trimazosin
	Nitrates/nitroglycerin (high dose)
	Angiotensin-converting enzyme inhibitors
	Phosphodiesterase inhibitors
	Nitroprusside
	Flosequinan

VASODILATORS

The vasodilators may be classified as **ventodilators, arterial dilators,** or **balanced-type vasodilators** (Table 26).

The rationale for vasodilation in the management of congestive heart failure is based on the increased arteriolar vasotone that occurs. This initiates a vicious circle in which cardiac function is further depressed by an increase in afterload and in resistance to ejection.

Vascular tone is regulated by the cytosolic calcium level, the interaction of calcium and calmodulin with myosin light-chain kinase, and the subsequent myosin light-chain phosphorylation, which promotes the interaction of myosin with actin and finally leads to contraction.

Receptor-dependent vasodilation may also take place in a more indirect way through the presynaptic modulation of the release of neurotransmitters such as norepinephrine and acetylcholine. In addition to its effects on postsynaptic receptors, norepinephrine stimulates the presynaptic alpha$_2$-receptor, thereby inhibiting further transmitter release. Moreover, the activation of other presynaptic receptors such as the muscarinic cholinergic, dopaminergic, purinergic, serotoninergic, and histaminergic receptors leads to diminished norepinephrine release and subsequent vasodilation.

A number of vasodilators, such as acetylcholine, bradykinin, adenine nucleosides, thrombin, histamine, or serotonin, need an **intact vascular endothelium** in order to exert their effects. For example, stimulation of endothelial cholinergic receptors cause the release of **endothelium-derived relaxing factors (EDRF)**, which may involve arachidonic acid formation and compartmentalization via the lipoxygenase pathway. EDRF, which is identical to **nitric oxide**, activates guanylate cyclase and enhances the formation of cyclic guanosine monophosphate (cyclic GMP) in smooth muscle. Tetranoic acid (a vasoconstrictor), thromboxane A$_2$ (a vasoconstrictor), and prostacycline (a vasodilator) are formed through the lipoxygenase pathway.

The vasodilating properties of captopril or hydralazine (antihypertensive agents) are mediated by the formation of EDRF or prostaglandin, or both. On the other hand, the vasodilating properties of nitroprusside (an antihypertensive agent) result directly from the formation of cyclic GMP (see also Figures 19, 34, and 62).

VASODILATORS: EFFECTS ON CARDIAC OUTPUT (CO)	
Drugs	**CO**
Venous vasodilators	
Isosorbide dinitrate	0/+
Arterial vasodilators	
Hydralazine	+
Minoxidil	+
Nifedipine	+
Diltiazem	+
Mixed arterial-venous vasodilators	
Prazosin	+
Captopril	+
Enalapril	+
Lisinopril	+
Abbreviations: + = increase; − = decrease; 0 = no change	

VASOPRESSIN

(Pitressin)

The second hormone that originates from the posterior pituitary gland is **antidiuretic hormone**, or **vasopressin**. It has the following amino acid sequence.

$$\begin{array}{c} \text{Gln–Asn–Cys–Pro–Arg–Gly} \\ \quad\quad\quad | \quad\quad\quad | \\ \text{Phe------Tyr} \end{array}$$

With the exception of two amino acids, vasopressin resembles oxytocin in structure. Oxytocin contains leucine and isoleucine, and vasopressin contains phenylalanine and arginine. The sites of synthesis, storage, and release of vasopressin are identical to those described for oxytocin. Many agents alter the secretion or action of vasopressin, and these are listed in Figure 94.

The loss of the neurosecretory neurons that make up the neurohypophysis eliminates the secretion of vasopressin, and this produces diabetes insipidus. Some of the various causes of **neurogenic diabetes insipidus** are:

Acquired
Idiopathic
Trauma (accidental or surgical)
Tumor (craniopharyngioma, metastasis, or lymphoma)
Granuloma (sarcoid or histiocytosis)
Infectious (meningitis or encephalitis)
Vascular (Sheehan's syndrome, aneurysm, or aortocoronary bypass)
Familial (autosomal dominant)

Another form of diabetes insipidus is a vasopressin-insensitive or **nephrogenic diabetes insipidus,** and it stems from the following causes:

Acquired
Infectious (pyelonephritis)
Postobstructive (prostatic or ureteral)

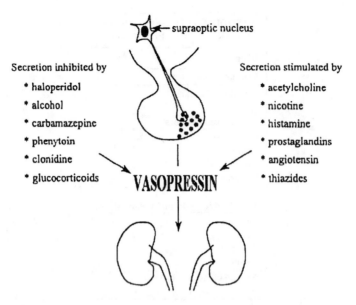

FIGURE 94   Many agents alter the secretion or actions of vasopressin.

    Vascular (sickle cell disease or trait)
    Infiltrative (amyloid)
    Cystic (polycystic disease)
    Metabolic (hypokalemia or hypercalcemia)
    Granuloma (sarcoid)
    Toxic (lithium, demeclocycline, or methoxyflurane)
    Solute overload (glucosuria or postobstructive)
Familial (X-linked recessive)

Agents that cause the **syndrome of inappropriate antidiuretic secretion** consist of:

    Carbamazepine
    Chlorpropamide
    Clofibrate
    Cyclophosphamide
    Haloperidol
    Monoamine oxidase inhibitors
    Nicotine
    Oxytocin
    Phenothiazine derivatives
    Thiazide diuretics
    Tricyclic antidepressants
    Vincristine

Vasopressin may be administered either subcutaneously or intramuscularly. It has a duration of action of 2 to 8 hours. Vasopressin tannate (Pitressin tannate) is a suspension and should be injected intramuscularly only. It has a duration of action of 2 to 3 days. **Desmopressin acetate** (DDAVP) is used topically. **Lypressin** (Diapid) is administered as an intranasal spray. All these agents may be used in the treatment of central diabetes insipidus (vasopressin sensitive).

VENLAFAXINE HYDROCHLORIDE

(Effexor)

Venlafaxine, an antidepressant blocking the uptake of serotonin, dopamine, and norepineph-rine (75 mg p.o. daily), is used in the treatment of depression. Venlafaxine has no significant affinity for muscarinic cholinergic, histaminergic, or alpha$_1$-adrenergic receptors. Venlafaxine is as efficacious as tricyclic antidepressants and trazodone; however, because it has fewer side effects, it is better tolerated (see Tables 3 through 5).

VERAPAMIL HYDROCHLORIDE

(Calan, Calan SR, Isoptin, Isoptin SR, Verelan)

Verapamil (80 mg p.o. q. 6 to 8 hours) is indicated in the management of Prinzmetal's or variant angina or unstable or chronic, stable angina pectoris; **verapamil** (0.075 to 0.15 mg/kg IV push over a two-minute period) is indicated in the treatment of supraventricular tachy-arrhythmias; **verapamil** (240 to 480 mg p.o. daily) is indicated in the prevention of recurrent paroxysmal supraventricular tachycardia; **verapamil** (240 to 320 mg p.o. daily) is indicated in the control of ventricular rate in digitalized patients with chronic atrial flutter and/or fibrillation; and **verapamil** (80 mg p.o. t.i.d.) is indicated in the management of hypertension.

Verapamil blocks both activated and inactivated calcium channels. Thus, its effect is more marked in tissues that fire frequently, those that are less completely polarized at rest, and those in which activation depends exclusively on the calcium current, such as the sinoatrial and atrioventricular nodes. It is therefore not surprising that verapamil has marked effects on these tissues. Atrioventricular nodal conduction and effective refractory period are invariably prolonged by therapeutic concentrations. Verapamil usually slows the sinoatrial node by its direct action, but its hypotensive action may occasionally result in a small reflex increase of sinoatrial nodal rate (Figure 95).

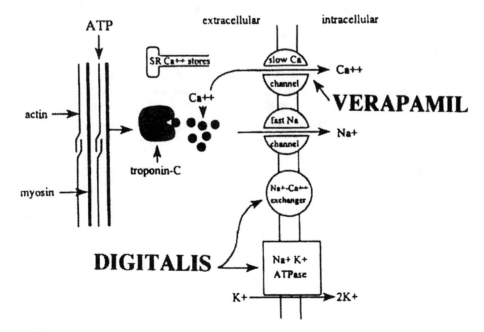

FIGURE 95 Verapamil is used in the management of Prinzmetal's or variant angina. ATP = adenosine triphosphate; SR = sarcoplasmic reticulum.

Verapamil can suppress both early and delayed depolarizations and may antagonize slow responses arising in severely depolarized tissue.

Verapamil causes peripheral vasodilation, which may be beneficial in hypertension and peripheral vasospastic disorders. Its effects upon smooth muscle produce a number of extra-cardiac effects (see Figure 95 Table 20).

Verapamil's cardiotoxic effects are dose-related and usually avoidable. A common error has been to administer intravenous verapamil to a patient with ventricular tachycardia misdiagnosed as supraventricular tachycardia. In this setting, hypotension and ventricular fibrillation can occur.

Verapamil's negative inotropic effects may limit its clinical usefulness in damaged hearts. Verapamil can lead to atrioventricular block when used in large doses or in patients with partial atrioventricular block. This block can be treated with atropine, beta receptor stimulants, or calcium. In patients with sinus node disease, verapamil can precipitate sinus arrest.

Verapamil is absorbed rapidly and completely from the GI tract after oral administration; however, only about 20 to 35% of the drug reaches systemic circulation because of the first-pass effect. Verapamil is N-methylated to norverapamil, which is an active metabolite. The half-lives of calcium blocking agents increase in hepatic cirrhosis and in older patients.

Verapamil is contraindicated in patients with severe hypotension (systolic blood pressure below 90 mmHg) of cardiogenic shock, because of the drug's hypotensive effect; in patients with second- or third-degree AV block or sick sinus syndrome (unless a functioning artificial ventricular pacemaker is in place), because of the drug's effects on the cardiac conduction system; in patients with severe left ventricular dysfunction (indicated by pulmonary wedge pressure above 20 mmHg and left ventricular ejection fraction below 20%), unless heart failure results from supraventricular tachycardia, because the drug may worsen the condition in patients with ventricular dysfunction or AV abnormalities who are receiving beta-adrenergic blocks, because of the drug's negative inotropic effect and inhibition of the cardiac conduction system.

Concomitant use of verapamil with adrenergic receptor **beta blockers** may cause additive effects leading to congestive heart failure, conduction disturbances, arrhythmias, and hypotension.

Concomitant use of oral verapamil with **digoxin** may increase serum digoxin concentration by 50 to 75% during the first week of therapy. Concomitant use with antihypertensives may lead to combined antihypertensive effects, resulting in clinically significant hypotension. Concomitant use with drugs that attenuate alpha-adrenergic response (such as prazosin and methyldopa) may cause excessive blood pressure reduction. Concomitant use with **disopyramide** may cause combined negative inotropic effects. Use with **quinidine** to treat hypertrophic cardiomyopathy may cause excessive hypotension; with **carbamazepine** may cause increased serum carbamazepine levels and subsequent toxicity; with **rifampin** may substantially reduce verapamil's oral bioavailability. Verapamil therapy may inhibit the clearance and increase the plasma levels of **theophylline**. Overdosage of verapamil causes heart block asystole and hypotension.

VERCURONIUM BROMIDE

(Norcuron)

Vercuronium, a nondepolarizing neuromuscular blocking agent (0.08 to 0.10 mg/kg IV), is indicated as an adjunct to anesthesia to facilitate intubation and to provide skeletal muscle relaxation during surgery or mechanical ventilation. Vercuronium prevents acetylcholine from binding to receptors on the motor endplate, thus blocking depolarization. Vercuronium exhibits minimal cardiovascular effects and does not appear to alter heart rate or rhythm, systolic or diastolic blood pressure, cardiac output, systemic vascular resistance, or mean arterial pressure. It has little or no histamine-releasing properties (see also Figure 92).

Vercuronium is an intermediate-acting nondepolarizing muscle relaxant. It has a wide margin of safety and does not produce undesirable hemodynamic effects. Its onset of action is similar to atracurium's but not as short as succinylcholine's.

VIDARABINE
(Adenine Arabinoside; ARA-A)

Vidarabine, an antiviral agent (10 to 15 mg/kg/day for 5 to 10 days), is indicated for the treatment of herpes simplex virus encephalitis, neonatal herpes simplex virus infections, and herpes zoster in immunosuppressed patients. In addition, vidarabine (ophthalmic ointment: 3% vidarabine monohydrate [equivalent to 2.8% vidarabine]) is indicated in the treatment of acute keratoconjunctivitis and recurrent epithelial keratitis due to herpes simplex virus types 1 and 2, or superficial keratitis caused by herpes simplex virus which has not responded to topical idoxuridine or when toxic or hypersensitivity reactions to idoxuridine have occurred.

Vidarabine is an inhibitor of viral DNA synthesis. Cellular enzymes phosphorylate vidarabine to the triphosphate, which inhibits viral DNA polymerase activity in a manner that is competitive with deoxyadenosine triphosphate. Vidarabine triphosphate is incorporated into both cellular and viral DNA, where it may act as a chain terminator. Vidarabine triphosphate also inhibits ribonucleoside reductase, RNA polyadenylation, and S-adenosylhomocysteine hydrolase, RNA polyadenylation, and S-adenosylhomocysteine hydrolase (SAHH), an enzyme involved in transmethylation reactions. Resistant variants due to mutations in viral DNA polymerase can be selected *in vitro*.

The main metabolite, arabinosyl hypoxanthine (Ara-Hx) has approximately 1/20 the activity of vidarabine. In renal impairment, the excretion of Ara-Hx is decreased requiring dose adjustment. Allopurinol, a xanthine oxidase inhibitor, may interfere with the metabolism of vidarabine (see also Figure 5).

Vidarabine has caused nausea, vomiting, anorexia, diarrhea; decreased reticulocytes, hemoglobin, hematocrit, WBC, and platelets; and tremor, dizziness, headache, hallucinations, confusion, psychosis, and ataxia. These side effects are more pronounced in patients with impaired hepatic or renal functions.

VIGABATRIN
(VGB, Sabril)

Vigabatrin is a new antiepileptic drug used for treatment of partial and secondarily generalized tonic-clonic seizures. Vigabatrin acts as an irreversible substrate for GABA transaminase that leads to elevated brain GABA levels. Adverse effects on the nervous system include drowsiness and fatigue, primarily during the first weeks of treatment (Figure 96).

VINBLASTINE
(VLB)

Vinblastine (initially 3.7 mg/m^2) is indicated in the treatment of frequently responsive malignancies such as generalized Hodgkin's disease (stages III and IV, Ann Arbor modification of the Rye staging system) and lymphocytic lymphoma (nodular and diffuse, poorly differentiated); histiocytic lymphoma; mycosis fungoides (advanced stages); advanced testicular

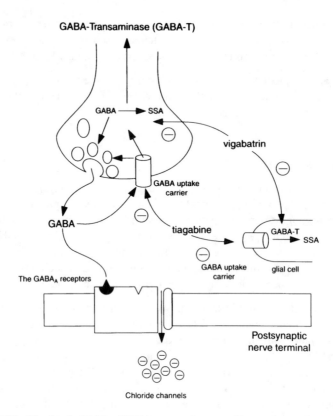

FIGURE 96   Vigabatrin inhibits GABA transaminase and has anticonvulsant properties.

carcinoma; Kaposi's sarcoma, and Letterer-Siwe disease (histiocytosis X). Less frequently, the drug is used in responsive malignancies such as choriocarcinoma resistant to other chemotherapy and breast cancer unresponsive to surgery and hormonal therapy.

Vinblastine is an alkaloid derived from vinca rosea, the periwinkle plant. Its mechanism of action involves depolymerization of microtubules, which are an important part of the cytoskeleton and the mitotic spindle. The drug binds specifically to the microtubular protein tubulin in dimeric form; the drug–tubulin complex joins to the forming end of the microtubules to terminate assembly, and depolymerization of the microtubules then occurs. This results in mitotic arrest at metaphase, dissolution of the mitotic spindle, and interference with chromosome segregation.

The combination of vinblastine and mitomycin C has caused shortness of breath and bronchospasm. Vinblastine reduces the level and hence the effectiveness of phenytoin requiring increased dosage. Vinblastine produces nausea and vomiting and marrow depression as well as alopecia (see Figure 2).

VINCA ALKALOIDS

The vinca alkaloids (vinblastine, vincristine, and vindesine), which bind to tubulin, block mitosis with metaphase arrest. Vinca alkaloids are used for the following types of cancer:

Acute lymphoid leukemia. In the induction phase, vincristine is used with prednisone.
Acute myelomonocytic or monocytic leukemia. Cytarabine, vincristine, and prednisone.
Hodgkin's disease. Mechlorethamine, Oncovin (vincristine), procarbazine, and prednisone (MOPP).

Nodular lymphoma. Cyclophosphamide, Oncovin (vincristine), and prednisone (CVP).

Diffuse histiocytic lymphoma. Cyclophosphamide, Adriamycin (doxorubicin), vincristine, and prednisone (CHOP); bleomycin, Adriamycin (doxorubicin), cyclophosphamide, Oncovin (vincristine), and prednisone (BACOP); or cyclophosphamide, Oncovin (vincristine), methotrexate, and cytarabine (COMA).

Wilm's tumor. Dactinomycin and vincristine.

Ewings' sarcoma. Cyclophosphamide, dactinomycin, or vincristine.

Embryonal rhabdomyosarcoma. Cyclophosphamide, dactinomycin, or vincristine.

Bronchogenic carcinoma. Doxorubicin, cyclophosphamide, and vincristine.

The chief toxicity associated with vinblastine use is bone marrow depression. The toxicity of vincristine consists of paresthesia, neuritic pain, muscle weakness, and visual disturbances. In addition, both vinblastine and vincristine may cause alopecia (see Figure 2).

VINCRISTINE SULFATE
(VCR:LCR)

Vincristine (1.4 to 2.0 mg/m^2) is indicated in the treatment of acute leukemia and in combination therapy for Hodgkin's disease, non-Hodgkin's malignant lymphomas (lymphocytic, mixed-cell, histiocytic, undifferentiated, nodular, and diffuse types), rhabdomyosarcoma, neuroblastoma, and Wilm's tumor. In addition, vincristine has been used in the treatment of idiopathic thrombocytopenic purpura, Kaposi's sarcoma, breast cancer, and bladder cancer. The intrathecal administration of vincristine is fatal.

Vincristine is an alkaloid derived from vinca rosea, the periwinkle plant. Its mechanism of action involves depolymerization of microtubules, which are an important part of the cytoskeleton and the mitotic spindle. The drug binds specifically to the microtubular protein tubulin in dimeric form; the drug-tubulin complex adds to the forming end of the microtubules to terminate assembly, and depolymerization of the microtubules then occurs. This results in mitotic arrest at metaphase, dissolution of the mitotic spindle, and interference with chromosome segregation.

Within 15 to 30 minutes following IV administration, >90% of the drug is distributed from blood into tissue where it remains tightly, but not irreversibly, bound. Penetration across the blood-brain barrier is poor. The liver is the major excretory organ; about 80% of an injected dose appears in the feces, and 10 to 20% in the urine. Hepatic dysfunction may alter the elimination kinetics and augment toxicity, which limits its use to short courses. It occasionally produces bone marrow depression (see Figure 2).

VITAMINS: THEIR COENZYMATIC FUNCTIONS	
Fat-Soluble Vitamins	
A, retinol	Rhodopsin, visual cycle, night vision
K, menadiol	Blood clotting factors II, VII, IX, and X
D, calciferol	Calcium and phosphorous homeostasis
E, tocopherol	Antioxidant, glutathione oxidase
Water-Soluble Vitamins	
C, ascorbate	Antioxidant, regulation of intracellular oxidation-reduction potentials, hydroxylation reactions which require copper or iron
B$_1$, thiamin	Oxidative decarboxylation of amino acids, transketolase
B$_2$, riboflavin	Flavin mononucleotide and flavin adenine dinucleotide, essential for oxidative systems and oxygen transport

B$_3$, pantothenic acid	As CoA precursor, necessary for acyl transfers
B$_5$, niacin	Endogenous source for tryptophan; component of NAD and its phosphorylate, NADP; assists in hydrogen transfer of glycolysis, fatty acid synthesis, and tissue respiration
B$_6$, pyridoxine	Nitrogen metabolism: transamination, racemization, decarboxylation, cleavage, synthesis, dehydration, and desulfhydration
B$_{12}$, cyanocobalamin	Methylation of homocysteine to methionine, conversion of methyl malonyl CoA to succinyl CoA
Biotin	Cofactor for some carboxylases; acetyl CoA carboxylase, pyruvate carboxylase, β-methylcrotonyl carboxylase, and methylmalonyl carboxylase
Folic acid	Transport of single carbon fragments, especially nucleic acid synthesis and metabolism of some amino acids

VITAMINS

Vitamins are organic dietary substances necessary for the maintenance of normal metabolic function. Only small amounts of the vitamins are required for normal health. In the body, they act as components of the important enzyme systems which catalyze the reactions by which protein, fat, and carbohydrate are metabolized. Some of the vitamins (e.g., vitamin K) may be formed by bacteria in the gut, while vitamin D is synthesized by exposure of the skin to sunlight. With these exceptions, the vitamins must be ingested in the food, and restricted diets or disorders of the gastrointestinal tract, interfering with absorption, lead to vitamin deficiency. When pronounced, such deficiencies give rise to easily recognizable clinical syndromes (**beriberi, pellagra, rickets, scurvy**) which have long been recognized. Milder forms of avitaminosis are much more common and also give rise to disability and ill-health.

The fat-soluble vitamins are A, D, E, and K. The water-soluble vitamins are thiamine (vitamin B$_1$), riboflavin, nicotinic acid (niacin) and nicotinamide, pyridoxine (vitamin B$_6$), pantothenic acid, biotin, para-aminobenzoic acid, choline, inositol and other lipotropic agents, ascorbic acid (vitamin C), the riboflavonoids, folate, and vitamin B$_{12}$ (see Figures 97 and 98).

VITAMIN A
(Retinol) (Aquasol A)

Vitamin A, a fat-soluble vitamin, is indicated for severe vitamin A deficiency with xerophthalmia.

VITAMIN E
(Alpha Tocopherol) (Aquasole E, CEN-E, Eprolin Gelseas, Episilan-M, E-Vital, Pheryl-E 400, Tocopher-Caps, Vita-Plus E, Vitera E)

Vitamin E, a fat-soluble vitamin, is used in vitamin E deficiency in premature infants and in patients with impaired fat absorption (including patients with cystic fibrosis) and in biliary atresia.

VITAMIN K DERIVATIVES

MENADIOL SODIUM DIPHOSPHATE
(Synkayvite)

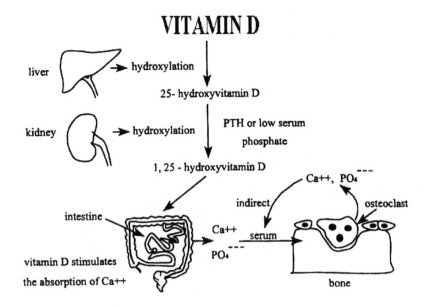

The activation of vitamin D and its action on calcium regulation

FIGURE 97 Vitamins D_3 and D_2 are produced by ultraviolet irradiation of animal skin and plants, respectively. The precursor of vitamin D_3 in skin is 7-dehydrocholesterol, or **provitamin D**. In humans, the storage, transport, metabolism, and potency of vitamins D_2 and D_3 are identical, and the net biologic activity of vitamin D *in vivo* results from the combined effects of the hydroxylated derivatives of vitamins D_2 and D_3.

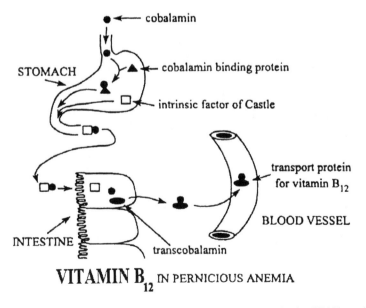

FIGURE 98 Both **vitamin B_{12}** and **folic acid** are essential for the synthesis of DNA, and this process is impaired in patients with megaloblastic anemia.

PHYTONADIONE

(Aquamephyton, Konakion, Mephyton)

Vitamin K derivatives are used in treating hypoprothrombinemia secondary to vitamin K malabsorption or drug therapy, or when oral administration is desired and bile secretion is inadequate; in hypoprothrombinemia secondary to vitamin K malabsorption, drug therapy, or excess vitamin A; hypoprothrombinemia secondary to the effect of oral anticoagulants; prevention of hemorrhagic disease in neonates; differentiation between hepatocellular disease or biliary obstruction as a source of hypoprothrombinemia; prevention of hypoprothrombinemia related to vitamin K deficiency in long-term parenteral nutrition; and prevention of hypoprothrombinemia in infants receiving less than 0.1 mg/liter vitamin K in breast mild or milk substitutes (see also Table 16).

VOMITING CAUSED BY ANTINEOPLASTIC AGENTS		
Severe Vomiting	**Moderate Vomiting**	**Mild Vomiting**
Cisplatin	Carboplatin	Bleomycin
Cyclophosphamide	Carmustine	Chlorambucil
Cytarabine	Cyclophosphamide	Cytarabine
Dacarbazine	Dactinomycin	Etoposide
Mechlorethamine	Daunorubicin	Fluorouracil
Streptozocin	Doxorubicin	Hydroxyurea
	Idarubicin	Melphalan
	Ifosfamide	Methotrexate
	Lomustine	Paclitaxel
	Mitomycin	Plicamycin
	Mitoxantrone	Thioguanine
	Pentostatin	Vinblastine
	Procarbazine	Vincristine

The incidence and severity of vomiting depends on the dosage and route of administration of antineoplastic agents. Intravenous **ondansetron** (Zofran) plus dexamethasone and lorazepam is the most effective treatment available for prevention of severe vomiting due to antineoplastic agents (see also Figure 64).

WARFARIN SODIUM
(Coumadin Panwarfin, Sofarin)

Warfarin (initially 10 to 15 mg p.o. for three days) is indicated as an anticoagulant in pulmonary emboli, deep-vein thrombosis, myocardial infarction, rheumatic heart disease with heart valve damage, and atrial arrhythmias.

In the presence of cardiac arrhythmias, when the heart is beating rapidly but inefficiently, the formation of clots in atrial appendages is common. When converting to a normal sinus rhythm, the clots may be freed and become lodged in vital organs. To avoid this, patients with arrhythmias may be treated with anticoagulants before and after conversion of the arrhythmia to a sinus rhythm.

The oral anticoagulants are antagonists of vitamin K. Coagulation factors II, VII, IX, and X and the anticoagulant proteins C and S are synthesized mainly in the liver and are biologically inactive unless 9 to 12 of the amino-terminal glutamic acid residues are carboxylated. The gamma-carboxyglutamate residues confer Ca^{2+}-binding properties on these proteins that are essential for their assembly into an efficient catalytic complex. This reaction requires carbon dioxide, molecular oxygen, reduced vitamin K, and a precursor form of the target protein containing a propeptide recognition site. It is catalyzed in the rough endoplasmic reticulum by a 758-residue protein that has been purified, cloned, and characterized. Carboxylation is directly coupled to the oxidation of vitamin K to the epoxide.

Reduced vitamin K must be regenerated from the epoxide for sustained carboxylation and synthesis of biologically competent proteins. Warfarin is rapidly and completely absorbed from the GI tract. It is highly bound to plasma protein, especially albumin; the drug crosses the placenta but does not appear to accumulate in breast milk. Warfarin is hydroxylated by the liver into inactive metabolites. Metabolites are reabsorbed from bile and excreted in urine. Duration of action is 2 to 5 days — more closely reflecting the drug's half-life.

The use of anticoagulants is contraindicated in the presence of active hemorrhage, potential hemorrhage (acid-pepsin disease), and hemorrhagic disorders (hemophilia).

Anticoagulants should be used with extreme caution in patients with traumatic injuries to the central nervous system or the eyes because it is very difficult to control hemorrhage in these areas.

Anticoagulant therapy during pregnancy is indicated for the treatment and prophylaxis of venous thromboembolic disease and systemic embolism associated with valvular heart disease or prosthetic heart valves. However, there are special problems that need to be considered when deciding on optimal anticoagulant therapy in pregnant women. Heparin does not cross the placenta and is probably safe for the fetus. However, long-term heparin therapy is occasionally associated with maternal hemorrhage and rarely with symptomatic osteoporosis. Coumarin derivatives cross the placenta and are potentially teratogenic, particularly in the first trimester. Neonatal hemorrhage is a risk if warfarin is administered to the pregnant mother near term.

The possible existence of an aneurysm must be considered in an untreated hypertensive patient.

Anticoagulant therapy should be monitored carefully in patients with severe hepatic or renal failure, vitamin K deficiency, or alcoholism, and those with arthritis who are taking acetylsalicylic acid in large quantities. Furthermore, anticoagulants are extensively metabolized and their metabolites excreted, which can have an important bearing in patients suffering from renal disorders.

The incidence of interactions between the oral anticoagulants and other drugs, especially barbiturates, salicylates, and phenylbutazone, are numerous and at times may be life threatening. All aspects of the pharmacokinetics may be involved.

Various drugs can **augment the properties of oral anticoagulants** in a variety of ways:

By displacing **extensively bound anticoagulants** from the plasma albumin (e.g., chloral hydrate, clofibrate, and phenylbutazone)

By inhibiting **hepatic microsomal enzymes** (e.g., chloramphenicol and clofibrate)

By reducing the **availability of vitamin K** (e.g., anabolic steroids and broad-spectrum antibiotics)

By inhibiting **clotting factor synthesis** (e.g., anabolic steroids and salicylates)

There are also a number of agents that can **diminish the response to oral anticoagulants**, and they accomplish this by the following means:

By inhibiting **absorption of anticoagulants** (e.g., griseofulvin and clofibrate)

By inducing **hepatic microsomal enzymes** (e.g., barbiturates, ethchlorvynol, and gluethimide)

By stimulating **clotting factor synthesis** (e.g., vitamin K)

These interactions have not been reported to occur with regard to heparin, however.

WILSON'S DISEASE: TREATMENT OF

Wilson's disease is an autosomal recessive disorder of copper metabolism that produces neurologic and hepatic dysfunction. The gene defect has been localized to the long arm of chromosome 13. While the precise nature of the biochemical abnormality in Wilson's disease is unknown, its pathogenesis appears to involve decreased binding of copper to the transport protein ceruloplasmin. As a result, large amounts of unbound copper enter the circulation and are subsequently deposited in tissues, including the brain, liver, kidney, and cornea. There are four drugs used in the treatment of Wilson's disease. These are zinc, which blocks intestinal absorption of copper, penicillamine and trientine, both of which are chelators that increase urinary excretion of copper, and **tetrathiomolybdate** which forms a tripartite complex with copper and protein, and can block copper absorption from the intestine, or render blood copper nontoxic.

WOUND INFECTION AND SEPSIS IN SURGICAL PATIENTS: TREATMENT OF

Nature of Operation	Pathogens	Recommended drugs
Clean		
Cardiac		
Prosthetic valve, coronary artery bypass, other open-heart surgery, pacemaker implant	*Staphylococcus epidermidis, S. aureus, Corynebacterium,* enteric Gram-negative bacilli	Cefazolin or cefuroxime or vancomycin
Noncardiac thoracic	*S. aureus, S. epidermidis,* streptococci, enteric Gram-negative bacilli	Cefazolin or cefuroxime or vancomycin

Nature of Operation	Pathogens	Recommended drugs
Vascular		
Arterial surgery involving the abdominal aorta, a prosthesis, or a groin incision	*S. aureus, S. epidermidis,* enteric Gram-negative bacilli	Cefazolin or vancomycin
Lower extremity amputation for ischemia	*S. aureus, S. epidermidis,* enteric Gram-negative bacilli, clostridia	Cefazolin or vancomycin
Neurosurgery		
Craniotomy	*S. aureus, S. epidermidis*	Cefazolin or vancomycin
Orthopedic		
Total joint replacement, internal fixation of fractures	*S. aureus, S. epidermidis*	Cefazolin or vancomycin
Ophthalmic	*S. aureus, S. epidermidis,* streptococci, enteric Gram-negative bacilli, *Pseudomonas*	Gentamicin or tobramycin or neomycin-gramicidin/polymyxin B, cefazolin
Clean-Contaminated		
Head and neck		
Entering oral cavity or pharynx	*S. aureus,* streptococci, oral anaerobes	Cefazolin or clindamycin ± gentamicin
Abdominal		
Gastroduodenal	Enteric Gram-negative bacilli, Gram-positive cocci	High risk only: cefazolin
Biliary tract	Enteric Gram-negative bacilli, enterococci, clostridia	High risk only: cefazolin
Colorectal	Enteric Gram-negative bacilli, anaerobes	Oral: neomycin + erythromycin base Parenteral: cefoxitin or cefotetan
Appendectomy	Enteric Gram-negative bacilli, anaerobes	Cefoxitin or cefotetan
Gynecologic and Obstetric		
Vaginal or abdominal hysterectomy	Enteric Gram-negative, anaerobes, Gp B strep, enterococci	Cefazolin or cefotetan or cefoxitin
Cesarean section	Same as for hysterectomy	High risk only: cefazolin
Abortion	Same as for hysterectomy	First trimester, high risk only: aqueous penicillin G or doxycycline Second trimester: cefazolin
Dirty Surgery		
Ruptured viscus	Enteric Gram-negative bacilli, anaerobes, enterococci	Cefoxitin or cefotetan ± gentamicin or clindamycin + gentamicin
Traumatic wound	*S. aureaus,* Gp A strep, clostridia	Cefazolin

XAMOTEROL
(Carwin)

Xamoterol (200 mg t.i.d.) has been shown to improve left ventricular systolic and diastolic function in most patients with mild to moderate heart failure. Xamoterol (±)-N-[2-[[2-hydroxy-3-(p-hydro-xyphenoxy)propryl]amino]ethyl]-4-morpholine carboxamide, is a beta$_1$-adrenoreceptor partial agonist with a pK$_a$ of 8.2 (see also Figure 27).

In the normal heart during exertion, xamoterol increases the force of myocardial contraction and the rate of myocardial relaxation and lowers left ventricular filling pressure, whereas the drug has little effect on the heart rate at rest. At high levels of sympathetic stimulation (e.g., with strenuous exercise) xamoterol reduces heart rate. Improved myocardial performance is maintained during submaximal exercise. There is no evidence of down-regulation of the beta$_1$-adrenoreceptors during prolonged administration of the drug.

Approximately 9% of an oral dose of xamoterol is absorbed from the gastrointestinal tract. The low absorption rate of the drug results from its hydrophilic nature, which limits penetration of the gastrointestinal wall to the bloodstream, but not absorption from extensive hepatic phase I metabolism. The only metabolism appears to be sulfate conjugation of the 4-hydro group, occurring primarily in the gut wall after oral administration and in the liver after intravenous administration. Xamoterol is cleared from the blood by renal excretion, and some tubular excretion may be involved. After oral administration, 56% of the conjugate, which is pharmacologically inactive, is excreted in urine. There is no evidence of enterohepatic circulation.

XANTHINE OXIDASE INHIBITORS

Gout is a hyperuricemic state (>6 mg/dl) that is effectively diagnosed through the detection of monosodium urate crystals in the synovial fluid of the involved joint. Conditions causing hyperuricemia include: the excessive synthesis of uric acid, the excessive synthesis of purine — precursor to uric acid, a high dietary intake of purine (shellfish, organ meat, anchovies, and wild game), diminished renal excretion of uric acid, and tissue destruction following injury or therapeutic irradiation.

Numerous agents, when used in therapeutic doses, can also cause hyperuricemia. This includes an analgesic dose of aspirin, thiazide diuretics, nicotinic acid, chronic consumption of alcohol and antineoplastic agents.

If left untreated, the hyperuricemic state may precipitate an acute attack of gout, which first appears in metatarsal phalangeal joints. Ultimately tophaceous deposits form in the joints and soft tissues such as the kidneys. The hyperuricemic state may be corrected either by inhibiting the synthesis of uric acid by allopurinol or by enhancing the elimination of uric acid by uricosuric agents.

Allopurinol (**Zyloprim**) reduces the synthesis of uric acid by inhibiting the activity of xanthine oxidase, according to the scheme shown in Figure 5).

The reduction in the uric acid pool occurs slowly. Because xanthine and hypoxanthine are more soluble than uric acid, they are easily excreted.

Allopurinol not only is used in treating the hyperuricemia associated with gout, but also in the secondary hyperuricemia associated with the use of antineoplastic agents. However, allopurinol may interfere with the metabolism of antineoplastic agents such as **azathioprine** and **6-mercaptopurine**.

XANTHINES

(Caffeine, Theobromine and Theophylline)

In a number of plants used in different parts of the world to form beverages and condiments, there are found the xanthine compounds, **caffeine, theobromine,** and **theophylline** (Theocin), which are also employed in therapeutics, and have, therefore, acquired a double importance as drugs and as articles of diet.

Caffeine, theobromine, and theophylline are purine derivatives closely related to the xanthine bodies found in the urine and tissues of animals. Xanthine is 2:6 dioxypurine; caffeine is 1:3:7 trimethylxanthine; theobromine is 3:7 dimethylxanthine; and theophylline is 1:3 dimethyl-xanthine.

These all resemble each other in most points of their pharmacological action, but they differ markedly in the relative intensity of their action on various functions. Thus caffeine is the most potent central nervous system stimulant of the group; theobromine exerts the greatest action on the muscles; and theophylline is the most effective diuretic and coronary dilator. Theobromine has comparatively little effect on the central nervous system, while theophylline has no action on the muscles.

Coffee is not used in medicine but is of great dietetic importance. The coffee bean contains about 1 to 2% caffeine, and a cup of coffee is equivalent to 0.1 to 0.2 g of caffeine along with some volatile substances, such as **furfuralcohol**, produced by the roasting; these have been called Coffeon and resemble the volatile oils in their action.

Tea leaves contain more caffeine than the coffee bean, but since a relatively smaller quantity of leaves is used in preparing tea, this beverage contains slightly less caffeine than does coffee. In green tea there is a considerable quantity of a volatile oil which also passes into the infusion, and the flavor of black tea also arises from volatile substances (**theon**). Both black and green tea contain about 7% tannic acid, but this is extracted only slowly. The bitter taste in tea that has been prepared too long is due to the tannic acid.

The wakefulness and the relief from fatigue produced by tea and coffee are undoubtedly due to the caffeine contained in them. On the other hand, the feeling of well-being and comfort produced by coffee after a full meal is similar to the carminative effects of the volatile oils and appears to be due to the local action in the stomach of the volatile constituents of coffee. There is a widespread belief that excessive tea-drinking disturbs gastric digestion, and this has generally been attributed to the tannic acid contained in it. It is not unlikely that the caffeine and theophylline may also play a part in this gastric action by causing irritation of the mucous membrane. Excessive consumption of tea or coffee may produce, in addition to digestive disturbances, increased nervousness, excitability, tremor, palpitation, and insomnia — effects directly due to the caffeine content of these beverages.

Chocolate contains theobromine (0.5 to 1%) instead of caffeine, and a large amount of fat (cacao-butter, 15 to 50%), starch, and albumins as well. The theobromine does not possess the stimulant action of caffeine on the nervous system, and chocolate may therefore be taken without producing wakefulness. The starch and fat are assimilated by the tissues so that chocolate is a true food.

XYLOMETAZOLINE HYDROCHLORIDE
(Chlorohist-LA-Neo-Spray Long Acting, Neo-Synephrine II, Otrivin)

Xylometazoline (spray 1% solution to nasal mucosa every 8 to 10 hours) is used as a nasal decongestant. Xylometazoline acts on alpha-adrenergic receptors in nasal mucosa to produce constriction, thereby decreasing blood flow and nasal congestion (see also Figure 27).

Xylometazoline is contraindicated in patients with narrow-angle glaucoma, because the drug may increase intraocular pressure, and in patients receiving tricyclic antidepressants, because of the potential for adverse cardiovascular effects.

Xylometazoline should be used with caution in patients with hyperthyroidism, cardiac disease, hypertension, diabetes mellitus, or advanced arteriosclerosis.

Y

YELLOW FEVER VACCINE
(YF-Vax)

This viral vaccine is used for primary vaccination.

YOHIMBINE HYDROCHLORIDE
(Yohimex)

Yohimbine, an alpha$_2$-adrenergic receptor blocking agent has no medical indications. Urologists have used yohimbine in determining the nature of male erectile impotence; and internists have used it successfully (18 mg/day) to treat impotence associated with vascular or diabetic origins.

Yohimbine, an indolalkylamine alkaloid, is chemically similar to reserpine. It is the principal alkaloid of the bark of the West African *Corynanthe yohimbe* tree and is also found in *Rauwolfia serpentina*. It is believed to have properties similar to rauwolfia alkaloids.

Yohimbine is primarily an alpha$_2$-adrenergic blocker. It blocks presynaptic alpha$_2$-adrenoreceptors causing release of norepinephrine, and hence has been used in the treatment of postural hypotension (see also Figure 27).

Symptoms of dizziness and syncope due to postural hypotension may result from dehydration, blood loss, and myocardial disease. However, the most important cause of chronic recurrent symptomatic postural hypotension is failure of the autonomic nervous system. The drug treatment for postural hypotension is difficult because the response varies and tolerance to drugs develops. Patients with autonomic abnormalities may suffer symptoms after eating, and this further hampers treatment (Table 24).

Z

ZACOPRIDE

In addition to agents that stimulate or irritate the stomach, many other factors may be responsible for inducing emesis centrally. The central control of vomiting is vested in two areas:

- The **vomiting center**, which is located in the lateral reticular formation in the midst of a group of cells governing such activities as salivation and respiration.
- The **chemoreceptor trigger zone**, which is a narrow strip along the floor of the fourth ventricle located close to the vomiting center (see also Figure 73).

The functions of these two areas are distinct but interdependent.

The vomiting center is activated by impulses that originate from the gastrointestinal tract and other peripheral structures. In addition, there are unidentified tracts that extend from the cerebral cortex to the vomiting center, such that emotional trauma and unpleasant olfactory and visual stimuli may cause nausea and vomiting.

Stimulation of the **vestibular apparatus** that responds to movements of the head, neck, and eye muscles may also cause nausea and vomiting by stimulating the vomiting center. On the other hand, circulating chemicals, toxins, virus, and ions may provoke nausea and vomiting by first stimulating the **chemoreceptor zone for emesis,** which in turn stimulates the vomiting center.

The nausea and vomiting associated with circulating physical agents (radiation therapy and virus particles) and chemical agents (toxins and cancer chemotherapeutic agents) are treated with phenothiazine derivatives such as chlorpromazine, perphenazine, prochlorperazine, promethazine, triethylperazine, and triflupromazine. These agents block the dopamine receptors in the **area postrema**.

A new class of antiemetic agents, the serotonin antagonists, has been identified. These agents could be clinically useful in a wide range of areas. Selective antagonists of the serotonin (5-hydroxytryptamine) type 3 (5-HT$_3$) receptor, such as **batanopride, granisetron, ondansetron,** or **zacopride**, have proved in early clinical trials to be potent antiemetic agents in patients undergoing cytotoxic chemotherapy. Their efficacy has been shown to be comparable or superior to that of conventional phenothiazine antiemetics. The toxic effects observed so far with these agents have been modest (see also Figure 64).

ZALCITABINE
(Dideoxycyctidine, ddC (Hivid)

Zalcitabine, a potent nucleoside analog inhibitor of reverse transcriptase with antiviral properties, is used in patients with advanced human immunodeficiency virus (HIV) infection (CD4 count below 300 cells/mm^3) who have demonstrated significant clinical or immunologic deterioration. It is approximately tenfold more potent than zidovudine (AZT) and causes reversible peripheral nephropathy (see Figure 99).

ZIDOVUDINE

(Zaidothymidine; AZT; Retrovir)

Zidovudine (200 mg every 4 hours) is indicated in the management of patients with HIV infection who have evidence of impaired immunity. Trimethoprim-sulfamethoxazole, pyrimethamine, and acyclovir may be necessary for the management or prevention of opportunistic infections.

Zidovudine (3'-azido-3'-deoxythymidine, commonly referred to as AZT) is a thymidine analog with antiviral activity against HIV-1, HIV-2, human T lymphotropic (or leukemia) virus (HTLV)-I, and other retroviruses. Low concentrations (<0.001 to 0.04 microgram/ml) inhibit acute HIV-1 infection in human T-cell lines and peripheral blood lymphocytes. Zidovudine is less active in human monocyte-macrophages or quiescent cells but inhibits HIV replication in human brain macrophages. Zidovudine is also inhibitory for HBV and EBV.

Low concentrations of zidovudine inhibit human myeloid and erythroid progenitor cell growth (0.3 to 0.6 microgram/ml) and blastogenesis in peripheral blood mononuclear cells.

Following diffusion into host cells, the drug is initially phosphorylated by cellular thymidine kinase. The rate-limiting step is conversion to the diphosphate by thymidylate kinase, so that high levels of the monophosphate but much lower levels of di- and triphosphates are present in the cells. Zidovudine triphosphate, which has an intracellular $t_{1/2}$ of elimination of 3 to 4 hours, competitively inhibits reverse transcriptase with respect to thymidine triphosphate (TTP). Because the 3'-azido group prevents the formation of 5'-3'-phosphodiester linkages, zidovudine incorporation causes DNA chain termination (Figure 99). Zidovudine monophosphate also is a competitive inhibitor of cellular thymidylate kinase, causing reduced intracellular levels of TTP. This effect may contribute to its cytotoxicity and enhance antiviral effects by decreasing the competition for zidovudine triphosphate. The antiviral selectivity of zidovudine is due to its greater affinity for HIV reverse transcriptase than for human DNA polymerases, although low concentrations inhibit DNA polymerase gamma (see Figure 99).

Resistant mutants with 10- to over 100-fold decreases in susceptibility have been recovered from treated patients and can be produced by site-directed mutagenesis of the reverse transcriptase. Resistance is associated with point mutations leading to amino acid substitutions at multiple sites in reverse transcriptase, particularly codons 41, 67, 70, 215, and 219. Resistance mutations appear sequentially, and multiple ones are required to confer high-level resistance.

Zidovudine is rapidly absorbed from the GI tract with peak serum concentrations occurring within 30 to 90 minutes. It binds to plasma proteins to the extent of 35 to 40%. Zidovudine is rapidly metabolized in the liver to the inactive 3'-azido-3'-deoxy-5'-0-beta-D-glucopyranuronosylthymidine (GAZT), which has an apparent elimination half-life of one hour. Zidovudine undergoes glomerular filtration and active tubular secretion. Coadministration of zidovudine with agents such as dapsone, pentamidine, amphotericin B, flucytosine, vincristine, vinblastine, Adriamycin, and interferon with potential to cause nephrotoxicity or cytotoxicity to hematopoietic elements, enhance its risk of adverse effects. Probenecid will inhibit the renal excretion of zidovudine.

Fluconazole, acetaminophen, aspirin, or indomethacin competitively inhibits the glucuronidation of zidovudine, increasing the risk of causing agranulocytosis. The major toxicities of zidovudine are granulocytopenia and anemia. The risk of hematologic toxicity increases with lower CD4 counts, more advanced disease, higher zidovudine doses, and prolonged therapy. Severe headache, nausea, emesis, insomnia, and myalgia occur commonly during initiation of zidovudine therapy.

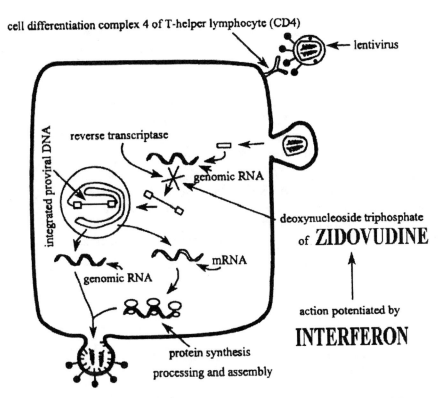

cell differentiation complex 4 of T-helper lymphocyte (CD4) ← lentivirus

reverse transcriptase

integrated proviral DNA

genomic RNA

deoxynucleoside triphosphate of **ZIDOVUDINE**

mRNA

genomic RNA

action potentiated by

INTERFERON

protein synthesis

processing and assembly

FIGURE 99   Patients with a clinical diagnosis of AIDS should undergo long-term therapy with **zidovudine** (AZT, 1,200 mg q. 4 hrs). **Acyclovir** may potentiate the beneficial effects of AZT. In addition, patients should be treated prophylactically for *Pneumocystis carinii* pneumonia; such regimens include **sulfadoxine** and **pyrimethamine** (Fansidar), **dapsone**, or aerosolized **pentamidine**. **Dextran sulfate** is also useful because it blocks the binding of HIV to target cells (see also Figure 3).

ZINC
(Medizinc, Orazinc, Scrip Zinc, Verazine, Zinc 15; Zinc 220, Zincate, Zinkaps-220)

ZINC SULFATE (OPHTHALMIC)
(Eye-Sedophthalmic, Op-Thal-Zin)

Zinc (200 to 220 mg p.o. t.i.d.) is used in zinc-deficiency state and as an adjunct in ulcers, acne, ear granulomata, rheumatoid arthritis, hypogeusia, anosmia, vitamin A therapy, and acrodermatitis enteropathica. In addition, zinc has antiinfective properties and hence as an ophthalmic solution (1 to 2 drops) is used twice a day. Zinc sulfate ophthalmic solution exhibits astringent and weak antiseptic activity, which may result from precipitation of protein by the zinc ion and by clearing mucus from the outer surface of the eye. This drug has no decongestant action and produces mild vasodilation.

Zinc, which serves as a cofactor for numerous enzymes, facilitates wound healing, normal growth rates, and normal skin hydration, and helps maintain the senses of taste and smell.

Adequate zinc provides normal growth and tissue repair. In patients receiving total parenteral nutrition with low plasma levels of zinc, dermatitis has been followed by alopecia. Zinc is an integral part of many enzymes important to carbohydrate and protein mobilization of retinal-binding protein.

Zinc sulfate is absorbed poorly from the GI tract, only 20 to 30% of dietary zinc is absorbed. After administration, zinc resides in muscle, bone, skin, kidney, liver, pancreas, retina, prostate, and, particularly, red and white blood cells. Zinc binds to plasma albumin, alpha-2 macroglobulin, and some plasma amino acids including histidine, cysteine, threonine, glycine, and asparagine.

Major zinc stores are in the skeletal muscles, skin, bone, and pancreas. After parenteral administration, 90% of zinc is excreted in the stool, urine, and sweat. After oral use, the major route of excretion is secretion into the duodenum and jejunum. Small amounts are also excreted in the urine (0.3 to 0.5 mg/day) and in sweat (1.5 mg/day).

Concomitant use of oral zinc with tetracycline will impair antibiotic absorption. When zinc sulfate ophthalmic solution is used with sodium borate, precipitation of zinc borate may occur; glycerin may prevent this interaction. Zinc sulfate ophthalmic solution has a dehydrating effect on methylcellulose suspensions, causing precipitation of methylcellulose. Zinc sulfate ophthalmic solution may also precipitate acacia and certain proteins.

Parenteral use of zinc sulfate is contraindicated in patients with renal failure or biliary obstruction.

ZOLPIDEM TARTRATE
(Ambien)

Zolpidem, an imidazopyridine (10 mg p.o. at bedtime), is used in short-term management of insomnia (see also Table 8).

ZOPICLONE

Zopiclone, the first compound of the cyclopyrrolone class to be marketed, possesses anticonvulsant, anxiolytic, muscle relaxant, and sedative properties. It causes no dependence and no rebound insomnia. Zopiclone interacts with gamma-aminobutyric acid (GABA) receptors (see Figure 40). It is rapidly absorbed from the gastrointestinal tract, and with an oral dose of 7.5 mg, it produces a peak plasma concentration of 50 to 80 microgram/liter. Zopiclone becomes metabolized to N-demethylzopiclone (inactive) and zopiclone N oxide (active). Zopiclone exhibits a high affinity for benzodiazepine binding sites in the cerebral cortex, hippocampus, and cerebellum, but does not interact with the peripheral benzodiazepine binding sites.

Index

D

E

H